DIAGNOSTIC AND SURGICAL ARTHROSCOPY OF THE SHOULDER

DIAGNOSTIC AND SURGICAL ARTHROSCOPY OF THE SHOULDER

LANNY L. JOHNSON, MD
Clinical Professor, Department of Surgery
Michigan State University
East Lansing, Michigan

With **1139** *illustrations*

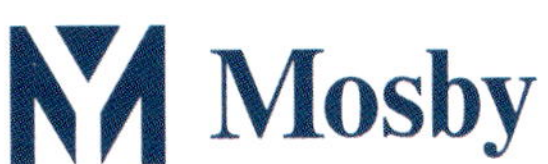

St. Louis Baltimore Boston Chicago London Philadelphia Sydney Toronto

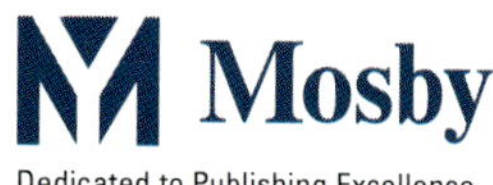

Sponsoring Editor: James R. Ryan
Developmental Editor: Emma Underdown
Project Manager: Carol Sullivan Wiseman
Production Editor: David S. Brown

Printed in the United States of America.

Mosby–Year Book, Inc.
11830 Westline Industrial Drive, St. Louis, MO 63146-3318

Library of Congress Cataloging in Publication Data

Johnson, Lanny L., 1933-
Diagnostic and surgical arthroscopy of the shoulder / Lanny L. Johnson.
p. cm.
Includes bibliographical references and index.
ISBN 0-8016-2400-2
1. Shoulder joint—Endoscopic surgery. 2. Shoulder joint—-Abnormalities—Diagnosis. 3. Arthroscopy. I. Title.
[DNLM: 1. Arthroscopy—methods. 2. Shoulder—pathology. 3. Shoulder—surgery. 4. Shoulder Joint—surgery. WE 810 J67d]
RD557.5.J64 1993
617.5′72059—dc20
DNLM/DLC 92-49312
for Library of Congress CIP

93 94 95 96 97 CL/WA 9 8 7 6 5 4 3 2 1

This text is
dedicated to my nurse,

RUTH BECKER, L.P.N.

Ruth is a great friend to me, my wife Mary Ann, and my daughters Charlotte and Autumn.

Ruth has been a loyal, trustworthy, consummate professional and co-worker for the past 24 years. It has been said that if she retired, I would have to quit. Probably so.

Eternal thanks, Ruth.

Preface

The purpose of this book is to help surgeons help patients with shoulder problems. As we enter the decade of the 1990s, arthroscopic surgery plays a major role in the care of patients with shoulder problems. An American Academy of Orthopedic Surgeons survey in 1991 showed 42% of respondents performed shoulder arthroscopy.

Shoulder arthroscopy represents a merging of the interests of two groups of orthopedic surgeons. One group includes those surgeons with established interest and knowledge in conventional shoulder surgery. The other group is composed of those orthopedic surgeons who developed arthroscopic surgical skills in the care of patients with knee joint problems. The shoulder surgeons provided the knowledge base. The knee joint arthroscopists contributed the technical aspects. The blending of the knowledge base with the technological advancements resulted in the present development of arthroscopic surgery of the shoulder.

Not surprisingly, the same controversial issues that played out in the 1970s with conventional knee surgeons and the arthroscopists was repeated in the 1980s concerning shoulder surgery. The established shoulder surgeon learned arthroscopic techniques. The arthroscopic knee surgeon learned about shoulder problems.

I approached arthroscopic surgery of the shoulder with knee joint arthroscopic technical skills. Like most orthopedic surgeons of my era, I had no formal training in shoulder surgery. My fellowship was in hand surgery. I started private practice in 1967, treating fractures and dislocations of the shoulder girdle. Eventually, I stopped taking patients with shoulder problems for two reasons: I knew very little about the shoulder and I was interested in the knee, sports injuries, and total joints.

I performed my first shoulder arthroscopy using local anesthesia with a Needlescope for diagnostic purposes in 1974. I was surprised how much could be seen with the arthroscope. I started saying, "Someone with some knowledge should get interested in shoulder arthroscopy." As it turned out, someone without shoulder knowledge got interested. I started performing diagnostic shoulder arthroscopy at the request of other surgeons and eventually advanced to surgical procedures.

This text summarizes how I practice and care for patients with shoulder problems. This text reports my entire shoulder practice, from patient encounter in the office, through clinical assessment, to arthroscopic findings, surgical techniques, and results. I have reviewed my experience so the reader will not have to learn by trial and error. I illustrate my arthroscopic observations so others may confirm or correct. I demonstrate the application of basic surgical principles to arthroscopic shoulder surgery.

Much of the book is a "how-to-do" book for practical success in using arthroscopic surgical techniques to care for orthopedic patients. This emphasis is necessary, because in the absence of technical skills the remainder of the discussion becomes as it has been so appropriately stated: academic. I have tried to give attention to detail in this text as one would in surgery. Successful arthroscopic surgery of the shoulder requires the relentless pursuit of attention to detail.

My observations at recent continuing education course motor skills laboratories convince me that a review, emphasis, and update on basic arthroscopic surgical principles should not be eliminated. In fact, lack of knowledge of basic arthroscopic skills is the main reason these attendees are incapable of performing arthroscopic surgery even on a plastic model or cadaver shoulder. These surgeons cannot attempt demanding surgical techniques without a basic understanding of the principles learned by their predecessors in the 1970s. Therefore no apologies are made for the repetitious, detailed emphasis on technique in this text.

Repetition of some material is intentional. Some text and illustrations are repeated in order to accommodate the reader. Most readers will not read cover to cover but will look up various topics. The repetition of text eliminates turning pages from chapter to chapter when reading about an instrument to see how it is used, or when reading about a technique to turn pages to see what instrument is recommended. The subject matter in Chapter 5 on surgical principles is repeated in subsequent chapters with an emphasis on the specific anatomical area, glenohumeral, subacromial, or acromioclavicular.

Presently, two major forces are pushing arthroscopic shoulder surgery forward at a fast pace. Foremost is the increasing numbers of orthopedic surgeons performing, inventing, and reporting on this area of orthopedic surgery. The second factor is the rapidly developing technological advances. As a result, this text includes a final chapter on the future.

I hope this text lays the foundation for future authors' contributions. The ultimate goal is rendering better care to those patients with shoulder problems.

Lanny L. Johnson, M.D.
East Lansing, Michigan

Acknowledgments

I am grateful to those surgeons who have years of experience in the care of patients with shoulder problems for being so tolerant of me and other arthroscopic surgeons as we entered this area of interest. These surgeons have freely shared their knowledge with us.

Foremost among that group for me was Charlie Rockwood. He was one of the first established shoulder surgeons to recognize the value of arthroscopy. Charlie brought balance to the use of the arthroscope in shoulder conditions. If he had not, his prophecy, "the arthroscope is a tool of the devil," may have come true. He has politely, but very directly, admonished me, while providing insight and encouragement. We are good friends, although he may still not believe the arthroscope could be used for a divine purpose.

My appreciation goes to each member of the East Lansing Orthopedic Association: Michael Austin, Dave Detrisac, Gregory Uitvulgt, and Kenneth Morrison. We have collaborated on patient care, instructional courses, and publications. Dave Detrisac deserves special thanks for his book *Arthroscopic Anatomy of the Shoulder*. He worked late at night and on weekends to document and clarify some uncharted ground.

Ruth Becker, L.P.N., my surgical assistant since 1968, has been the most important member of the arthroscopic team. In addition, those who work at Ingham Medical Center's arthroscopy suite know the meaning of team work and tolerance. In 1991 these team members were Cindy Everett, R.N., Director; Diana Many, S.T.; Julie Murray, R.N.; Sandy Sinkovitz, R.N.; Sue Harris, L.P.N.; Cindy Walker, R.N.; Sally Lopez, Unit Secretary; Jackie Friar, R.N.; Stan Krawczyk, C.S.T.; Anna Filice, O.R. Assistant; and Barb Tranberg, R.N.

Andrew Pittsley's programming skills have been essential to my computerized medical record and research program. His frequent assistance when I was lost in simple word processing during the writing of this manuscript is appreciated.

My appreciation is also extended to Bellinda Bays, my research associate. She has diligently tracked our patients. She has performed the computer searches necessary for the clinical reports and has assisted with the construction of this text.

Both Richard Fitzler and Dori Farnsworth contributed to the artwork and I thank them for their renditions.

My first impression of Emma Underdown's work on this book as Developmental Editor was less than favorable. She edited the manuscript. I felt like she was sterilizing my style, when she was really correcting my English. Early on I gave her the same appreciation one gives a dentist while he or she is drilling on your teeth. I have changed my opinion to one of appreciation. She has truly contributed to the production of this text.

I want to acknowledge both potential and/or real conflicts of interest concerning my commercial relationships. These exist with the following corporations: Smith and Nephew-Dyonics, Inc.; Instrument Makar, Inc.; Information Health Network, Inc.; and Biologic, Inc.

P.T.L.

Contents

DIAGNOSTIC AND SURGICAL ARTHROSCOPY OF THE SHOULDER

CHAPTER

1 The Clinical Practice of Shoulder Arthroscopy

Arthroscopy of the shoulder is gaining acceptance in present-day orthopedics.[19] Just as established knee surgeons were hesitant to use arthroscopy in the 1970s, so were the shoulder surgeons of the 1980s. We know now what happened to arthroscopic knee surgery. We are now about to learn what this surgical method will do for shoulder surgery. How did it get started? Who did the first shoulder arthroscopy? What is the state of the art in shoulder arthroscopy? How are these techniques applied to the shoulder? What are the pitfalls of shoulder arthroscopy? What must the surgeon know about shoulder problems to successfully apply these methods? What are the principles of arthroscopy that must be embraced for a beneficial outcome? A brief historical review of the development of arthroscopy in general will be helpful to the surgeon approaching shoulder arthroscopy.

HISTORICAL BACKGROUND

Knee arthroscopy was first performed in Japan by Professor Kenji Takagi in 1918 using the urological cystoscope.[100] In 1921, Eugen Bïrcher of Germany used gas for arthroscopy, often performing the procedure with the patient under local anesthesia.[13] In 1925, Phillip Kreuscher, an American, first reported arthroscopic meniscectomy.[63] In 1931, Michael Burman at New York Hospital for Joint Diseases reported arthroscopic inspection of both the knee and the shoulder in cadavers[18] (Fig. 1-1). Like so many other events in medicine, a seed was planted, but a germination period was necessary before growth of shoulder arthroscopy started. Dr. Masaki Watanabe, a student of Takagi, developed various size arthroscopes and demonstrated technique in many joints, including the shoulder.[101,102]

In the late 1960s Robert Jackson in Toronto,[55] Ward Cassells[22,23] in Wilmington, Delaware, and the late Dick O'Connor of West Covina,[78,79] California visited Watanabe. These three surgeons brought the ideas and techniques of Watanabe to North America. Their presentations on arthroscopy of the knee were greeted with little more than curiosity. Other first generation arthroscopists included John Joyce, John McGinty, Royer Collins, Kenneth DeHaven, Robert Metcalf, and myself in the United States. The European pioneers were Harold Eikelaar of the Netherlands,[34] Jan Gillquist of Sweden,[42] A. N. Henry of Great Britain,[51] and W. Glinz of Switzerland.[43] A progression was made from diagnostic arthroscopy to application of arthroscopic techniques to most of the established open surgical procedures of the knee.

Pioneers were considered misled. Perhaps they did not know what they were doing. Sometimes the word crazy was used. Arthroscopy was viewed as a fad or at best a passing phase in orthopedics like ostemer or the hanging hip operation. It was considered unnecessary because its opponents could see better by cutting the knee open. Others thought it was harmful in that the arthroscope often scratched the joint. Interestingly, this criticism of superficial joint damage usually came from a surgeon who specialized in total joint replacement. Stronger criticisms included labels like unnecessary, unethical, and even immoral surgery. If that was not bad enough, many of the procedures were categorically deemed MALPRACTICE. It is no wonder that there were few pioneers.

It was unique that arthroscopy developed outside of academia. Unlike the development of total joint replacement, the training programs were not involved. Knee arthroscopy was popularized by surgeons in private practice without existing reputations, and it was unlikely that they would gain one with this procedure in those days.

Throughout the 1970s very few surgeons performed arthroscopy of the knee, let alone the shoulder. At that time arthroscopy was not professionally or economically threatening to the surgical community. It was thought that the arthroscopic surgeon was looking for a practice niche.

Yet the pioneers persisted. The medical profession changes by evolution, not revolution. Much to my surprise

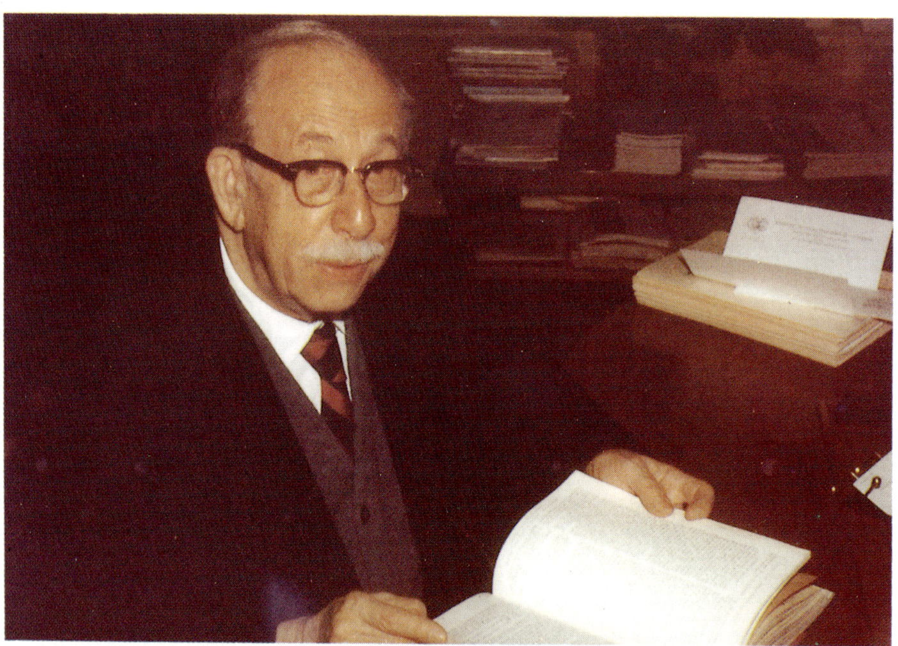

FIG. 1-1 Dr. Micheal Burman, 1901-1975. His vision for arthroscopy was demonstrated in cadaver experiments in 1931. (Courtesy Serge Parisien.)

the sports medicine sector of orthopedics was slow in accepting and learning arthroscopy. Nonetheless, it was in the sports arena that arthroscopy found the exposure it needed. In the 1970s a man on the street could more easily grasp the value of arthroscopy than most orthopedists. He read about its benefit each day in the sports pages. Athletes, trainers, and surgeons alike were expounding the procedure, and reporting less morbidity, same day surgery, and a quick recovery.

Public opinion affects a surgeon's market share, and patients began to seek out those who would perform knee surgery by arthroscopy. Patients would not believe any doctor who tried to explain that knee arthroscopic surgery would not work or that a torn cartilage was too big to pull out through a scope. Thus established knee surgeons were prodded to accept and learn arthroscopic techniques.

Now, some 20 years later, arthroscopic surgery of the knee is accepted standard in orthopedic surgery. As our experience with the knee grew, practitioners and the public began seeing the value of applying the principles of arthroscopic surgery to other areas, such as the shoulder. Despite proven successes, skeptics remain. Just last year, I was telling a sage and renown knee surgeon that there was some reluctance on the part of the established shoulder surgeons to accept the value of arthroscopy to the shoulder. He replied, "I don't understand that, arthroscopy should be good for the shoulder. I am still not sure of its place in knee surgery."

This perspective of pioneers of arthroscopy of the knee joint is important as we hear about and watch our colleagues that are developing an interest and skills in arthroscopic surgery of the shoulder.

THE DEVELOPMENT OF SHOULDER ARTHROSCOPY

I performed my first shoulder diagnostic arthroscopy in 1974. This was followed by periodic referral cases throughout the 1970s as I did not have a shoulder practice. The acceptance of shoulder arthroscopy was first reflected in the results of a survey of the American Academy of Orthopaedic Surgeons (AAOS) Educational Committee in 1978. That report indicated that arthroscopy of joints other than the knee was performed by only 7% of the respondents, but the specific incidence of shoulder arthroscopy was not available. According to an independent survey in 1981, only 5% of orthopedic surgeons performed arthroscopy of joints other than the knee. By 1983, 26% of orthopedic surgeons reported that they performed arthroscopy on joints other than the knee. No specific numbers were available for the shoulder.

The shoulder joint became a focus of interest for the arthroscopic surgeon for several reasons. One was socioeconomic. As more surgeons performed arthroscopy on the knee, there was a dilution of the potential patients for knee arthroscopy. At the same time there was a large patient population with shoulder problems. In that the shoulder patient presented a diagnostic enigma to most orthopedic surgeons, arthroscopic inspection was reasonable. Subsequently, just like the knee experience, arthroscopic techniques were applied to established shoulder surgical procedures. The growth of shoulder arthroscopy in the '80s is faster than that of the knee in the '70s because the surgeon did not have to learn arthroscopic techniques, but only transfer known technical skills from the knee to the shoulder. Also, patients have become accustomed to requesting arthroscopy as the method of treatment, if possible. The modern emphasis on outpatient surgery with cost savings is another impetus for arthroscopy.

An AAOS survey in 1990 showed that 81% of 14,185 respondent orthopedic surgeons perform arthroscopy; 42% (5958) of those surgeons perform arthroscopy of the shoulder.[61] Shoulder arthroscopic procedures account for 12% of all arthroscopies; knee, 81%; ankle, 4%; elbow, 2%; and wrist, 2%. This report also indicated that 93% of arthroscopies of any kind are performed on an outpatient basis.

Shoulder arthroscopy had its pioneers. They included, among others, the following alphabetical group: James R. Andrews, Birmingham, Alabama; Louis U. Bigliani, New York, New York; Richard Caspari, Richmond, Virginia; David A. Detrisac, East Lansing, Michigan; Harvard Ellman, Los Angeles, California; James C. Esch, Oceanside, California; Gary M. Gartsman, Houston, Texas; ; Michael R. Gross, Omaha, Nebraska; Leslie S. Matthews, Baltimore, Maryland; Stephen S. Snyder, Van Nuys, California; Russell R. Warren, New York, New York; Masaki Watanabe, Japan; A.M. Wiley, Toronto, Canada.

Utilization and Potential for Overutilization

The experience of arthroscopic utilization in the knee joint went from no one doing the procedure to almost everybody doing it in a short period of time. This now has happened with shoulder arthroscopy.

This development has caused an interesting twist in patient management. Since many patients now ask for arthroscopy, the doctor in good conscience must often talk many patients out of this procedure when their condition is not suitable. However, for those surgeons of another persuasion, a patient request means additional surgical cases. I know of one Mid-Western clinic in which a surgeon performed 80 operations on every 100 new patients in 1984 and 104 arthroscopies on every 100 new patients in 1985. The operations were performed within an average of 21 days from the initial visit. No case went unscoped, undiagnosed, or unbilled. Colleagues with the same type of practice in the same clinic performed surgery at one half this rate. Did they lack clinical diagnostic skills? Were they withholding treatment? I think not.

The potential for overutilization of arthroscopy continues. The indication for arthroscopy must be clearly defined and must include the expectation of patient benefit.

Organized Medicine

The International Arthroscopy Association was formed in 1974. Requirements for membership were state medical licensure and the ability to fill out a one page application and sign your name to a check for $50. A survey taken a few years later showed that 20% of the membership not only had never attended a society meeting, but had yet to perform arthroscopy.

The Arthroscopy Association of North America (AANA) was formed in 1982. The AANAs membership requirements are more stringent. They go beyond requiring attendance at meetings and performing arthroscopic surgery. The numbers and types of procedures are considered. The applicant's past and potential contributions to the society are weighed. AANA now has over 900 members.

Continuing Education

At first, the only educational experience available to the surgeon interested in shoulder arthroscopy was to personally visit one of the few knee arthroscopists who were transferring techniques to the shoulder joint.

The educational experience was broadened with continuing education courses by individuals, AANA, and AAOS. Still, the training programs were slow to react. This was due in part to a lack of interest by training program chairpersons. Only 20% of program chairpersons were involved in arthroscopic training by 1983.

The educational programs were initially didactic, with motor skill laboratories finally gaining popularity. Howard Sweeney developed the first knee model simulator for the motor skills laboratory. Models now exist for the shoulder. Because arthroscopy is technically intensive, motor skill laboratories continue to be included in most continuing education courses. Companies that market instrumentation offer motor skill experiences. One company has constructed a permanent motor skill laboratory; AANA plans a similar facility in Chicago, Illinois.

The educational process experience in the '70s with the knee has repeated itself in the '80s for the shoulder. The arthroscopist with knee joint skills started to explore the possibility in the shoulder in practice. Likewise, the shoulder surgeon explored arthroscopic techniques to the shoulder. One group went to arthroscopic meetings; the other went to shoulder meetings. The majority of registrants at recent conventional shoulder surgery courses have been arthroscopists. They attend these courses to learn about shoulder problems and open surgery with plans to utilize arthroscopy in their patient management. There is a demand for education and use of arthroscopic techniques in the shoulder. In the mid 1980s, over 1000 orthopedists attended seminars in our city (East Lansing, Michigan) in a period of 18 months. Now topics on arthroscopy are commonly integrated with meetings on the shoulder joint.

The practicing surgeon's continuing educational process will go on and arthroscopic surgery of the shoulder will be integrated into the practice of orthopedic surgery. Video tapes are helpful for learning technique. Journal articles emphasize concepts and results.

Medical Literature

To properly utilize arthroscopic techniques for patient care, one must study problems of the shoulder. I direct your attention to three recent textbooks on shoulder surgery, without which knowledge the mere performance of arthroscopy is without a firm foundation. These texts are: Neer CS II: *Shoulder Reconstruction*; Rockwood and Matsen: *The Shoulder*; and Rowe CR: *The Shoulder*.[73,90,92]

A review of initial publications on arthroscopy of the shoulder has more than a historical interest. The review of such material should help the shoulder arthroscopist to avoid various pitfalls and gain an appreciation of how problem solving occurred in shoulder arthroscopy.[21,24,25,94,103]

CLINICAL ASSESSMENT OF THE PATIENT WITH A SHOULDER PROBLEM

The orthopedic surgeon is commonly confronted with patients having shoulder problems, including many diagnostic enigmas and therapeutic challenges.

Like most orthopedic surgeons, I had no formal training in shoulder surgery. Therefore I am not able to write based on years of clinical experience in care of patients with shoulder problems, but I can only bring to your attention those resources I have uncovered or developed during my own learning experience. It is also important to realize that patients choose doctors before doctors have a chance to select patients, so my patient population is skewed toward those conditions treatable by arthroscopy. The reader should keep that in mind while reading the following discussion to evaluate the patient presenting with a shoulder problem.

Medical History

The modern practice of orthopedic surgery today requires a comprehensive medical record. Both government and insurance industry demands for these data are increasing. The information is used for billing purposes, outcome studies, and eventually treatment and physician evaluation. The orthopedic surgeon also has record keeping requirements for billing purposes and medical malpractice risk management. The process of collecting this information is annoying to the patient and laborious for the surgeon. During every health care encounter the patient must report the same information, a time-consuming and repetitive process. In my practice I have looked for ways to facilitate this tedious process for the patient, while making sure I get from them all the information I need.

We are well into the information age. Data collection can no longer be based on recall and recorded only by the physicians' handwriting.[47,57] Information must be collected by protocol, which requires a data collection form to jog the surgeon's memory. The simplest means is to collect the data on a form by making checkmarks, circling, and writing notes. I initiated a computerized medical record in my practice in 1980. This proprietary computerized medical record software* has been continually improved and expanded. Many surgeons have copied my shoulder forms for their use (see Chapter 4).

The emerging technology of interactive video is utilized to collect the data points on these multitudes of medical history questions at the time of first office visit (Fig. 1-2). Out-of-town patients are sent printed forms with the same questions so their case can be evaluated to assess whether the trip to our clinic would be beneficial.

The questionnaire asks the usual questions on demographics, present illness, past medical history, and review of systems. Specific questions relate to the shoulder itself. The process identifies and records the patient's chief complaint and the joint or joints involved. Previous arthroscopic or open surgery is documented. The absence of symptoms localized to the shoulder suggests an arthritic, cardiac, or neurovascular disease. Often the shoulder diagnosis is obvious by the history alone, such as in fractures and dislocations in referral patients with accompanying medical documents. Conditions such as acute calcific tendinitis or acromioclavicular (AC) joint degeneration with accompanying x-ray changes rarely test the diagnostic acumen of the physician.

The cause of many other shoulder disorders are not so obvious.[49] Discomfort in and about the shoulder joint is often vague and undefined by patients. Nonetheless, the problems interfere with their well-being, their activities of daily living, their work, their recreation, and occasionally their professional athletic endeavors. More specific information on shoulder problems includes the onset and location of pain, its frequency, and its relationship to specific activities. All these facets aid in diagnosis and management.

The interview must uncover the existence of grinding, catching, "going-out" sensations, and especially any limitations in daily activity. The assessment also includes questions about range of motion limitation, numbness, and circulatory problems.

Upon its completion, the information gathered in this form is generated into a written rough copy that is reviewed by both the patient and the surgeon (Fig. 1-2, *C*). Space is available on the rough copy for further notation by the surgeon at the time of patient evaluation. The amended form is eventually constructed into a final form of the patient's medical history and stored on hard disc within the computer.

---

*Benevolent Dictator, Information Health Network, 2950 Mt. Hope, Okemos, MI 48864, 1-800-443-0613

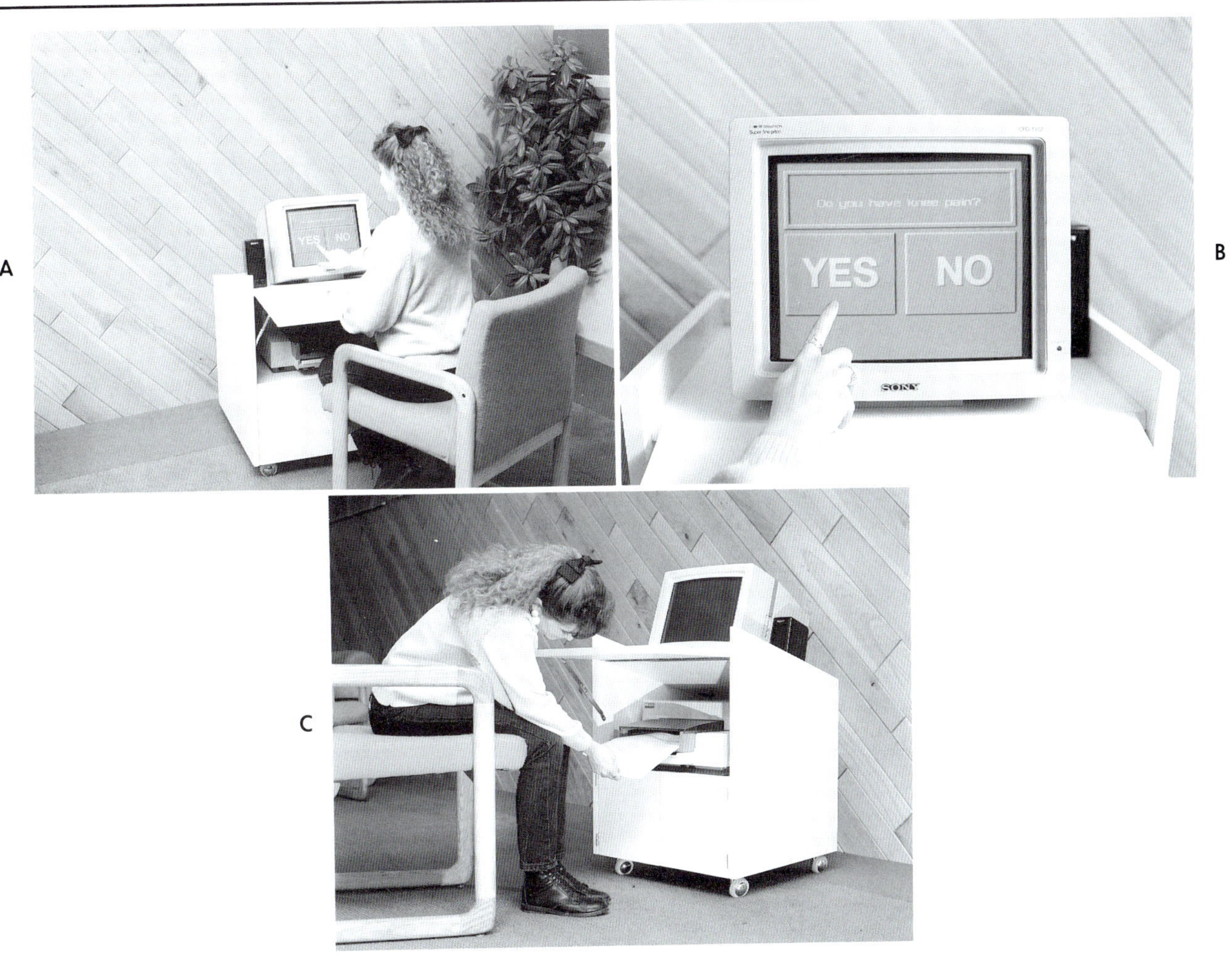

FIG. 1-2 Interactive video is used to collect the patient history. Proprietary software is used to generate a medical record. Patients sit before the television touch screen and answer medical historical questions.

A Patient sits in front of touch screen and cabinet that holds the computer.

B Close up of the touch screen as patient gives response. Note that no typing skills on keyboard are needed.

C Patient reaches into cabinet to retrieve typed narrative of just completed medical history.

Physical Examination

The reader is directed to publications by expert shoulder surgeons on the physical examination.[50,73,75,90,92]

I have organized the physical examination of the shoulder to parallel the classic examination of the heart. The examination involves inspection, palpation, manipulation, percussion, and auscultation.

My physical examination form is presented in Appendix A. The examiner fills in the form while performing the examination. The completed form is later input by office personnel into the computer.

Inspection. The examiner's inspection of the patient starts with any opportunity for observation. The chance observation of the patient entering the waiting room, filling out forms, entering the examination room, or removing a coat or shirt may provide valuable information on the daily routine. The patient's facial expression during the physical examination can also signal a problem.

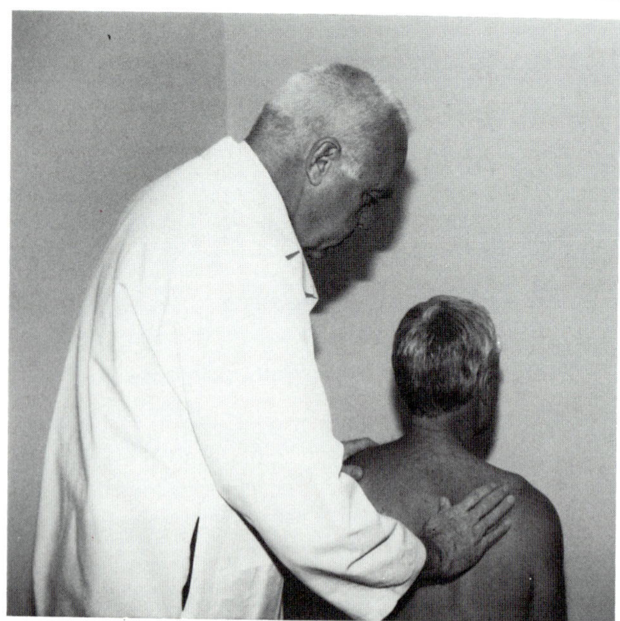

FIG. 1-3 Physical examination. The patient is sitting in position so that examiner may approach patient from all sides.

During the formal examination, the patient should be sitting in such a position that the examiner may walk around the patient (Fig. 1-3). The inspection should be done from both the anterior and posterior approach, and at some distance from the patient, to better observe areas of asymmetry or atrophy. It is important to watch the patient get out of a chair and move about the room so as to check the posture of the upper extremity. Is the patient wearing a sling or protecting the extremity at his or her side? Is he or she supporting the arm with the opposite hand?

The position or attitude in which the shoulder is held is important. Specifically, the contour of the shoulder joint can indicate whether the patient is hunching the shoulder or whether the humeral head is depressed. Are bony or tumor prominences present (Fig. 1-4, *A*)? Has atrophy occurred? Muscle atrophy may be better evaluated by inspection rather than palpation (Fig. 1-4, *B*). Comparing one shoulder to the other will reveal any asymmetry. Any discoloration from either a contusion or inflammation should be noted. Are any scars present that might indicate a previous injury or surgery? Inspection includes the bony prominence, the AC joint, and the scapula for prominence or winging. Prominence of the scapular spine may result from supraspinatus, infraspinatus, or trapezius muscle atrophy. Suprascapular nerve injuries are frequently overlooked in the differential diagnosis of shoulder pain.[11,14,33,50]

In watching the motion of the shoulder and its elevation, it is important to observe how much motion is contributed by the glenohumeral or scapular thoracic articulation. Initially, the glenohumeral joint comes into motion, and then with further abduction the scapular thoracic motion contributes to the elevation of the arm. The patient who has ankylosis of the glenohumeral joint or a rotator

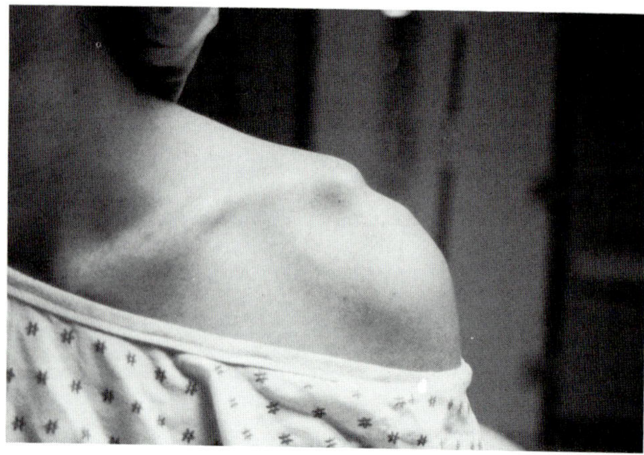

A

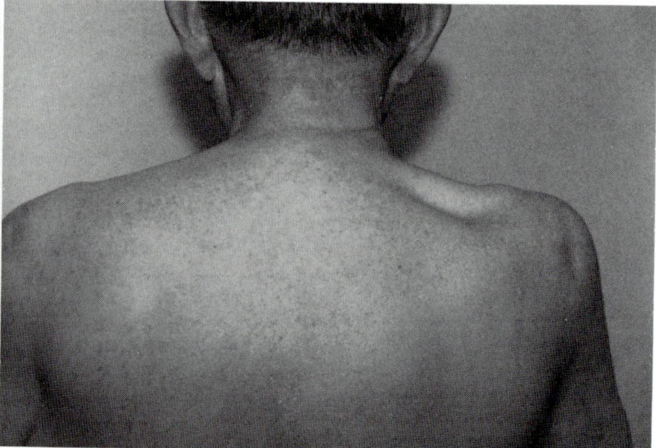

B

FIG. 1-4 Inspection.

A Bony prominence: The anterior view of right shoulder shows prominent end of clavicle representing old acromioclavicular separation.

B Muscular atrophy: The atrophy of the supraspinatus muscle in this patient is obvious by inspection from posterior.

cuff tear tends to hunch or elevate the scapulothoracic area without any change in its glenohumeral relationship on abduction.

Palpation. The patient is first instructed to identify, on palpation, the area of greatest tenderness. Is this area on the surface and palpable, or is it in a deeper area? Palpation of the area can also indicate induration, scars, redness, edema, or increased heat. The subcutaneous area might be indurated or might be the site of tumor (commonly a lipoma) or a cyst.

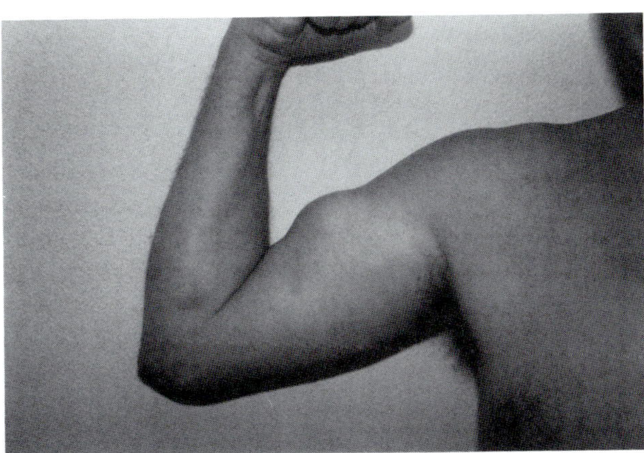

FIG. 1-5 The long head of the biceps tendon is prominent after spontaneous rupture. The patient may not recall this has happened. Another scenario of rupture is shoulder pain followed by sudden relief and the appearance of a "knot" in the arm.

The area of muscle, fascia, and ligaments is next to be considered. Is any rupture in the musculature present? In particular, the biceps tendon should be evaluated (Fig. 1-5). Atrophy may be evident in the deltoid or supraspinatus area. Does the patient have any tenderness around the trapezius or cervical musculature? Areas about the parascapular musculature in the rhomboids can be examined for so-called trigger points that are not related to the glenohumeral or AC joint.

The muscles should also be palpated during contraction. Is there any weakness present? Is muscular function impeded because of pain?

The area of the coracoclavicular ligament is palpated as is the humeral head from beneath and lateral (Fig. 1-6). One can palpate each of the bones and the prominence that make up the shoulder girdle: the sternum, the clavicle, the humerus, and the scapula. Are they tender to palpation? The examination should also include the area of the neck and spine and the adjacent parascapular area. The coracoid process and the adjacent AC joint can also be palpated. Palpation of the glenohumeral joint, the AC joint, or the sternoclavicular joint may show thickening caused by synovitis or osteophytes.

Manipulation. During this part of the examination, the physician can further manipulate the patient's neck to determine active range of motion, extension, flexion, and rotation. One can discern whether any motion of the neck produces shoulder pain and whether deep palpation behind the clavicle causes any pain or radiation in the area of the brachial plexus.

The sternoclavicular and AC joints have been examined by direct palpation. With midclavicular manual pressure, the joints at either end of the clavicle are indirectly

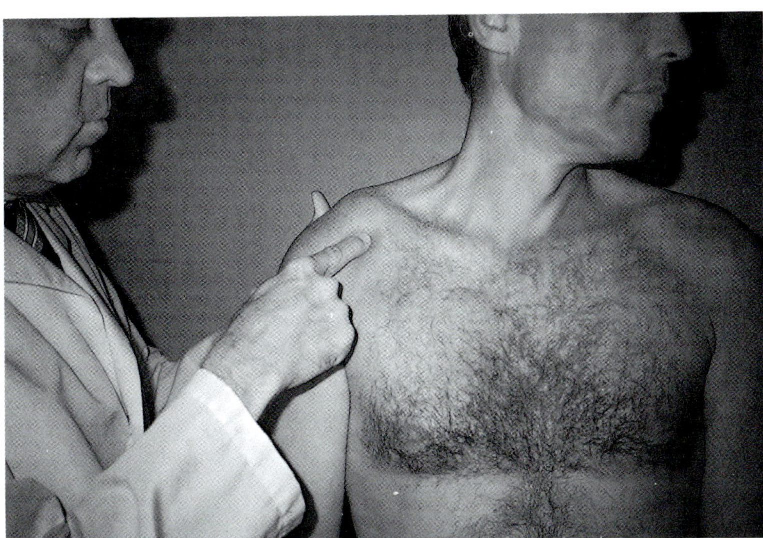

FIG. 1-6 Palpation of coracoclavicular ligament.

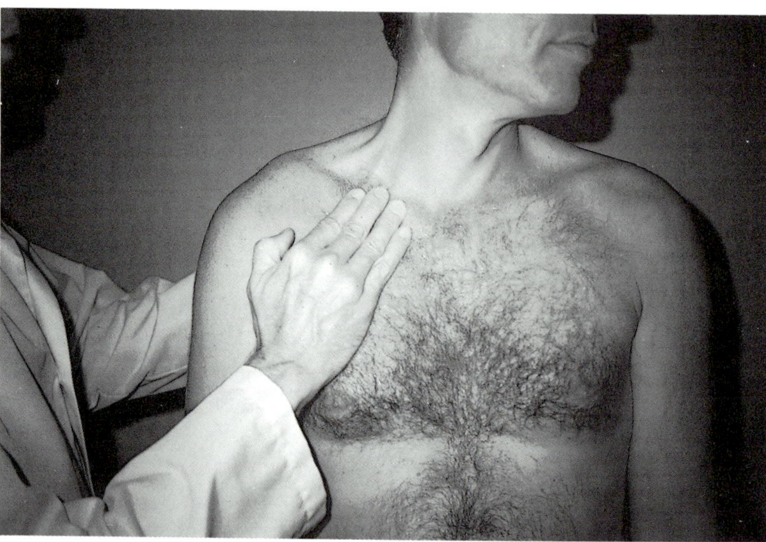

FIG. 1-7 Pushing on clavicle away from sternoclavicular joint will cause pain at involved joint.

evaluated for tenderness. This is accomplished by grasping the clavicle with thumb and fingers and pushing in and out and up and down in an attempt to elicit discomfort away from the area of manipulation. This test is positive if it produces discomfort at either end of the clavicle (Fig. 1-7) Remote force on the clavicle may produce pain at the abnormal joint. This finding is correlated with that of direct joint palpation.

Separation of the AC joint is best determined by having the patient hang the dependent arm at the side while the examiner secures the upper extremity. The patient voluntarily pushes down against the examiner's resistance. The clavicle will ride up in the separated shoulder as the scapula is actively depressed (Fig. 1-8). This test has been a more reliable test for me than simple weighted x-ray films in determining AC joint separation.

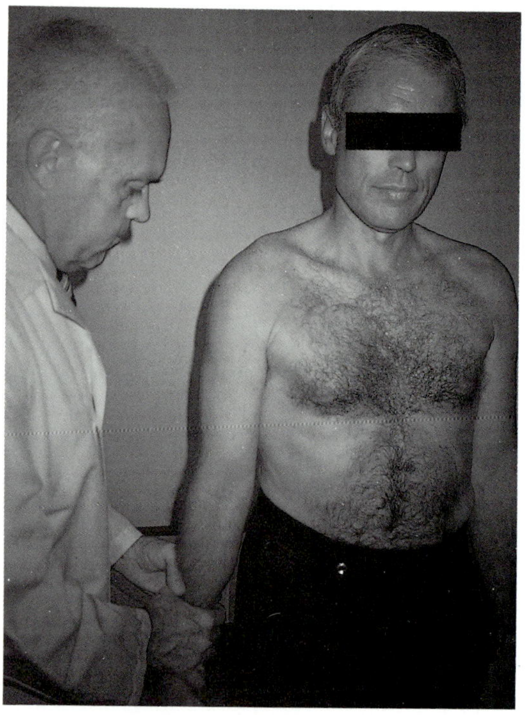

FIG. 1-8 Test for AC joint separation. Patient actively depresses arm against resistance. AC joint is then palpated for displacement.

Range of motion measurements. Opportunities for error in these measurements abound. The patient's initiative or lack thereof may influence active range of motion. Loss of range of motion occurs with aging, and older women have less motion than older men.[9] Pain, ankylosis, or muscle weakness may restrict the patient's ability to move the shoulder. Trunk rotation or leaning will affect the measurement. The base line can be the perpendicular or the patient's thoracic spine. Marked curvature or the spine makes this benchmark an estimate at best. It seems to me that the examiner is making estimates in space even when a goniometer is utilized. To me, shoulder measurements of range of motion are subject to variability and error. They are at best estimates.

Nonetheless, I still measure and record range of mo-

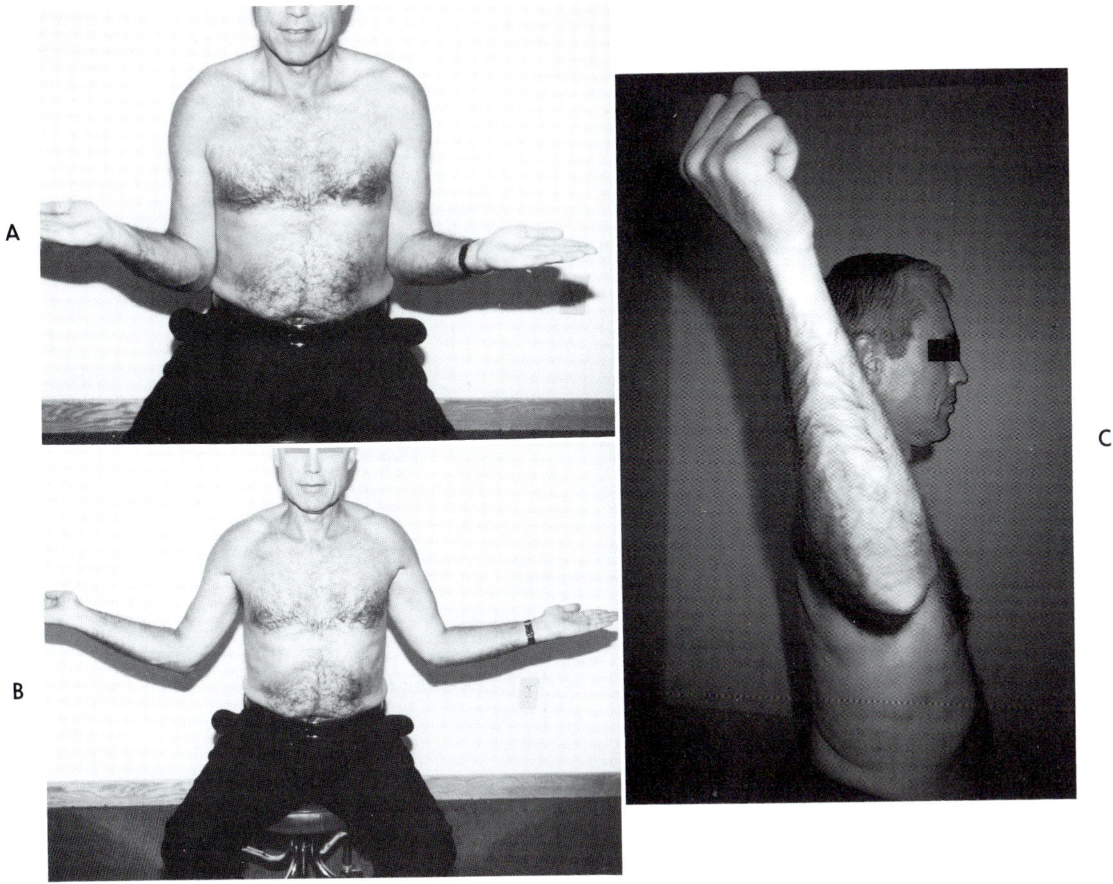

FIG. 1-9 Physical measurement of external rotation.

A Adduction/external rotation: CORRECT METHOD: Proper arm position is full adduction when external rotation is measured.

B WRONG METHOD: False postitive increased measurement in external rotation is achieved when arms abduct away from the trunk.

C Abduction/external rotation: The starting position of the arm is at 90 degrees abduction. From this point maximal active external rotation is achieved. This position simulates the cocked position for throwing.

tion with a goniometer. Simultaneous comparison measurements reduce the tendency to false recordings caused by trunk rotation or leaning (Fig. 1-9; see also Fig. 1-11). Motion of the opposite shoulder provides a control for comparison. The active voluntary ranges of motion of the shoulder should be compared to the passive (Fig. 1-9).

External rotation is measured in two starting positions: with the arm adducted and then abducted to 90 degrees. First, the patient should hold the elbow at the side in adduction, prior to initiating external rotation (Fig. 1-9, *A*). A false increase in external rotation occurs when the patient moves the arm off the trunk. All patients require instruction during this test to avoid erroneous measurements (Fig. 1-9, *B*). The starting position for the second test is 90 degrees abduction, neutral flexion/extension before external rotation. This later motion is the preparatory position for throwing (Fig. 1-9 *B*). The second examination for external rotation may not be performed properly in rotator cuff disease or frozen shoulder, because the patient cannot easily achieve abduction, extension, and external rotation. The patient with these disorders achieves false external rotation by unconsciously bringing the arm into flexion to achieve external rotation. To standardize this measurement, I assist the patient in first gaining maximal abduc-

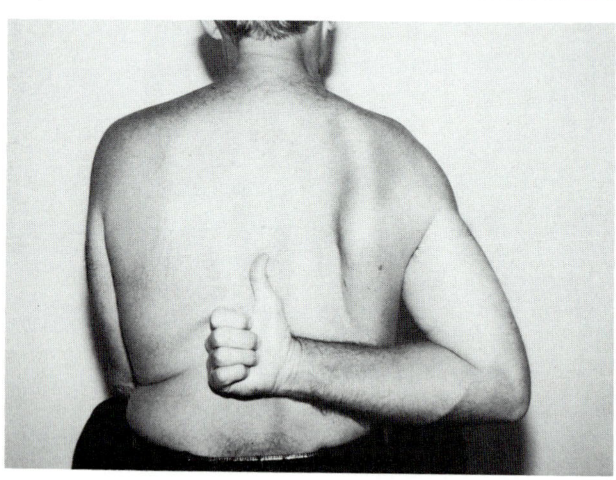

FIG. 1-10 Measurement for internal rotation is recorded by how far the patient can place his or her thumb up the spine.

tion before any attempt at external rotation. In the most severe cases the patient can neither fully abduct, extend or externally rotate the arm. In addition, when shoulder instability exists, this second test of range of motion in the abducted external rotation position may be limited by apprehension, pain, or contracture. Comparisons of active and passive external rotation are possible under anesthesia if the patient comes to surgery. The examination under anesthesia determines the presence of a fixed glenohumeral contracture. (See Chapter 8.)

Since virtually all patients can bring their hand over across their abdomen, internal rotation can be better assessed by how far they can reach the hand up behind the back. The extent of this motion is recorded by the bony landmark touched with the tip of the thumb (Fig. 1-10).

The extent of elevation includes both shoulder joint and scapular motion, so often the examiner must stabilize the scapula to assess actual glenohumeral motion. Shoulder elevation is measured in a different plane than shoulder abduction (Fig. 1-11). Active glenohumeral joint motion can be evaluated during elevation of the shoulder (Fig. 1-11, *A*). A patient with a limited range of motion frequently can pull the arm higher when coming up in adduction and flexion in the sagittal plane than when coming up

A

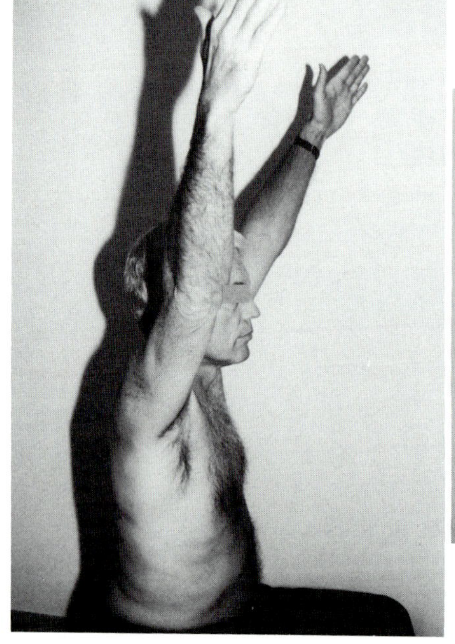

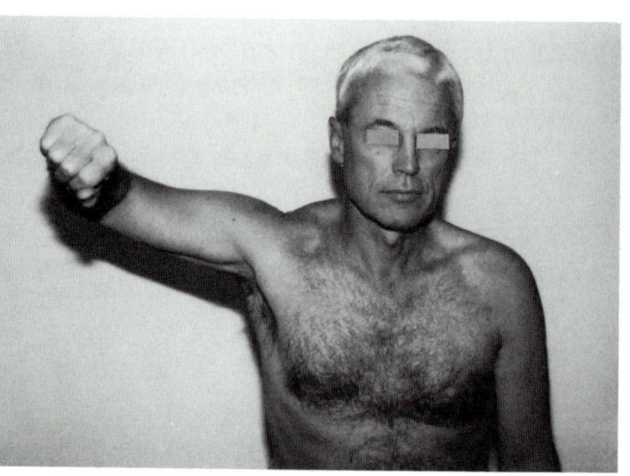

B

FIG. 1-11 Measurement of shoulder elevation.

A Shoulder elevation is measured in the plane of the scapular (that is, slight forward flexion), followed by combination of elevation and abduction.

B After achieving full elevation the patient is instructed to bring the arm into extension and slowly lower the arm. This maneuver will produce pain at this position in a patient with rotator cuff disease.

in the coronal plane with the arm out in extension and abduction. This is especially true of a patient who has rotator cuff problems at the supraspinatus attachment. After full elevation in the sagittal plane, the patient is asked to lower the upper extremity in the coronal plane (with the arm out to the side) (Fig. 1-11, *B*). Pain or weakness occurs at 90 degrees of abduction. Supporting the patient's arm until past this point or even stopping the action is often required. This sign indicates a rotator cuff problem.

The grip strength can be measured with the use of a Jamar dynamometer (Fig. 1-12).

Impingement. Signs of impingement syndrome on the anterior side of the joint can be elicited as described by Neer (Fig. 1-13).[67,74] The abducted arm is brought into adduction, and the area of the coracoacromial ligament is palpated (Fig. 1-14). The greater tuberosity comes into contact with the anterior acromion and coracoacromial ligament. If the maneuver produces symptoms, this area of the rotator cuff has likely undergone pathological changes. I like to have the patient reproduce the freestyle swimming motion to evaluate impingement. I first take them through the motion with the thumb down, and then with the thumb up. The thumb down position brings the supraspinatus tendon insertion and the greater tuberosity under the acromion; this reproduces the impingement. Auscultation should accompany impingement testing. Correlation is

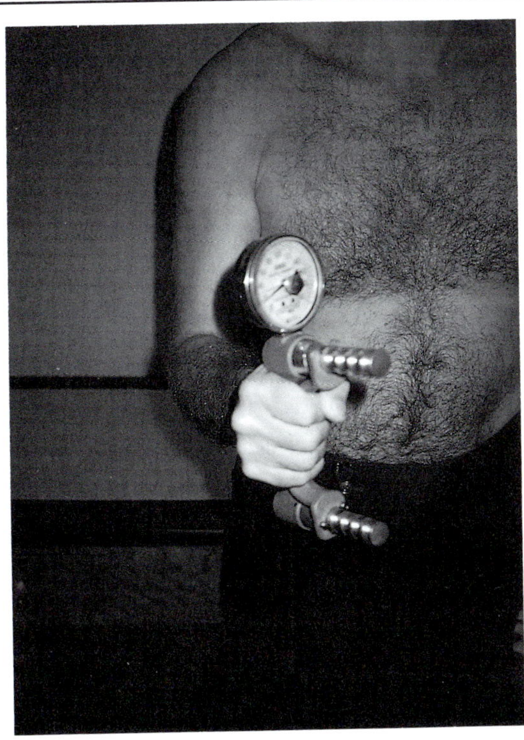

FIG. 1-12 Jamar Dynanometer for measuring grip strength.

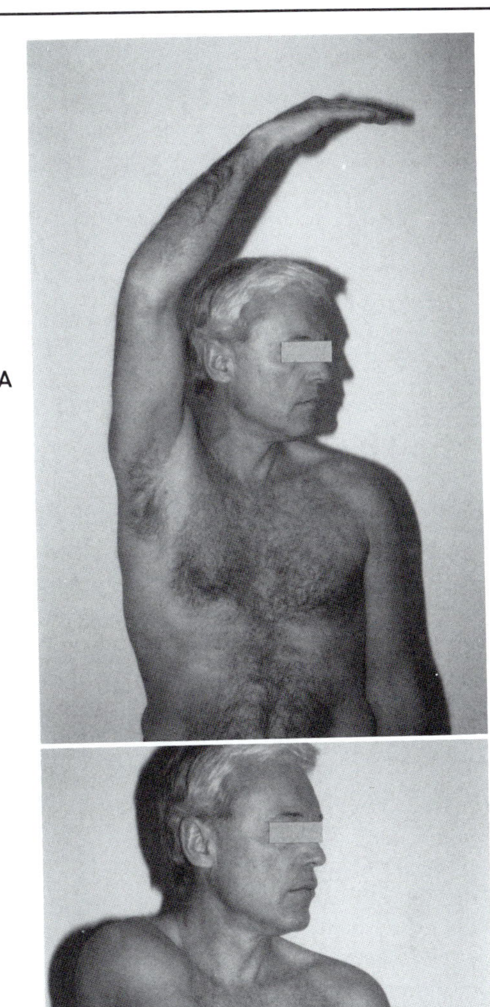

A

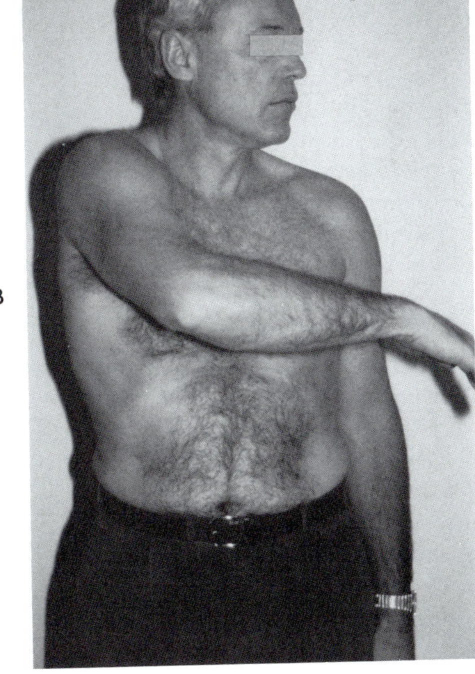

B

FIG. 1-13 Elevation for impingement.

A Patient is performing arm elevation in adducted postion that produces discomfort of impingement.

B Patient internally rotates and adducts the arm.

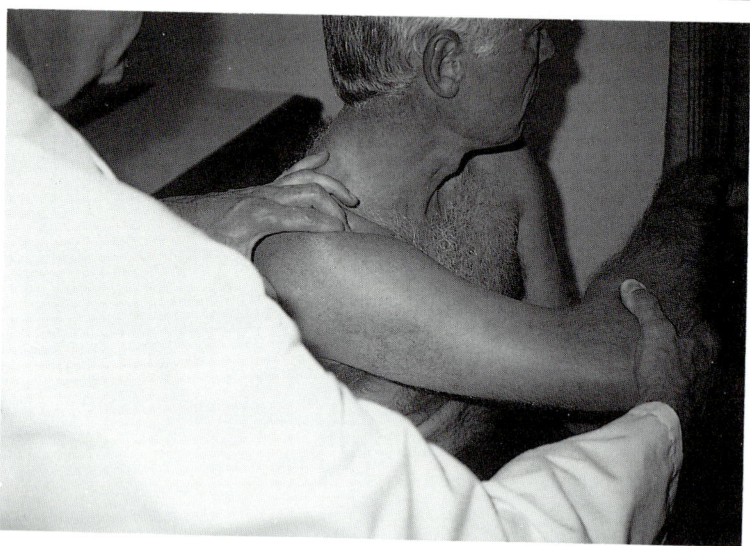

FIG. 1-14 Physical examination for anterior humeral impingement on acromion and coracoacromional ligament.

possible with plain film x-rays. The outlet view may confirm an acromial bony spur (Fig. 1-15). Areas of erosion under the acromion should be present at arthroscopy to confirm impingement diagnosis (Fig. 1-16).

Instability. Testing for instability requires a variety of tests. The tests combine the examiner's palpable sensation and observation of the patient's reaction by muscular guarding or expression of apprehension. The first examiner and the first attempts often yield the greatest information because the patient may have involuntary muscular guarding. Any subtle anterior, posterior, and inferior glenohumeral subluxation must be determined. The examiner must gain the patient's confidence and perform a gentle test looking for subtle motion. Attempts at frank dislocation are not necessary and should be avoided. The examiner must support the patient's arm while producing the various gentle forces (Fig. 1-17). Furthermore, the examiner must determine the aspect of voluntary and involuntary instability, since the voluntary type has a greater propensity for psychological problems and poor outcome from attempts at surgical repair.

These instability tests are repeated with the patient under anesthesia, but without the benefit of watching the patient's reaction.

The downward pressure test was described by John Feagin.[91] In this test the examiner and the patient are both standing (Fig. 1-17). The patient's elbow is positioned on the examiner's shoulder. Then the examiner gently depresses the abducted humerus and watches for the patient's reaction, either by muscular resistance or by facial expression. Care should be taken to limit the maneuver to subluxation, not actual dislocation, of the patient's shoulder.

A posterior subluxation can be diagnosed by bringing the patient's arm into abduction and 90 degrees of flexion. With counterpressure against the scapula, the surgeon pushes on the elbow to try to drive the humerus out posteriorly (Fig. 1-18). Next, the patient is asked to reproduce this maneuver. Those with voluntary subluxation can repeat this test at will; those without voluntary subluxation cannot. Every patient should have the chance to do this on his or her own. This opportunity will sort out the patients who have a learned muscular contracture that is considered voluntary in nature.

The patient sits to test anterior–posterior passive motion. The scapula is controlled with the examiner's forearm (Fig. 1-19).

Another apprehension test is performed with the patient in the supine position. This test has been popularized by Frank Jobe of Los Angeles.[56] The patient's arm is placed at 90 degrees abduction and external rotation while the examiner applies anterior force to keep the shoulder reduced (Fig. 1-20, *A*). The examiner quickly removes the hand from the humeral head. The production of pain results in a positive sign for anterior instability (Fig. 1-20, *B*).

Another method of checking glenohumeral instability uses the examination table as a fulcrum (Fig. 1-21). The patient is placed in the supine position. The examiner controls the elbow and forearm with one hand, while placing force on the proximal humerus with the other hand.

Fowler has described a relocation test.[39] The patient is placed in the supine position near the edge of the examination table. The examiner holds the patient's elbow so that the arm is at 90 degrees abduction and external rotation. A

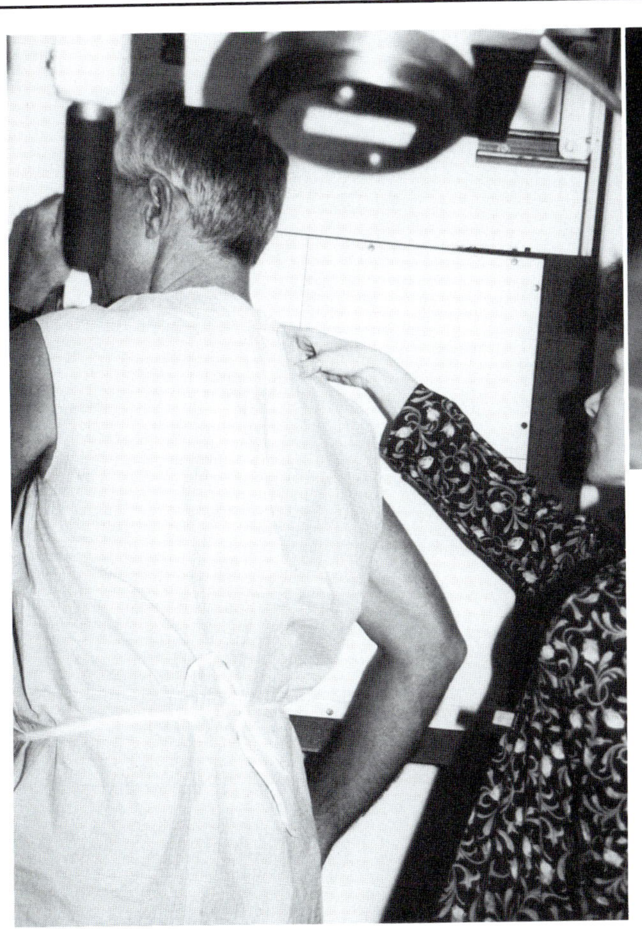

A

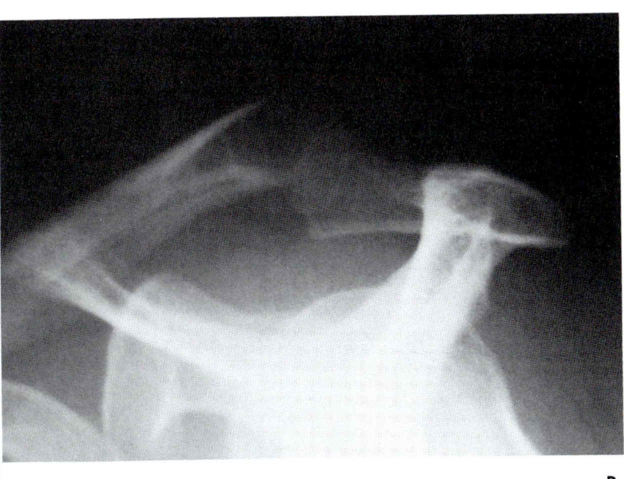

B

FIG. 1-15 X-ray film of acromial arch outlet.

A Patient is positioned for acromial arch view.

B Abnormal x-ray acromial prominence below level of the clavicle.

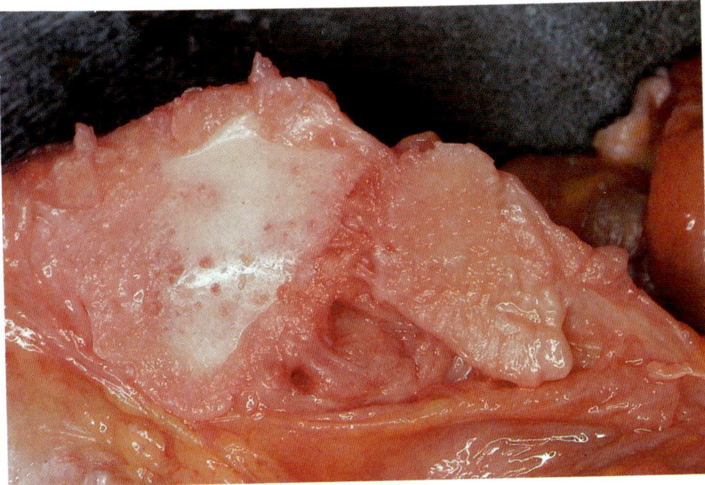

FIG. 1-16 Gross pathological specimen illustrates erosion of soft tissue under acromion and bone exposed.

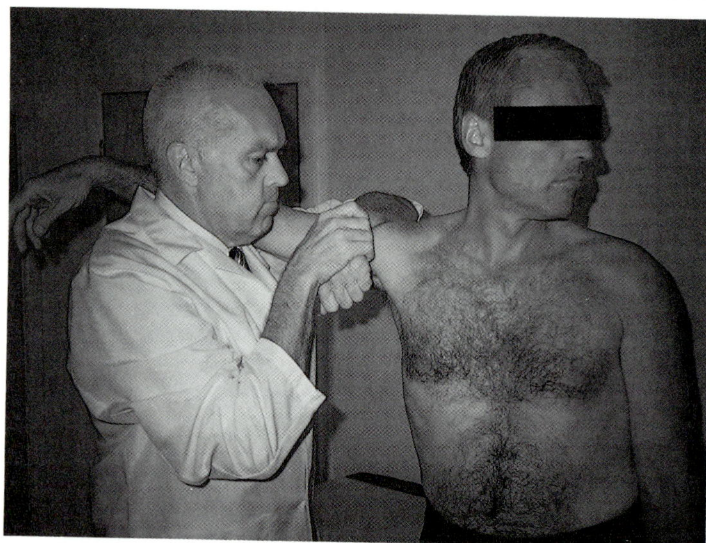

FIG. 1-17 Anterior–inferior instability testing: Both the patient and the doctor are standing. Downward pressure is applied to the patient's shoulder.

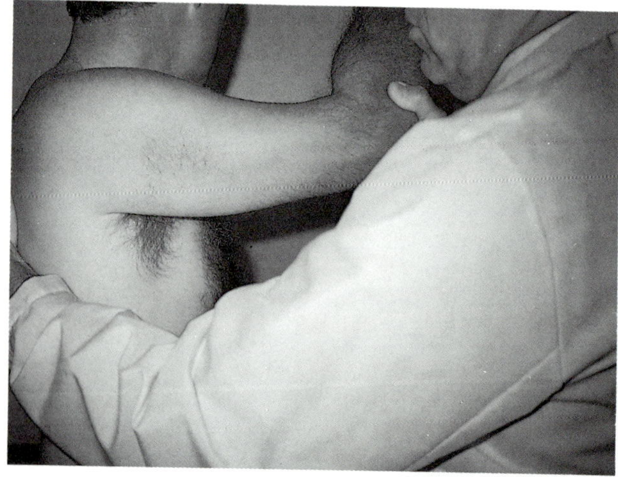

FIG. 1-18 Posterior instability testing: Physical examination for posterior dislocation.

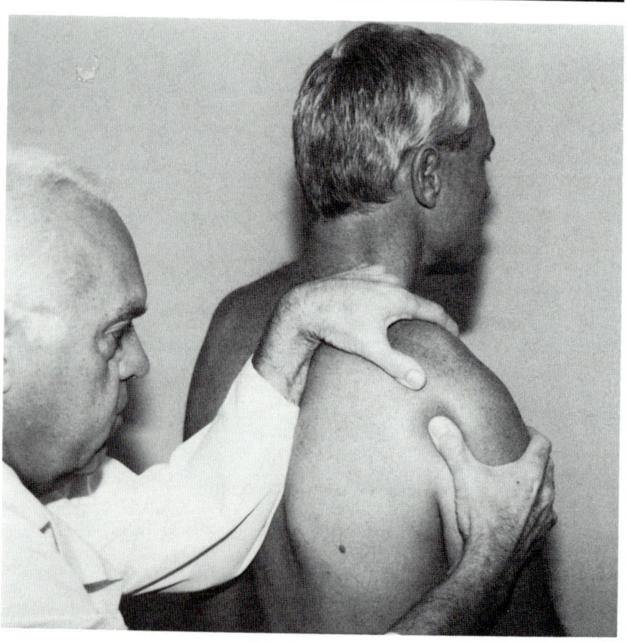

FIG. 1-19 Anterior instability testing: Examination for glenohumeral instability requires the examiner to control the scapula with forearm and hand while producing passive motion with other hand.

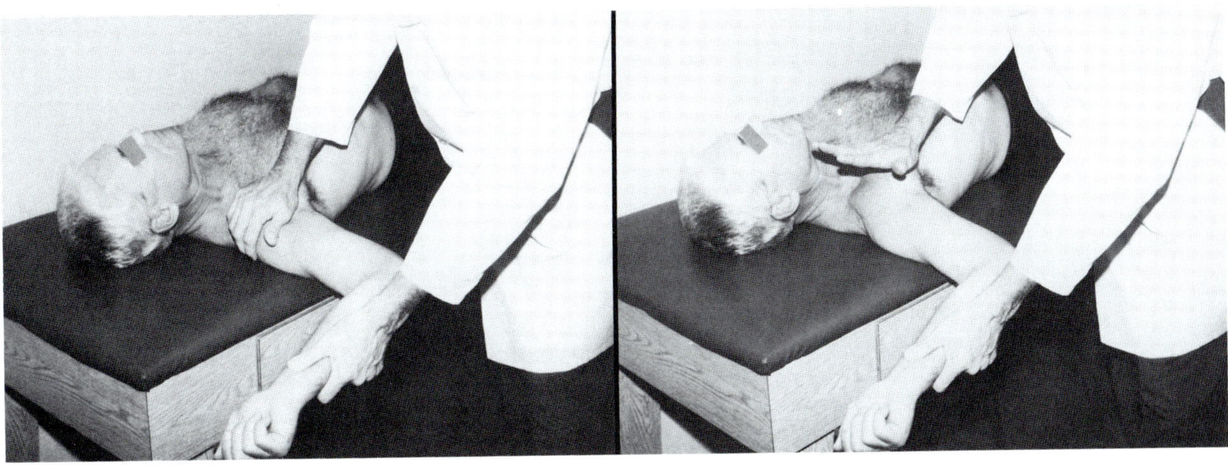

A B

FIG. 1-20 Apprehension testing.

A Arm is placed at 90 degrees abduction and external rotation. Examiner applies anterior force to keep shoulder reduced.

B Pain after examiner removes hand indicates anterior instability.

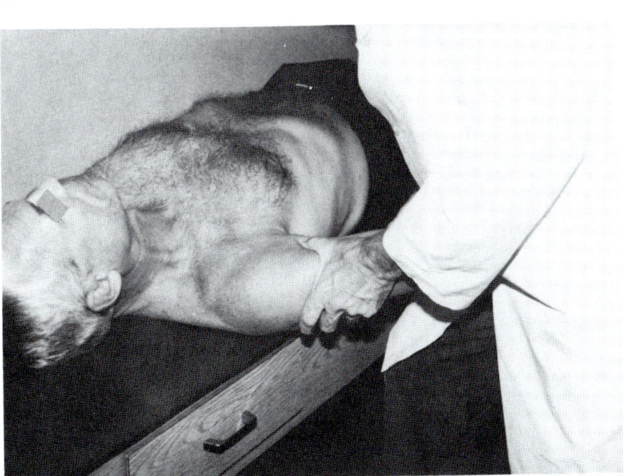

FIG. 1-21 Another anterioposterior testing method: The patient is supine and the scapula is controlled with table as a fulcrum.

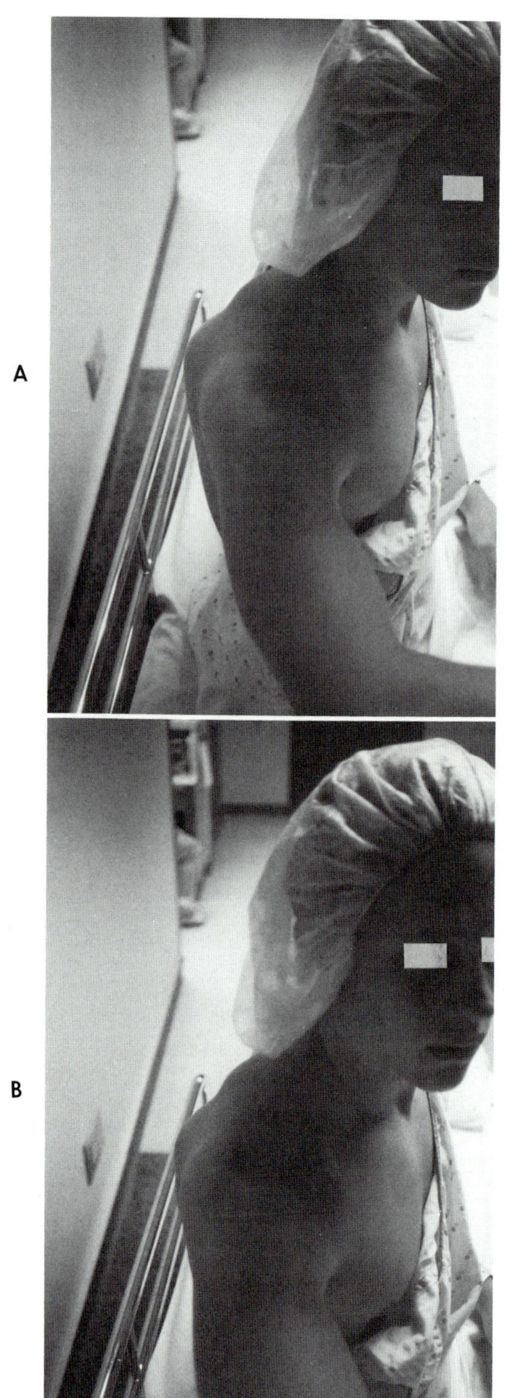

FIG. 1-22
A Patient makes voluntary movement that subluxes the glenohumeral joint.
B Reduction occurs with relaxation and extension of arm.

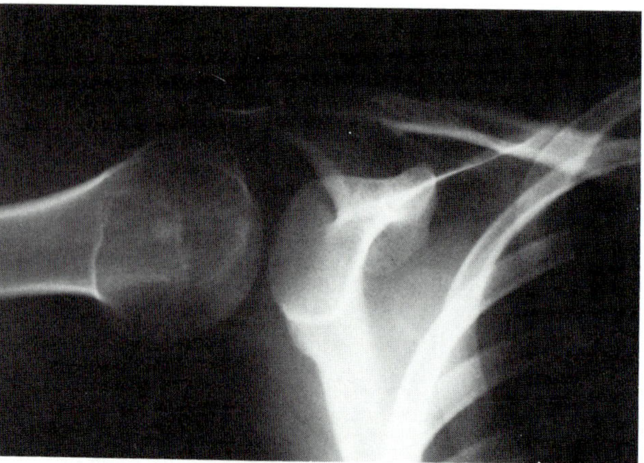

FIG. 1-23 X-ray film taken in anterior-posterior position and in axillary view to demonstrate subluxation.

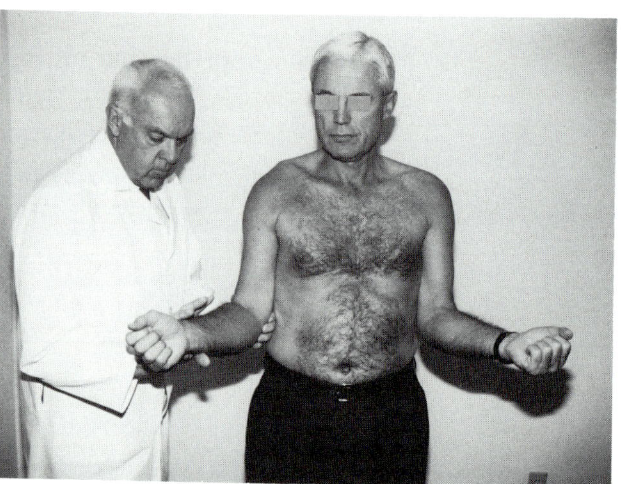

FIG. 1-24 Muscle strength testing: External rotation strength is tested with arm adducted. The patient with large full-thickness rotator cuff tear often shows weakness with this test.

posterior force is applied to the proximal humerus. The test is positive when the patient's apprehension is relieved, as the anteriorly displaced shoulder is reduced by the posterior pressure.

In addition to passive manipulation testing for shoulder instability, the patient should be encouraged to demonstrate voluntary movements that could reproduce the abnormality (Fig. 1-22). This is especially important for a patient with a hyperelastic joint who demonstrates anterior, posterior, or (rarely) inferior voluntary subluxation of the joint. X-ray films are taken as the patient holds a voluntary position of subluxation. Images of the patient's other side and the same side in a reduced position are com-

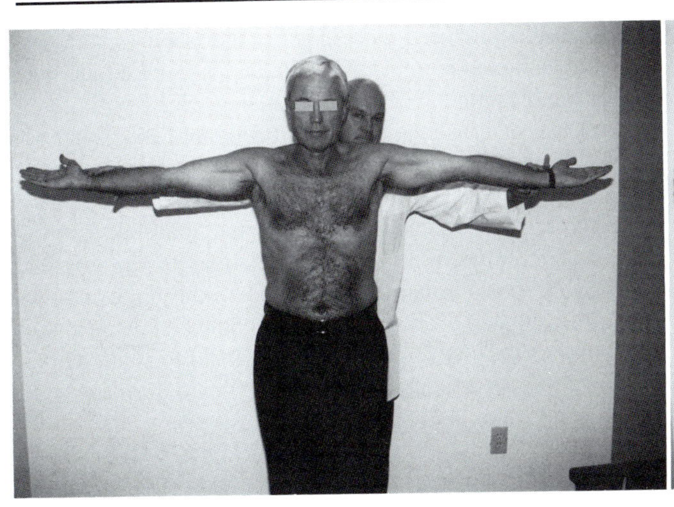

A

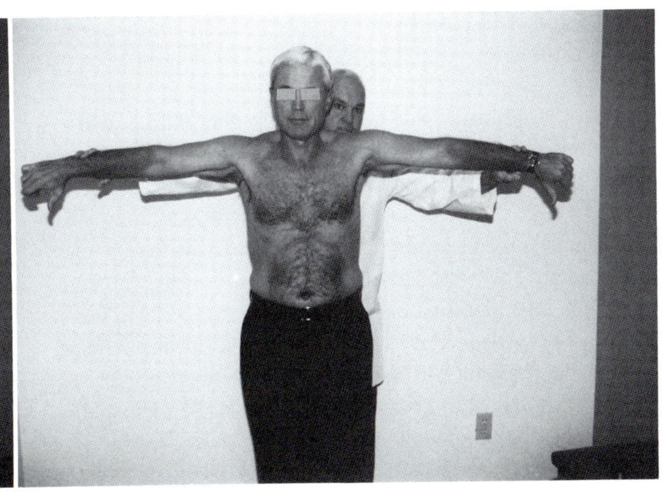

B

FIG. 1-25 Muscle testing in abduction: Both arms are tested simultaneously.
A First test is with patient's palms up for anterior cuff muscles.
B The second test is with patient's thumbs down for posterior cuff muscles.

pared. Anterior–posterior and axillary positions are necessary for comprehensive appraisal (Fig. 1-23).

Some patients can produce the sulcus test just by relaxing. This sign is positive when the humerus is inferiorly distracted from the acromion, producing a depression between the two bones. Other patients can produce this sign with voluntary muscular motion. The sign also occurs in deltoid paralysis. Passive force on the arm by the examiner may demonstrate the subtle sulcus sign. It may also be present when patient is placed in skin traction at time of arthroscopy (see Chapter 8).

The opposite shoulder should be tested in the same manner for the benefit of comparison. The examiner should be aware that both shoulders are involved in 24% of cases.[80]

Muscle strength. Testing the musculature around the shoulder for power is combined with observation and correlation of the patient's expression of discomfort. I test for motor power with the patient standing if possible (Figs. 1-24 and 1-25). This allows me to move around and about the patient to expedite the testing.

Strength testing is performed from different starting positions. With the patient's arms at the side, I test flexion, extension, adduction, abduction, and internal and external rotation power (Fig. 1-24).

The second starting position is with the arms extended at 90 degrees abduction and neutral flexion. I first test with the patient's palm up for anterior rotator cuff and then with the thumbs, down for posterior rotator cuff (Fig. 1-25).

The third starting position has the patient abduct the shoulder to 90 degrees and neutral flexion/extension position, plus flex the elbow to 90 degrees. The examiner's hand is placed upon the patient's wrist for resistance to active elevation and external rotation. This maneuver tests combined abduction external rotation strength and sensitivity (Fig. 1-26).

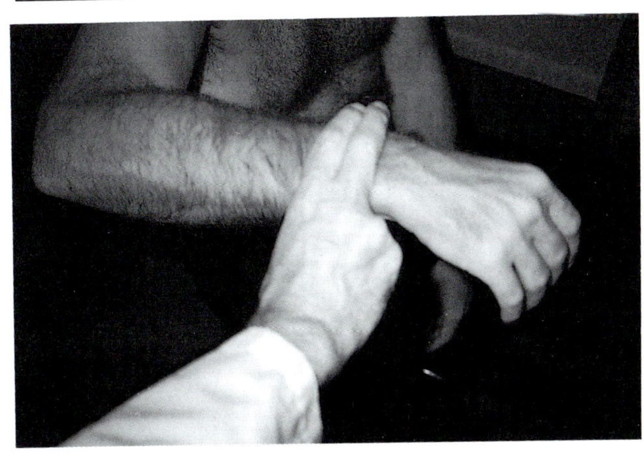

FIG. 1-26 Physical examination to put stress on supraspinal area, testing for possible weakness or tear.

Neurovascular assessment. A routine neurological test should direct the examiner's attention to cervical nerve root compression or peripheral nerve injury.

Circulatory problems that produce shoulder region symptoms include congenital abnormalities, compression syndromes, shoulder hand syndrome, sympathetic dystrophy, or even cardiac muscular ischemia.[77] Simple palpation (diminished pulse) or even auscultation (bruit) should detect a problem. Doppler testing may be helpful.

The Adson maneuver, in which the patient takes the chin to the opposite side and the neck goes into extension with contraction of the scalene musculature on the effected side, may decrease the patient's pulse. Also, traction on the arm with the head leaning the opposite way may point out a neurological impingement syndrome in the subclavicular area. The presence of radial pulse serves as a benchmark for postoperative assessment.

Another Adson test may be performed on the wrist arteries. The patient makes a fist. The examiner compresses both the radial and ulnar artery at the wrist. The patient unclenches the fist; first one, then the other vessel is released. The previously blanched palm becomes red with restoration of blood flow. If no filling occurs or filling is delayed when the radial artery is released, then a blockage may be presumed. The same would be true for the ulnar artery.

Percussion. Gentle percussion by tapping, not actually palpating, the top of the patient's head tests for nerve compression in or radiation from the cervical spine.[49] Also, gentle percussion on the scapula, clavicle, or sternum, and even on areas around the humerus, can indicate bony sources of discomfort. Percussion is performed along peripheral nerves when testing for a Tinel's sign.

Auscultation. Auscultation adds considerable insight to the patient's shoulder problem. Listening provides an opportunity to correlate the noises to the pain the patient has experienced. The examiner must learn how to discern the crepitus produced by both active and passive motion of the glenohumeral joint. Auscultation is carried out with both the examiner and patient standing. The arm is internally and externally rotated to produce the noise, first actively and then passively, with the examiner's ear against the shoulder (Fig. 1-27).

When subsequently inspecting the joint by arthroscopy, the surgeon can make correlations to the physical findings. These opportunities provide a means of improving the surgeon's examination and clinical skills. Auscultation enables the surgeon to distinguish separated labrum tears, fine degenerative arthritis, synovitis, rotator cuff tear, and some impingement problems.

Examination Following Local Anesthetic Injection. The injection of local anesthetic assists in determining the origin of shoulder pain.[68] The AC joint is palpable and easily injectable (Fig. 1-28).

Anesthetic is injected into the subacromial space to relieve pain of impingement so that motion and muscle strength can be evaluated in the absence of pain.

Anesthetic is injected into the glenohumeral joint when an intraarticular lesion is suspected. A second observation is possible with glenohumeral fluid injection. The normal joint volume is decreased to less than 20 ml in frozen shoulder.

It should be noted that a full-thickness rotator cuff defect will allow anesthetic agent to move to both spaces and not give selective clues to the origin of pain.

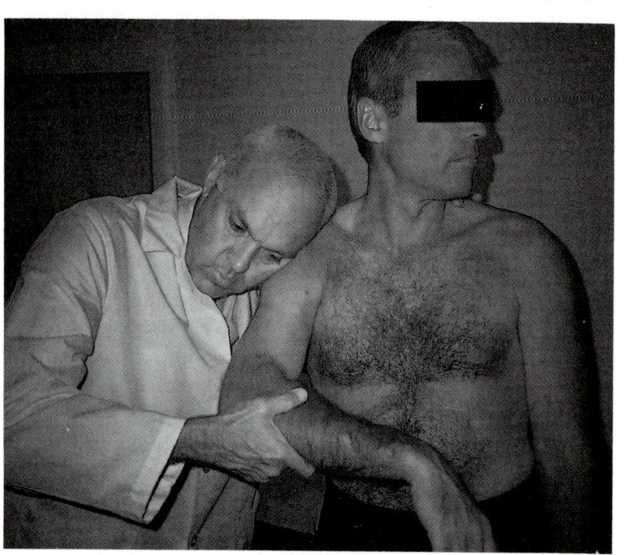

FIG. 1-27 Auscultation of shoulder.

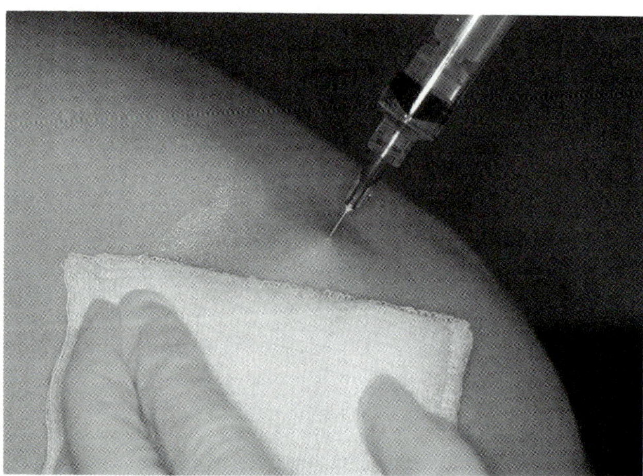

FIG. 1-28 Local anesthetic injection: The use of local anesthesia assists the examiner to determine the source of pain. The AC joint source of symptoms can be removed with injection of local anesthetic agent.

Shoulder Imaging

Photographs. Photographs, both prints and 35 mm slides, are the best means of recalling physical abnormalities. The prints may be placed in the permanent medical record, while slides are useful for scientific presentations. The arthroscopic surgical findings are routinely recorded and stored by photographic methods.

Television. The recording of patient physical findings, including motion, may be recorded and stored on videotape. The decreasing price of television cameras and their smaller sizes make this a viable alternative for patient function documentation.

Plain Film X-Rays. Plain film x-rays are taken to confirm or discover diagnoses. The clinical impression should determine the request for plain film x-ray views. I do not have one routine x-ray series. I do not start with a "routine AP and lateral x-ray." No one x-ray series will cover all cases, unless unnecessary films are taken. After review of the initial x-ray films, additional views may be requested. My initial request is directed toward the most likely diagnosis.

If calcific tendonitis is suspected, then internal and external rotation anterior–posterior films are requested to locate the position of the deposit without superimposition of bone over the calcium deposit (Fig. 1-29).

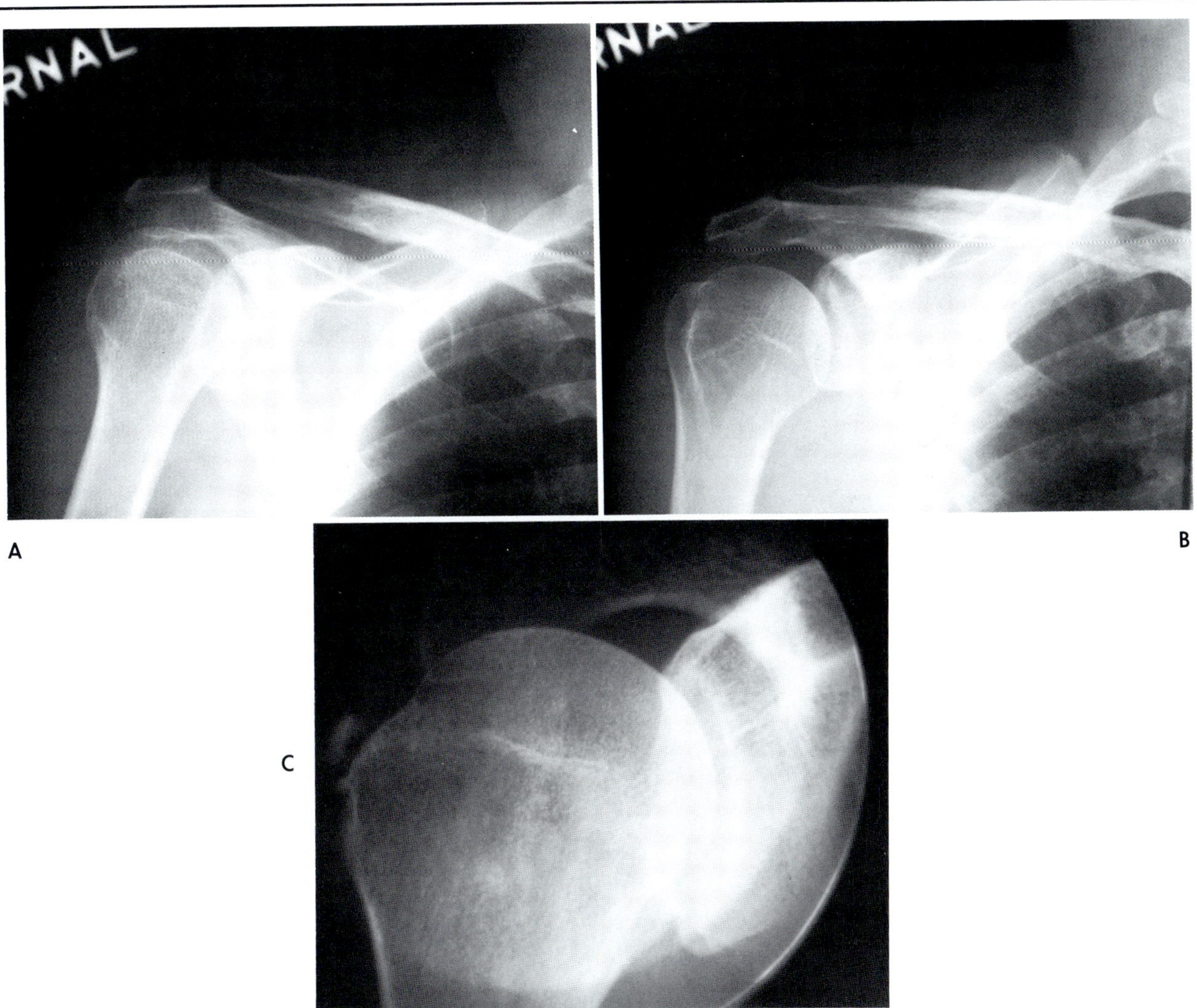

FIG. 1-29 Internal and external rotation film.

A Internal rotation.

B External rotation.

C Calcific tendonitis: Plain film x-ray taken in AP direction, but with shoulder internally rotated shows the calcium deposit without being obscured by overlying bone.

If frozen shoulder or rotator cuff disease is suspected, then an arch or outlet view helps visualize an acromial spur with the associated impingement (see Fig. 1-15).[71]

The axillary view is important on a routine basis because it is the truest lateral view of the shoulder (Fig. 1-30). The transthoracic lateral view is not recommended for lateral projection because of the overlying thorax.

In glenohumeral instability cases, I request true anterior–posterior, axillary and Stryker views (Fig. 1-31). Comparing the problem shoulder to the opposite one is often helpful for interpretation of bony defect of humeral head on Stryker view (Fig. 1-32). This view will often show an os acromion that is not easily seen in other views (Fig. 1-33).[12,72]

The joint space is best seen with true anterior–posterior (Fig. 1-34, *A*). The apical oblique view of the shoulder demonstrates the anterior and inferior avulsion fracture associated with dislocation (Fig. 1-34, *B*).[40]

Rockwood's fracture series is recommended for trauma cases.[90] This series includes a scapular view (Fig. 1-35). Internal and external rotation films taken in the anterior to posterior postion have the potential to show avulsion fracture of greater tuberosity (Fig. 1-36).

X-ray films for the AC joint often require modification of technique, as this joint is a periphery of bone structure (Fig. 1-37). Stress x-ray films may be requested to obtain a permanent document of AC joint separation, but this diagnosis is best established by history and physical examination (see Fig. 1-8). X-ray film confirmation of an AC joint separation can be performed with weight and/or traction. However, this test is generally not reliable, because the patient may guard the painful shoulder, giving a false negative test.

Cervical spine films are requested when degenerative arthritis is suspected as cause of the shoulder pain. Hawkins et al[49] have outlined tests to differentiate neck and shoulder pain.

A chest x-ray film is requested when Pancoast tumor or condition is suspected in the ribs.

Text continued on p. 25.

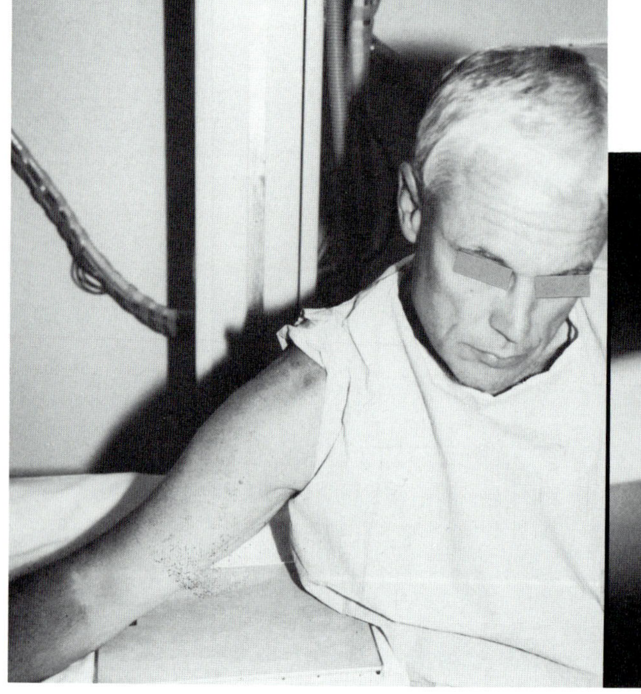

A

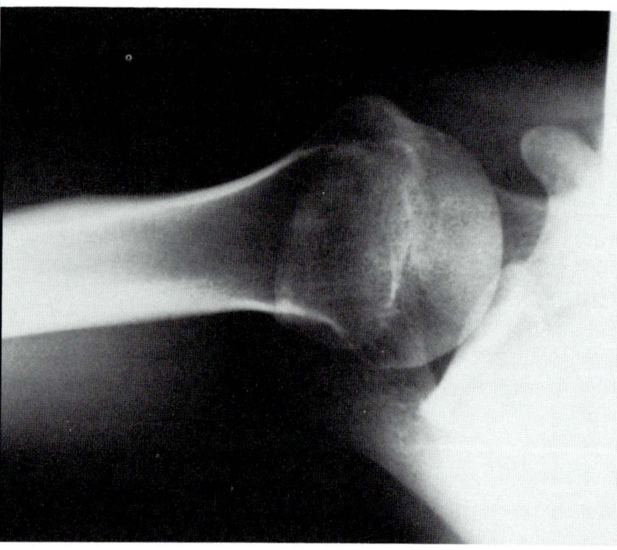

B

FIG. 1-30 Axillary view.

A Patient is positioned for axillary view x-ray.

B Axillary view provides true lateral view of joint.

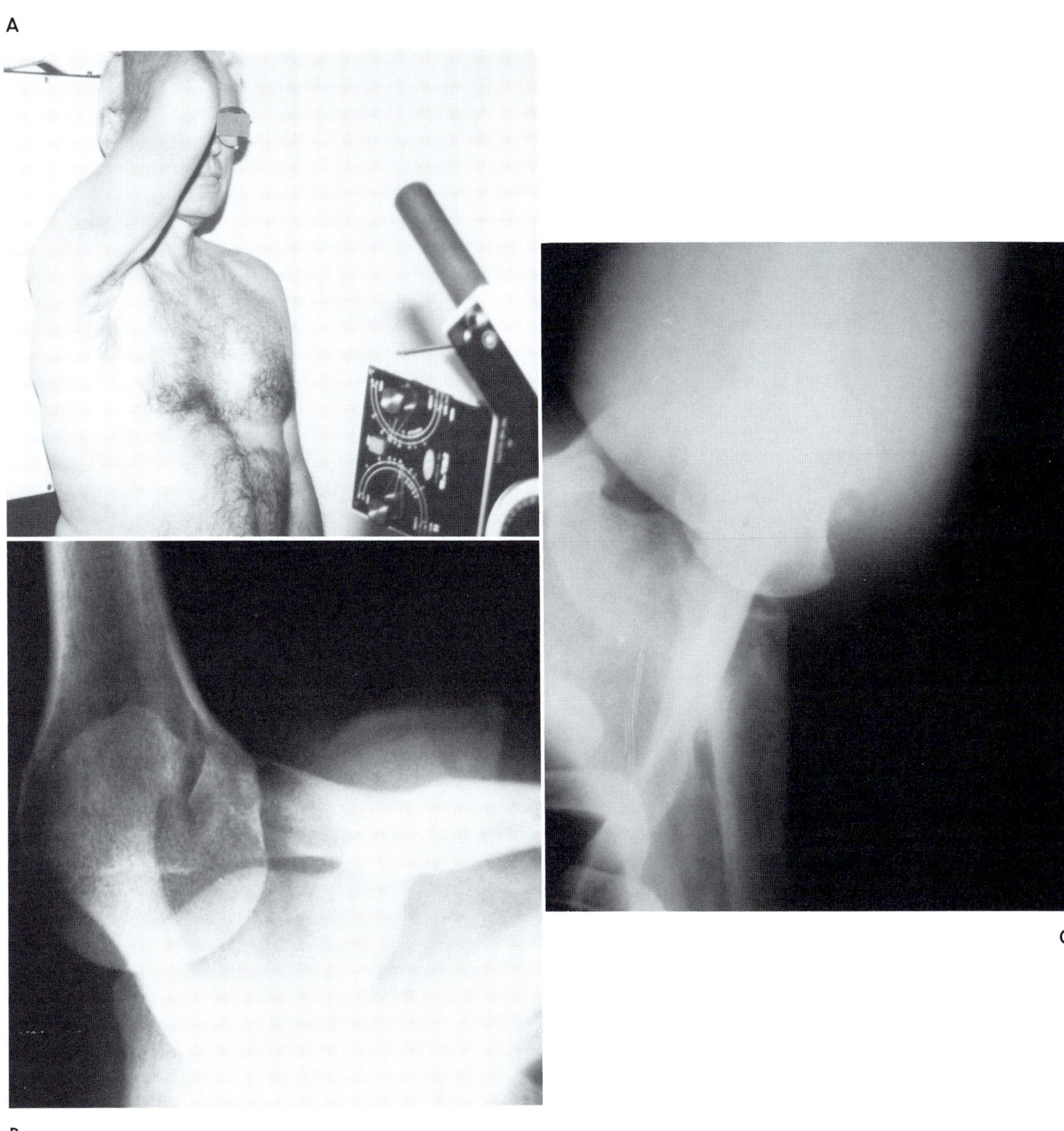

FIG. 1-31 Stryker view.

A Patient is positioned for x-ray.

B Normal Stryker view shows round humeral head.

C Large Hill-Sach lesion indents posterior–lateral humeral head.

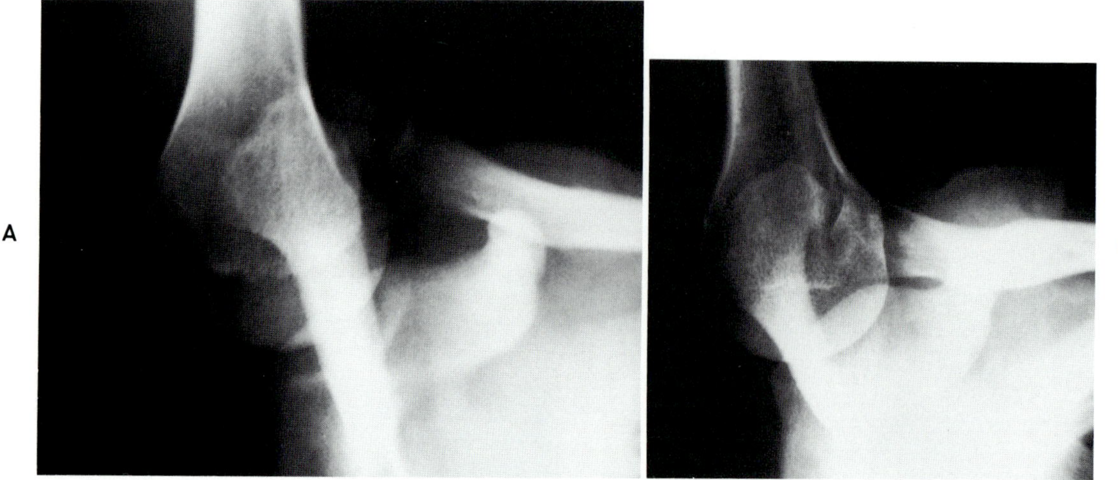

FIG. 1-32 Comparison of right and left shoulders is best way to demonstrate the Hill-Sachs compression fracture on Stryker view x-rays. The left shoulder x-ray film has been reversed for exact comparison.

A Right shoulder with Hill–Sachs lesion.

B Left film reversed for comparison.

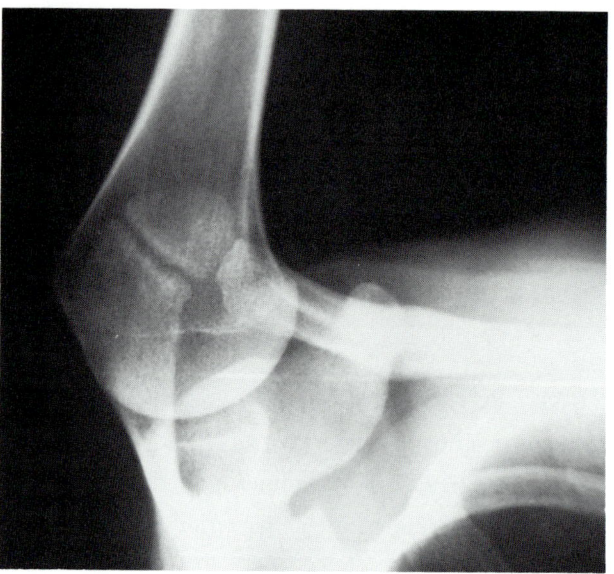

FIG. 1-33 Os acromion. The Stryker view often shows the congenital anomaly of os acromion.

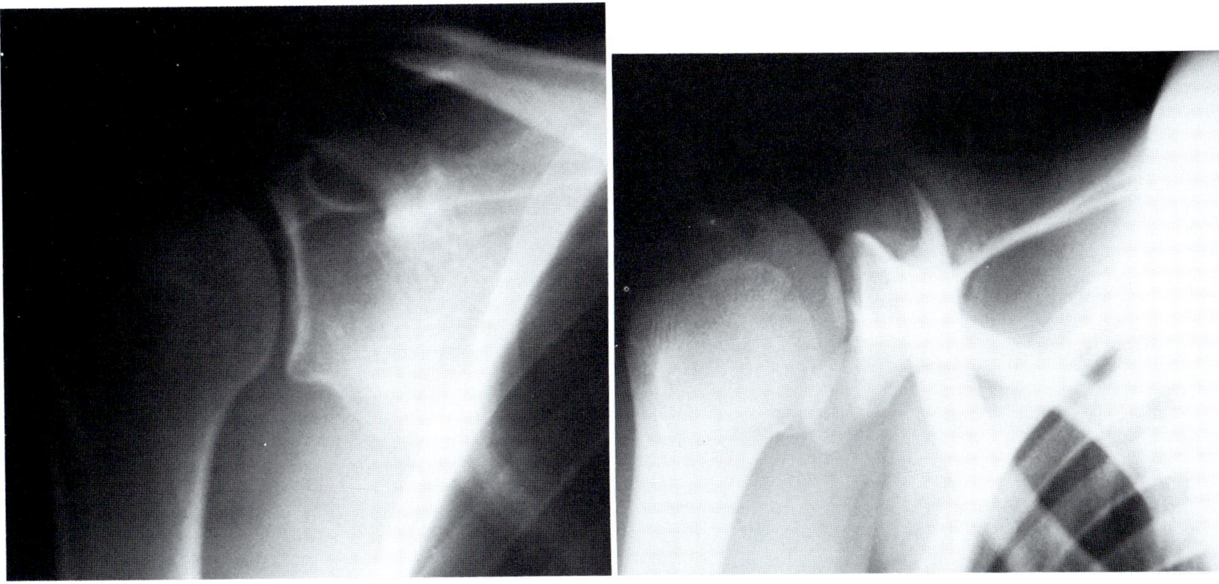

FIG. 1-34 Anterior–posterior views.

A True anterior–posterior shows joint space open.

B Apical oblique view: This projection shows the anterior avulsion fracture associated with anterior traumatic dislocation.

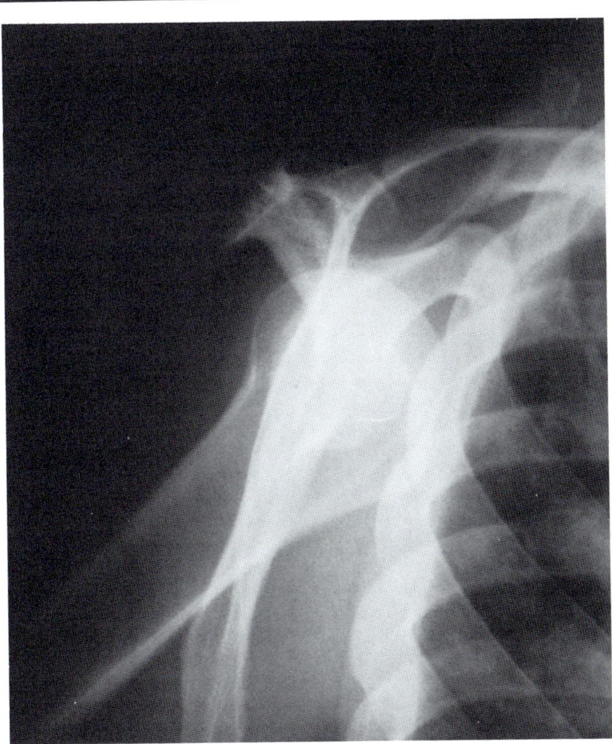

FIG. 1-35 Scapular tangential view. This is best manner to visualize the scapula without overlying projection of thorax.

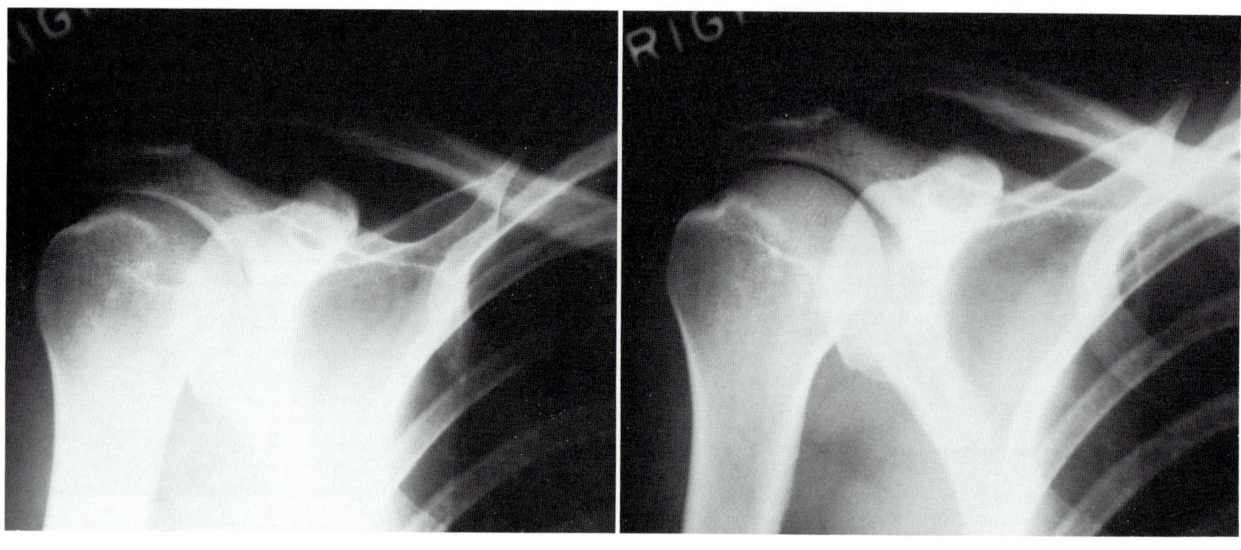

A B

FIG. 1-36 Internal and external rotation plain films. These projections are normal and may show both avulsion fracture of greater tuberosity and calcium deposits.

A Internal rotation.

B External rotation.

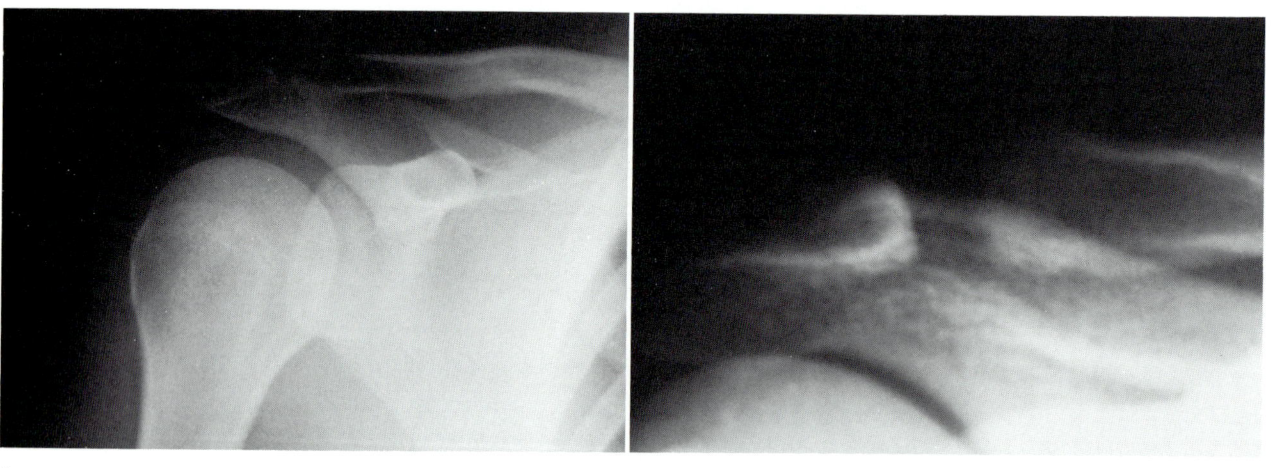

A B

FIG. 1-37 AC joint.

A Overview of entire shoulder region. The AC joint is normal on this film.

B Close viewing required to see AC joint. Widening of this space occurs with mensical injury.

Arthrogram. The arthrogram is most valuable when it shows a rotator cuff tear (Fig. 1-38),[28,46,62,87] but false negative arthrograms are common. If the actual tear is small or filled with a clot, scar tissue, or a thin synovial covering, the flow of the dye is blocked. As in knee joint arthrography, the usefulness of shoulder arthrograms decreases as the surgeon's clinical judgment and his or her arthroscopic skills improve.

Referral patients frequently have had arthrograms. I rarely request the test when clinical signs indicate that an operative lesion is present. The diagnostic arthroscopy is very sensitive and reliable.

I do use the arthrogram in the patient with both loss of motion and strength. The arthrogram will differentiate a rotator cuff tear from a frozen shoulder or a cuff tear that accompanies frozen shoulder. This knowledge helps with preoperative planning and advising on the magnitude of anticipated surgery and length of convalescence.

Computed Tomography (CT) Arthrogram. This test has been most valuable in assessing labral tears (Fig. 1-39).[10,60,76,88,96]

Bone Scan. The bone scan is a sensitive test that is especially useful in preoperative planning for the patient with global shoulder involvement (Fig. 1-40). The reactivity of the bone scan shows the exact localization of joint involvement, whether the shoulder joint, the cervical spine, or the AC area. The correlation of clinical symptoms with this information at the time of diagnostic arthroscopy avoids overlooking potential significant lesion. The bone scan is helpful in determining the site and extent

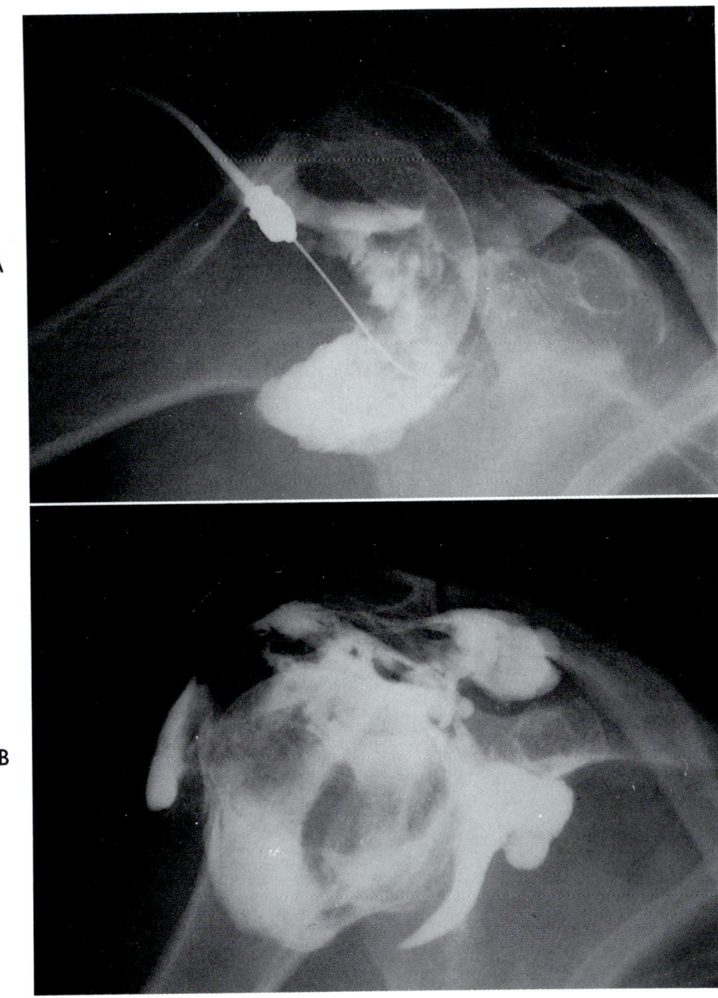

FIG. 1-38 Arthrogram of rotator cuff tear.

A Initial injection shows dye in glenohumeral space.

B Dye extravasation into subacromial bursa demonstrates tear. Note dye in bicipital groove and subscapularis bursa.

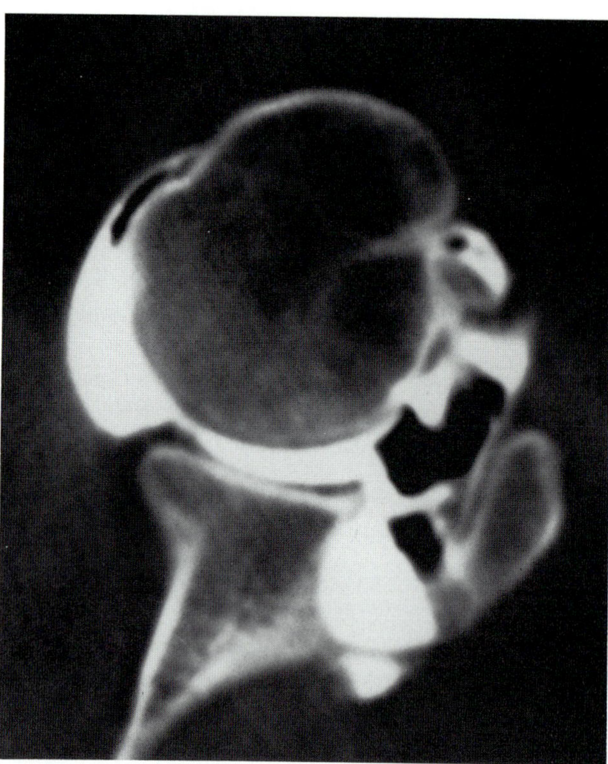

FIG. 1-39 Computed tomography (CT) arthrogram. This close illustration shows the air in the joint anterior above and below the normal extension of the middle glenohumeral ligament attachment to the glenoid labrum.

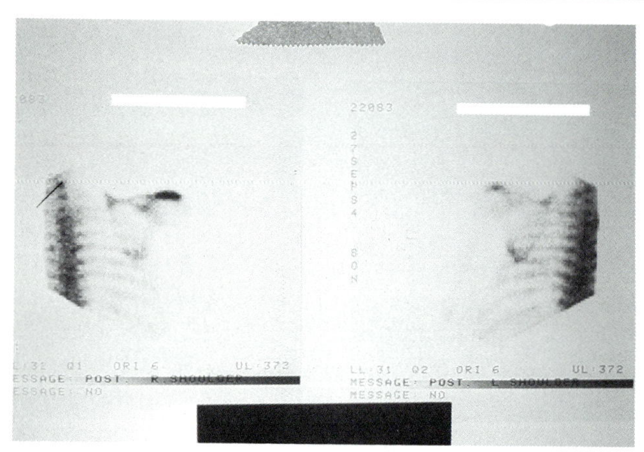

A

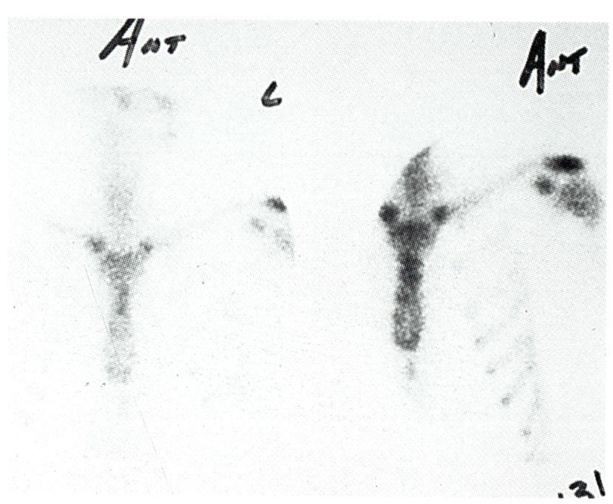

B

FIG. 1-40 Bone scan.

A Increased activity localized in right AC joint as compared to the opposite side. In addition, no uptake in the glenohumeral joint occurs on either side.

B Increased activity in glenohumeral joint is not as intense as the AC joint and the coracoid process.

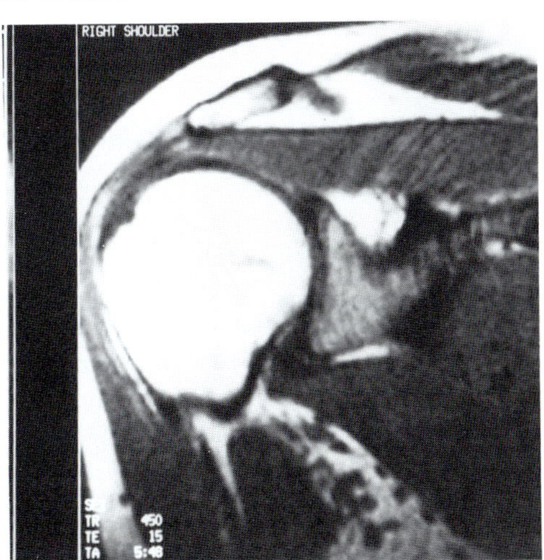

FIG. 1-41 Magnetic resonance imaging (MRI). MRI provides means of observing not only rotator cuff tears, but tumor and osteonecrosis.

of resection in debridement procedures. For example, if the AC joint has a normal bilateral bone scan, the acromioplasty is restricted to the anterior acromion and coracoacromial ligament. If the AC joint shows increased uptake, then resection extends from the underside of the acromion and into the AC joint.

In difficult diagnostic problems or previously operated joints, the benefit of bone scan localization is important. The bone scan is a very sensitive test that shows the localization of increased vascularity. Vascularity may increase in the AC joint to the exclusion of the acromion or glenohumeral joint, which indicates the problem is primarily in the AC joint. If the acromion alone has increased uptake and the glenohumeral joint and AC joint are normal, then the test correlates best with impingement syndrome.

The bone scan may be beneficial in evaluating medicolegal or workmen's compensation problems. If the bone scan of a patient with chronic problems is negative and the history, physical examination, and x-ray results are negative, it is highly unlikely that an intraarticular pathological problem would be identifiable, let alone treatable.

MRI. My experience with magnetic resonance imaging (MRI) in shoulder joint problems is limited because the major insurance carrier in Michigan has not approved MRI for payment in routine shoulder problems. Nonetheless, MRI is a valuable adjunct in the evaluation of shoulder problems, especially aseptic necrosis and tumors and can be obtained on special requisition.

The use of MRI in the care of patients with rotator cuff disease creates a management problem because of the high degree of sensitivity to discover lesions in the tendon (Fig. 1-41).[54,88] The MRI reports often overstate the magnitude of the lesion when compared to the clinical evaluation. The existence of the lesion on MRI is not in itself an indication for surgery, arthroscopic or otherwise. Therapeutic decisions still must be made on the clinical significance of the patient's problem.

Ultrasound. Ultrasound is a readily available, noninvasive and inexpensive diagnostic imaging test.[15,27,29-32] Sonography has limited value in screening patients for rotator cuff tears.[83] However, a positive reading is more reliable than a negative one.[69] Furthermore, the clarity of the image is less than that of MRI. Ultrasound may be of benefit when performed and interpreted by an experienced person.[52]

My own experience with sonography is limited. Ultrasound is not so readily available in my community and I believe other tests have greater benefit.

DIAGNOSTIC ARTHROSCOPY

Arthroscopy provides direct visualization.* Although an image is visualized, it is not considered an imaging procedure in the usual sense. Arthroscopy provides direct evidence as opposed to circumstantial. Even after the physician has clinically ruled out the possibility of a shoulder girdle problem being cervical arthritis, neurovascular compression, shoulder-hand syndrome, and even coronary artery disease, the problem in the shoulder joint may still present a diagnostic dilemma. The condition may be empirically labeled as being in one of various diagnostic groupings, such as bursitis, tendinitis, rotator cuff degeneration, or even impingement syndrome. In spite of a thorough history-taking, physical and x-ray examinations, MRI, and bone scan, including the findings from an examination under anesthesia, the surgeon often remains limited to circumstantial evidence for the diagnosis. Arthroscopy's direct evidence is limited to the intraarticular and bursal structures.

Diagnostic arthroscopy should precede or accompany most surgery on the shoulder joints. Diagnostic arthroscopic inspection allows visualization of the glenohumeral joint to an extent not possible by the largest arthrotomy or even by disarticulation. When arthrotomy of the glenohumeral joint is performed, the open surgical exposure alters and distorts the anatomy to such an extent that the benefit of "insight," which is offered by arthroscopy, is lost. The dynamics of motion and the various anatomical relationships can be studied by arthroscopy. The diagnostic accuracy of arthroscopy prevents empirical surgical decisions and often prevents unnecessary surgery.

*5, 16, 53, 58, 59, 64, 66

OPERATIVE ARTHROSCOPY

Beyond its exacting diagnostic capabilities in the shoulder, as with the knee joint, various arthroscopically monitored surgical procedures offer the patient decreased morbidity, shorter hospitalization, more pleasing cosmetic results, and more exacting surgical debridement and repair.[35] Arthroscopic glenohumeral ligament reconstruction can be an example of this type of procedure.* In addition, conventional major operative procedures have been replaced successfully by arthroscopic debridement alone or repair in certain rotator cuff tears.[6] Arthroscopically monitored anteroinferior acromioplasty has also been performed with good results.†

I have used arthroscopy to identify and treat a number of pathological conditions that could not otherwise have been as easily diagnosed or surgically managed. Both accuracy and technical ease are possible when arthroscopic methods are mastered.

At present, operative arthroscopy of the shoulder includes synovectomy and debridement procedures like loose body removal, resection of glenohumeral labral tears, subacromial bursectomy, and acromioplasty. Reconstructive procedures include labral repairs, glenohumeral ligament repair, and rotator cuff repair. Furthermore, it is now possible to delineate shoulder lesions, even to the small area of the AC joint, with meniscectomy, synovectomy, and chondroplasty. Arthroscopic resection of the distal end of the clavicle is also possible.

COMBINED PROCEDURES

Although some procedures are performed entirely by arthroscopy, in some circumstances arthroscopy can be combined with open procedures. Arthroscopic acromioplasty combined with mini-incision rotator cuff repair is a good example.[84]

OUTPATIENT SURGERY

Most shoulder arthroscopic procedures are routinely performed on an outpatient basis. Patients undergoing bony debridement, as in glenoid preparation for glenohumeral ligament reattachment or acromioplasty, may experience enough pain to require overnight admission. Most patients are discharged with oral pain medication.

Unanticipated admissions occur because of pain requiring injectable anesthetics or as a result of postanesthetic vomiting. Although postoperative bleeding is a common cause of unexpected admission, it is rare following shoulder arthroscopy.[44] The likelihood of unanticipated admission is related more to the type of anesthesia and magnitude of the surgical procedure, rather than the patient's medical condition.[44] Arthroscopic procedures fit well with the societal push for decreased cost of treatment with use of same day surgery facilities.

Routine orders are used for both outpatient recovery and inpatient hospital admission (Fig. 1-42).

POSTOPERATIVE MANAGEMENT

The postoperative management following shoulder arthroscopy is specific to the disease and procedure. I have postoperative written instruction forms that we give to each patient (Fig. 1-43).

The surgical incisions for arthroscopy are puncture wounds. The incisions are covered with a simple bandage to absorb any fluid leakage that accumulates during the procedure. This dressing is changed to Band-Aids the following day.

Pain medication consists of Tylenol #3 if the patient has no allergy to codeine. Otherwise, Talwin or Darvon is given. In anticipation of more severe pain or for a patient with a low pain threshold, Vincodin is given. A prescription is written for 40 tablets or capsules, but rarely is this amount consumed. One tablet is used every 3 to 4 hours as necessary to control pain.

Postoperative pain is minimal following arthroscopy. In fact, an independent study on the effectiveness of various types of oral pain medication involved the arthroscopy patients at our medical center. The arthroscopy patient model was actually found unsuitable because of the minimal pain and requests for medication. The use of arthroscopic patients in this study was abandonded and the experience was not published.

COMPLICATIONS IN SHOULDER ARTHROSCOPY

Complications of arthroscopic surgery of the shoulder in my patients have been minimal, including the use of metallic staples.[58] My patients have not experienced infection, serious bleeding, permanent articular cartilage injury, permanent nerve injury, adhesions, or reflex sympathogenic dystrophy.

The Arthroscopy Association of North America (AANA) has reported the combined experience of a group of arthroscopic surgeons. A 3.3% incidence of complication follows shoulder metal staple capsulorrhaphy for glenohumeral ligament repair.[97,98] Other authors have reported on arthroscopy complications in the knee, but did not include the shoulder.[95]

In an AANA study, one complication occurred with rotator cuff repair with a metal staple.[98,99] This was grouped with all acromioplasty procedures, for a complication rate of 1.1%. The other acromioplasty complications were reflex sympathic dystrophy.

Complications related to juxtaarticular metallic implants have been reported following open surgery.[89,106]

Complications with metal staples in both open and arthroscopic surgery appear to be related to placement in or adjacent to the joint, so that articular cartilage injury re-

*20, 37, 45, 48, 58, 65, 70
†2, 3, 35-38, 41, 81, 84, 86

PHYSICIAN'S ORDERS		INGHAM MEDICAL CENTER — LANSING, MICHIGAN
		SAME DAY SURGERY ROUTINE POST-OP ORDERS
______	1	Routine vital signs
______	2	Clear liquid diet, advance as tolerated post nausea
______	3	Up with assistance
______	4	IV: Discontinue present IV when patient tolerates fluids and vital signs are stable
______	5	Weight bearing status: _____ NWB _____ PWB _____ FWB _____ As Tolerated. _____ Crutches _____ Walker _____ Immobilizer _____ Sling
______	6	Discharge when vital signs stable, tolerating fluids and pain controlled.
______	7	Return to office
______	8	Other:
		MEDICATIONS
 ______ ______ ______ ______ ______	1	Analgesics: Demerol _____ mg IM q 3-4 hrs PRN (unless allergic) Tylenol #3. 1-2 tabs P.O. q 3-4 hours PRN Percocet _____ tabs P.O. q 3-4 hours PRN Talwin NX _____ mg P.O. q 3-4 hours PRN Other:
 ______ ______ ______	2	Antiemetics: Compazine _____ mg IM q 4-6 hours PRN Tigan _____ mg IM q 4-6 hours PRN Other:
______	3	Other Medications:

DATE: __________ TIME: __________ PHYSICIAN'S SIGNATURE: ______________________________

FIG. 1-42 Postoperative routine orders.

A Outpatient.

Continued.

PHYSICIAN'S ORDERS | **INGHAM MEDICAL CENTER** | **LANSING, MICHIGAN**

STANDARD PRACTICE—96 hr. stop order on all narcotics, sedatives, hypnotics, antibiotics, and anticoagulants unless otherwise specified by the physician.

PEDIATRICS ONLY—24 hr. stop order on all injectable mercurial diuretics, and anticoagulants.

POST-OP KNEE, FOOT, HAND, ARM, SHOULDER AND LEG (EXCEPT ARTHROSCOPIC AND TOTAL KNEE)

DOCTOR(S)
Standing Orders for the Department of Orthopedics

	AUTHORIZATION IS GRANTED TO SUPPLY BY NON-PROPRIETARY NAME AS PER FORMULARY POLICY UNLESS CHECKED HERE.	
✓	**ORDER NO.**	**PHYSICIAN'S ORDERS AND SIGNATURES**
		Patient Allergic To:
	1	Follow routine Orthopedic Nursing Care for the post-surgical patient.
	2	Cl. liq. diet if no N/V and bowel sounds active. Resume normal pre-op diet as tolerated. NPO if N/V.
	3	Protime daily for patients 40 and older DHS.
	4	Rehab Services: a. P.T. for routine post-op ambulation with the weight-bearing status as indicated below. b. O.T. for ADL evaluation and Rx when appropriate.
	5	Activity: Please check appropriate entry. a. Elevate extremity with Trendelenburg position. If casted or has bulky dressing elevate with pillows also. b. May be up ad lib with the following weight-bearing status: _____ NWB _____ PWB _____ FWB _____ As Tolerated. c. Affected upper extremity—may be up ad lib with: d. _____ Sling _____ Immobilizer
	6	Cut Cast PRN as indicated: a. _____ BiValve _____ Med/Lat _____ Ant/Post b. Split: _____ ANT _____ MED _____ RADIAL _____ DORSAL _____ POST _____ LAT _____ ULNAR _____ VOLAR c. CUT COTTON
	7	Fleets enema PRN for constipation/straight catheterize PRN for distension or distress
		MEDICATIONS
	1	a. Demerol _________ mg IM q 3-4 hrs, PRN x 5 days (unless allergic) b. Demerol _________ mg IV q 2-4 hrs, PRN x 24 hrs (unless allergic) c. Phenergan _________ mg IM q 3-4 hrs, PRN with Demerol (unless allergic) d. OR: MS _________ mg, IM, q 3-4 hrs PRN x 5 days (unless allergic)
	2	a. Tylenol #3, 1-2 tabs, P.O. q 3-4 hrs PRN, DHS. b. Talwin NX 50 mg tabs, 1-2 P.O., q 3-4 hrs PRN, DHS if allergic to above oral pain meds.
	3	Patient under 70 Coumadin 10 mg, P.O., tonight, NONE TOMORROW. Coumadin 5 mg, P.O., beginning day-after-tomorrow and continuing DHS. Patients 70 and older—Coumadin 5 mg. P.O., tonight: NONE TOMORROW. Coumadin 2.5 mg. P.O., beginning day-after-tomorrow and continuing DHS. OMIT DAILY COUMADIN IF PROTIME IS GREATER THAN 20 AND NOTIFY PHYSICIAN.
	4	Mylanta 30 cc P.O., PRN, DHS (Order must be recopied for Pharmacy to fill).
	5	Emete-con 50 mg, IM q 3-4 hrs. PRN for relief of N/V if N.P.O. fails.
	6	Tylenol 650 mg q 3-4 hrs, PRN DHS (unless allergic).
	7	Restoril _________ mg P.O. at H.S. PRN (MRx1) DHS for sleep
	8	MOM 30 cc P.O. at H.S. PRN DHS (unless at risk for bowel obstruction or ileus)
	9	Peri-colace 1 capsule; p.o. q day PRN (unless at risk for bowel obstruction or ileus)
	10	Dulcolax Supp. 1 rectally, PRN for relief of constipation.
	AUTHORIZATION OF PATIENT AS TEACHING CASE IS AUTOMATIC UNLESS CHECKED HERE.	

CHECK APPROPRIATE ORDERS IN (✓) COLUMN.

DATE: __________ TIME: __________ PHYSICIAN'S SIGNATURE: ____________________

FIG. 1–42, cont'd Postoperative routine orders. **B** Inpatient.

POSTOPERATIVE
PATIENT INFORMATION
SHOULDER SURGERY

Your shoulder operation was performed using the arthroscopic surgical technique. The inside of your joint was viewed using a small telescope attached to a television system. The surgery was performed with miniature instruments.

The diagnosis was ____________________

We removed ____________________

We released ____________________

We repaired ____________________

We also performed ____________________

WOUNDS: The arthroscopic surgery was performed through two or more small puncture wounds. There are no skin stitches to be removed. In some cases, a small strip of surgical tape was used to close the wounds. The tape strips may be removed 7 to 10 days following surgery. They come off easily when wet and may be removed during bathing.

A conventional incision was necessary to complete the surgical repair of the ____________________.

The wounds should be kept clean and dry. The skin and wounds may be cleansed with a wash cloth and soap and water. It is not necessary to apply an antiseptic. The wounds are usually sealed in 48 hours and healed in 10 to 14 days.

The wounds may be sore and show bruising over the next several days. This is due to a leakage of fluid or a small amount of blood from the joint that stayed under the skin. It will eventually disappear and does not require any special care.

DRESSING: The wounds were covered with a soft dressing. The dressing absorbs any leakage of fluid. The amount of fluid leakage can be considerable, since your shoulder joint was distended with sterile fluid during the operation. Some of the residual fluid is absorbed by the body and the remainder leaks onto the dressing. Both pathways are normal.

Blood may also stain the dressing. This is normal. Any continued bleeding, especially bright red blood, is reason to seek medical attention. Call us(517/351-7450).

The dressing may be changed anytime, usually the day after surgery. If drainage persists, an absorbent dressing should be applied. When the drainage has stopped, the wounds may be covered with bandaids.

BATHING: You may safely shower 48 hours following surgery. Soaking the wound areas should be delayed until the skin is healed.

PAIN/MEDICATION: Patients often wonder why they hurt when the surgery was performed through small, arthroscopic puncture wounds. In spite of the small size of the external wounds, major surgery was performed inside the joint. You should receive a prescription for pain pills upon leaving the hospital. Please inform us of any known drug allergy.

A prescription is usually written for Tylenol with codeine. Codeine may produce nausea, vomiting, headache and/or a fine skin rash. If any of these symptoms develop, the medication should be stopped and you should contact our office for an alternate medication.

GENERAL PRECAUTIONS: Postoperative problems may be recognized by

- UNUSUAL PAIN NOT RELIEVED BY PAIN MEDICATION
- A TEMPERATURE ELEVATION OF 101 DEGREES FAHRENHEIT OR ABOVE
- CHEST PAIN
- SHORTNESS OF BREATH
- CONTINUOUS COUGHING, ESPECIALLY WITH SHOW OF BLOOD
- HEART IRREGULARITIES
- PROGRESSIVE SWELLING OF ARM OR HAND
- BLEEDING
- NUMBNESS
- LOSS OF MOVEMENT IN HAND AND/OR FINGERS
- LOSS OF CIRCULATION

If any of these symptoms are observed, or you have any question concerning their significance, you should seek medical attention at our office (517/351-7450), with your local physician, or even an emergency room, if necessary.

POSITION OF THE UPPER EXTREMITY (ARM): Your arm has been place in a ____________________. It should remain in this for ______ days/weeks. It may be removed for bathing, but the arm should not be moved. This may require another person's assistance while showering or bathing so that the surgical repair is not disturbed.

ACTIVITY: You may use your hand, wrist and elbow within the limits permitted by your sling or splint. In fact, you should make a fist and tighten your muscles every hour, as this reduces swelling. Minor adjustments in the arm position may be made, so long as you remain comfortable.

MEDICAL RECORD: A medical record is filed at Ingham Medical Center and at our office. A copy will be forwarded to the referring physician, when identified, and to you, or anyone you designate, upon written request.

OFFICE APPOINTMENT: You should call our office today to schedule an appointment for ______ days/weeks from now. Our telephone number is 517/351-7450.

Thank you,

Lanny L. Johnson, MD

NOTE: Although this is a postoperative form, it is specific for your condition unless otherwise noted during the course of your treatment.

3/88

FIG. 1-43 Routine written postoperative patient instructions.

sults.[93] In my experience, problems with subsequent "loosening" and migration of staples resulted from the failure to secure the arthroscopic staple during initial implantation. In my cases of loose staples, I reviewed the original videotape. Invariably, the tape showed previously unrecognized failure of implantation. I suspect this is the problem with other surgeons' techniques as well. The immediate postoperative x-ray film may show the position of the staple resting near the glenoid, but it is interpreted as being in bone. The staple is being held during this short interval by the soft tissue. Subsequent x-ray films show the change in position. The observer erroneously thinks the staple was initially secured and then loosened. Anyone who has tried to remove a securely implanted staple knows spontaneous loosening is unlikely. They are difficult to remove from the glenoid, even after a long time.

The complication rate for debridement of the glenoid rim in Small's report was 0.5%[97].

No neurovascular injuries were reported in Small's series, but I have seen referral patients who have sustained this type of injury. Andrews and others have reported neuroplaxia following arthroscopic surgery of the shoulder when traction, not suspension, was applied.[7,8,82] Cadaver studies show the greater forces applied (25 pounds) resulted in greater strain on nerves.[61a] Intraoperative monitoring by somatosensory evoked potentials has been suggested to avoid neuropraxia.[85]

INTRAOPERATIVE

The most common intraoperative complication is extravasation of fluid and swelling. Extravasation decreases mobility of instrumentation. No evidence indicates that pressures become high enough to produce compartment syndrome.[26] Instrument breakage is possible, but this has not occurred in my experience.

Vascular complications are rare. I have inadvertently lacerated the cephalic vein during the skin puncture. In such cases I ligate the vessel and have seen no resultant problems. The use of a pulse oximeter for monitoring digital pulse has been recommended during shoulder arthroscopy to avoid vascular compromise.[1] Burkhart reported a subclavian deep venous thrombosis following arthroscopy of the shoulder.[17] The patient also had compressing mass of Hodgkin's disease.

Injury to the neurovascular structures of the arm is possible if instruments are passed medial to the coracoid process.[104,105] The suprascapular nerve is at risk with transscapular drilling for reconstructive procedures.[33] The acromial branch of the coracoacromial artery may be lacerated during acromioplasty.

IMMEDIATE POSTOPERATIVE

I have not recognized any immediate postoperative complications. None of my patients have experienced cardiopulmonary complications. Anderson et al reported three cases of pulmonary edema following knee arthroscopy, but none were thought to be of fluid absorption etiology.[4]

Transient paresthesia is rare. This may be caused by the forearm wrap and suspension of the upper extremity. An occasional patient has complained of irritation of the superficial radial nerve at the wrist. This was caused by compression from the forearm elastic wrap.

LATE POSTOPERATIVE

I have noted no postoperative infection, bleeding, or neurovascular injury following arthroscopic or combined surgery of the shoulder. I have seen postarthroscopic acromioplasty result in frozen shoulder in two young men and one middle-aged woman. They were timid about early active motion exercises. The men required manipulation and intensive physical therapy for recovery. The woman reponded to physical therapy.

Arthroscopy is a safe procedure. Complications are avoided by awareness of their potential and attention to surgical detail.

CLINICAL DECISION MAKING

Decision making starts with the initial patient encounter and continues throughout the examination, imaging, arthroscopy and the post operative period. Patient care is one continuous involvement in decision making. The patient should be an active participant in the preoperative decision making. This requires the physician to inform the patient with illustrations and expected outcomes. The patient must understand the pros and cons of testing and treatment before proceeding.

Once the operative procedure is commenced the patient is no longer an active participant. However, the surgeon's knowledge of the patient and the patient's objectives are paramount. The intraoperative decisions rest with the surgeon.

This text will provide information and illustration to assist the surgeon's decision making in anatomy, pathology, and arthroscopic treatment modalities for shoulder problems.

REFERENCES

1. Agel J, Levy IM: The use of a pulse oximeter for the monitoring of digital pulse during shoulder arthroscopy, *J Arthroscopy Relat Surg* 4(2):124-125, 1988.
2. Altcheck DW et al: Arthroscopic acromioplasty, *Arthroscopy* 4(2):145, 1988.
3. Altcheck DW et al: Arthroscopic acromioplasty, *J Bone Joint Surg* 72A (8):1198-1207, 1990.
4. Anderson AF, Alfrey D, Libscomb AB Jr: Acute pulmonary edema, an unusual complication following arthroscopy: a report of three cases, *J Arthroscopy Relat Surg* 6(3):235-237, 1992.
5. Andrews JR: Personal communication, 1982.
6. Andrews JR, Broussard TS, Carson WG: Arthroscopy of the shoulder in the management of partial tears of the rotator cuff: a preliminary report, *Arthroscopy* 1:117, 1985.

7. Andrews JR, Carson WG Jr: Shoulder joint arthroscopy, *Orthopaedics* 6:1157, 1983.
8. Andrews JR, Carson WG Jr, Ortega K: Arthroscopy of the shoulder: Techniques and normal anatomy, *Am J Sports Med* 12:1-7, 1984.
9. Bassey EJ et al: Flexibility of the shoulder joint measured as range of abduction in a large representative sample of men and women over 65 years of age, *Eur J Appl Physiol* 58(4):353-360, 1989.
10. Beltran J et al: Rotator cuff lesions of the shoulder: evaluation by direct sagittal CT arthrography, *Radiology* 60:161-165, 1986.
11. Bigliani LU et al: An anatomical study of the suprascapular nerve, *Arthroscopy* 6(4):301-305, 1990.
12. Bigliani LU et al: The relationship between the unfused acromial epiphysis and subacromial impingement lesions, *Orthop Trans* 7:138, 1983.
13. Bïrcher E: Beitrag sur Pathologie und Diagnose der Meniscusverletzungen (Arthroendoskopie), *Beitr Klin Chir* 127:239, 1922.
14. Black KP, Lombardo JA: Suprascapular nerve injuries with isolated paralysis of the infraspinatus, *Am J Sports Med* 18(3) May-June:255-258, 1990.
15. Bretzke CA et al: Ultrasonography of the rotator cuff: normal and pathologic anatomy, *Invest Radiol* 20:311-315, 1985.
16. Bunker TD: Shoulder arthroscopy, *Ann Roy Coll Surg* 71:213-217, 1989.
17. Burkhart SS: Deep venous thrombosis after shoulder arthroscopy, *J Arthroscopy Relat Surg* 6(1):61-63, 1990.
18. Burman MS: Arthroscopy or the direct visualization of joints: an experimental cadaver study, *J Bone Joint Surg* 13:669-95, 1931.
19. Caspari RB: Arthroscopy—an orthopaedic subspecialty or a technique, *Arthroscopy* 7(4):390-393, 1991.
20. Caspari RB: Arthroscopic reconstruction for anterior shoulder instability, *Tech in Orthop* 3(1)59-66, 1988.
21. Caspari RB: Shoulder arthroscopy: a review of the present state of art, *Contemp Orthop* 4:523, 1983.
22. Cassells SW: *Arthroscopy: diagnostic and surgical practice*, Philadelphia, 1984, Lea and Febiger.
23. Cassells SW: Arthroscopy of the knee joint: a review of 150 cases, *J Bone Joint Surg* 53A:287, 1971.
24. Cofield RH: The future of shoulder surgery, *Orthopedics* 11(1):179-181, 1988.
25. Cofield RH: Arthroscopy of the shoulder, *Mayo Clin Proc* 589:501, 1983.
26. Cohn L, Lee YF, Tooke SM: Intramuscular compartment pressures during shoulder arthroscopy, *Arthroscopy* 5(2):159, 1989.
27. Collins RA et al: Ultrasonography of the shoulder, *Orthop Clin North Am* 18:351, 1987.
28. Craig EV: The Geyser sign and torn rotator cuff: clinical significance and pathomechanics, *Clin Orthop* 191:213-215, 1984.
29. Crass JR, Craig EV: Noninvasive imaging of the rotator cuff, *Orthopedics* 11(1):57-64, 1988.
30. Crass JR et al: Ultrasonography of the rotator cuff, *Radiographics* 6(5) Nov:941-953, 1985.
31. Crass JR, Craig EV, Feinberg SB: Ultrasonography of rotator cuff tears: a review of 500 diagnostic studies, *J Clin Ultrasound* 16:313-327, 1988.
32. Crass JR et al: Ultrasonography of the rotator cuff: surgical correlation, *J Clin Ultrasound* 12:487-493, 1984.
33. Drez D, Proffer D: Suprascapular nerve anatomy and relationship to the glenoid. Paper presented at American Academy of Orthopedic Surgeons, Anaheim, California, March 1991.
34. Eikelarr HR: *Arthroscopy of the knee*, Groningen, Netherlands, 1975, Royal United Printers.
35. Ellman H: Shoulder arthroscopy: current indications and techniques, *Orthopedics* 11(1):45-51, 1988.
36. Ellman H: Arthroscopic subacromial decompression: analysis of 1 to 3 year results, *Arthroscopy* 3(3):173-181, 1987.
37. Ellman H: Arthroscopic subacromial decompression, *Orthop Trans* 9(1)Sp:48, 1985.
38. Esch JC et al: Arthroscopic subacromial decompression: results according to the degree of rotator cuff tear, *Arthroscopy* 4(4):241-249, 1988.
39. Fowler P: Swimmer problems, *Am J Sports Med* 7:141-142, 1979.
40. Garth WP Jr, Slappey CE, Ochs CW: Roentgenographic demonstration of instability of the shoulder, the apical oblique projection, *J Bone Joint Surg* 66A:1450-1453, 1984.
41. Gartsman GM: Arthroscopic acromioplasty for lesions of the rotator cuff, *J Bone Joint Surg* 72A (2): 169-180, 1990.
42. Gillquist J, Hagberg G, Oretorp N: Arthroscopy in acute injuries of the knee joint, *Acta Orthop Scand* 48(2):190, 1977.
43. Glinz W: Arthroscopic partial meniscectomy, *Helv Chir Acta* 47:115, 1980.
44. Gold BS et al: Unanticipated admission to the hospital following ambulatory surgery, *JAMA* 21(262) Dec:3008-3010, 1989.
45. Gross M, Fitzgibbons TC: Shoulder arthroscopy: a modified approach, *Arthroscopy* 1(3):156-159, 1985.
46. Hall FM: Arthrography: past, present and future, *Amer J Radiol* 149:561-563, 1987.
47. Haralson RH III: Computerized information retrieval and medical education for orthopedists, *JBJS* 70A (4):624-629, 1988.
48. Hawkins RB: Arthroscopic stapling repair for shoulder instability: a retrospective study of 50 cases, *Arthroscopy* 5(2):122-128, 1989.
49. Hawkins RJ, Bilco T, Bonutti P: Cervical spine and shoulder pain, *Clin Ortho* 258(9):142-146, 1990.
50. Hawkins RJ, Hobeıka P: Physical examination of the shoulder, *Orthopedics* 6(10):1270-1278, 1983.
51. Henry AN: Arthroscopy in the management of internal derangements of the knee. From The knee joint, *Excerpta Medica*, Amsterdam, New York: American Elsevier, 1974:120-125.
52. Holder J, Fretz CJ, Terrier F et al: Rotator cuff tears: correlation of sonographic and surgical findings, *Radiology* 169:791-794, 1988.
53. Hurley JA, Anderson TA: Shoulder arthroscopy: its role in evaluating shoulder disorders in the athelete, *Am J Sports Med* 18(5):480-483, 1990.
54. Iannotti JP, Zlatkin MB, Esterhai JL, Kressel HY, Dalinka MK, Spindler KP: Magnetic resonance imaging of the shoulder: Sensitivity, specificity and predictive value, *J Bone Joint Surg* 73A:17-29, 1990.
55. Jackson RW, Dandy DJ: *Arthroscopy of the knee*. New York: Grune and Stratton, 1980.
56. Jobe F: Personal communication, 1990.
57. Johnson LL: A rationale for systematized record keeping and improved documentation, *Arthroscopy* 3(4):258-264, 1987.
58. Johnson LL: *Arthroscopic surgery: principles and practice*, St Louis, 1986, Mosby–Year Book.
59. Johnson LL: Arthroscopy of the shoulder, *Orthop Clin North Am* 11(2):197-204, 1980.
60. Kinnard P et al: Assessment of the unstable shoulder by computed arthrography, *Am J Sports Med* 11:157, 1983.
61. Kitay W: More than 1,000,000 arthroscopies a year, *Am J Arthroscopy* 1(10):5, 1991 (editorial).
61a. Klein AH et al: Measurement of brachial plexus strain in arthroscopy of the shoulder, *Arthroscopy* 3(1): 45–52, 1987.
62. Kneisl JS, Sweeney HJ, Paige ML: Correlation of pathology observed in double contrast arthrotomography and arthroscopy of the shoulder, *Arthroscopy* 4(1):21-24, 1988.
63. Kreuscher PH: Semilunar cartilage disease: plea for early recognition by means of arthroscope and early treatment of this condition, *Illinois Med J* 47:290, 1925.
64. Lilleby H: Shoulder arthroscopy, *Acta Orthop Scand* 55(5):561-566, 1984.
65. Maki N: Personal communication, 1991.

66. Matthews LS, Vetter WL, Helfet DL: Arthroscopic surgery of the shoulder, *Adv Orthop Surg* 7:203, 1984.
67. McLaughlin HL: Rupture of the rotator cuff, *J Bone Joint Surg* 44A:979-983, 1962.
68. Mikhail S, de Lerman L: Painful shoulder and lidocaine test, *Surg Rounds Orthoped* (8):45-46, 1989.
69. Miller CL et al: Limited sensitivity of ultrasound for the detection of rotator cuff tears, *Skeletal Radiol* 18(3):179-183, 1989.
70. Morgan C: Arthroscopic transglenoid bankart suture repair, *Operative Techniques in Orthopedics* 1(2) April:171-179, 1991.
71. Morrison DS, Bigliani LU: The clinical significance of variations in acromial morphology, *Orthop Trans* 11:234, 1987.
72. Mudge MK, Wood VE, Frykman GK: Rotator cuff tears associated with os-acrominale, *J Bone Joint Surg* 66A:427-429, 1984.
73. Neer CS II: *Shoulder reconstruction,* Philadelphia, 1990, WB Saunders.
74. Neer CS II: Impingement lesions, *Clin Orthop* 173:70, 1983.
75. Nelson MC et al: Evaluation of the painful shoulder, *J Bone Joint Surg* 73A(5):707-716, 1991.
76. Nottage WM, Duge WD, Fields WA: Computed arthrotomography of the glenohumeral joint to evaluate anterior instability: correlation with the arthroscopic findings, *Arthroscopy* 3(4):273-276, 1987.
77. Nuber GW et al: Arterial abnormalities of the shoulder in athletes, *Am J Sports Med* 18(5) Sept-Oct:514-519, 1990.
78. O'Connor RL: *Arthroscopy,* Philadelphia, 1977, JB Lippincott.
79. O'Connor RL: Arthroscopy in the diagnosis and treatment of acute ligament injuries of the knee, *J Bone Joint Surg* 56A:33, 1974.
80. O'Driscoll SW: Contralateral shoulder instability following anterior repair, *JBJS* 73-B:941-946, 1991.
81. Ogilvie-Harris DJ, Boynton E: Arthroscopic acromioplasty: extravasation of fluid into the deltoid muscle, *Arthroscopy* 6(1):52-54, 1990.
82. Ogilvie-Harris DJ, Wiley AM: Arthroscopic surgery of the shoulder: a general appraisal, *J Bone Joint Surg* 68B:201-207, 1986.
83. Pattee GA, Snyder SJ: Sonographic evaluation of the rotator cuff: correlation with arthroscopy, *Arthroscopy* 4(3):15-20, 1988.
84. Paulos LE, Franklin JL: Arthroscopic shoulder decompression: development and application: a five year experience, *Am J Sports Med* 18(3):235-244, 1990.
85. Post M, Cohen J: Impingement syndrome—A review of the late stage II and early stage III lesions, *Orthop Trans* 9(1):48, 1985.
86. Raggio CL, Warren RF, Sculco T: Surgical treatment of impingement syndrome: 4 year follow-up, *Orthop Trans* 9(1):48, 1985.
87. Resnick D: Shoulder arthrography, *Radiol Clin North Am* 19:243-252, 1981.
88. Resnick D, Niwayama G: *Diagnosis of bone and joint disorders,* ed 2, Philadelphia, 1988, WB Saunders.
89. Rockwood CA Jr: Migration of pins used in operations on the shoulder. *J Bone Joint Surg (Am)* 72(8):1262-1267, 1990.
90. Rockwood CA Jr, Matsen FA III: *The shoulder,* Philadelphia, 1990, WB Saunders.
91. Rokous JR, Feagin JA, Abbott HG: Modified axillary roentgenogram: a useful adjunct in the diagnosis of recurrent instability of the shoulder, *Clin Orthop* 82:84, 1972.
92. Rowe CR: The shoulder, New York, 1988, Churchill Livingstone.
93. Sachs RA, Riehl B, Lane JA: Arthroscopic staple capsulorraphy: a long term followup, *Arthroscopy* 7(3):324, 1991.
94. Schonholtz GJ: *Arthroscopic surgery of the shoulder, elbow, and ankle,* Springfield, Ill, 1988, Charles C Thomas.
95. Sherman OH et al: Arthroscopy—no problem surgery, *J Bone Joint Surg* 68A:256-265, 1986.
96. Shuman WP et al: Double-constrast computered tomography of the glenoid labrum, *Am J Radiology* 141:581-584, 1983.
97. Small NC: Complications in arthroscopic surgery performed by experienced arthroscopists, *J Arthroscopy Relat Surg* 4(3):215-221, 1988.
98. Small NC: Complications in arthroscopy: the knee and other joints, *Arthroscopy* 2:253-258, 1986.
99. Smith CF et al: The carbon dioxide laser: a potential tool for orthopedic surgery, *Clin Orthop* 242:43-50, 1989.
100. Takagi K: The classic arthroscope, *Clin Orthop* 167:6, 1982 (from J Jap Orthop Assoc 1939).
101. Watanabe M: *Arthroscopy of small joints,* Tokyo, 1985, Igaku Shoin.
102. Watanabe M, Takeda S, Ikeuchi H: Atlas of arthroscopy, ed 3, Tokyo, 1979, Igaku Shoin.
103. Wiley AM, Older JW: Shoulder arthroscopy: investigation with a fiberoptic instrument, *Am J Sports Med* 8:31-38, 1980.
104. Wolf EM: Arthroscopic anterior shoulder capsulorraphy, *Techniques Orthop* 3(1):67-73, 1988.
105. Wolf EM: Arthroscopic anterior staple capsulorrhaphy. *Arthroscopy* 4(2):142, 1988.
106. Zuckerman JD, Matsen FA: Complications about the glenohumeral joint related to the use of screws and staples, *J Bone Joint Surg* 66A:175, 1984.

CHAPTER

2

Creating the Optimal Operating Environment

Visitors are always surprised at the optimal environment in which the arthroscopic surgical procedures are performed at Ingham Medical Center, Lansing, Michigan. The arthroscopic suite is a separate surgical unit within a general hospital setting. The suite was designed to service the special needs of arthroscopic surgery. We have two operating rooms (one with a glass wall for viewing), a recovery room, and all the ancillary support systems in one location (Fig. 2-1). The operating rooms are specially designed for arthroscopic surgery and include television monitors (Fig. 2-2). The personnel have primary responsibility to arthroscopic surgery, and the surgeons have block anesthesia time.

Guests to our facility immediately reflect on their own situation, which in comparison they describe as less than optimal. They want to know how we obtained such a nice facility. I inform them that we used to work in circumstances similar to theirs and faced all the same problems. I tell visitors that this environment did not just happen.[3] The ideal operating environment is created only by the initiative and persistence of the surgeon with cooperation from the administration staff. Only too often, orthopedic sur-

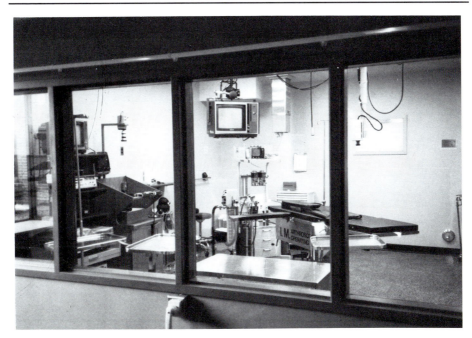

FIG. 2-1 Arthroscopy surgical suite at Ingham Medical Center, Lansing, Michigan, as seen from viewing room.

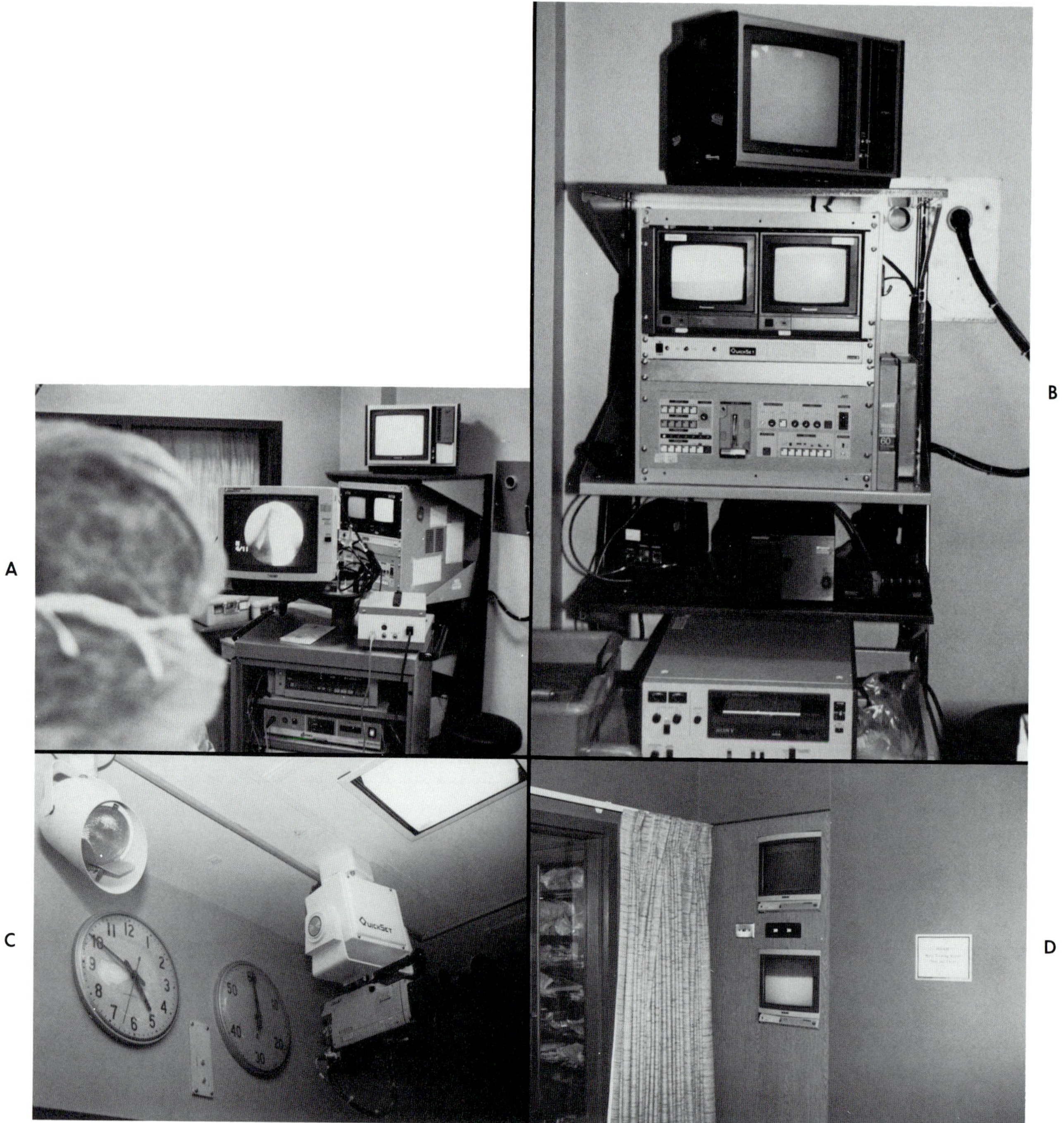

FIG. 2-2 Operating room equipped with television.

A Surgeon viewing image off television monitor to perform the surgery.

B Television console with monitors, mixers, and recorders. A Polaroid slide or print camera is attached to video.

C Wall mount television camera photographs the outside view of the surgery. This image can be electronically mixed with the arthroscopic view with an editing system in the operating room.

D Viewing room has monitors for both operating rooms.

geon-arthroscopists' requests for a proper environment are met with a lack of understanding from administrators, some bewilderment on the part of the operating room personnel, and hostility from staff orthopedists who have no interest in arthroscopic surgery. Fortunately, these attitudes are changing.

To create the optimum environment, the hospital must be willing to invest money.[5,6] The start up for arthroscopy is expensive because of the unique instrumentation: arthroscopes, television, motorized and miniature instruments, etc. The surgical staff must actively participate in organizing and creating the environment that facilitates this type of surgery. The ultimate responsibility for creating the operating room environment, however, rests with the surgeon. The orthopedist who uses arthroscopic surgical techniques must organize, plan, and insist on the proper environment to maximize his or her skills in the care of the patient. This is not a one-time task, but a continuous effort. Attention to the proper environment continues throughout the surgeon's practice lifetime.

Subspecialization now is common in orthopedic surgery, including arthroscopy. In the past an orthopedic surgeon was expected to perform surgical procedures in whatever operating room, at whatever time, might be available. In addition, it was customary to work with a different untrained assistant for every surgical procedure. Today many procedures are recognized as requiring a superb level of coordination and skill to achieve success. A specialized surgical environment is no less important for the arthroscopic surgeon than it is for the cardiac surgeon or organ transplant team. This chapter discusses how we have worked together as a successful team to create an environment and staff dedicated to arthroscopic procedures.

A DEDICATED ARTHROSCOPIC SURGEON

The arthroscopic surgeon must be dedicated to arthroscopy. It is not a surgical field for dabblers. Caspari has recently suggested that arthroscopy is indeed an orthopedic subspecialty. To enjoy success in arthroscopy, the surgeon must first prepare for this surgical experience as outlined in Chapter 5. The surgeon must embark on both an educational and essentially a promotional effort on behalf of both himself or herself and arthroscopic surgery within the institution. The surgeon must assume a position of leadership and responsibility in creating the proper environment. If the operating room environment—be it personnel, hospital, or equipment—is not suitable, then it is the surgeon's responsibility, not someone else's, to encourage changes.

Success in arthroscopic surgery requires that the surgeon have previously prepared the environment and trained the staff. During surgery, the surgeon must concentrate intensely to treat pathological intraarticular structures through miniature incisions in restricted joint spaces. Once the procedure is underway, neither time nor attention is available for planning or organization.

The care of the patient is directly related to the leadership role that the surgeon takes in creating the ideal environment. If the surgeon is lax in personal discipline, the other people in the operating room will take this approach. If the surgeon is disciplined, careful, and attentive and works with dispatch, this approach will be reflected in the staff and the environment.

The surgeon's attitude will condition the working relationships of those in the environment and how well the operation will be performed. Arthroscopic surgery, more so than any other orthopedic discipline, requires a great deal of patience. One cannot force one's way through it. I have often said, "If things are not going fast enough for you arthroscopically, then slow down." In some situations it is a good idea to stop altogether, even for 5 minutes. If the surgeon has been operating under frustrating circumstances, a rest period allows him or her time to regroup, reconsider another surgical approach, plan the conclusion, or even abort the procedure.

Last, but certainly not least important, the surgeon must be confident that his or her technical skills are equal to the anticipated level of surgery. Nothing is more discouraging to the surgeon, alarming to the personnel, and potentially injurious to the patient than an operation on a condition or in an anatomical area that is beyond the surgeon's training or experience. I liken this to skiing out of control: it is risky. I believe that every surgeon should operate at a level that is below his or her ability, so that if any unforseen problem occurs an extra capacity is available to meet the challenge. Like skiing under control, arthroscopy can be enjoyable and safe!

A DEDICATED HOSPITAL ADMINISTRATION

The hospital administration should be apprised of the specialized needs of arthroscopic surgery, both the financial commitment and the commitment of operating room personnel. Administrators usually come to a greater understanding when the surgeon talks in terms of patient volume and cash flow. If the necessary capital expenditures are not made or the proper personnel assembled, then arthroscopic surgery will be performed in a competing institution. Administrators do understand the consequences of this alternative.

Educating the administrators will be necessary. They should know that the arthroscopic surgical procedure will be—if it is not already—the most common procedure within orthopedics. If orthopedics is a major specialty within a hospital, arthroscopy and its combined procedures are likely the most common operative procedures performed within the operating room suite. Administrators can rapidly calculate this fact in terms of cash flow, especially when they understand that arthroscopy brings a large outpatient volume and its potential cost effectiveness. This factor is especially convincing with today's medical economic reimbursement policies. Furthermore, recent legislative and administrative actions by group health carriers have accelerated the use of outpatient surgery. Thus the hospital has a financial incentive to deliver outpatient arthroscopic surgery.

A DEDICATED ARTHROSCOPIC SURGICAL TEAM

Assembling the team is the responsibility of the arthroscopic surgeon(s). Arthroscopic surgery requires assembling a surgical team that does only this type of surgery and is devoted to its success.The surgeon is the team leader.

The anesthesiologist and staff must be willing and able to manage their responsibilities in an outpatient environment (see Fig. 2-30).

Assembling a model team may require a major effort to "sell" the procedure to the hospital personnel. Usually the first arthroscopic procedures performed at an institution consume more time than those done by previous methods. Both colleagues and staff must be educated to the ultimate patient benefits that arthroscopic methods provide.

Recruitment of the team starts with other orthopedic surgeons. If they have the same interest, you may consider forming a coalition. Only in recent years have enough orthopedic surgeons been interested in arthroscopic surgery to make this possible. A coalition has both benefits and disadvantages. One of the benefits is the safety found in numbers. In addition, coordination of operating room scheduling, personnel, and organization is possible with a group effort. Each surgeon brings information from his/her experience and from continuing education meetings. A disadvantage is that getting agreement from all the surgeons concerning how something ought to be done, what ought to be purchased, and especially what their "perceived needs" are may be difficult. (The concept of "perceived needs" means that the uninitiated, inexperienced arthroscopist will project his or her needs based on previous nonarthroscopic experience or concepts. Having had no actual arthroscopic experience, these surgeons can only "perceive" their needs. Consultation with experienced arthroscopists can reshape perceived needs before actual purchases are made.)

Some resistance may be forthcoming from the operating room supervisor and personnel. People tend to resist change. One way to encourage the operating room personnel to change is to communicate the idea of the adventure and excitement of something new and better. For example, the use of television during arthroscopic surgery has helped encourage staff interest and participation.

Personnel Selection

For simple, direct-viewing, diagnostic arthroscopy, an untrained assistant might be sufficient, although less than desirable. For more advanced technical procedures, the operating room staff must be both knowledgeable and interested in arthroscopic surgery. By choice or by personality, some individuals have no interest in arthroscopy. They should not be enlisted because they will not be of benefit to either the surgeon or the patient.

The arthroscopic surgeon needs specialized team support because arthroscopic surgery is a procedure as demanding as any performed in the hospital. A successful arthroscopic service demands a proper environment with interested, actively participating, knowledgeble personnel. The primary motivating factor that draws all the personnel together is patient benefit.

The best way to select people for the arthroscopic surgical team is on a volunteer basis. If arthroscopic surgery is being introduced at a hospital, I suggest renting instructional videotapes from the American Academy of Orthopaedic Surgeons (AAOS) or the Arthroscopy Association of North America (AANA). These materials, which show the surgical techniques in action, will both encourage and educate the staff. The videotapes can also be used for inservice training. A number of individuals may participate in the early arthroscopic cases. After their exposure, the surgeon may select the arthroscopic surgical team. The personalities of the potential team members and the surgeons must be compatible.

Unfortunately, operating room supervisors traditionally want every individual in the operating room to know every possible surgical procedure and discipline. Their reasoning, of course, is to provide ample coverage for all procedures in case of an off-hours emergency. In practice, emergencies remain a crisis situation. The search for cabinet keys and surgical equipment still goes on. The preparation of the operating room still takes time. There is therefore no actual benefit to the traditional point of view. Most emergency procedures are performed under less than optimal conditions in spite of multispecialty experience, with the loss of daily benefit of a team approach.

I recommend that teams be created of people with similar interests working in special areas: general surgery, urology, ENT, and so on, with limited overlap where practical. The hospital administration does not think twice about having an organ transplant team or a cardiac surgical team. A team could just as easily be established for arthroscopic surgery.

The arthroscopic surgical team will take time to develop. The type of person to recruit should have a keen interest in arthroscopic surgery. The desire to learn and a spirit of cooperation create a pleasant environment. Skills develop with time and experience.

Arthroscopic surgery is not a simple technique to learn, and thus the initial cases will consume more time than procedures performed conventionally. This should not discourage the participants; the procedures will be performed more rapidly as they gain experience.

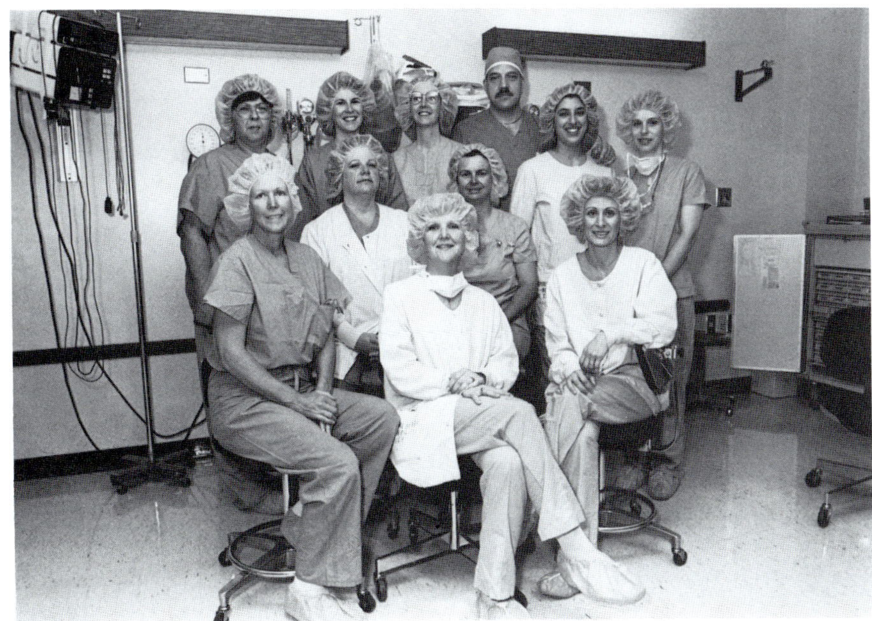

FIG. 2-3 Ingham Medical Center's arthroscopic team in 1991. Seated left to right: Diana Many, S.T.; Julie Murray, R.N.; Sandy Sinkovitz, R.N.; Sue Harris, L.P.N.; Cindy Walker, R.N. Standing left to right: Sally Lopez, unit secretary; Cindy Everett, R.N., Director, Jackie Friar, R.N.; Stan Krawczyk, C.S.T.; Anna Filice, O.R. assistant;Barb Tranberg, R.N.

The Model Team

At the Ingham Medical Center, the hospital adminstration honored our request for a surgical team dedicated to arthroscopic surgery (Fig. 2-3). Once assigned to the arthroscopic suite, the staff does not rotate through various surgical subspecialties. Team members have the added benefit of no night call. This provides a very highly skilled and efficient team. The hospital benefits by the cost effectiveness.

Emphasis is on each person's primary responsibilities, and overlap of assignments is minimized. All team members have a position and an assignment (Fig. 2-4). All resources—the power sources, the tables, and the people—should be in the same position for every case. Each instrument should be in the same location and on the same table for every case (Fig. 2-5). Thus arthroscopy lends itself to the establishment of a protocol. When each procedure is carried out in a similar manner, each team member anticipates each step. The experience is far more satisfying and success is more certain. Staff anticipation and participation is a pleasure to be a part of and to observe. During the operation the team should function in a coordinated and cooperative manner. Many simultaneous activities require the attention of each team member, and numerous details attract the attention of the surgeon. The surgeon directs this orchestra and expects its members to be in tune and on cue; otherwise there is discord.

These patterns of responsibility, as outlined below and carefully observed, result in extreme efficiency and optimal patient care.

Surgical Assistants. Ideally the assistants are specialists in arthroscopy.[2] Their job descriptions are individualized to circulating nurse, first assistant, and second assistant, but cooperation provides for overlapping responsibilities. The surgical assistants are usually hospital employees. My assistant, Ruth Becker, L.P.N., has worked for me for the past 23 years. She is truly an expert and specialist at arthroscopic surgery. I often joke that if Ruth retires, so do I. She assists in the office, with scheduling, and with patient management. If a woman can be a "right hand man," she has been just that.

The assistants care for the instrumentation. Proper handling and care of endoscopic equipment increases its longevity. With careful handling, some instrumentation can last many years.

The circulating nurse. The foremost responsibility of the circulating nurse is the patient's welfare. The circulating nurse converses with the patient who is under local anesthesia. Talking with the patient contributes to his or her assurance and relaxation by allaying any anxiety or fears.

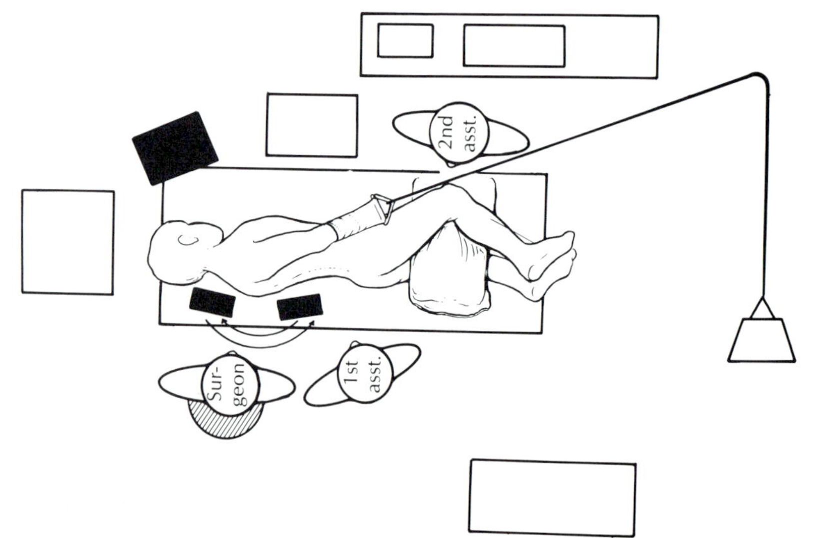

FIG. 2-4 Room layout for shoulder arthroscopy.

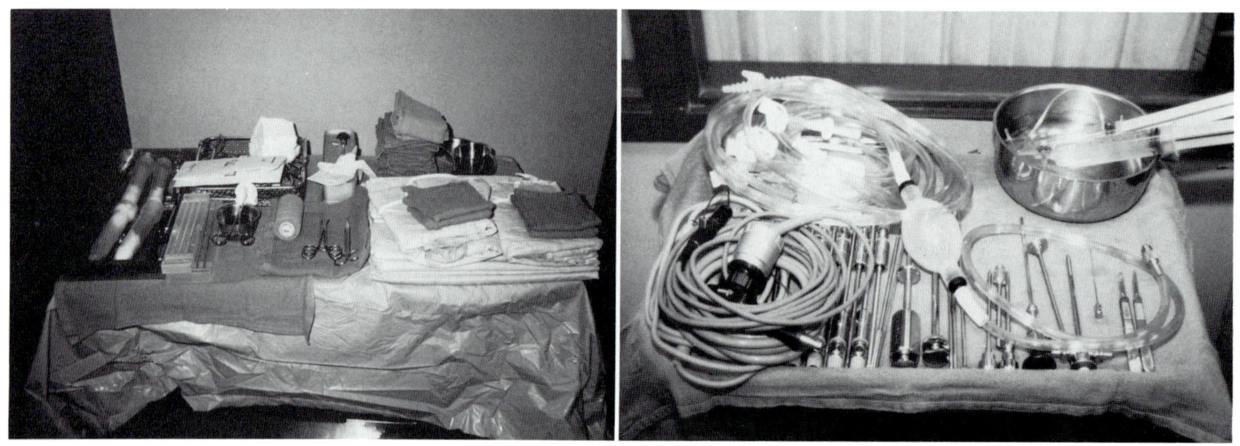

A

B

FIG. 2-5 Instrument table layout for arthroscopic surgery.

A Back table preparation.

B Instrument Mayo stand.

The circulating nurse also assists the anesthesiologist during administration of regional or general anesthesia and supports the surgical team.

The circulating nurse's duties are as follows:

Preparation for the procedure

1. Opens sterile supplies and dispenses to sterile field.
2. Ties scrub nurse's gown.
3. Dispenses Betadine solution.
4. Dispenses sterile water to rinse Cidex from instruments.
5. Interviews patient and *confirms surgical extremity.*
6. Brings patient into operating room.
7. Assists anesthesiologist with induction.
8. Assists with positioning patient.
9. Applies suction to Olympic vacuum bag.
10. Assists with suspension of upper extremity.
11. Positions arthroscopic tables.
12. Attaches light guide to light source.
13. Connects television cable.
14. Positions instrumentation foot pedal.
15. Positions Bovie and foot pedal.
16. Positions and connects suction tubing.
17. Positions and connects fluid reservoirs.
18. Ties gowns of surgeon and first assistant.

During the procedure

1. Monitors fluid reservoirs.
2. Applies pressure to saline bags when requested.
3. Fills out OR records.
4. Manages outflow bottles and suction.
5. Manages fluids on floor.

Following the procedure

1. Replaces power source pedal to top of arthroscopic table.
2. Unplugs shaver and abrasion cords and turns off power box.
3. Disconnects suction and places specimen into specimen bag.
4. Disconnects light source.
5. Moves television and power sources to the side.
6. Moves saline IV pole off to the side.

After dressings are applied:

7. Assists with removal of suspension.
8. Assists with application of sling/immobilizer.
9. Moves patient to recovery room cart.
10. Transports patient to recovery room.
11. Completes OR records.
12. Logs in pathological specimen and adds formalin.

The first assistant. The responsibilities of the first assistant during set-up are to bring equipment to the back table, ensure that all instruments are available in the operating room suite (both sterile and sterile-wrapped in the cupboards), and assist in preparing and draping the patient. During arthroscopy the first assistant must control the arthroscope to assist with the inflow and outflow systems, oversee the second assistant, and assist the surgeon. At the conclusion of the case, the first assistant participates in taking down the instruments. The delicate arthroscopes should be carefully placed in trays for cleansing and sterilization.

At the end of each week the first assistant prepares the arthroscope for gas sterilization. After each arthroscopic examination, the first assistant carefully cleans the arthroscope with saline solution and then alcohol and places it in activated dialdehyde solution of Cidex. He or she cleans the instrumentation with soap and forced water with brushing.

The duties of the first assistant include the following:

Preparation for the procedure

1. Brings all instruments:
   a. To back table.
   b. Sterile-wrapped in cupboard.
2. Assists in set-up of tables.
3. Assists in positioning of patient.
4. Assists in suspension of the upper extremity.
5. Organizes and positions arthroscopic Mayo stand.

During the procedure

1. Controls arthroscope and attached television camera.
2. Oversees instrumentation coordination with second assistant.
3. Assists the surgeon.

Following the procedure

1. Assists with application of dressing.
2. Assists with removal of suspension.
3. Assists with application of sling or splint.
4. Assists with moving patient to gurney.
5. Organizes instrumentation.
6. Cleans instruments.
7. Prepares instruments for next case.

The second assistant. The second assistant is responsible for setting up the back table, the Mayo stand, and the skin preparation materials, as well as assisting in preparation of the patient. This person is responsible for positioning of the Mayo stand and attachment of the suction tubing and motorized instrument cables. At the end of the procedure the second assistant places the arthroscope and the knife blade in Cidex solution, readies the steam autoclaving tray, and assists in removing and stripping the operating room of laundry and waste to prepare the appropriate materials for gas and/or steam autoclaving.

The second assistant addresses the following:

Preparation for the procedure

1. Scrubs clean.
2. Gowns and gloves self and others on the team.
3. Organizes back table.
4. Prepares surgical preparation table.
5. Drapes Mayo stand.
6. Arranges instruments on Mayo stand on front of patient.

7. Prepares sterile draping for upper extremity.
8. Prepares sterile tubing, Gravity Assist, and connectors for fluids.
9. After instruments have soaked 10 minutes, rinses Cidex from instruments.
10. Gowns and gloves surgeon.
11. Assists in draping patient.
12. Brings Mayo stand into position.
13. Runs fluid tubing through holes in drape and hands off to circulating nurse.
14. Hands to circulating nurse the light cable to connect to light source.
15. Hands motorized instrumentation cable for circulating nurse to connect to power source.

During the procedure

1. Passes instruments to surgeon.
2. Regulates outflow of suction to maintain proper distention.

Following the procedure

1. Breaks down draping and assist surgeon with dressing.
2. Gathers instruments for first assistant to wash.
3. Follows usual procedure for turning room over for next case.

A DEDICATED ARTHROSCOPIC OPERATING SUITE

Diagnostic arthroscopy by direct viewing is possible in an operating room equipped for general surgical procedures. Advanced arthroscopic surgery, however, demands a more elaborate and specific environment. The general operating room may accommodate the unique needs of arthroscopic techniques, but modifications are usually necessary. The room lighting must be dimmable. The electrical outlets must be abundant, with isolated, dedicated lines. Electrical and radio wave frequency interference must be eliminated. Accommodation must be made for the suspended fluid reservoirs, fluid pumps, suction outflow, collection bags for specimens, and fluid spillage. A provision must be made for intraoperative television, with special stands, outlets, and connections (Fig. 2–2).

Because arthroscopic surgery has so many special requirements, I recommend a dedicated room. The Ingham Medical Center administration had the foresight 10 years ago to establish an arthroscopic surgery suite (see Fig. 2-1). It includes two operating rooms, one with an observation/viewing room. A recovery room, nurses' station, nurses' offices, instrumentation and sterilization rooms, and storage and locker facilities are adjacent to the suite. An outpatient holding area and waiting room were placed next to the suite to facilitate patient transportation.

Despite this planning, deficiencies of the suite at Ingham Medical Center have developed over time. The small operating room size was in part caused by the remolding of existing space intended for OB/GYN. In addition, space and storage problems were created by the proliferation of arthroscopic equipment and the development of arthroscopy combined with various open procedures. So when planning such a suite, keeping in mind future developments and needs is wise.

The Observation Room

The observation/viewing room was built in response to the daily continuing education programs for in-service and visiting physicians, nurses, and administrators (see Fig. 2-1). The room is equipped with telephone for communicating and television monitors for simultaneous inside and outside viewing. The hospital has also used this room in public relations and promotional activities to provide a rather innocuous view of "high-tech" surgery for those involved in hospital development programs (i.e., fund raising).

The Operating Room

The operating room dedicated to arthroscopic surgery has many requirements to create the optimal environment. Every construction or remodeling decision should accommodate future change. Change is the one constant in arthroscopic surgery.

Construction Features. I suggest a minimum room size of 24 feet × 24 feet. The ceiling should be 16 feet high to accommodate a drop ceiling. This height allows for electrical and television cables as well as suspension systems (Fig.2-6). If the space above the drop ceiling is limited, any repairs or future revisions will be difficult.

The ceiling may serve as a mount for various suspension systems (Fig. 2-7). The television camera and monitor connections are commonly suspended, thus eliminating cables on the floor. Suspended systems facilitate personnel and patient movement within the room as well as cleaning. Permanent installation avoids the wear and tear of electronic equipment caused by handling.

An alternative method places all the equipment on one stand (Fig. 2-8). In this case, the cables should still connect via the ceiling to keep the room clear of cables for people movement.

Electrical system. Ideally the electrical system of an arthroscopic room or suite should be isolated from all other systems because microwave, electrocautery, or x-ray equipment running adjacent to or on the same circuits as the equipment in the suite will cause considerable interference with the video picture. Loss of visualization can stop an operation. The room should be lead-lined or be set off by distance and thick cement walls.

Radio wave frequencies (RF) can also affect the operating room video picture. Sources of the interfering radio waves are the emergency room's radio dispatch system and the arthroscopic lights. The electrical light sources

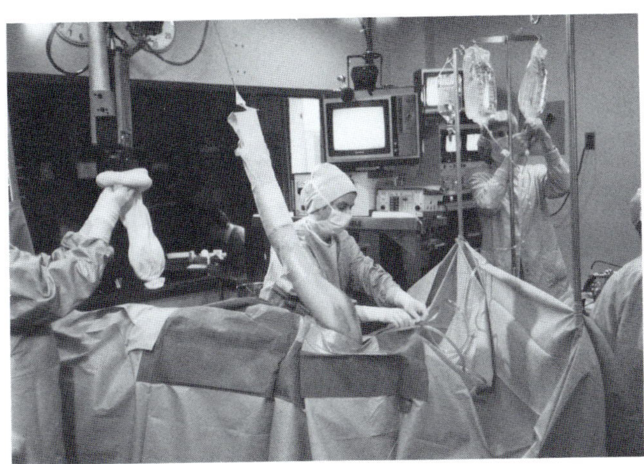

FIG. 2-6 Operating room has sufficient room for tables, poles, and television and ceiling high enough for cables. Each member of the arthroscopic team is performing his or her individual tasks.

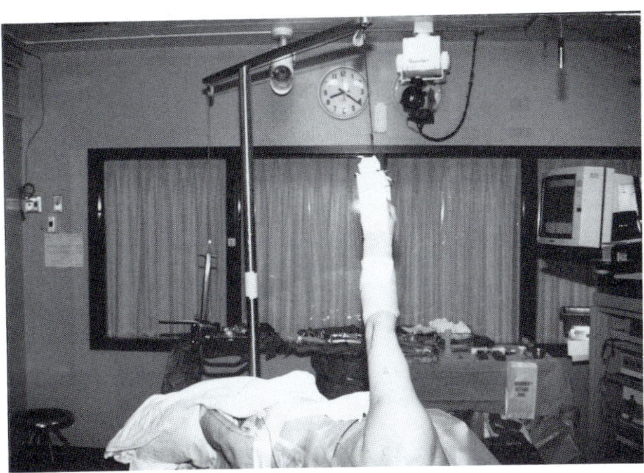

FIG. 2-7 High ceiling provides room for suspension equipment and cords.

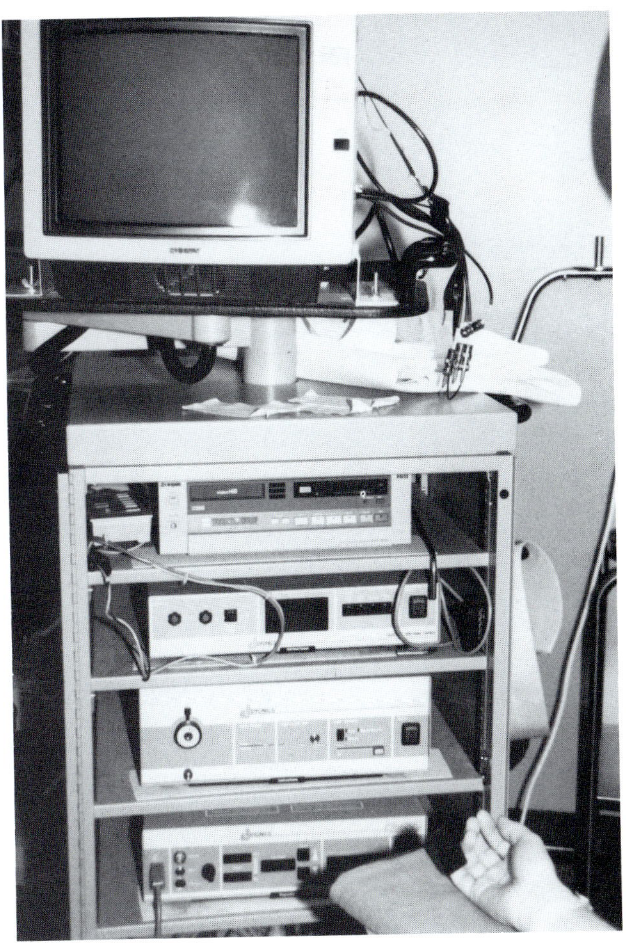

FIG. 2-8 The mobile operating room cabinet holds power sources and cantilevered television.

should be shielded from RF waves. Televsion systems must be constructed by the manufacturer to shield the units from radio wave interference.

Electrical cords should drop from the ceiling for a single connection to the power source at the table. This is preferable to cords running from side to side across the floor (see Fig. 2-7).

The power sources should be conveniently placed in front of the surgeon. They should also be of such design and style that they will offer easy recharging overnight or over the weekend.

Lighting. The operating room lights should be on a rheostat dimmer so that a spectrum of illumination is possible (Fig. 2-9, *A*,*B*, and *C*). The lighting system for arthroscopic procedures must not allow bright lights to reflect on the video monitor, which makes visualization more difficult. If an arthroscopic room has been designated, surgical spotlights should be available for the combined surgical cases (Fig. 2-9, *C*). If no surgical lighting exists, the light cable can be detached from the arthroscope and used as a light source during an open procedure. This source will be adequate for most surgeries (see also Chapter 3).

Air conditioning. The matter of supplying hot or cool air is taken for granted by architects and engineers. However, this does not constitute air conditioning. Calculations

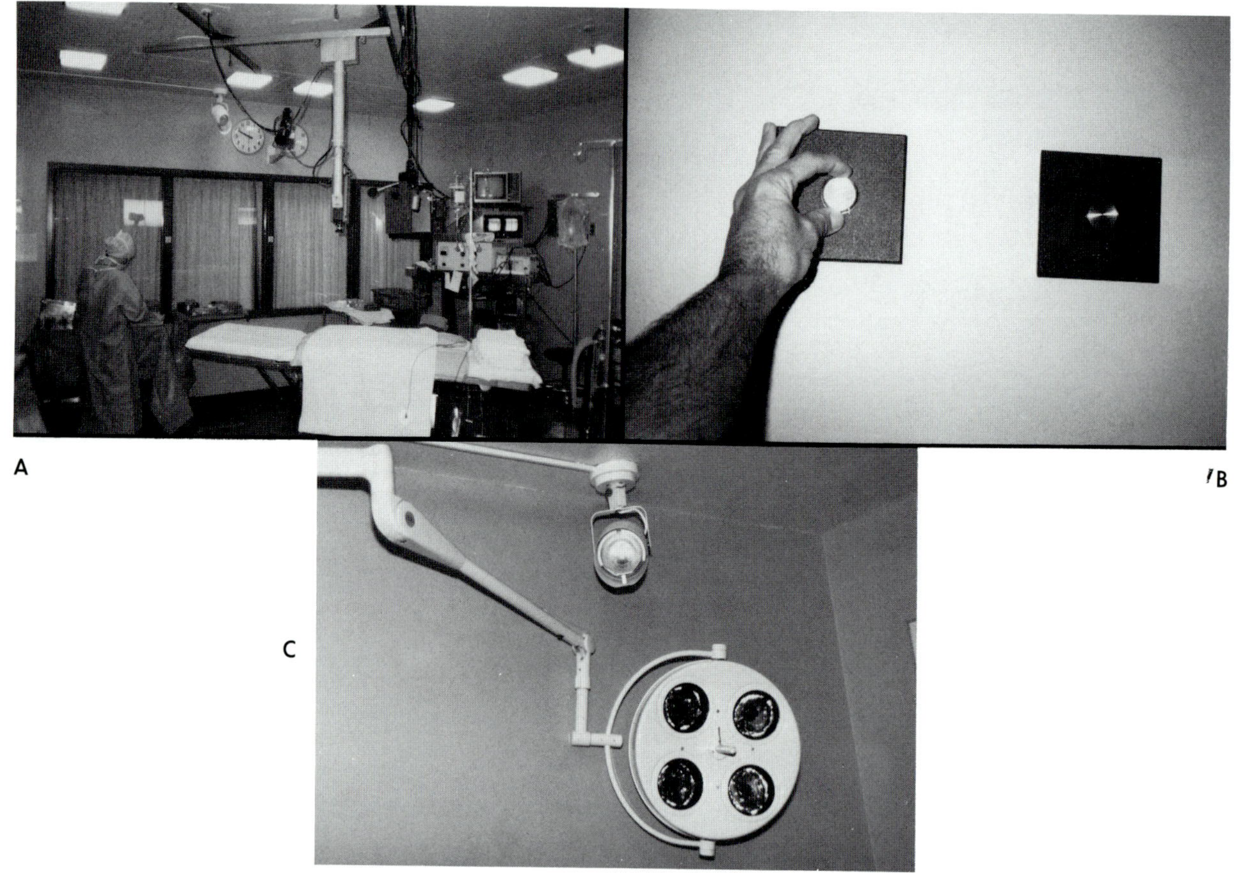

FIG. 2-9 **Lighting system.**

A **Ceiling lighting is diffuse.**

B **A rheostat system is necessary to reduce glare.**

C **Additional spot lights are necessary for open surgery and outside television flood lights.**

must also be made for the heat of people, lights, and power sources. Consideration must also be made for gown-covered personnel and the patient covered with surgical drapes.

The matter of hot or cool air supply is not as critical as the circulation or exchange of air, which is usually neglected. Air circulation is the most critical factor for a pleasant, comfortable environment. Humidity control is especially challenging in an arthroscopic suite because of the "water, water everywhere" syndrome experienced during this type of surgical procedure. A separate air circulation system allows for better control of these factors.

Floor. The floor should have a terrazzo surface (Fig.2-10). It should be as clear of cords as possible via the use of ceiling wiring. The direction of drainage should be away from or toward the end of the operating room table. Floor drains are not permitted by law in some states. Ideally the drain would be directly under the operating room table so that all the water flows to an area where no one is walking or standing.

Room Arrangement of Equipment and People. The furniture arrangement for shoulder arthroscopy should be constant. These arrangements may have to be modified for combined procedures.

Operating room table. The operating room patient table need not be elaborate; kidney rests, side tilting, and motorization are not necessary. The table should, however, have the capacity to be lowered more than the usual tables (27 inches from the floor). The requirement for going lower with the table is necessary in very large people. If the table will not lower, the involved shoulder may be above the surgeon's arm and eye level.

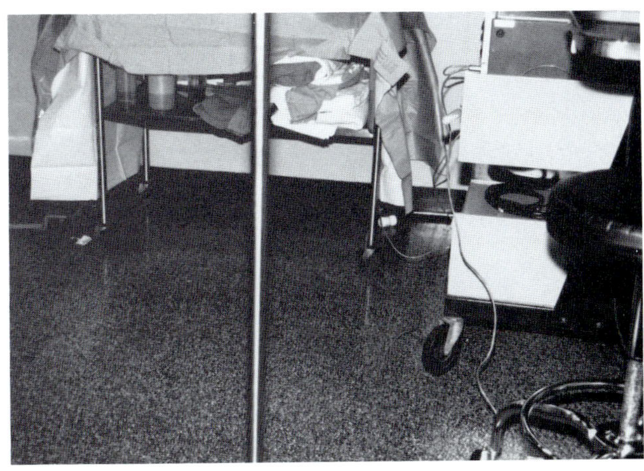

FIG. 2-10 The floor should be free of cords and wiring by use of ceiling mounts. Notice the one cord that hangs low and may cause a staff member to trip or pull out the plug.

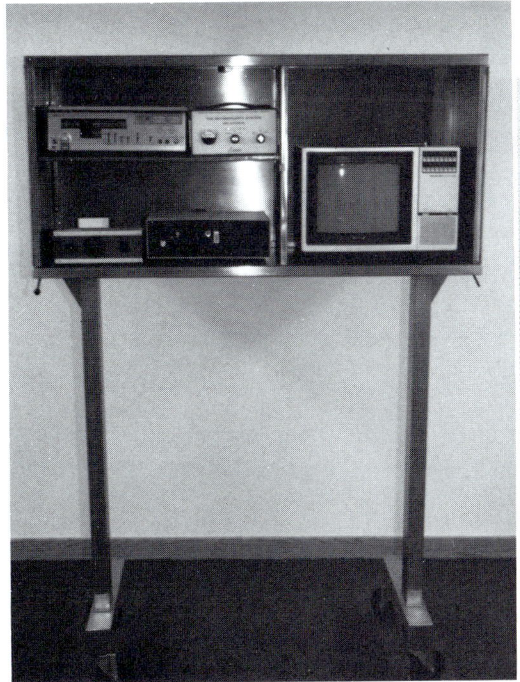

A

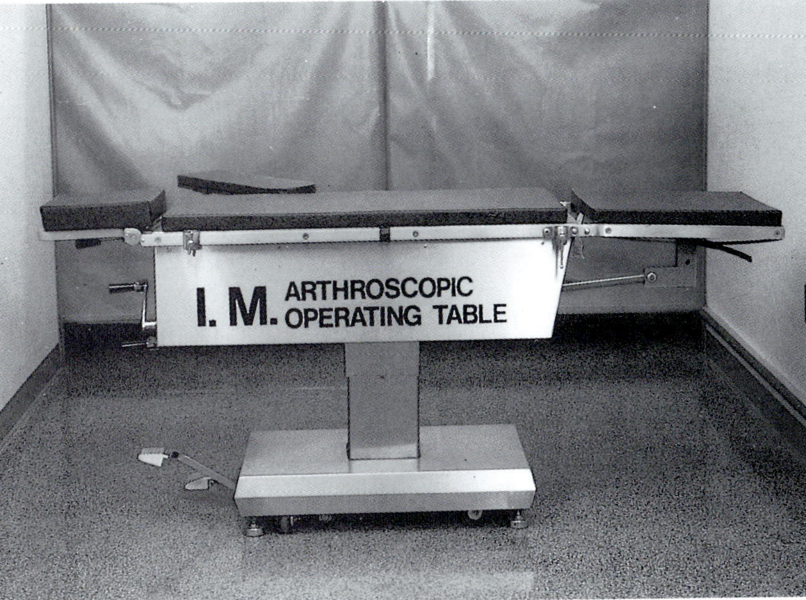

B

FIG. 2-11 Cabinets.

A Treasure chest cabinet that holds all equipment and can be locked.

B Surgicenter table.

Television monitor. Ideally the television monitor is suspended or cantilevered and movable, including side-to side, up-and-down, and rotating movements (see Fig. 2-8). The need for additional monitors for simultaneous editing, viewing by the anesthesiologist, or teaching purposes may be determined on an individual basis (see Fig. 2-2).

Cabinets. Mobile cabinets are needed for monitors and power sources. The first is an enlarged version of the original over-the-top table (Fig. 2-11, *A*). This cabinet also has locking doors for secure off-hours storage. The cabinet holds all power sources. It is especially adapted to handheld camera use and facilitates room-to-room changes.

The second cabinet, known as a Surgicenter, incorpo-

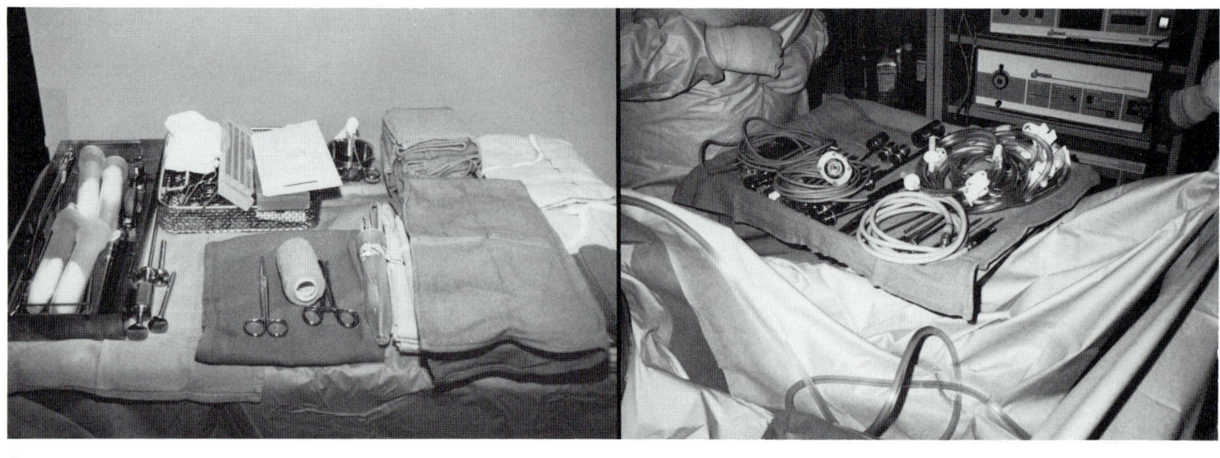

A B

FIG. 2-12 Tables.

A Back table.

B Surgical Mayo stand holding equipment before set up.

rates all of the necessary spaces and structures for a standalone system (Fig. 2-11, *B*). Constructed of stainless steel for operating room standards, it contains shelf space for all power sources. A suspension bar is cantilevered for television camera suspension. Mechanically operated poles are included for saline bag suspension. A mobile arthroscopic surgical center is very handy. Mounted on wheels, it can be moved from room to room or from storage without the need for carrying each piece of heavy equipment.

Another mobile cabinet has storage space for power sources and a cantilevered platform for a television monitor (see Fig. 2-8).

Tables. The back table is any customary stainless steel operating room table with wheels. It serves for initial instrument gathering and holds the less frequently used instruments and various trays and containers (Fig. 2-12, *A*).

One Mayo stand is used for shoulder arthroscopy. It is controlled by the second assistant and during the procedure is positioned in front of the patient (Fig. 2-12, *B*).

Position of personnel. The surgeon stands behind the patient. Each assistant stands in the same position for every case. The first assistant is behind the patient and to the side of the surgeon. The second assistant is on the opposite side of the table from the surgeon (see Fig. 2-4).

The surgeon may sit at the head of the table for open rotator cuff repairs. In this case, the surgeon's stool should sit securely on the floor. If it has rollers, a simple locking mechanism should be included. The seat should be firm. The stool must be secure, because it often serves as the platform against which the surgeon pushes to manipulate the extremity or anatomical structures. The wetness of the floor during arthroscopy increases the necessity for security. The stool should occupy little space and be easily movable with the surgeon's foot.

Positioning the patient. The patient is customarily placed in the lateral decubitus position (Fig. 2-13). An important next step is to move the patient posterior on the table. If this is not done, the surgeon's position and comfort is compromised. The surgeon must lean forward to do the surgery and the edge of the table will press uncomfortably against the surgeon's thigh.

The patient is secured with an Olympic Vac Pac and tape to the table. The Vac Pac is filled with styrofoam beads. Suction is applied to the bag, which changes the nature of the pad from soft to rigid. Padding is placed between the ankles to avoid pressure sores (Fig. 2-13, *C*). Suction remains attached to the Vac Pac to eliminate accidental deflation (Fig. 2-13, *D*).

Shoulder suspension system. At one time, we installed multiple pulleys in the ceiling for shoulder and elbow work. However, we now use a T-shaped double pulley system attached to the table (Fig. 2-14). The forearm is secured to one end, and the weight is attached to the other. The shoulder suspension system is also used in open rotator cuff repairs, as it holds the arm in an abducted position, eliminating the need for an assistant to do the same (Fig. 2-14, *A*). The suspension system attaches to the operating table by a Clark clamp (Fig. 2-14, *B*).

The desired shoulder abduction is achieved by placement of an upright proximally or distally at the foot of the table. Flexion or extension is achieved by rotating the upright, thereby moving the crossbar in an arc over the patient. Finetuning can be achieved by dropping or elevating the foot of the operating room table by increments via controls at the head of the table. The double pulley system provides safe, balanced suspension rather than traction.[1,4]

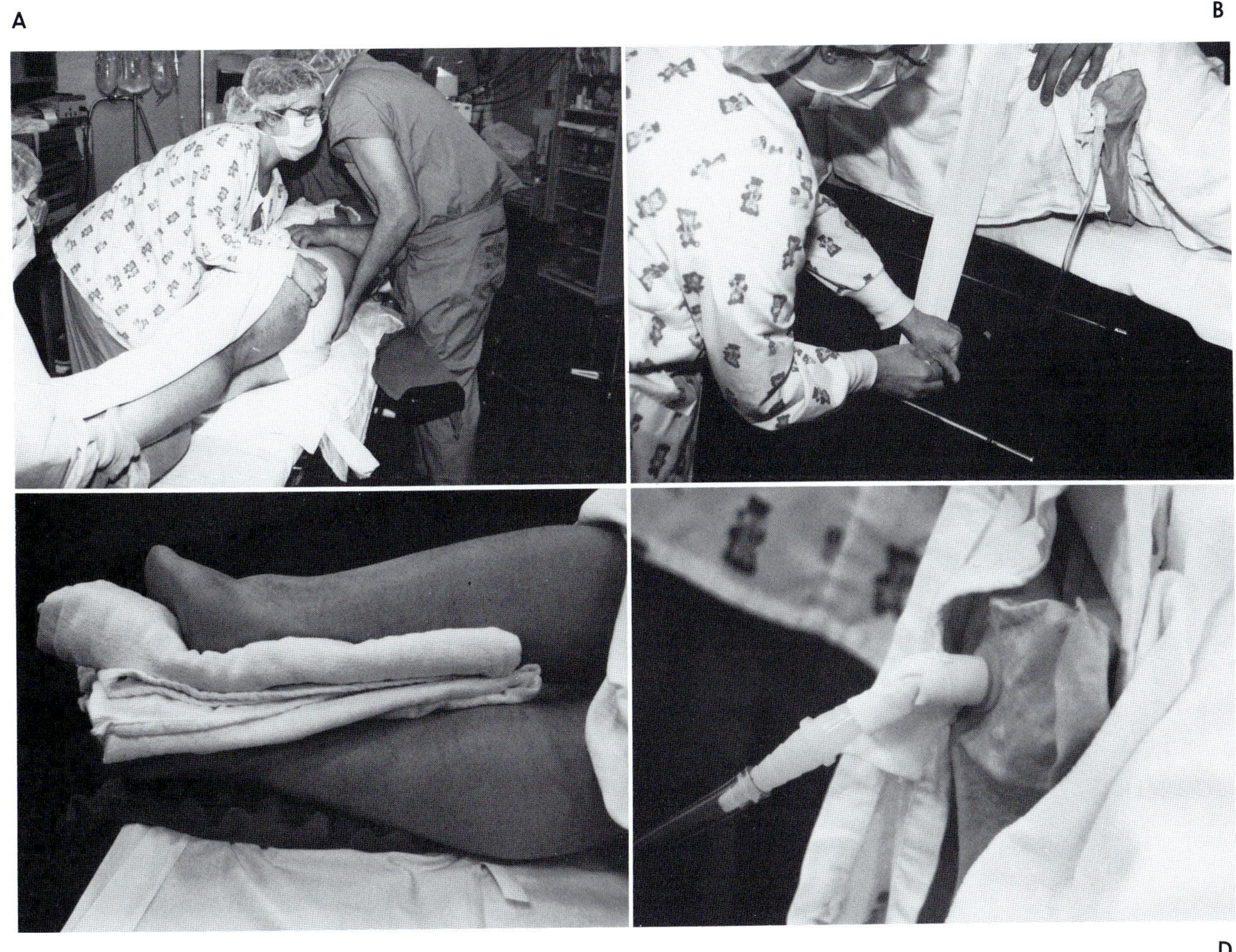

FIG. 2-13 **Positioning the patient.**

A The patient is moved to the opposite lateral decubitus position.

B After the patient is moved posterior on the table, he or she is secured to the table with tape over the pelvic area.

C Padding is used between the legs.

D The suction is attached to the Vac Pac and taped in place; constant suction is applied to avoid decompression.

A

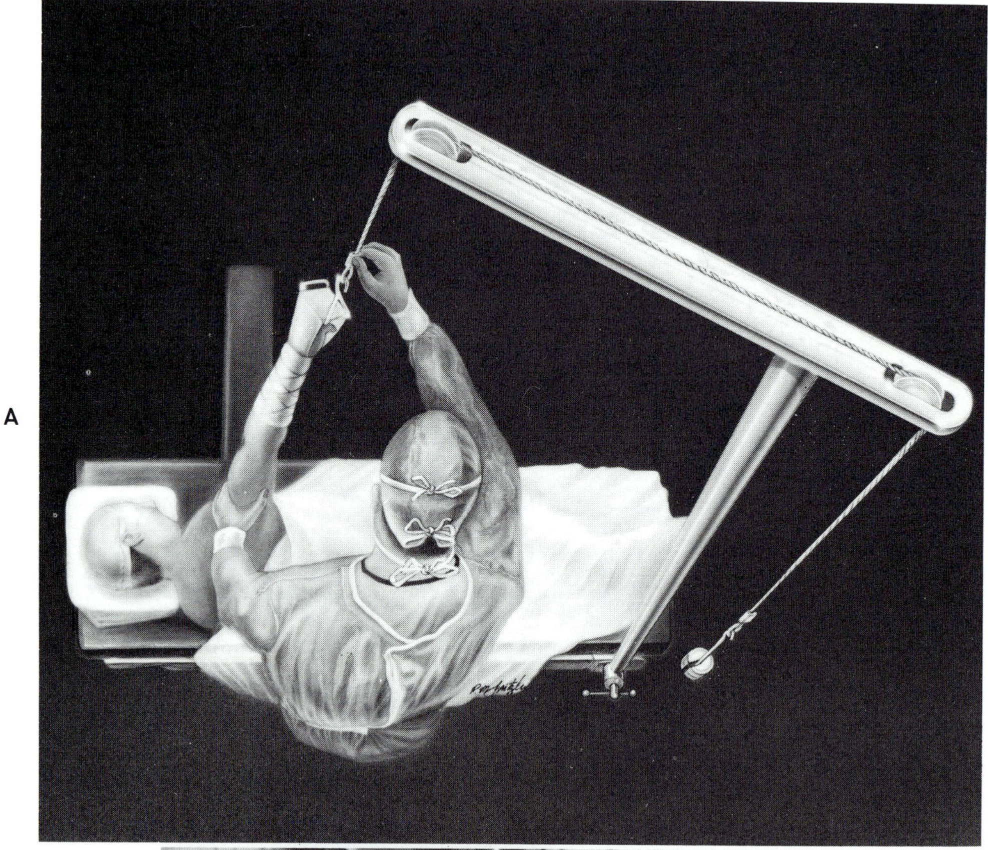

B

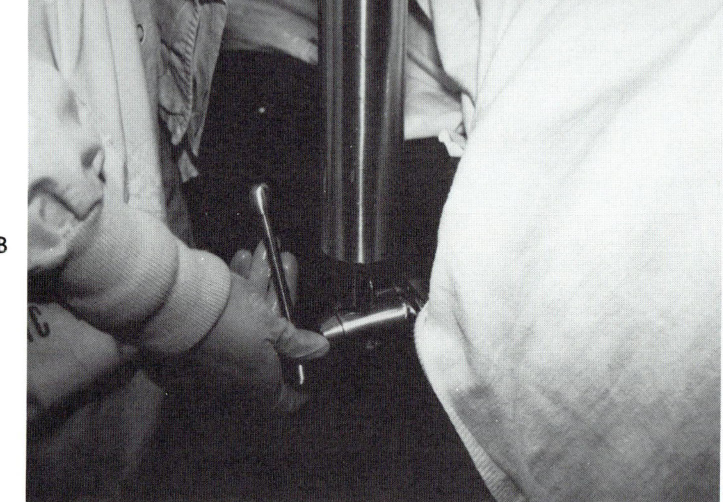

FIG. 2-14 **Shoulder suspension system.**

A **Drawing of system. (Courtesy Instrument Makar, Inc.)**

B **The upright pole is secured to the operating room table with a C-clamp to the side rail.**

Securing the upper extremity. The upper extremity is secured by wrapping the forearm with a strip of perforated tape, Ace wrap, and adhesive tape. I have applied this to my own arm in the same surgical position (Fig. 2-15, *A*) and can report this simple system is more comfortable than commercially available, more expensive attachments. The patient's arm is then raised. The metal frame is taped to the loop in the foam strip and also to the suspending cable (Fig. 2-15, *B*).

Draping. Arthroscopic draping must accommodate liquid leakage and spillage. The Surgikos Division of Johnson & Johnson has developed disposable draping packages for the shoulder. These packages were developed by my nurse, Ruth Becker (Fig. 2-16).

Draping commences after the patient is positioned and the arm is suspended. A clean towel is placed over the patient's head. An unsterile 3M plastic U-drape with adhesive is placed over the patient's head and sealed about the neck (Fig. 2-16, *A*). The disposable paper shoulder draping package provides a sterile two piece yoked drape with plastic adhesive. The larger drape is placed over the body. The upper drape is placed from superior to inferior to create a tight seal around the shoulder (Fig. 2-16, *B* and *C*). The arm is covered with a sterile towel, which is held with a 3M Coban elastic wrap (Fig. 2-17).

The commerical draping system is modified in two ways. Folds are placed in the drape over the pelvis so that pockets are formed to hold the arthroscope and instruments. This prevents them from falling on the floor (Fig. 2-18). A fold is made in the drape in front of the surgeon. This fold provides a collection pouch so that fluids are contained and directed to the opposite side of the operative field (Fig. 2-19). The draping is attached to the anesthesia poles in such a manner to direct the fluid into a bucket on the floor.

The Surgikos system has integrated loops that permit passage of cords of the power supply and light cables, as well as inflow/outflow tubing (Fig. 2-20).

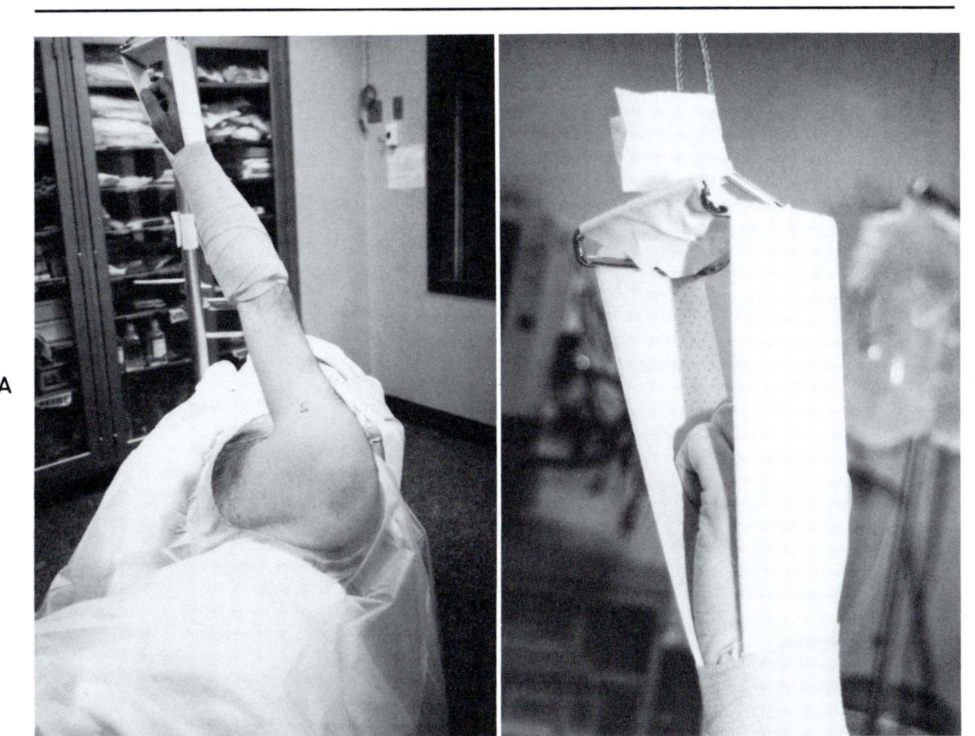

FIG. 2-15 Upper extremity suspension.

A Patient's upper extremity is suspended with perforated foam strip, Ace wrap, and adhesive tape.

B Close-up of the taping to prevent the metal bar or cable from pulling apart.

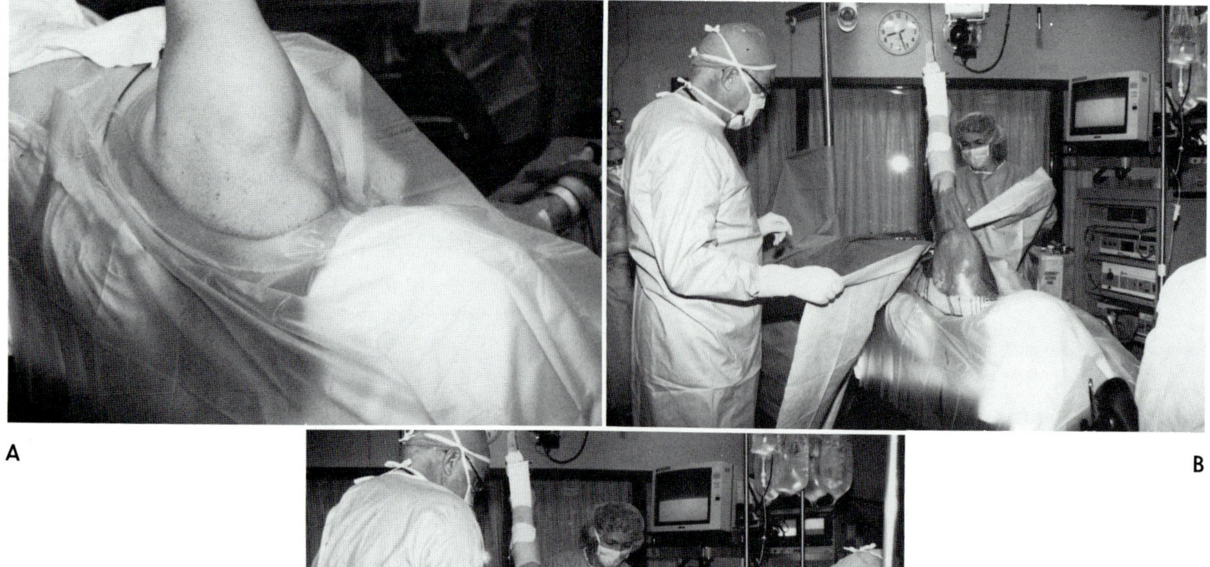

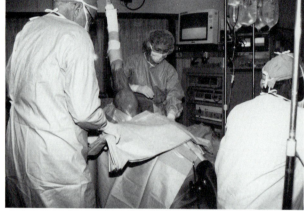

FIG. 2-16 Draping.

A A towel is placed over the patient's head and this is covered with 3M plastic U-shaped drape.

B The lower drape is secured to the suspension pole. Drape is drawn superiorly into the patient's axilla.

C A second horseshoe drape joins the inferior drape to surround the base of the shoulder.

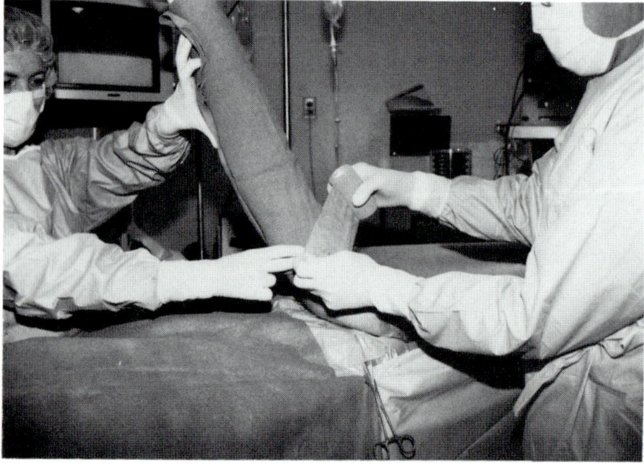

FIG. 2-17 A sterile towel covers the suspended forearm. Sterile Coban is wrapped from proximal to distal to secure the sterility.

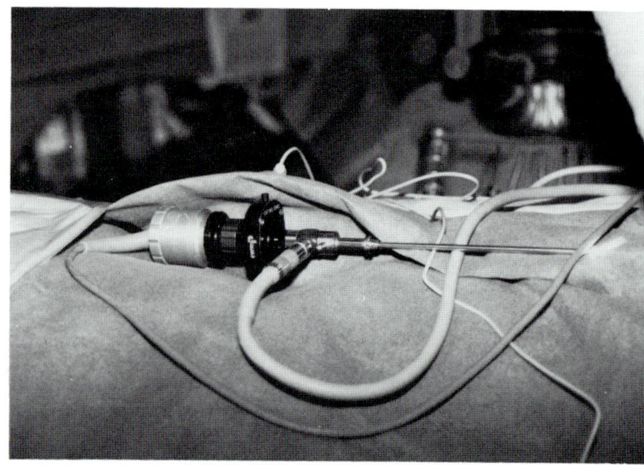

FIG. 2-18 An additional fold is made over the patient's pelvis to hold the arthroscope and surgical instruments.

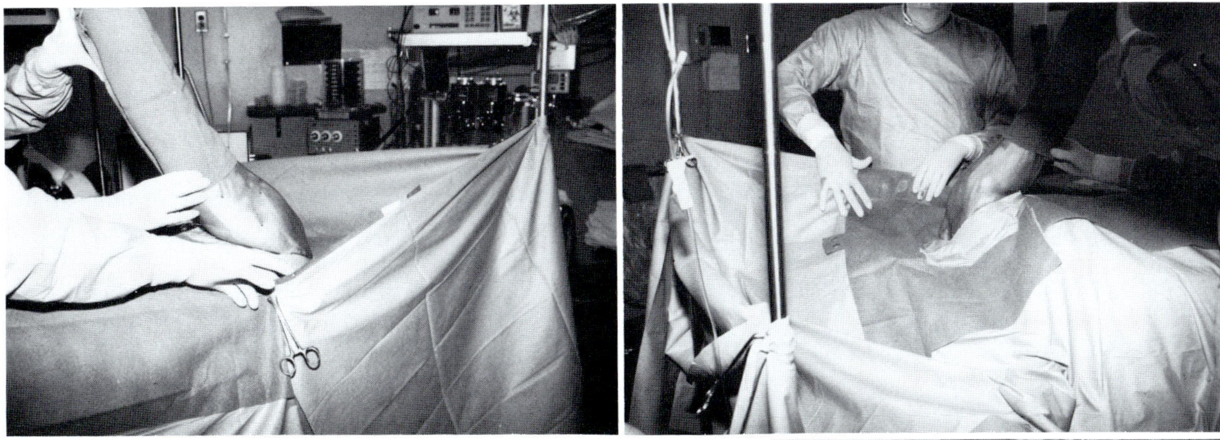

A B

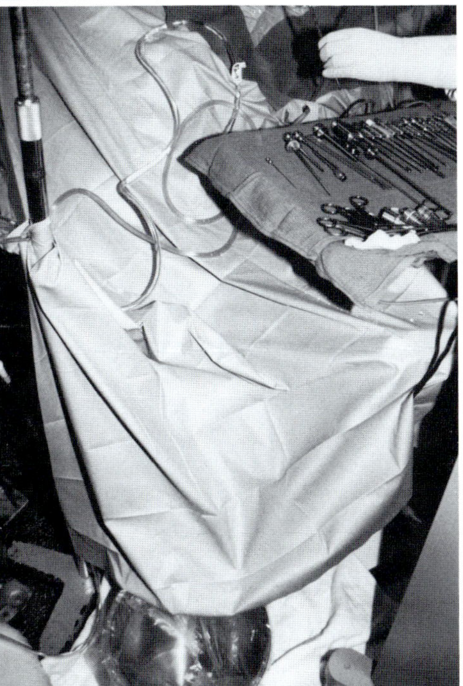

C

FIG. 2-19 Folding of drape to divert fluids.

A The drape is folded and clipped to the adjacent drape posterior to the shoulder. The drape provides a channel to divert fluid flow away from the surgeon and toward a bucket on the floor.

B View of diversion draping shows how fluid will flow away from the surgeon.

C View of draping from side of table opposite the surgeon shows how fluid will flow into bucket on the floor.

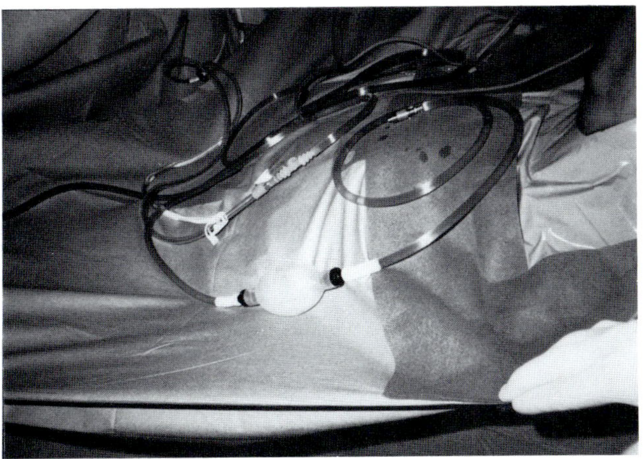

FIG. 2-20 The fluid tubes and power cords are held in place by paper loops on the drapes.

Fluid Management Systems

Fluid Reservoir. The sterile fluids are suspended by a weighted intravenous pole (Fig. 2-21).

Suction. Suction principles are important to arthroscopic motorized instrumentation. Suction is also used during diagnostic arthroscopy. Most modern operating rooms feature permanently installed suction systems. The suction in the operating room pressures must be measured, as the efficiency of the motorized system depends on adequate suction. Our Dyonics motorized system is calibrated for 14 to 16 inches of mercury, which is the suction used at Ingham Medical Center.

Whether a permanent or temporary suction system is used, the pressure should be known and regulated for arthroscopic work. The measurement is not taken end-on, but with an in-line gauge (Fig. 2-22). The gauge should be inserted in the system just outside the operative field for the best pressure measurement.

Collection bottles. A large collection system reduces the necessity for frequent emptying of bottles (Fig. 2-23). A small collection bag, or tobacco bag, can catch the specimen for pathologic analysis. The use of this bag avoids the need to strain large volumes of saline to collect the surgical specimen.

Fluid on the floor. Adequate drainage is paramount (see above). The use of disposable hyperabsorbant paper matting is most effective to handle extra water on the floor (Fig. 2-24). Not only does the matting collect and remove fluid, it collects debris that otherwise would be on the operating room floor.

Another method is the use of commerically available continuous suction device on the floor (Concept, Inc.). This plastic device is necessary only for long procedures with excessive spillage of water.

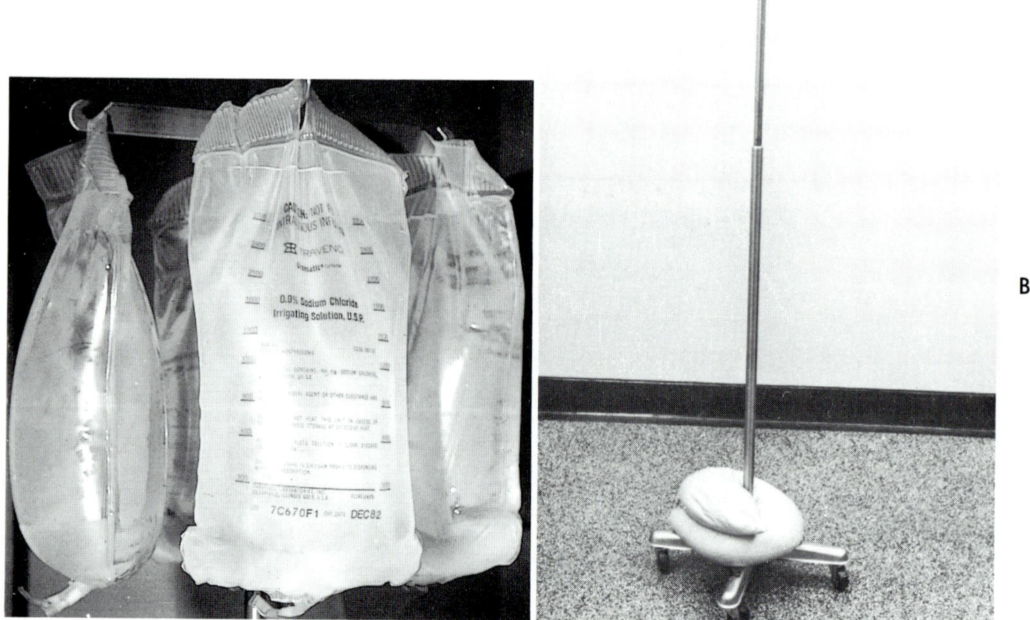

FIG. 2-21 Inflow system. Fluid reservoir consists of two 3-liter bags (A) suspended at least 1 m above the patient on a weighted IV pole (B).

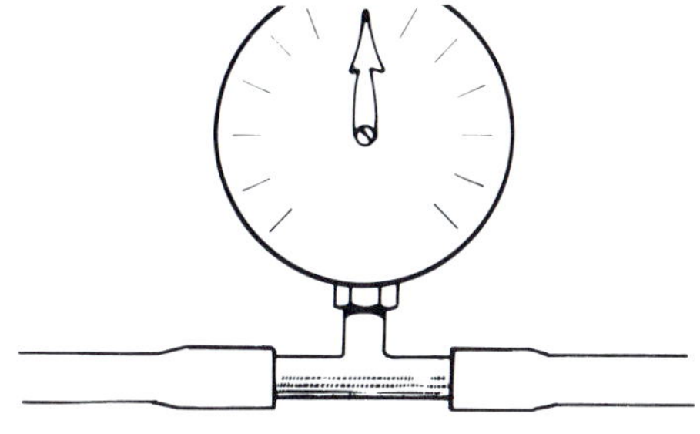

A

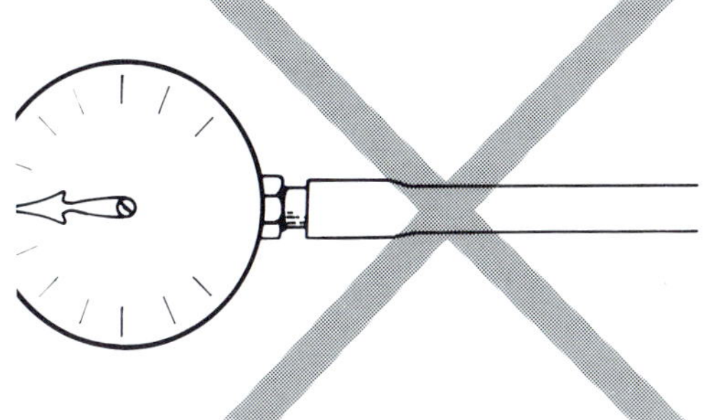

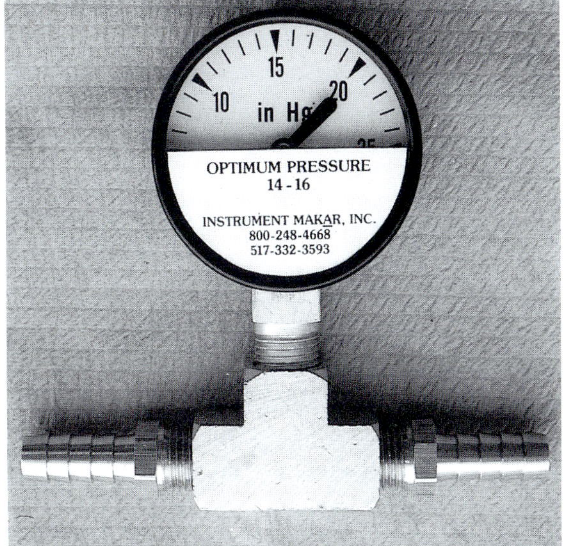

B

FIG. 2-22 **Suction measurements.**

A Diagram of in-line and end-on suction measurements.

B Instrument.

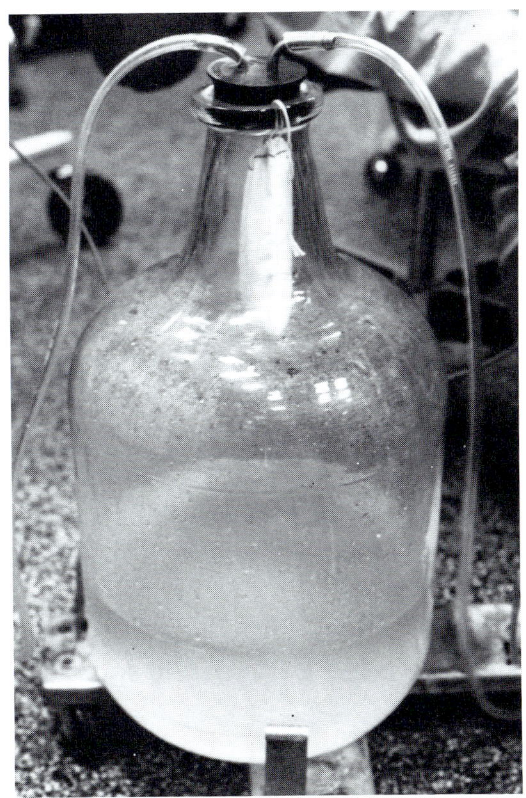

FIG. 2-23 **Collection bottle.**

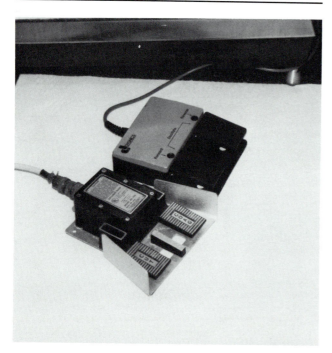

FIG. 2-24 Hyperabsorbent, disposable paper toweling on floor assists with fluid management. Matting is placed under surgeon's feet. Notice both the motorized instrument and electrocautery foot pedals in place on matting.

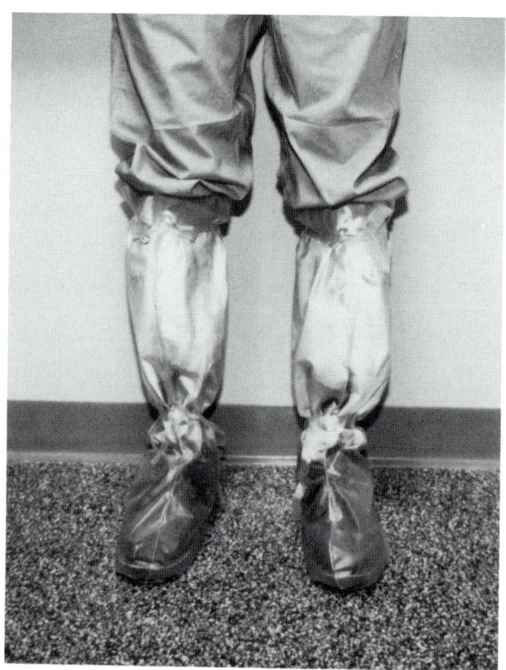

FIG. 2-25 Disposable plastic knee high boots provide both protection and comfort.

Protection of personnel from body fluids. With the increased incidence of acquired immunodeficiency syndrome (AIDS) and risk of hepatitis comes a renewed interest in sterile technique. One function of sterile technique is to protect the patient from germs on the operating team. The interest now includes protection of the doctor and staff from the patient's germs. Since fluids and fluid spillage is abundant in arthroscopy, water impervious gowns are necessary. Disposable plastic boots provide both comfort and protection (Fig. 2-25). An inexpensive disposable face shield is also indicated to reduce the risk of splashing fluids in operating room teams' eyes (Fig. 2-26).

Instrumentation's Role in the Environment. For a complete discussion of instrumentation in shoulder arthroscopy, see Chapter 3.

Clear image transmission. The bottom line of successful arthroscopic surgery is the ability to visualize. A good, clear image is a necessity for arthroscopic surgery. The factors involved in a good picture are not limited to the arthroscope. The maintenance of a clear, bright image requires constant checks on the many potential problem areas. The light source must be powerful and with a new bulb. The light cable must be of adequate size (5 mm in diameter and 6 ft long) and be without breaks and free from corrosion or debris at both ends. The arthroscope's fiberglass conduit should be uninterrupted and clean at both ends. The objective should be polished and without scratches or fracture. No disruption of the lens system alignment or seals should be present. The ocular should be inspected for dirt, dust, or water droplets, especially before it is coupled with the television camera. The camera must be properly focused. The result should be an optimal size of apparent image (focal length) on the television screen. The television must be clean, including the monitor screen.

Potential sources of diminished light are as follows:

1. Light source
   a. Bulb
2. Cable
   a. One end deficient
   b. Fibers
3. Arthroscope
   a. Fibers
   b. Objective lens
   c. Glass lens system
   d. Ocular
4. Television camera sensitivity
   a. Glass of scope connector
5. Television monitor

Organization of instruments. A list of the instruments used should be compiled. Instruments should be organized into groups according to their end-of-the-day stor-

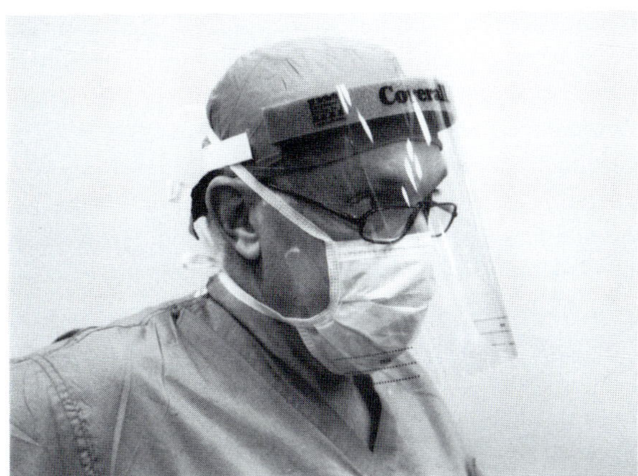

FIG. 2-26 A plastic face shield provides protection from fluid splashes and flying debris with use of oscillating saw.

age or means of sterilization. For example, the arthroscope and cannulas are put together for ethylene oxide gas sterilization. The hand-held and motorized instruments are in containers for another area. The less-used equipment is stored in a movable cabinet. The instrument list should include the exact place of storage.

A map of the operating room with the specific placement of instruments on Mayo stands should be mounted within the operating room for reference as the surgical team mobilizes the equipment for the surgical procedure (Fig. 2-27).

The final step in the organization process separates the instruments based on their frequency of use. The most-used instruments are kept closer to the operative field and grouped by type. For example, the arthroscope, cables, cannula, etc., are placed on one Mayo stand.

The following lists reflect the organization of instruments and are invaluable for training purposes and with substitute assistants. Each surgeon should construct his or her own similar list.

Instruments for operative field (by table)

1. Scissors (two)
2. No. 11 knife blade on No. 3 knife handle
3. No. 15 knife blade on No. 3 knife handle
4. No. 18 spinal needle
5. Dyonics cannulas, without side holes, and a sharp trocar
6. Blunt IAS trocar
7. Additional Dyonics cannulas without side holes; small and large
8. Probe
9. IM 761 knife blade
10. No. 64 Beaver blade on Beaver handle
11. IM knife holder
12. Switching sticks (two)
13. Wissinger rod
14. Stylet for cleaning debris from instruments
15. Arthroplasty cannula on sharp trocar
16. Arthroplasty cannula on blunt trocar

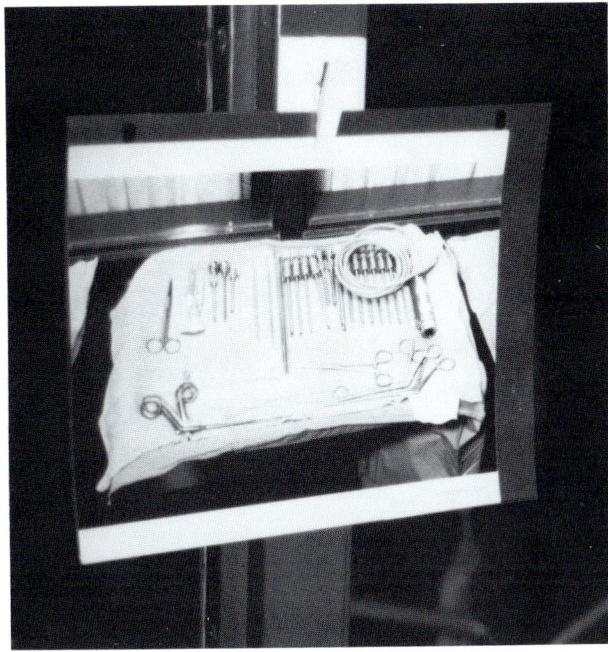

FIG. 2-27 Photographs of set up position of instruments on the tables are helpful to staff. They provide a check on types, numbers, and position of instruments.

Motorized instruments

1. Dyonics PS 3500 motor

Cutting heads

1. 3.5 mm meniscal cutter
2. 4.5 mm meniscal cutter
3. 5.5 mm meniscal cutter
4. 3.5 mm trimmer
5. 4.5 mm trimmer
6. 5.5 mm trimmer
7. Small and larger synovial Whisker

Arthroplasty heads

8. Medium burr
9. Large burr
10. Acromionizer
11. 4.5 mm regular synovial resector
12. 5.5 mm regular synovial resector
13. 3.5 mm full-radius synovial resector
14. 4.5 mm full-radius synovial resector
15. 5.5 mm full-radius synovial resector

Miscellaneous

1. Single inflow adaptor
2. Meniscus graspers (small and large)
3. Basket forceps, 2.7 mm angled
4. Variable-axis scissor/basket forceps
5. Basket forceps 3.5 mm straight
6. 3 × 4 inch gauze (under towel)
7. Basin
8. Dyonics light cord attached to scope
9. Large-jawed forceps
10. Gravity assist bulb and tubing

Arthroscopes

1. Storz cannula with modified sharp trocar
2. Storz scope with bridge
3. Sharp Storz trocar
4. 4.0 mm.; 0-degree inclined arthroscope
5. 4.0 mm; 90-degree inclined arthroscope

Instrument care. The care of instruments is a behind-the-scenes activity that is not so well appreciated until the surgeon is handed a dull instrument, the television camera or monitor does not work, the suction is off, or the suction tubes are clogged with debris.

Instrument care should be the responsibility of one person, preferably an employee of the owner of the instrumentation. Every individual on the arthroscopic team must be educated as to the importance of maintenance (Fig. 2-28). The kind of care required for arthroscopic surgical instruments, television equipment, suction and flow equipment, etc. cannot be handled adequately by a variety of people on a rotational basis or by someone who is not involved in arthroscopic surgery.

Problems will occur if no one at the hospital is specifically assigned to care for arthroscopic instrumentation. Replacement and repair costs will be exceedingly high, which is unnecessary; dollar savings will result from having a team or even one person care for the instrumentation.

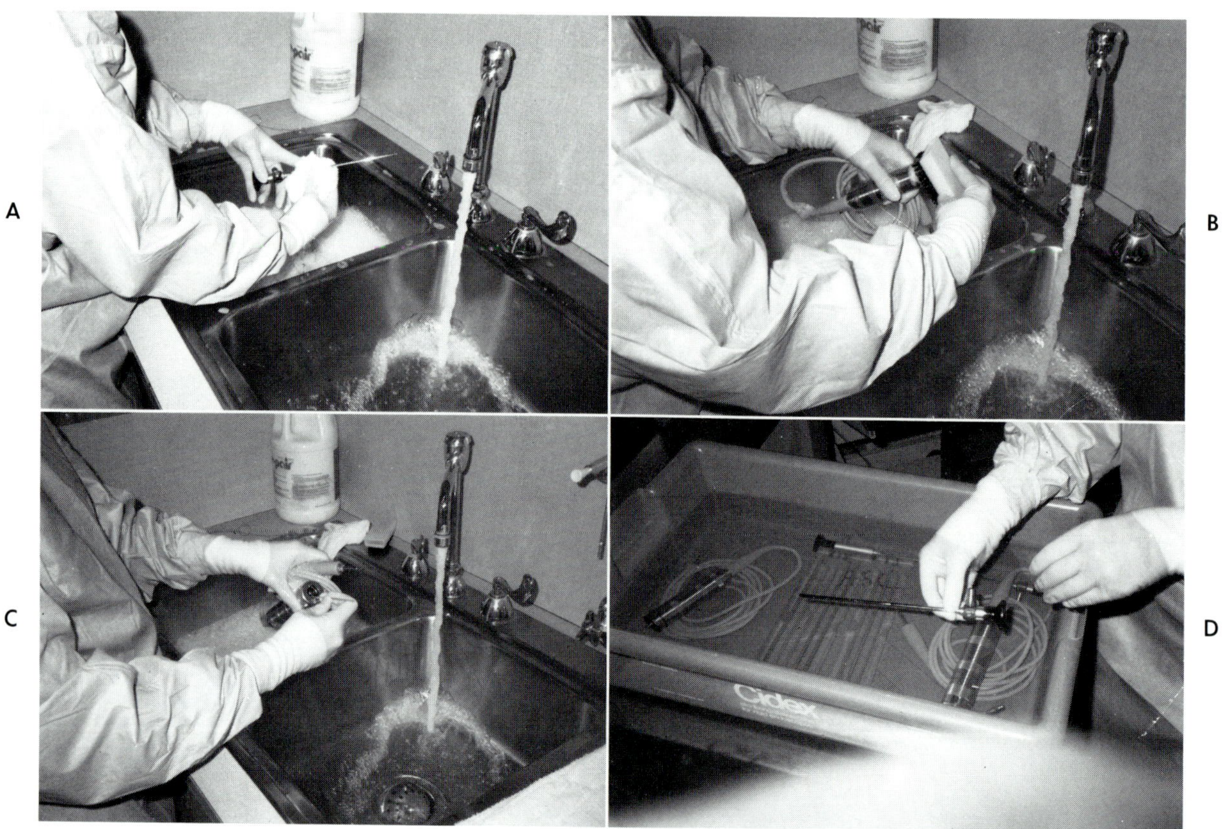

FIG. 2-28 Care of the instruments.

A Careful cleansing of arthroscope in soap and water.

B Brush scrubbing of hand and motorized instruments.

C Careful cleaning of recesses in instruments with cotton swabs.

D Cold-soak disinfectant for motors, knife blades, and arthroscopes.

The arthroscope, motors, and knife blades should be placed in Cidex solution between surgical case (Fig. 2-28, *D*). Such care decreases the handling of blades and lessens contact with other metal instruments, which dulls edges. Autoclaving itself does not dull edges.

Electric motors are autoclavable but hold heat. Motors are too hot to hold when they are first taken out of the autoclave. Thus autoclaving motors requires cooling and delays of the start of the next case.

Arthroscopes should be soaked between cases and subjected to gas sterilization at the end of each day. Steam autoclaving will injure the cement that holds the lens system. Sterilization of instruments is detailed in Chapter 3.

I own my instruments. My employee, Ruth Becker, LPN, cares for my instruments before, during, and after surgery. She prepares instruments for overnight storage or sterilization. In spite of this effort, we find instruments missing and breakage obviously due to droppage. The care of instruments is a continuous vigil.

Backup instruments. A backup instrument should be on hand for each piece of equipment used in arthroscopy. That includes motorized instruments, arthroscope, and television camera. I do not want to start a case without this benefit.

Storage and warehousing. A separate lockable storage case on wheels facilitates availability and security of expensive instruments and keeps instruments in one place (Fig. 2-29). The less frequently used or back-up instruments are kept in storage, sterile wrapped, and ready on request. This system eliminates searching from cupboard to cupboard or room to room at a crucial time during the arthroscopic procedure. The case also serves as a storage area at the end of the day.

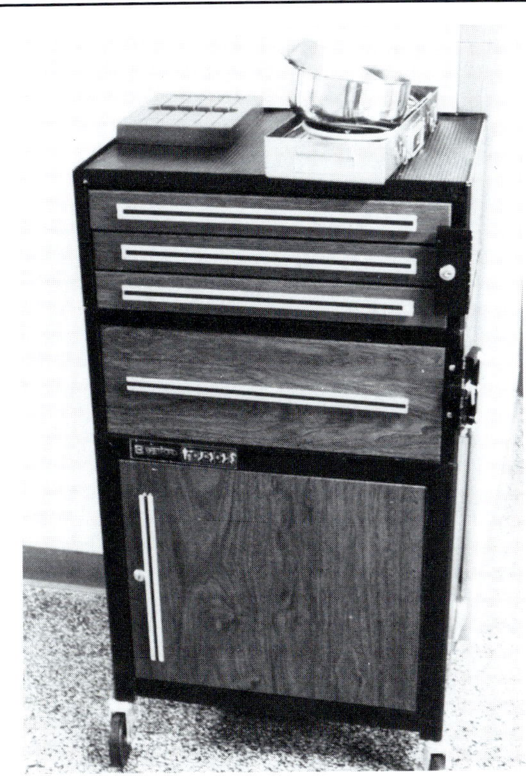

FIG. 2-29 Storage case for instruments.

A system to avoid losing or misplacing instruments is recommended. With such a system, any space that is not filled means an instrument is missing. A list of contents may be placed inside each drawer or door as a reminder.

In addition to the areas of table and case storage, it is important to consider a tertiary area in which to store certain instruments. From time to time, manufacturers' supplies or loaner services cannot meet the needs of our center. Therefore, we purchase extra arthroscopes, cables, and instrumentation that experience has shown may not be available on request. This method eliminates any disruption in the surgical schedule because we have backups on hand.

Central supply. The instrumentation is most vulnerable to damage in the hospital's central supply. The central supply area is usually situated away from the operating suite, yet the activities that occur there have great bearing on surgical activities. The work at central supply is accomplished by assembly line techniques, with the focus on the total project rather than individual care of instruments.

The surgeon is well advised to visit this facility. Education of the central supply staff will help prevent the mishandling of arthroscopic equipment. A videotape of arthroscopic procedures or the opportunity to observe live surgery reinforces the importance of their job.

CASE SCHEDULING

The use of the arthroscopic operating room is maximized when arthroscopic cases are scheduled in sequence. It is an additional benefit if one surgeon has successive cases. The interspersion of arthroscopic cases with other types of surgery in nondedicated suites requires longer down time between cases to make equipment changes. The operating room staff should schedule ample time for each case and for room changeovers. Alternating surgeons rather than one surgeon having series of cases is inefficient. Finally, the surgeon should not bracket himself or herself with other types of cases or office hour commitments. Changing types of surgery for the same doctor is no different than changing the room for a different surgeon. The length of arthroscopic surgery is variable and not exactly predictable, so an open-ended schedule removes the pressure of time. Because other surgeons on the staff, orthopedists or otherwise, wish to avoid delays within operating room schedules, arthroscopic cases should be scheduled with block time. This might be at the end of the day. Such scheduling is a courtesy to other members of the staff and a means of avoiding conflicts or resistance to arthroscopic surgery within the institution.

ANESTHESIOLOGIST

In our arthroscopy suite the anesthesologists and nurse anesthetists are an integral part of the arthroscopic procedures. In our facility the anesthesiologist participates not only in the preoperative medical evaluation of the patient but also in the control of discomfort following surgery, especially in reconstructive or combined surgical procedures (Fig. 2-30).

The anesthesiologist maximizes the outpatient procedures with his or her ability to manage same-day surgical cases. Proper skills reduce postoperative recovery time or nausea and vomiting. Regional anesthesia is used on patients with certain medical conditions. Often a stand-by anesthetic is requested to maximize local anesthesia. General anesthesia is given only if it becomes necessary as the procedure commences.

TROUBLESHOOTING THE ENVIRONMENT

Troubleshooting the environment is everyone's business. I emphasize THE RELENTLESS PURSUIT OF ATTENTION TO DETAILS. Attention to the details is an absolute necessity for success while exercising delicate, even frustrating arthroscopic techniques. Those who perform this surgery must give attention to the details in three categories: the obvious, the not-so-obvious, and the invisible factors (see box). Troubleshooting the environment never ends. For example, an obvious problem is that the television monitor has no image. The not-so-obvious underlying problem is that the monitor is not plugged in to the electrical outlet. An invisible factor is that electrical cord is not long enough to reach one of the two outlets in the room or that someone just tripped over the cord and unplugged it.

THE PATIENT

The patient becomes part of the environment when he or she enters the arthroscopy suite. The most important focus is the patient's care, comfort, and treatment. This can be facilitated in several ways. First, the patient should be given directions and a map of the hospital (Fig. 2-31). The entrance to the hospital and the designated parking areas

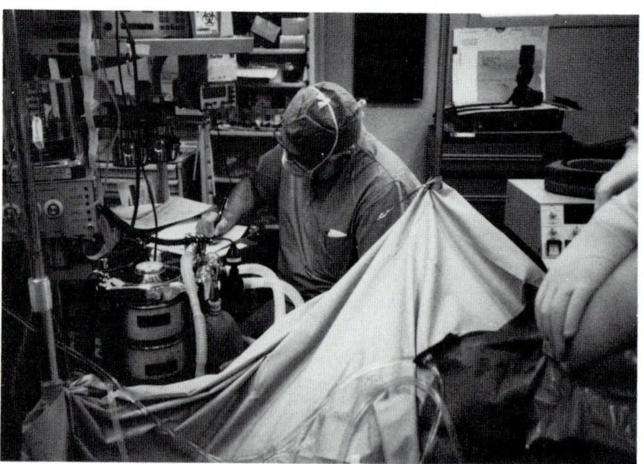

FIG. 2-30 The anesthesiologist is an important member of the team.

FACTORS IMPORTANT TO THE SURGICAL ENVIRONMENT

Obvious

- Patient
  - Evaluation
  - Preparation
  - Comfort
  - Confidence
- Surgeon
  - Knowledge
  - Comfort
  - Confidence
  - Leadership
  - Attitude
  - Technical skills
- Image transmission
  - Scope
  - Video
- Instruments
- Lighting
  - Room dimmer
  - Scope
- Draping

Not so obvious

- OR furniture
  - OR table
  - Other tables
    - Cast cart
  - Stool
- Power sources
- Tourniquet
- Suction
- Collection bottles
  - Tobacco bag
- Anesthesiologist
- Staff surgeons
  - Orthopedic
  - Others
- OR team approach
- Instrument care
  - Surgical
  - Television
  - Suction
- Floor

Unseen

- Administration
- Hospital policy
- Insurance
  - Hospital
  - Physician
- Central supply
- Outpatient service
- Physical therapy
  - Therapists
- X-ray
- Laboratory
- Electrical
  - Microwave
  - Radiowave
  - Bovie
  - Electrocautery
- Air conditioning

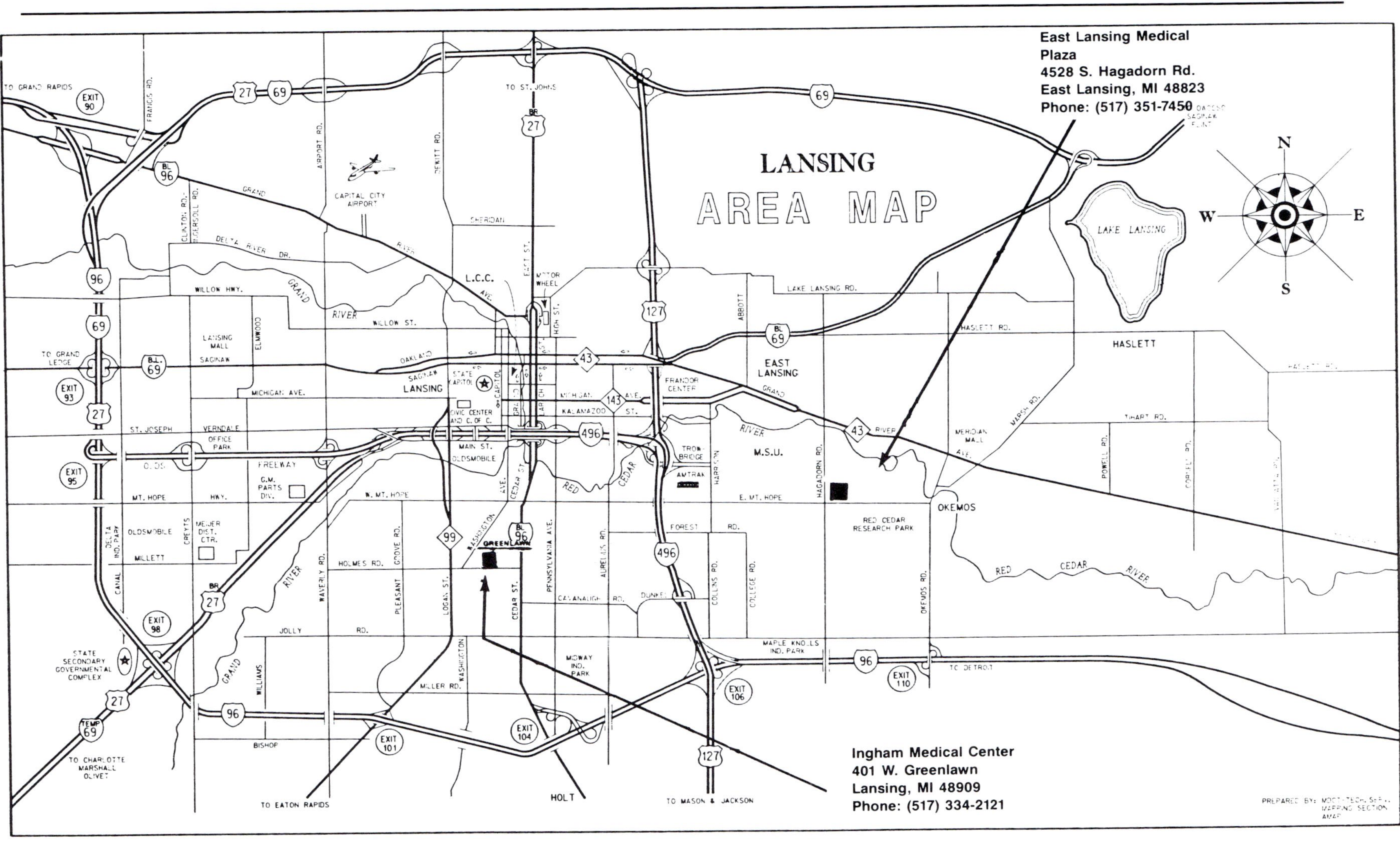

FIG. 2-31 Typical directional map to the office and the hospital.

CHAPTER

3 Instrumentation

Arthroscopy is an instrument-intensive surgical procedure.[16] The instruments are specialized for arthroscopy and vulnerable to damage because of their small size. The glass arthroscope can break. The arthroscope lens may become scratched or broken, thereby compromising the image (see Fig. 2-28). The small cutting surfaces on the instruments may become dull. Because of this fragility, a second similar instrument must be available to provide a backup in case of failure.

Arthroscopic instruments are expensive, and purchasing all the instruments requires is a major investment. The expense of instrumentation is reduced by better care, optimal function, and accountability. Proper care of instrumentation is absolutely necessary (see Fig. 3-68). These instruments cannot be dumped into a stainless steel tray, placed under hot water and soap, soaked, shaken, and sorted without being damaged. Careful maintenance is essential to optimal instrument condition to ensure satisfactory arthroscopic surgical technique.

I believe that a serious arthroscopist should have his or her own personal instruments. When instruments are shared, the care of the instruments is not optimal. They become dull or broken. Seeing through the abused arthroscope is difficult. Recognition that the equipment is defective may not occur until during the surgical procedure, in which the case the surgeon would simply have to make do. This situation is just not good enough.

If the hospital or clinic group insists on a common pool of instrumentation, it should include only the nonbreakable, nondulling tools, such as power sources, motors, probes, and television monitors. In this situation, each surgeon should be assigned an arthroscope and allotted cutting heads for motorized instruments, knife blades, and basket forceps. Each surgeon thus becomes responsible for and more interested in the care of the instruments. The gradual deterioration of instrumentation can be monitored. In addition, the hospital administration can monitor each surgeon's use or abuse for individual accountability and cost effectiveness. With this system, no surgeon's instrument abuse causes another an inconvenience. The adverse affects on patient care are minimized. The responsibility of instrument care is properly placed on the individual surgeon.

The purpose of this chapter is to discuss the various instruments the surgeon uses during diagnostic or operative arthroscopy. The variety of instruments available to the arthroscopic surgeon is truly amazing. Manufacturers have responded to the increased interest in arthroscopy with a gradual improvement in the image transmission devices and instruments available to the arthroscopic surgeon.

The physician entering the marketplace for arthroscopic instrumentation has to heed the old adage, "Let the buyer beware." Even taking advice from other surgeons can be misleading. A physician's relationship with the manufacturer may range from satisfied purchaser to consultant or ownership. Virtually no instrument or treatment idea develops without the input of an investigative surgeon. The surgeon may be the inventor or consultant, may serve on an advisory board, or may even hold stock in the parent company. When asking the advice of other physicians, the potential buyer should recognize that the most valid opinion would come from a *satisfied purchaser*.

I advise the surgeon who is considering the purchase of these instruments to evaluate them independently as carefully as possible through his or her own observations. One should talk with as many different people as possible; there is safety in many counselors. The salesperson should be allowed to detail the equipment carefully, and the surgeon should shop the marketplace for quality and price.

In 1984 the American Academy of Orthopaedic Surgeons (AAOS) recognized these possibilities for potential conflict of interest and instituted a voluntary commercial interest identification system at its meetings. The audience can be made aware of any possible commercial interest by an asterisk designation in the program. Surgeons making presentations are asked to indicate if the subject matter they are presenting is in any way related to a commercial interest. If the presenter agrees to it, an asterisk is placed by his or her name in the program. I support and cooperate with this method of open communication concerning these matters. Look for the asterisk (*); this text has one (see Chapter 2).

ARTHROSCOPIC INSTRUMENTATION

The unique environment of arthroscopic surgery places special demands on instruments. Arthroscopy differs from open surgery. It requires operating in a confined space via a two-dimensional image projected in space on a television monitor. To operate within these parameters is a challenge.

Development

The original arthroscopic instruments were adapted from equipment used in other endoscopic disciplines.[5] One of the original arthroscopes, the Watanabe No. 21, was so large it limited mobility within the joint and restricted visualization.[3,17] The first operative tools, basket forceps and operating arthroscopes, were adapted from gynecological laparoscopy.[8,9] At that time arthroscopy was laborious and limited to lavage, loose body removal, and resection of simple knee joint meniscal tears.

In 1975 I collaborated with the Dyonics Corporation to develop the first motorized instrument specifically designed for arthroscopic surgery (Fig. 3-1). The Intra-articular Shaver (1976) and the later Arthroplasty System (1980) provided a motorized arthroscopic surgical system now computerized as PS 3500 (Figs. 3-2 and 3-9, *A*).

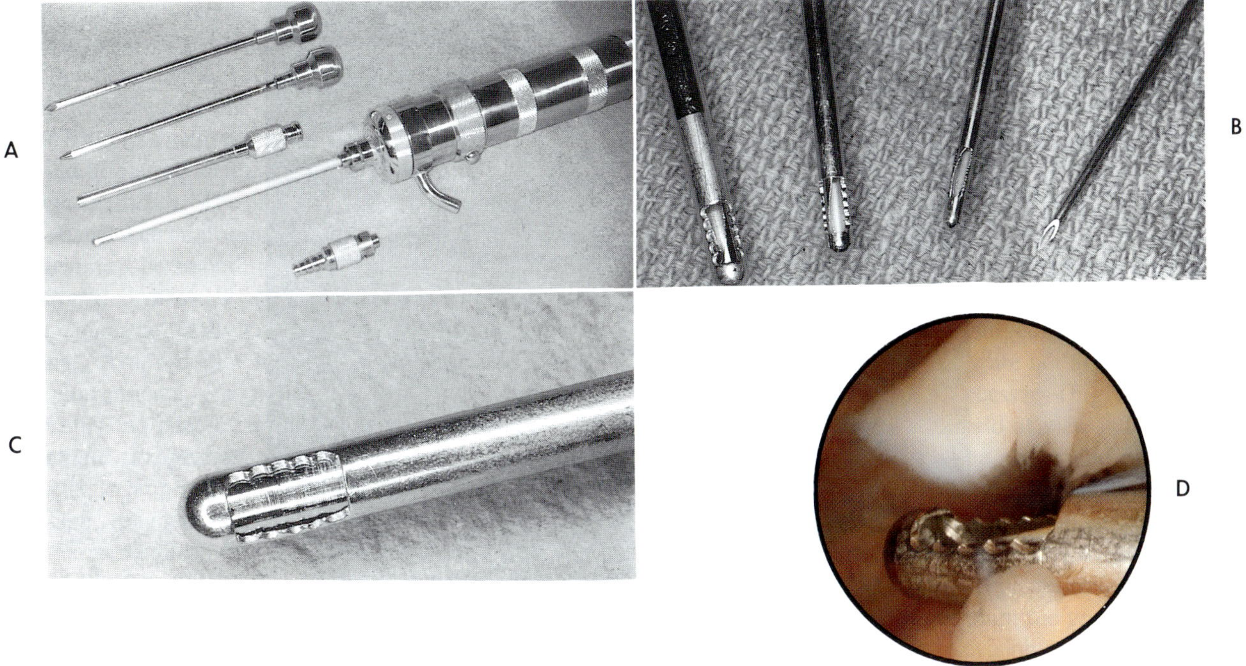

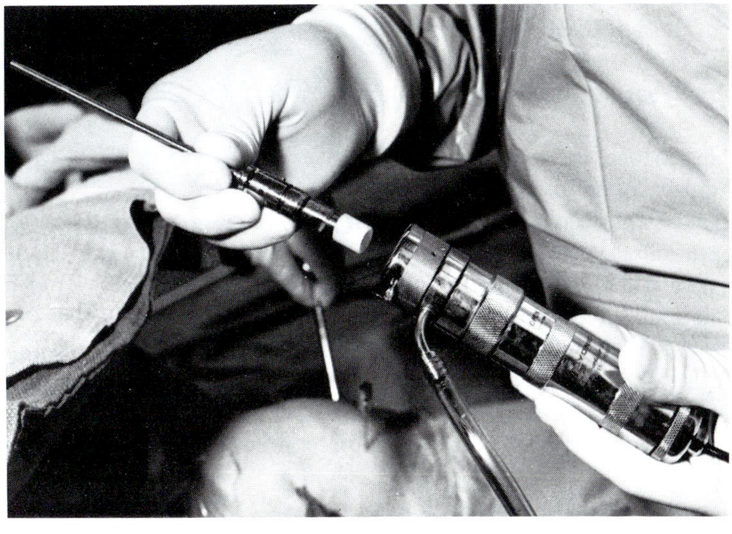

FIG. 3-1 Dyonics Intra-Articular Shaver System.

A Motor, drive shaft, and cannula system.

B Various cutting heads with No. 18 spinal needle to right for reference.

C Close-up of original shaver head.

D Arthroscopic view of original shaver cutting synovium.

E Intra-articular Shaver System has quick release from the crankcase to accommodate interchangeable heads. Instruments are manufactured by Dyonics, Inc., Andover, Mass.

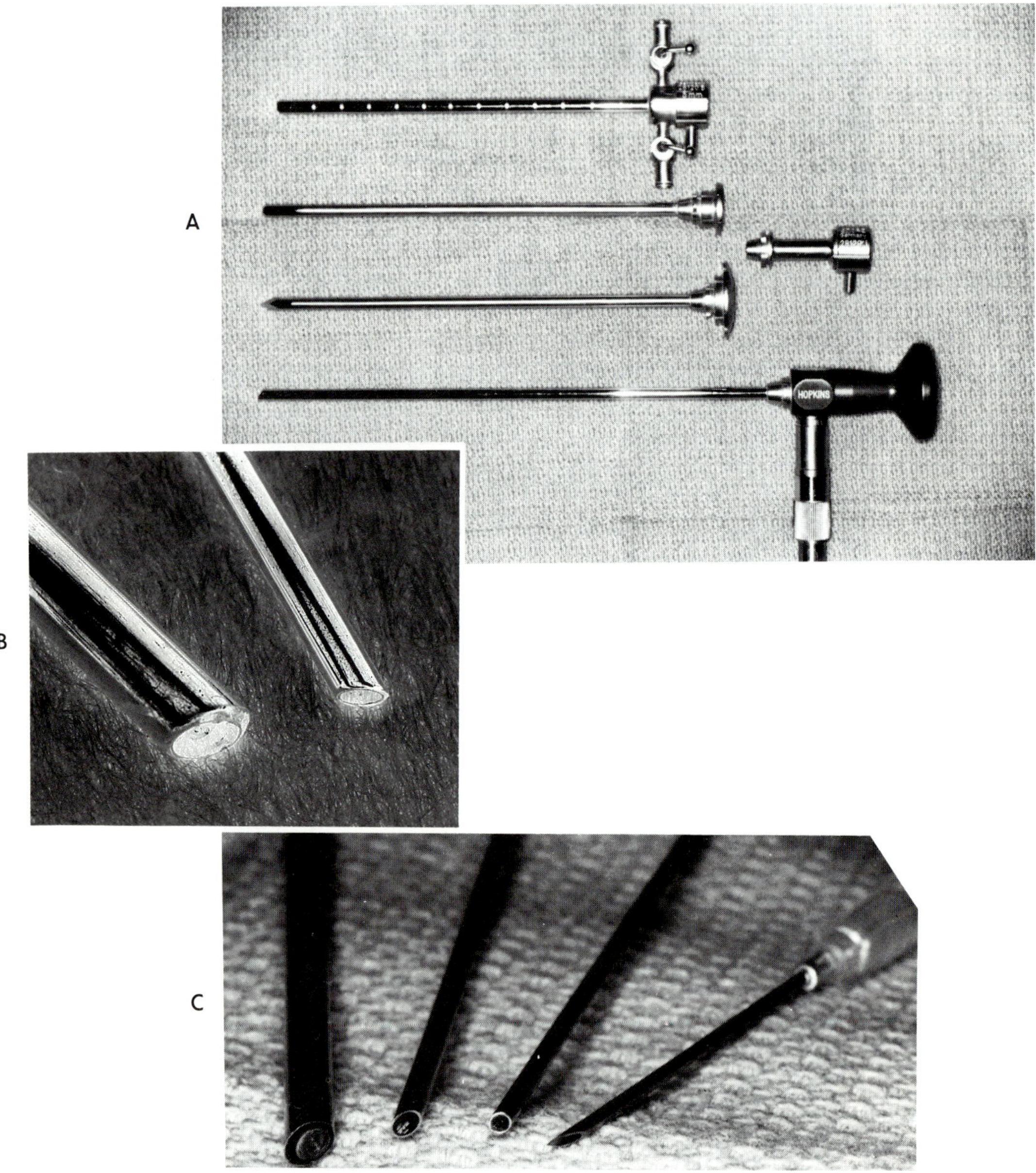

FIG. 3-3 **Standard arthroscopes.**

A Storz arthroscope, 4 mm, and cannula system.

B Storz rod-lens arthroscope is available in two sizes, with 2.7 or 4 mm telescope. Both provide excellent optical clarity.

C *Left to right,* 4 mm diameter Dyonics rod-lens endoscope; 2.2 mm Needlescope seen in end view; 1.7 mm Needlescope; No. 18 needle shown for relative size comparison.

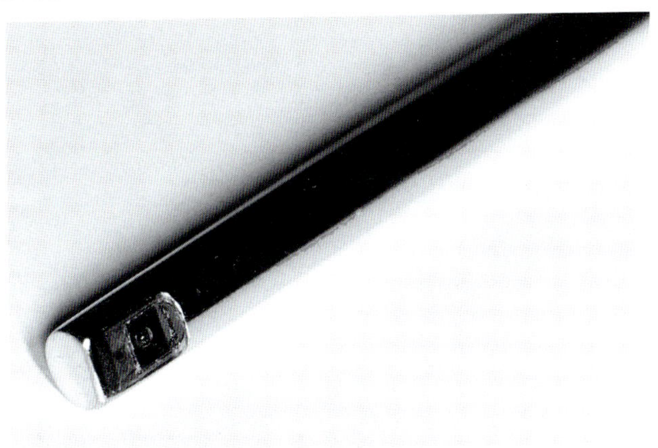

FIG. 3-4 90-degree arthroscope: Close up of angled lens.

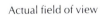

FIG. 3-5 Comparison: Field of view.

A Apparent field of view. Circles are different sizes, yet actual image is same. Larger circle gives impression of wider view, hence the designation "apparent" field of view. Actual field of view is same, but apparent view (size of circle) differs.

B Circles are same size, yet image in left circle is far greater than that taken from inset. Apparent fields of view are the same, but actual fields of view differ.

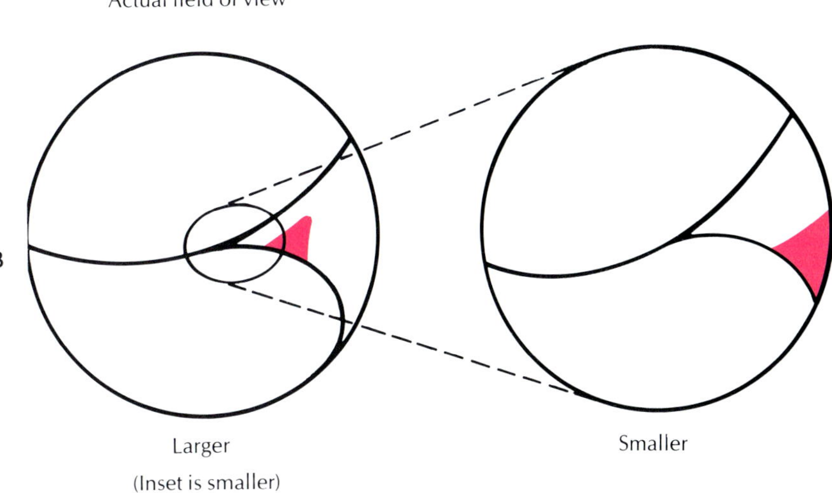

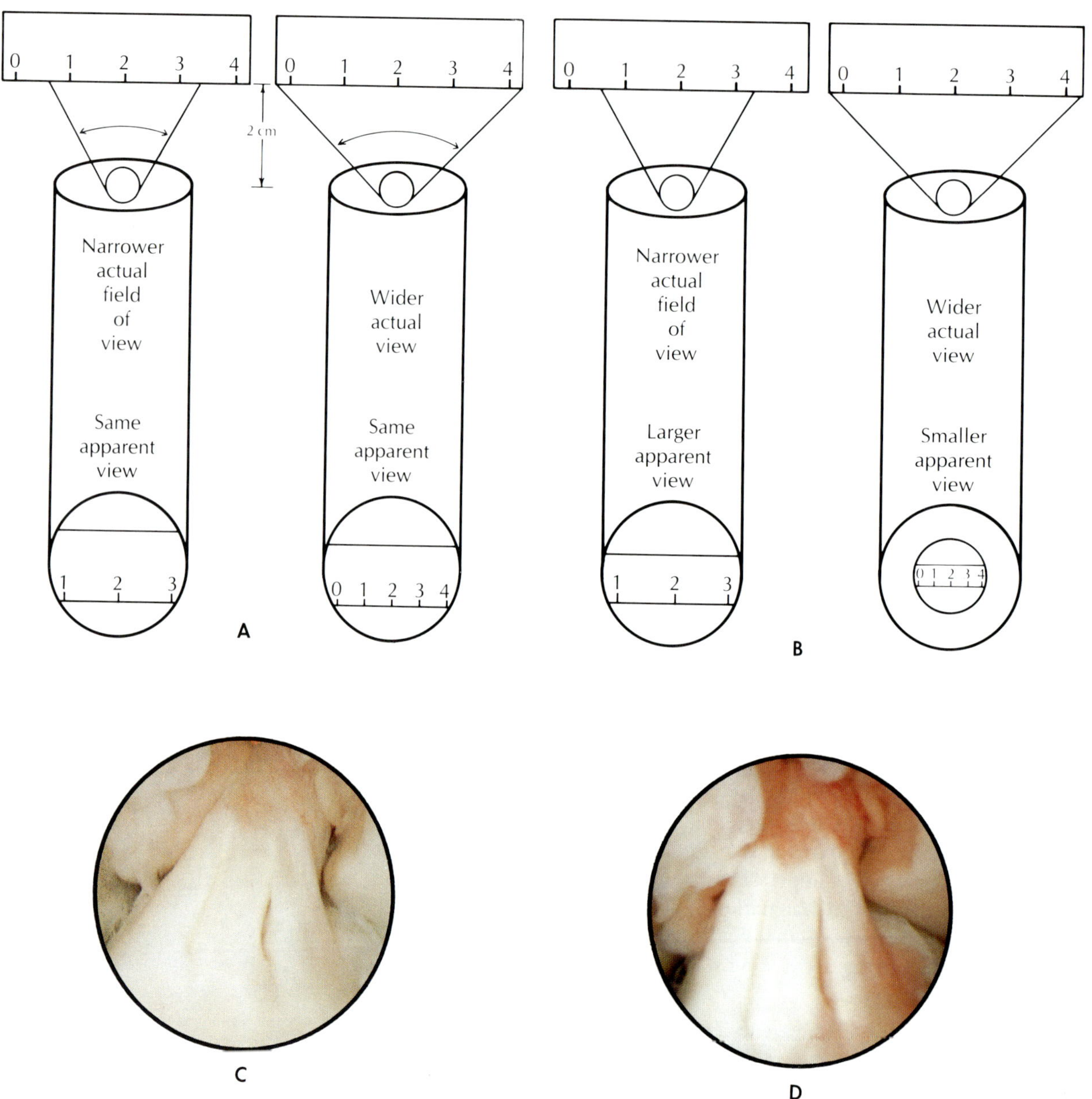

FIG. 3-6 Testing actual field of view.

A Diagram on left shows narrower actual field but equal apparent field of view. Illustration on right shows wider actual field of view, but same apparent field of view.

B Diagram on left shows narrower actual but larger apparent field of view. Diagram on right shows larger actual but smaller apparent field of view.

C Same apparent view as *D*. Larger actual view.

D Same apparent view (circle size) as *C*. Smaller actual view (close-up of *C*).

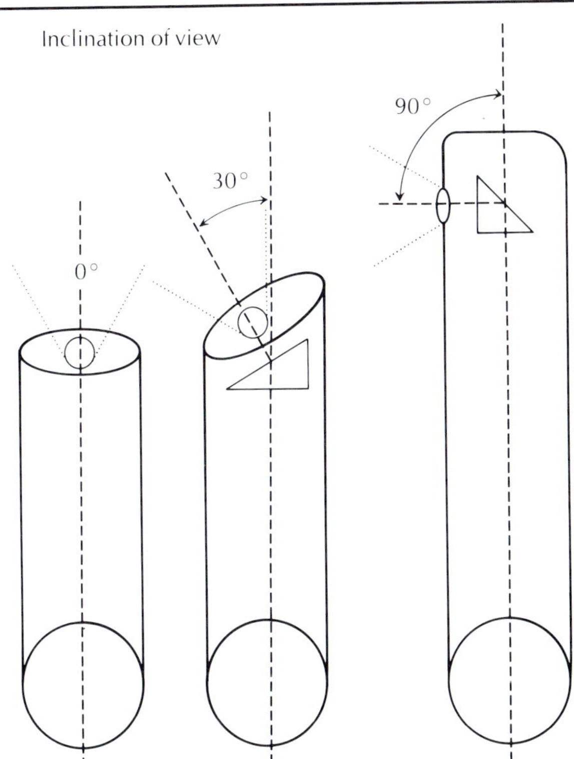

FIG. 3-7 Inclination of view. The 0-degree inclination views straight ahead. A 30-degree incline views on an angle deviated from axis of arthroscope. A 90-degree scope views at right angle to axis of arthroscope.

of view. The new Storz arthroscope encompasses an actual field of view of approximately 100 degrees in air.) Note that the field of view is reduced in fluid medium.

Various scopes can be compared. An arthroscope could have a very large apparent field of view (the large circle seen on the television) and an actual field of view of 35 degrees. The inspecting surgeon might be impressed with the large apparent field of view. On the other hand, an arthroscope could have a small apparent field of view (a small circle on the television), but an actual field of view of about 75 degrees—exceeding the actual field of view of the scope in the first example. The surgeon perceives the smaller circle as the smaller field of view; hence the designation apparent field of view.

The ideal circumstance is to have the largest apparent view possible without image irregularities at the periphery and a maximal actual (angle width) field of view that is evenly illuminated.

Inclination of View. The inclination of view is the angle of projection at the objective end of the arthroscope. Inclination is calculated by drawing a line along the axis of the arthroscope that intersects the line drawn from the center of the arthroscopic image to the objective end of the scope (Fig. 3-7). The incline may be straight or angled.

The 0-degree inclined, or straight-viewing, arthroscope is simple for orientation but not practical for operative arthroscopy. Direct viewing scopes will be important in the future for bone endoscopy (see Chapter 11).

Of the inclined views, the most common are 30, 70, 90, and 120 degrees. These angles permit visualization around corners. Most objects seen arthroscopically are to the side, above, or below the position of the arthroscope.

The most practical arthroscope for the shoulder is the 30-degree inclined view (see Fig. 3-3). When rotated, the 30-degree inclined view scope provides the best arthroscopic surgical exposure. During surgery, it allows eccentric placement of the arthroscope away from the approach of the surgical instruments. Mental adaption to the 30-degree inclined view is accomplished with some practice. Adaption to greater inclined views is more difficult. Change of the scope's position may result in disorientation. Scopes with a greater inclined view (70 and 90 degrees) are best used for single-placement, stationary viewing.

The 120-degree scope has no practical value in the shoulder.

Delivery of Light. Several factors affect the delivery of light and the subsequent visualization of the image. Two important factors are the amount of light on the object and the quality of the lens system transmitting light back to the ocular.

A large arthroscope has a greater capacity to hold glass fibers for carrying light to the object, resulting in a brighter image. A smaller endoscope has less space for fibers; therefore less light is delivered to the image because the light of origin is less. It does not matter how good the lens system is if the amount of light on the object is compromised.

The second factor in delivery of light is the quality of the lens system returning light from the object to the eye. The rod lens system is the highest-quality optical design for bringing light back to the eye.

Brightness is affected by the number of lenses in the endoscope. The greater the number of lenses, the more refraction there is to light transmission. An increased number of lenses also decreases the clarity of the image.

The higher the quality of glass, the higher the quality of the image. Although two endoscopes may have the same rod lens optical design, the design of the objective lens greatly affects the resultant imagery. Storz's objective lenses have a technological advantage for inclined view arthroscopes.

The arthroscope is affected by the technique or the workmanship during assembly. Mechanical security of the lenses and freedom from microscopic particles, accomplished in so-called clean rooms, may be necessary to achieve perfect imagery. Quality control is perfected only over years of manufacturer experience.

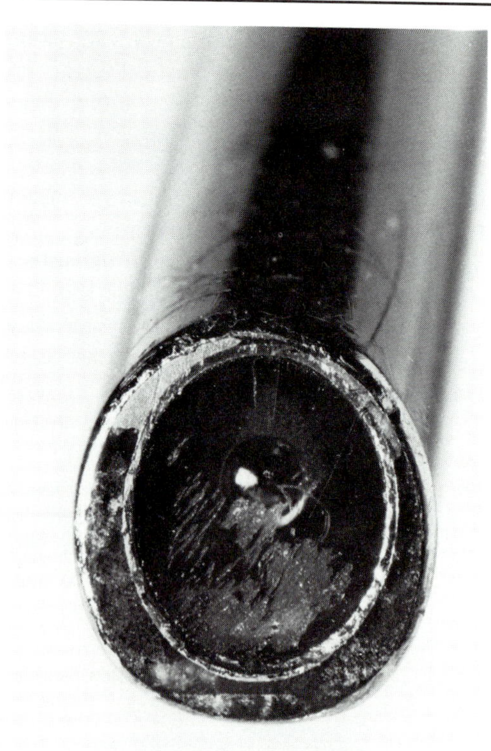

FIG. 3-8 Mechanically injured end of arthroscope may be salvaged by polishing or refurbishing.

Another issue is how the lenses are cemented in place. To date no cement is perfectly heat resistant. Manufacturers offer arthroscopes that are autoclavable, but image transmission capacity deteriorates when they are subjected to high levels of heat. In fact, the lens systems within the telescope can loosen, resulting in need for repair. Damage is possible by use, by autoclaving, or, of course, by dropping (see Care of Instruments in Chapter 2).

As an arthroscope ages it gives a yellow coloring to the image. The shelf life of an arthroscope should exceed 2 years without alterations in glass or cement.

Repairs

The most common cause of damage to the endoscope is injury to the ocular surface during arthroscopic surgery or instrumentation, by either banging, cutting, or scratching the end of the arthroscope (Fig. 3-8). When the ocular is damaged, three means of repair are possible depending upon the company's exchange policy. If the lens is only scratched, then inexpensive polishing is all that is required. If only the ocular lens is damaged, then replacement is a moderate expense. If the scope must be replaced, then many companies offer so-called exchange programs. An exchange program is one in which the new arthroscope is returned to the company, which sends an exchange arthroscope that has been refurbished. If the continuity of the transmission lens system is intact the ocular can be replaced at a minimum cost to the company. This savings is in part passed on to the purchaser with an exchange program. In this way one need not purchase a new arthroscope every time the lens cover suffers a scratch or crack. For the purchaser to maintain cost control, a determination should be requested of the extent of damage. Do not accept buying new scopes as replacements when refurbished ones are servicable.

Light Sources

Arthroscopy, like photography, depends on light. Many varieties of light sources are available in North America. Most hospitals have purchased several types for other endoscopic procedures, and most light sources produce light of adequate intensity for direct-view arthroscopy. The 150-watt bulbs produce a yellow hue light of low intensity. More powerful light sources have a 300- or 350-watt tungsten bulb, or metallic halogen or xenon arc as a source. The higher-intensity lights are necessary for proper illumination for photography and television viewing during arthroscopic surgery.

The modern light source models have built-in automatic gain controls coordinated with the television system (Fig. 3-9). They are color balanced for electronically generated pictures, but not for color slide photography, except those taken with an attached Polaroid system. The quality of the polaroid generated slide is not as clear as that taken with an attached 35 mm slide camera (Fig. 3-9, *C*).

A light bulb does not last indefinitely. Its intensity may start to decline even after 6 hours, when light is still coming from the source. The loss of level may not be recognized under direct viewing, but certainly would result in poor photographic documents. This often surprises the arthroscopist, who sees a good image by eye and then later sees a very dull videotape, movie, or photograph. One must remember that the eye is very forgiving and a better photographic instrument than any man-made arthroscope or television or any other type of camera. Light intensity variations are most easily appreciated when recording and viewing on television.

Warning: The high-intensity light sources are too bright for comfortable, and perhaps safe, direct viewing with the surgeons's eye on the arthroscope. A shading device or rheostat should be used for direct viewing. Some systems have a less powerful light source within the same unit to facilitate direct viewing (Dyonics 510).

Light Guides (Cables). A variety of light guides or light cables are available. All manufacturers make adapters

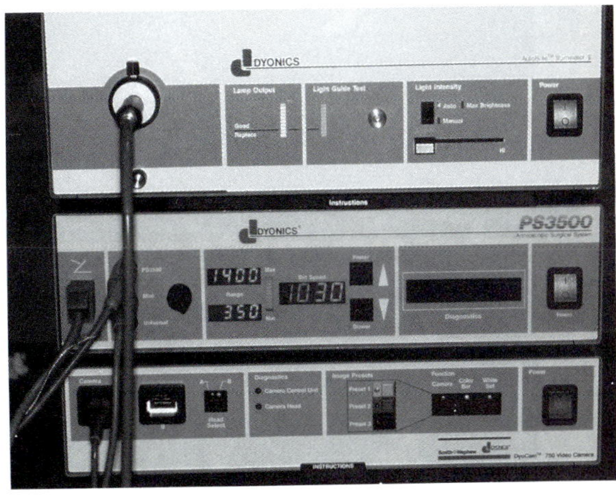

A

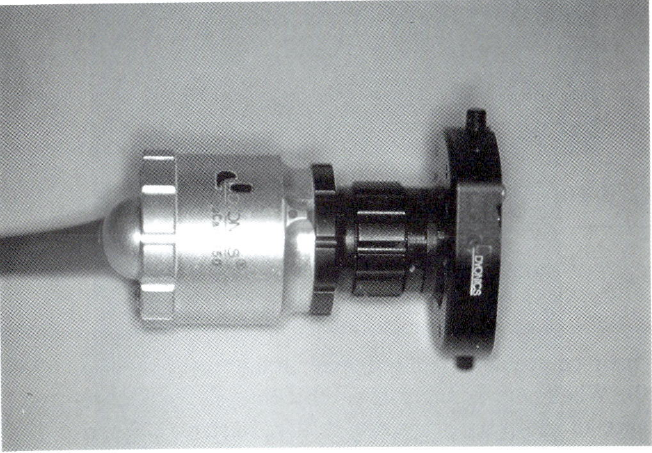

B

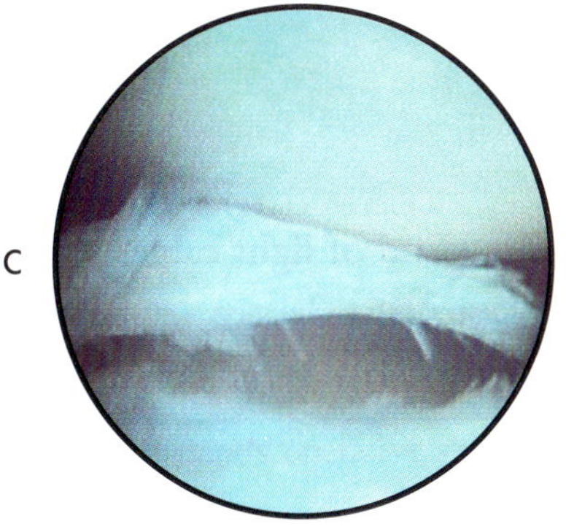

C

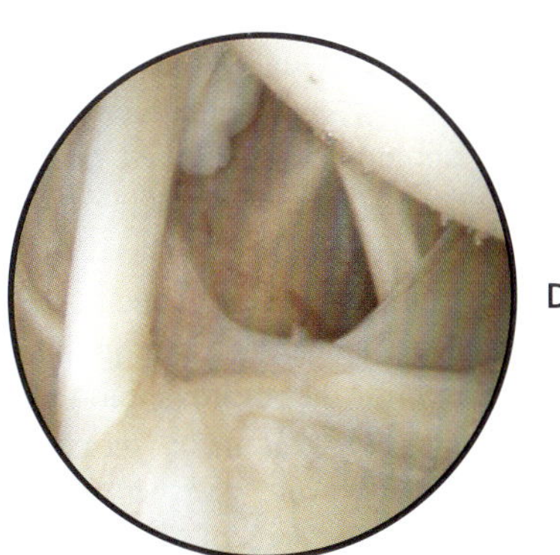

D

FIG. 3-9 Combined video system and balanced light source.

A The power sources are placed in cabinet. The light source is above. The motorized instrument power source is in the middle. The balanced light source is on the lower deck.

B Miniature video camera.

C Arthroscopic image typical of balanced light source and television camera is not as clear as this picture taken with attached 35 mm camera.

D Photo taken with 35 mm camera and lens attachment. This gives best quality photographic image.

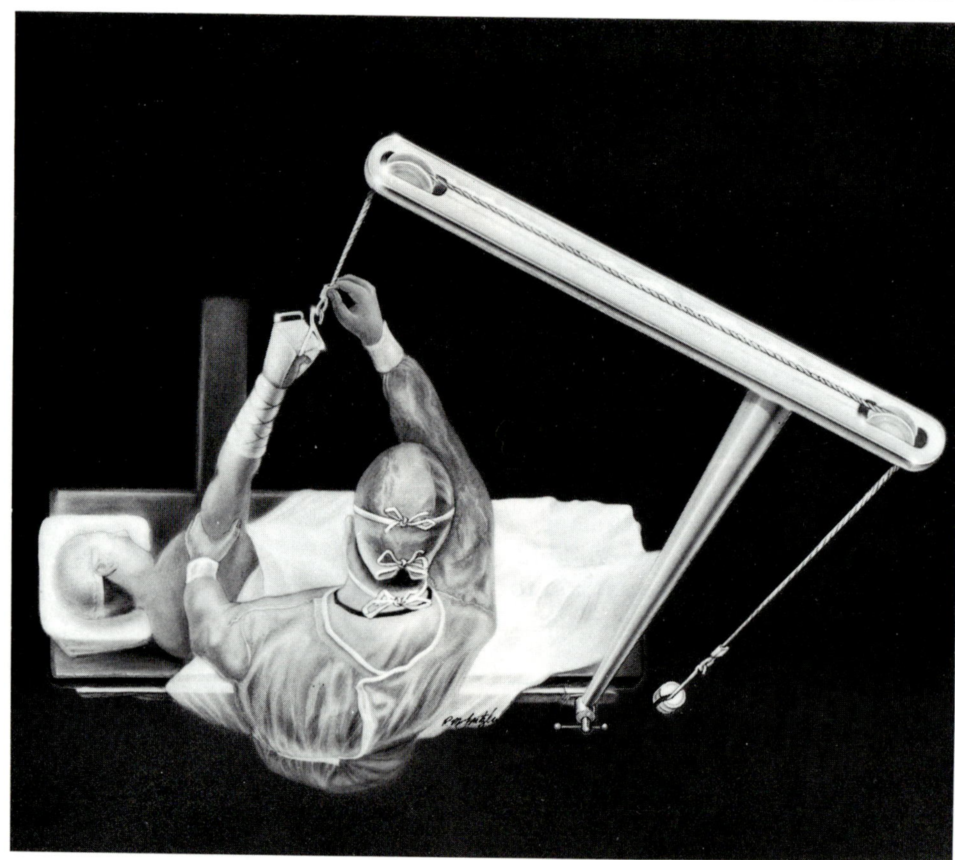

FIG. 3-14 Shoulder Suspension System. (Courtesy Instrument Makar, Inc.)

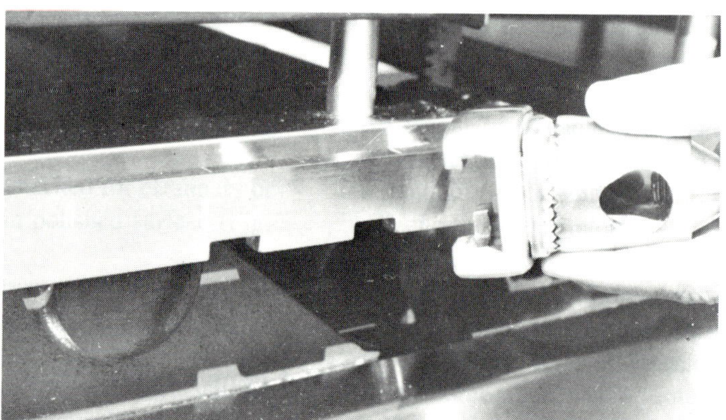

FIG. 3-15 Shoulder Suspension System. Clark attachment is generally used for stirrups suspension but also to accommodate surgical assistant and shoulder suspension.

FLUID MANAGEMENT EQUIPMENT

Fluid Reservoir

The fluid reservoir is commonly 6 liters of saline suspended at least 1 m above the patient (Fig. 3-16). Two plastic bag containers, each with 3 liters of fluid, produce this reservoir. A plastic bag permits manual squeezing of the bag for increased pressure as opposed to rigid bottles or containers. Smaller resevoirs require more frequent changing.

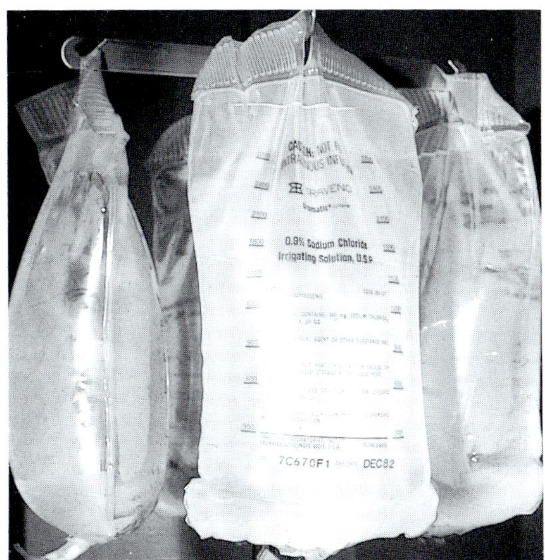

FIG. 3-16 Fluid reservoir: 6 liters of fluid suspended 1 m above patient.

Suspension Intravenous Pole

A weighted IV pole or other well-secured apparatus is necessary for safety with an elevated, heavy, suspended reservoir (Fig. 3-17). Remember, "a pint is a pound the world around."

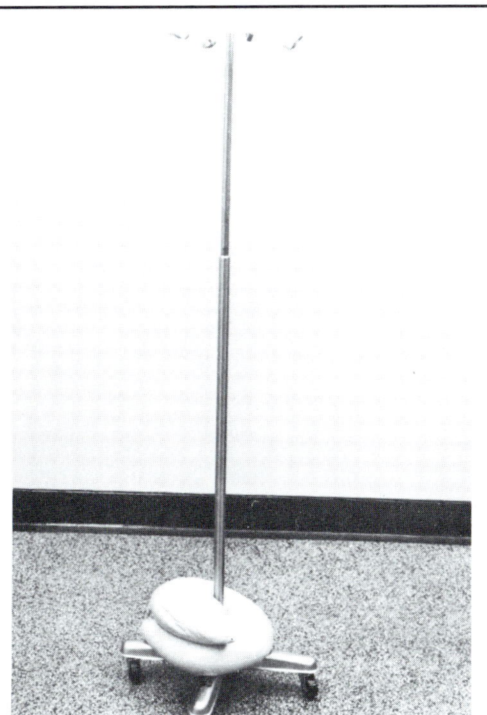

FIG. 3-17 IV pole: Weighted IV pole secured with sandbag.

Mechanical Pumps

In recent years, mechanical pumps have gained popularity by surgeons who have difficulty "seeing" or controlling fluid flows during surgical procedures (Fig. 3-18). I have used different manufacturers' pumps. I found them to be of no advantage over a gravity system. There are but two major disadvantages. One disadvantage is unrecognized continuous pumping and extravasation of fluids. The other problem is that in the two systems I tried, the volume recovery in the joint space was at a slower rate than a gravity system alone. I do not use electrically driven mechanical fluid infusion pumps.

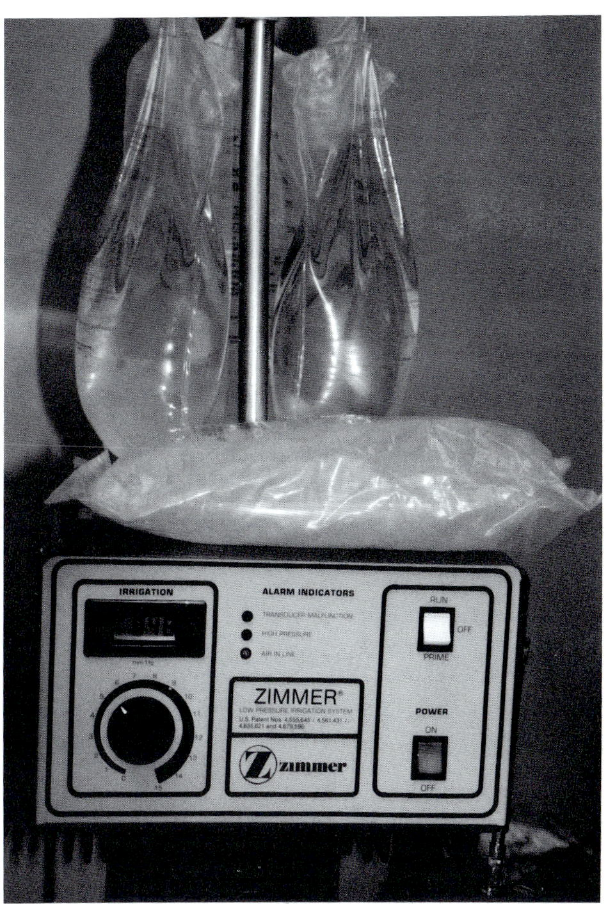

FIG. 3-18 Mechanical pump.

Gravity Assist System

Increased pressure or flow is needed during short intervals during shoulder arthroscopy, such as during acromioplasty. Increased pressure will also control bleeding by hydrostatic pressure, but bleeding is better controlled by electrocautery. I have met this intermittent need by developing a Gravity Assist Bulb with unidirectional valves (Fig. 3-19). This system connects in line to the gravity system. There is no diminution of gravity flow. When a short burst of fluid is needed the assistant squeezes the bulb. This system places a secondary reservoir next to the joint. Since the assistants physically participate in the increased flow, they are conscious of the volume being delivered. They inform the surgeon, and thus unrecognized extravasation does not occur. In the absence of this bulb, increased flow may also be met by having the circulating nurse squeeze the suspended plastic reservoir bags.

Tubing

The inflow tubing is sterile and Y shaped to control separate flows (Fig. 3-20). It is now available in 8-foot lengths. The longer tubing allows higher placement and displacement of the reservoir from the surgical field.

Cannulas

The inflow cannula is 4.2 mm inside diameter. The cannulas for shoulder arthroscopy should not have side holes (Fig. 3-21). The two small holes at the end of the cannula were designed to provide flow in knee arthroscopy. When the end of the cannula is unintentionally against the far wall of the knee joint, the side holes still allow flow. This idea is not as effective in the shoulder. The lack of space in the shoulder joint may result in the cannula partially backing out of the joint. If so, extra synovial leakage may occur through small side holes, even though the end of cannula is seen in the joint.

A

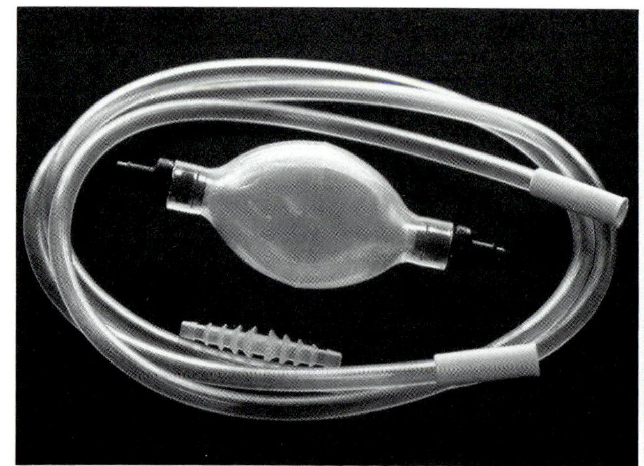

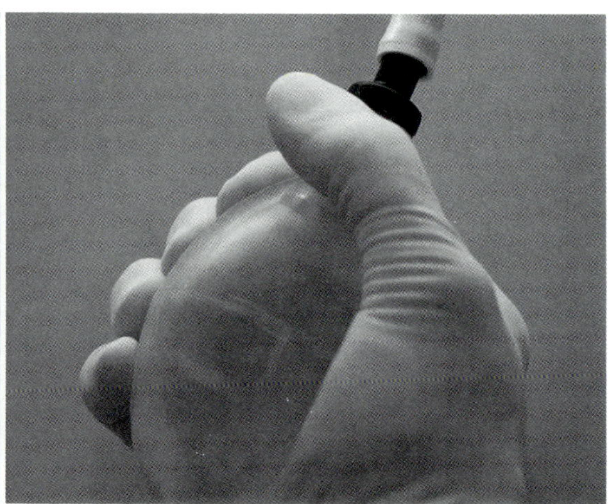

B

C

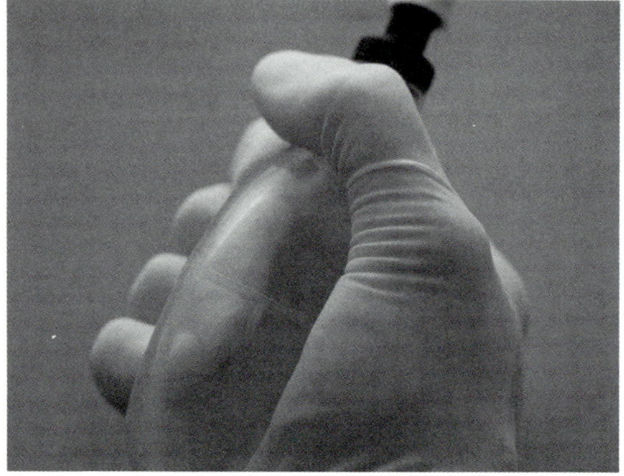

FIG. 3-19 Gravity assist.

A This instrument consists of a sterile compressible silastic bulb with calculated memory to reform after compression. There are unidirectional valves at each end to avoid backflow. The tubing connects to the gravity system. Both air and fluid may be delivered with this system.

B The assistant relaxes on bulb to distend. Gravity flow continues in the resting state.

C Intermittent squeezing of the bulb increases flow and pressure.

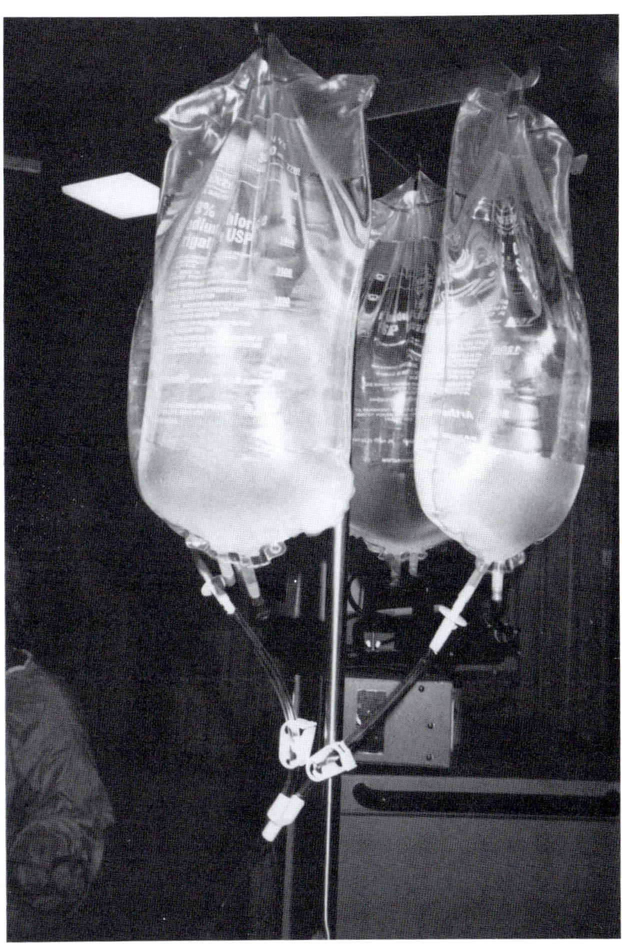

FIG. 3-20 Tubing.

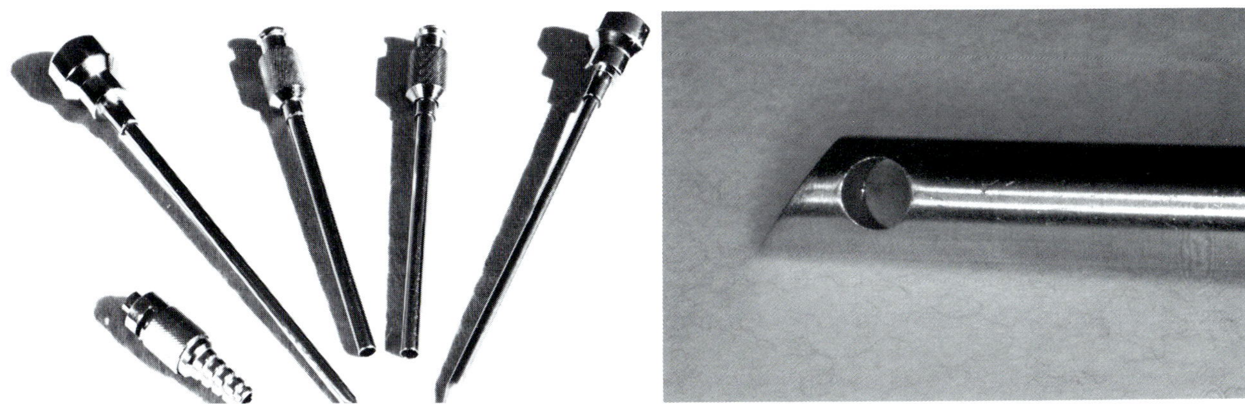

A B

FIG. 3-21 Cannulas.

A Inflow cannulas, obturators, and tubing adaptor.

B This cannula is not suitable for shoulders as it has side openings that may result in extravasation of fluid if the cannula backs out.

Adaptors

A small metal adaptor accommodates the connection of the plastic inflow tubing to the metal inflow cannula to provide a secure fit (Fig. 3-22, *A*). Alternately, the inflow can be connected directly to the arthroscope metal cannula. To facilitate placement of the inflow plastic tube, a small metal adaptor with a valve secures this fitting to the arthroscope spigot (Fig. 3-22, *B*). Direct attachment of the tube to the arthroscope is not tight and results in leakage.

Plastic adapters are used to connect fluid tubing to the gravity system or the inflow system. One is straight (Fig. 3-22, *C*), while the other is Y-shaped to accommodate two different fluids to be selected within the operative field (Fig. 3-22, *D*).

Outflow Tubing/Reservoir

The suction tube connects to the collection bottle. During the diagnostic phase this tube is connected to the arthroscope for cleaning the joint (Fig. 3-23). A large glass reservoir must be present for collection of fluids (Fig. 3-24). A small cotton collection bag avoids the necessity of straining the entire collection of fluid for a specimen.

Outflow Pressures

The suction may be central or generated by machine in the operating room. Ingham Medical Center has a central system. It has been measured as 14 to 16 inches of mercury (40 mm Hg) in-line pressure. Our Dyonics motorized instrumentation was calibrated on this pressure.

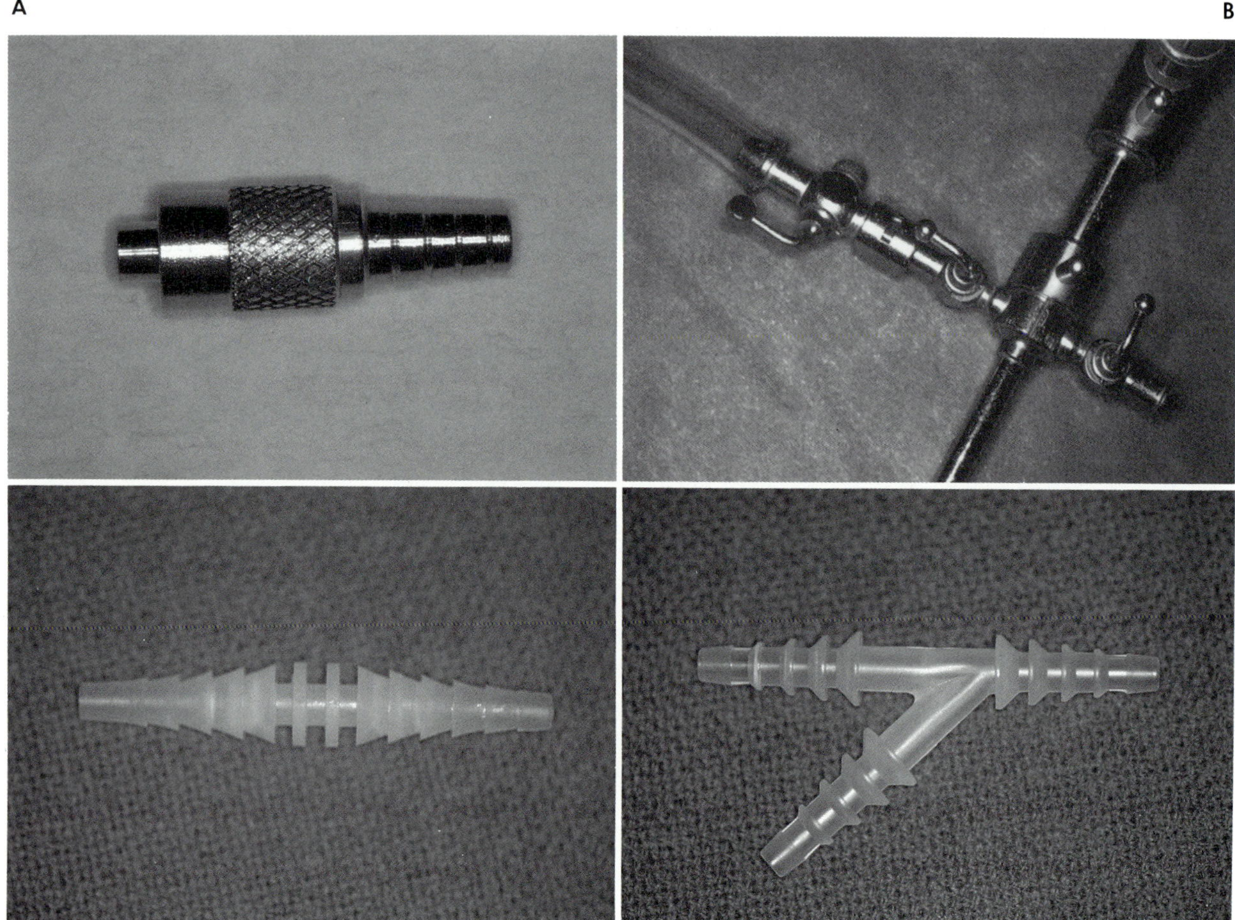

FIG. 3-22 Adaptors.

A Metal adaptor for tubing to the inflow cannula.

B An adaptor to attach tubing directly to the arthroscope cannula.

C Adaptor to connect plastic tubing.

D Adaptor to connect two different fluid sources.

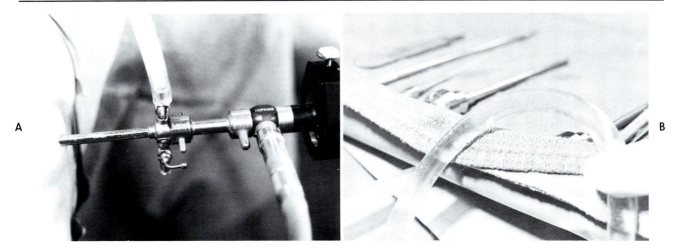

FIG. 3-23 Direct connection to arthroscope.

A Outflow on arthroscope during diagnostic phase.

B Suction tube showing pieces of debrided articular material being removed from joint.

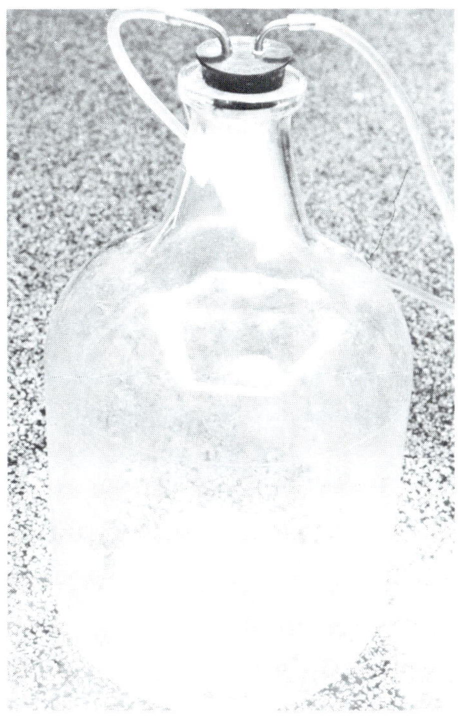

FIG. 3-24 Glass reservoir. Large collection bottle accommodates even longest procedure and abundant fluid use. Collection bag is placed in top of suction bottle; thus decanting of all fluid is not necessary at end of procedure.

The suction pressure should be calibrated to a specific motorized system. The revolutions per minute, window size, and tubing diameter affect efficiency. If the motorized instruments used are other than Dyonics, the instruction manual should be checked for calibration.

Pressure Gauge

The suction pressure should be measured in-line as opposed to end-on. A simple gauge is available for this calculation (Fig. 3-25). The end-on measurement gives a closed-system measurement, resulting in an unrealistic peak pressure (Fig. 3-26). The in-line pressure measures flow during actual conditions.

Manual Outflow Pressure Control

Variations in pressure can be created by the second assistant clamping the outflow tube with intermittent manual pressure on the inflow reservoir (Fig. 3-27). The same assistant who controls the inflow with Gravity Assist Bulb should monitor the outflow tubing.

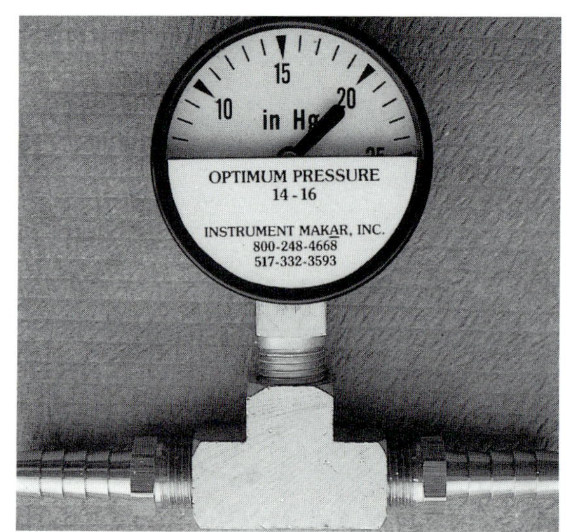

FIG. 3-25 Pressure gauge: Suction gauge placed in-line near operative field.

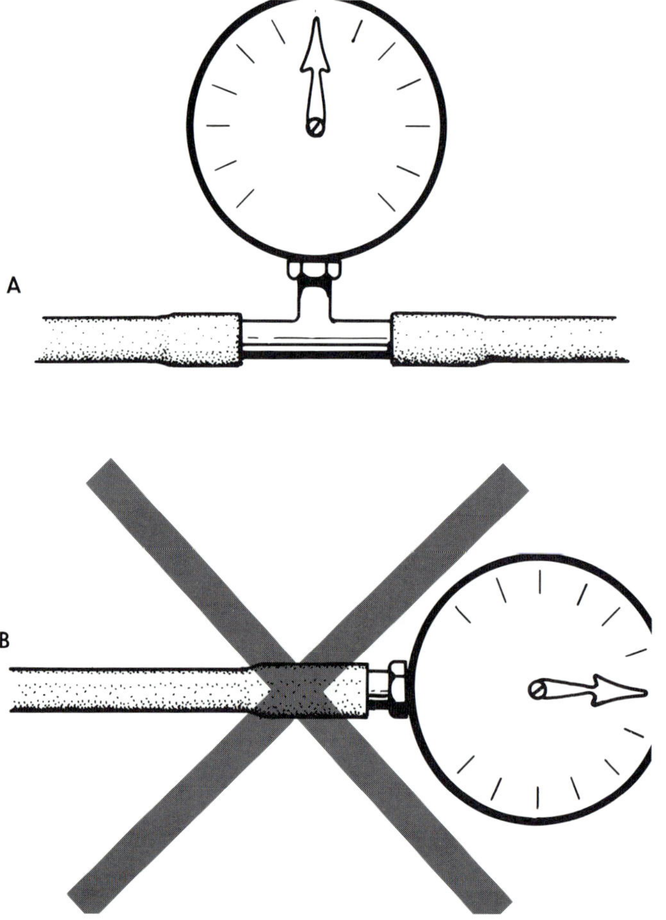

FIG. 3-26 End-on versus in-line pressure.

A In-line.

B End-on.

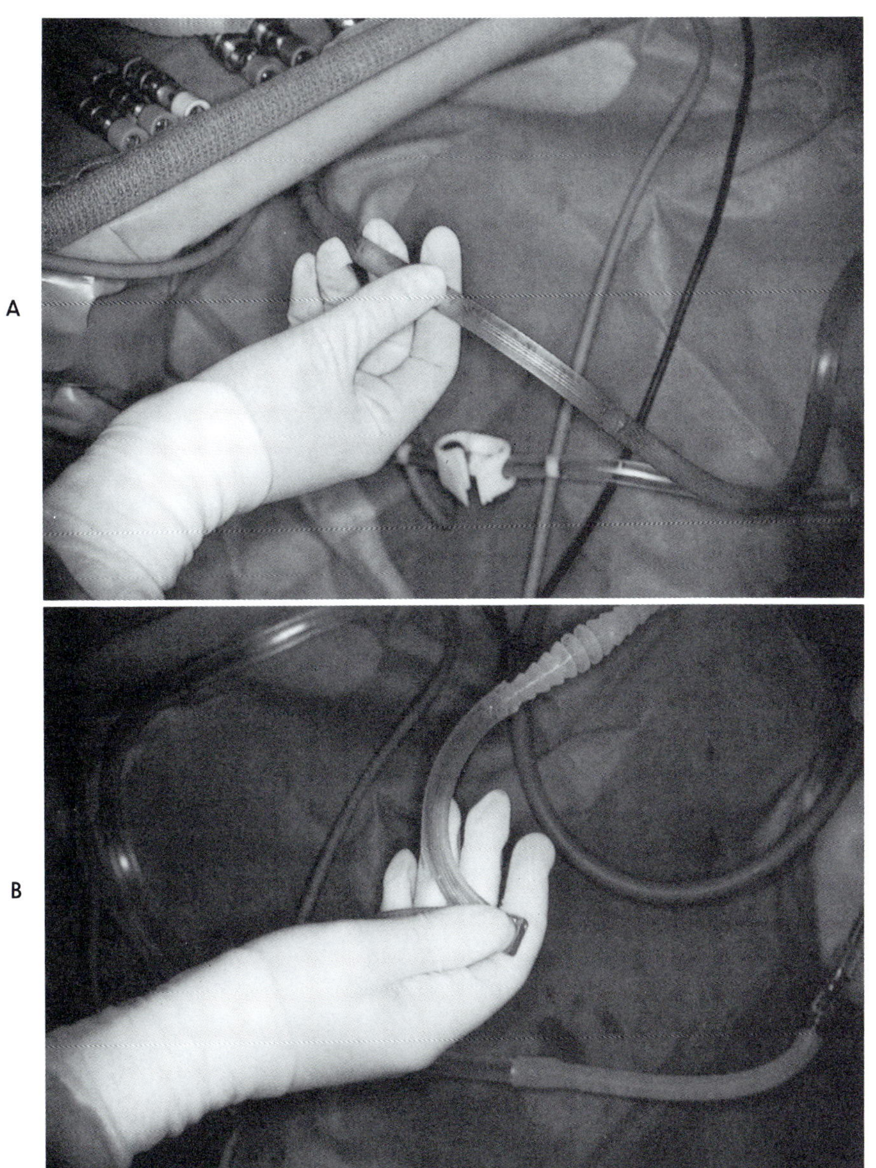

A

B

FIG. 3-27 Second assistant restricts outflow with bend in outflow tubing.

A Partial measured restriction.

B Clamped off to redistend joint.

CANNULA SYSTEM

A cannula system is essential for shoulder arthroscopy (see Fig. 3-21, *A*). The depth of the soft tissue surrounding the shoulder is greater than that in the knee joint. Safe and reliable passage and repeat passage of instruments is possible only by using cannulas for shoulder arthroscopy. The arthroscopic surgical system outlined in this text is predicated on the use of cannulas. The cannula system ensures joint penetration, but it maintains the intraarticular position. The use of cannulas minimizes trauma by minimizing passages through the tissues. Whenever possible, joint entries are made through the cannula to avoid trauma caused by repeated probing, pushing, or channelization.

Most arthroscopic instruments are designed to pass through cannulas. The knife blades as well as the Dyonics motorized instrumentation fit in and out through the cannula system. The cannula system may be interchangeable with the arthroscope cannula system.

The use of cannulas provides safety in case of intraoperative accident. If an instrument breaks, the cannulas provide a channel for fluid inflow and are positioned for fragment removal.

Dyonics cannulas come in two diameters (see Fig. 3-21). Each operative cannula comes with a sharp trochar and semi-sharp obturator. The sharp trochar is for skin and fascial penetration; the semi-sharp obturator is for joint entry. The appropriate size cannula depends on which surgical system is used.

The original calibration for the Dyonics IASS was made with a 4.5 mm ID cannula. I routinely use this cannula via the supraspinatus portal for operative shoulder arthroscopy. (See Chapter 5, Fig. 5-30, *D*.)

A cannula and obturator accompany the Ligamentous and Capsular Repair (LCR) system (see Fig. 3–56). It is too large in diameter (1.3 cm OD) to use to place instruments and maintain joint distention. This system was intended for delivery of various metallic or biodegradable staples, but can also be used for evacuation of loose bodies or debris.

Large obturators and cannulas, up to 1 cm in size, are useful in removal of large loose bodies or multiple loose bodies of osteochondromatosis (Fig. 3-28).

Switching Sticks

Switching sticks are merely two 9-inch rods, 4.0 mm OD (Fig. 3-29). Switching sticks facilitate the interchange of cannulas of different sizes or lengths while securing cannula position and avoiding further channelization or tissue trauma. When the operative cannula is in one position and the arthroscope is in another, the instrumentation can be removed from the cannula and the switching stick inserted. The arthroscope is removed from its cannula system, which is a different shape, size, and length. A switching stick is placed in the arthroscope cannula. The two switching sticks remain in the shoulder, looking very much like chopsticks. The cannulas are interchanged to their new positions over the switching sticks. The switching sticks are removed and replaced with the arthroscope and instrument. (For more details, see Chapter 5.)

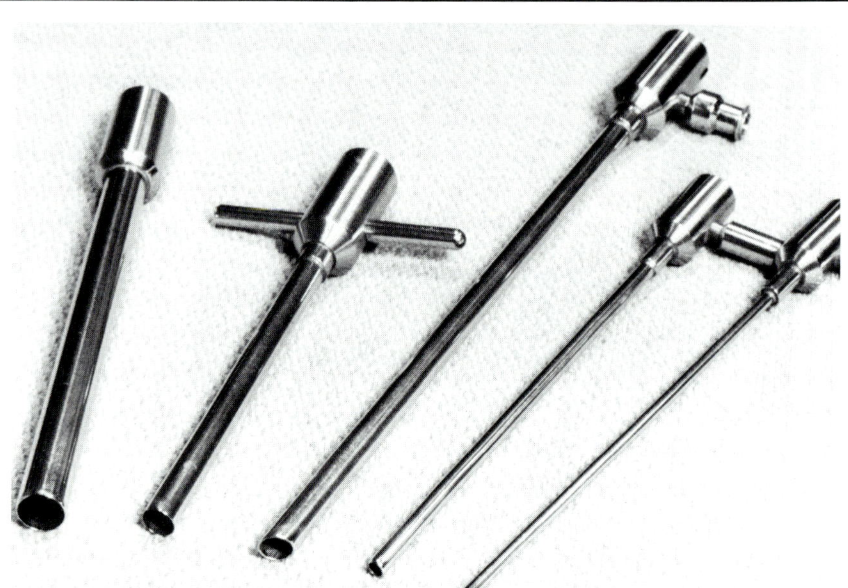

FIG. 3-28 Large operative cannulas for loose body removal. Cannulas vary in size from 8 mm *(left)* to 2 mm *(right)* OD. The latter holds a 1.7 mm Needlescope.

Wissinger Rod

In securing the surgical exposure, especially in the shoulder or the elbow joints, I had previously visualized from one side of the joint and then by trial and error placed a No. 18 spinal needle from the opposite side of the joint. After entering the joint I attempted to place a cannula along the same course. This was not always an easy maneuver.

Dr. H. Andrew Wissinger, during a visit with me in East Lansing, Michigan, observed the shortcomings of this method.[19] During a case, he recommended that the opposite portal be established from inside with a rod. I did it. It worked. Although Dr. Wissinger never specialized in shoulder arthroscopy, he made a valuable contribution to this aspect of orthopedic surgery (Fig. 3-30).

The Wissinger rod method involves placing the arthroscope and the cannula against the desired point of entry on the far wall of the joint, usually just superior to the upper margin of the subscapularis tendon (see Fig. 5-67). The cannula is held in place and the scope removed. The Wissinger rod is placed down the arthroscope cannula and out anterior under the skin. The skin is incised and an operating cannula is placed over the rod and into the joint. The rod is removed, and the scope is replaced in its cannula. The instrument is then placed in the cannula. Proper opposite-side cannula position is thus facilitated.

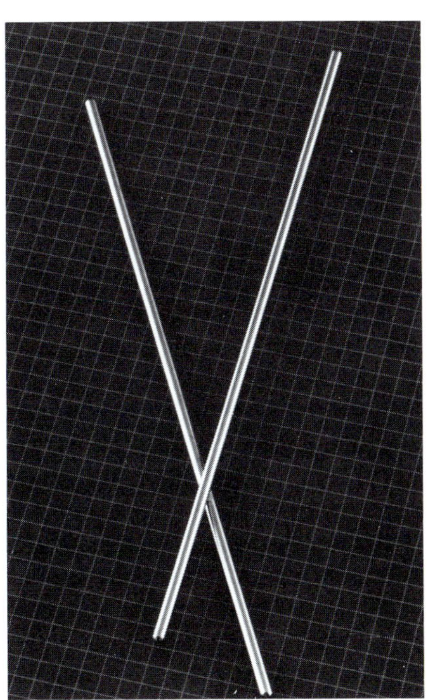

FIG. 3-29 Switching sticks.

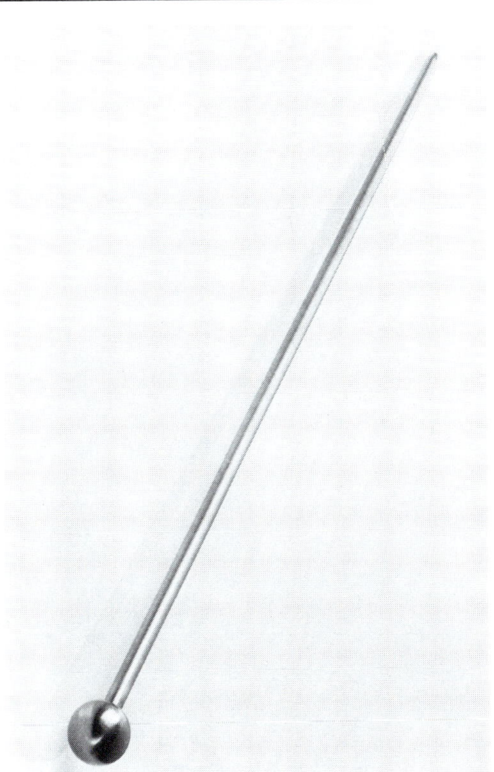

FIG. 3-30 Wissinger rod.

HAND INSTRUMENTS

Palpation Instruments

The instrument most commonly used to establish proper joint entry is the No. 18 spinal needle (Fig. 3-31). A 3-inch needle is used for the shoulder joint. A 6-inch needle may be needed in some cases. Even with multiple attempts at securing a proper position, tissue disruption is minimal. The spinal needle can then be used for intraarticular palpation of the anticipated operative sites.

The No. 18 spinal needle can be the "third hand" in the joint. With both the arthroscope and instrument in a confined space, the spinal needle, if properly placed transcutaneously, can hold tissue up, down, out of the way, or in place without obstructing view or surgical manipulation.

Probes. I prefer a probe that passes through cannulas (Fig. 3-32). Thus I can place the probe through the cannula and remove the cannula to avoid leakage of fluids. After entry, the cannula is removed from the probe to eliminate joint leakage. The cannula is then placed on the instrument table.

The probes can be either rigid or semimalleable. The rigid type is most commonly used. A semimalleable probe may be needed to reach certain areas not directly in line with the entry portal.

Anodized black or gold probes provide excellent visual contrast, especially if silver-metallic instruments are also in the visual field. Millimeter markings on the probe assist in estimation of anatomical or lesion size. The inflow cannula is convenient for palpation of the patellofemoral and suprapatellar areas.

A blunt obturator, with its larger size, may be best suited for palpation and manipulation of large defects or soft areas of articular cartilage.

Grasping Instruments

Miniature Forceps. A miniature forceps can be placed through a 2 mm OD cannula, or even transcutaneously through a small puncture wound for biopsy of synovial membrane or articular cartilage (Fig. 3-33). A synovial specimen can be obtained with the patient under local

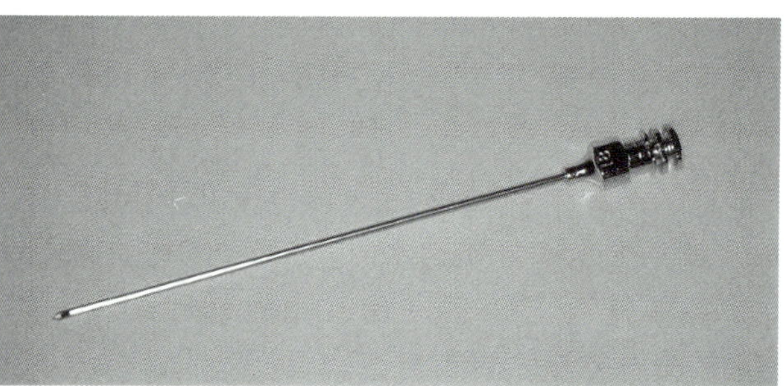

FIG. 3-31 No. 18 spinal needle.

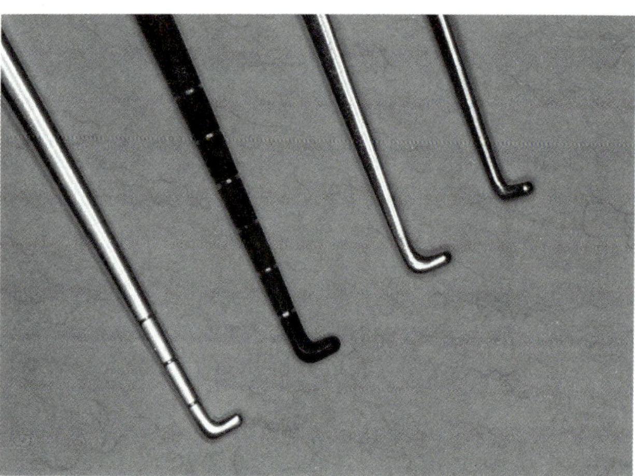

FIG. 3-32 Several kinds of probes exist. The gold and black anodized probe improves visualization in the joint. The probe may have 1 cm markings to estimate anatomical size within the joint. Plain metal probes come in regular and miniature size. *Left* to *right:* gold anodized, black anodized, regular metal, miniature metal.

anesthesia using the sense of palpation alone; however, direct visualization is surer. The specimens retrieved with a miniature forceps are of adequate size for histological evaluation.

The 2-mm forceps is used for intraarticular manipulation of suture within the joint. This instrument may be straight or curved (Fig. 3-33, *B*).

Schlesinger Forceps. A Schlesinger-type clamp was adapted from the neurosurgical instrumentation for arthroscopic surgery (Fig. 3-34). Originally this clamp was used for arthroscopic knee meniscectomy. Two sizes are available: 3.1 × 5.5 mm and 3.3 × 3.5 mm. The larger size comes in staight and angled design. These forceps may be used for removal of soft loose bodies. Because of its size, forceful grasping of hard or large pieces will cause instrument breakage, especially if rotation, angulation, and forceful traction are applied. The large forceps may be used as an adjunct in shoulder ligament repair for pulling up glenohumeral ligaments before internal fixation. The superior portal anterior to the acromion gives the proper plane of approach for this maneuver.

Breakage potential is less with the larger grasper. Breakage occurs at the pin, causing the grip to release. It is rare for the jaw of the grasper to fracture.

Two models are available, with and without a ratchet-holding device (Fig. 3-34). I prefer the control and release of the plain model. In some cases, however, the security of grasping with the ratchet model may be an advantage.

Loose Body Graspers. To accommodate the size of various loose bodies or foreign objects, pituitary forceps were modified with reverse teeth on the maxillary side and a cutout on the mandibular portion (Fig. 3-35). The reverse teeth reduce the chance of pinching the loose body out of the mechanism while grasping (the so-called watermelon-seed effect). The cutout on the mandibular jaw accommodates the configuration of the object. Because of its

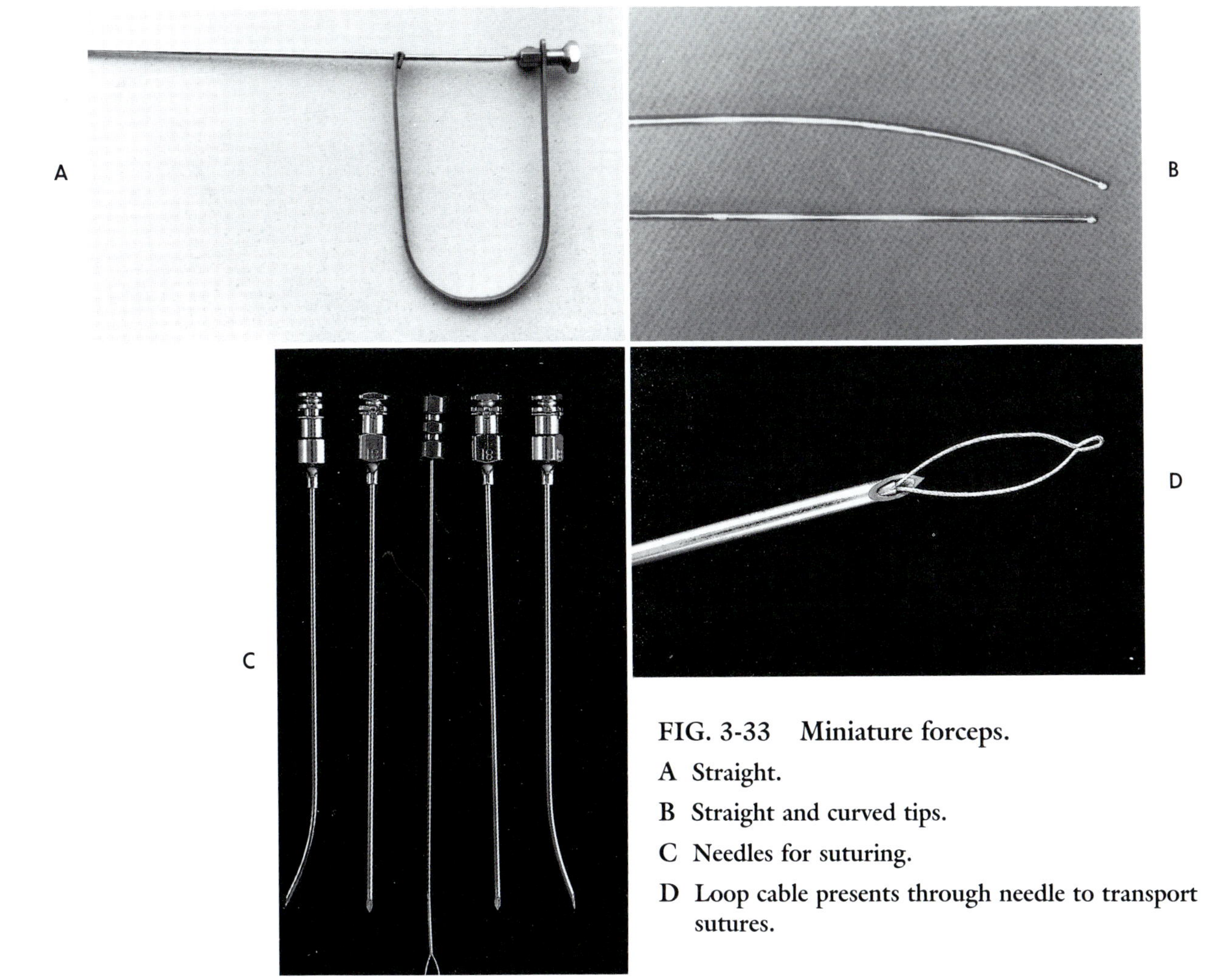

FIG. 3-33 Miniature forceps.
A Straight.
B Straight and curved tips.
C Needles for suturing.
D Loop cable presents through needle to transport sutures.

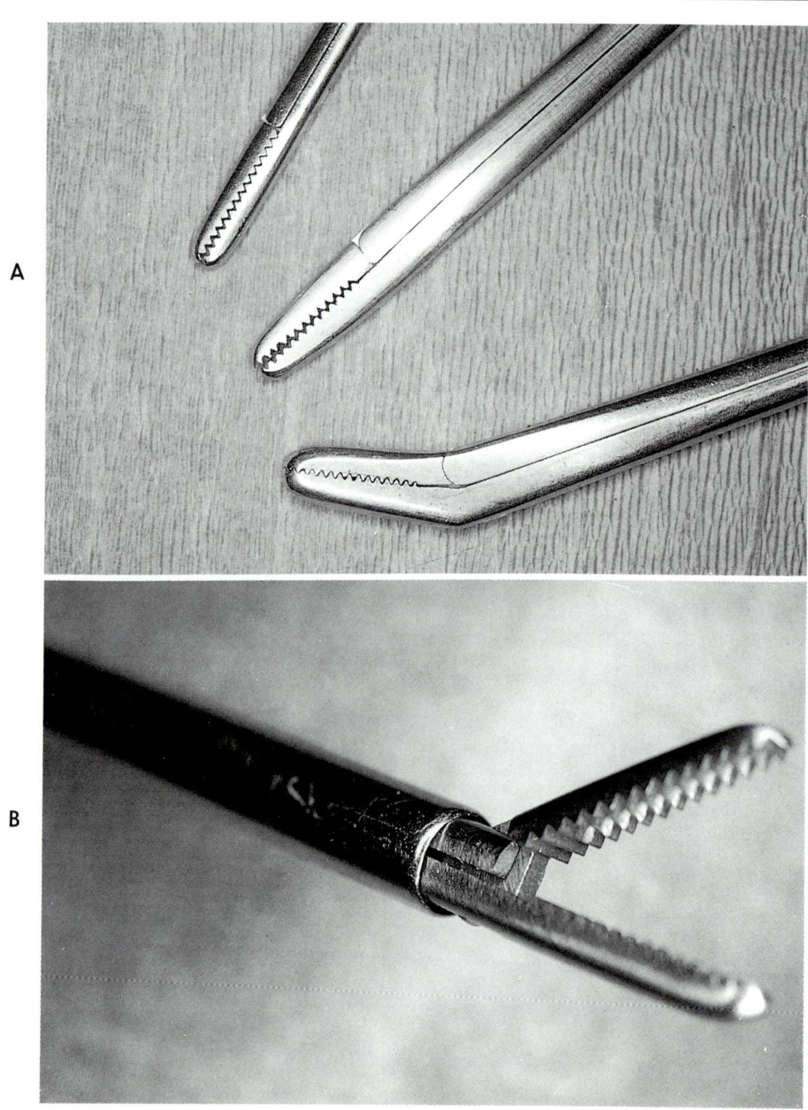

FIG. 3-34 Grasping forceps (Schlesinger clamp).
A Various shapes and sizes.
B Small size passes through cannula.

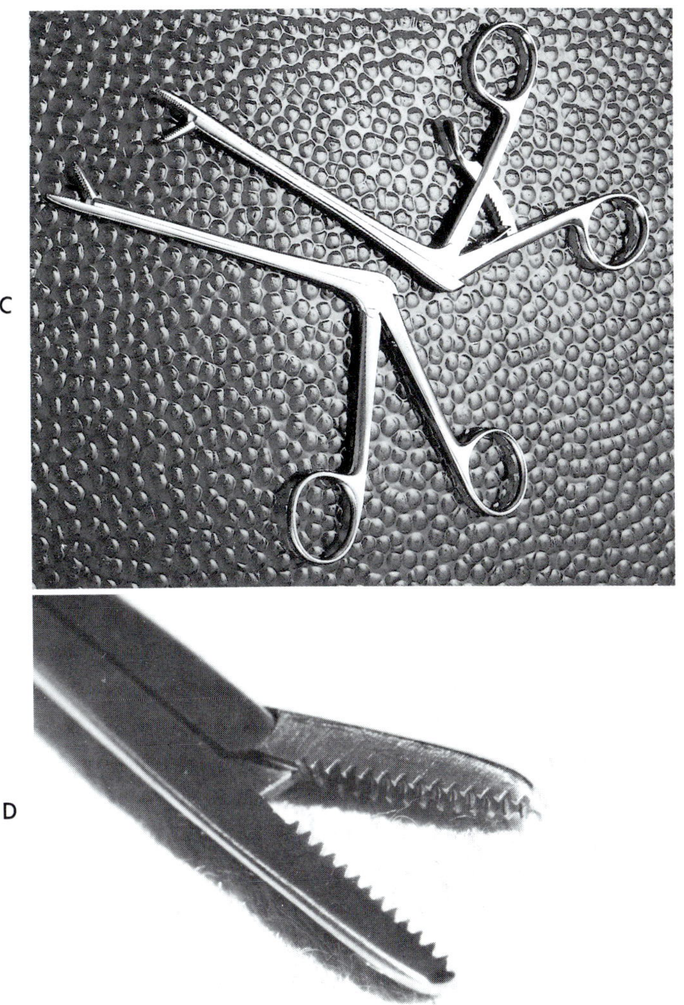

FIG 3-34, *cont'd* Grasping forceps (Schlesinger clamp).
C Two styles: with and without ratchet.
D Multiple tooth grasper.

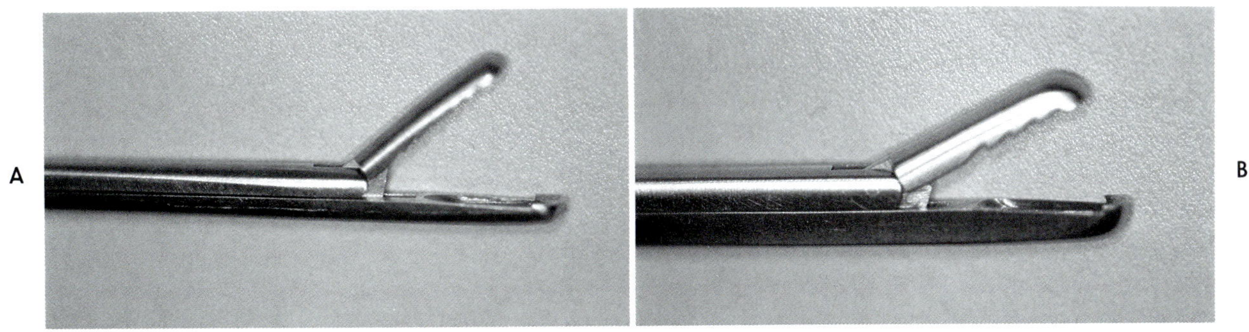

FIG. 3-35 Loose body graspers.
A Small forceps.
B Large "Jaws" forceps.

appearance and the popularity of the movie of the same name, the manufacturer chose to market this instrument under the name of Jaws.

Two model sizes are available: 6.5 × 3.5 mm and 4.0 × 3.2 mm (Fig. 3-35). The larger must be placed transcutaneously. The smaller has the advantage of being able to pass through the IASS cannula system; it is useful for multiple small objects. The small grasper is particularly effective in the shoulder, as it will pass through a cannula.

Retrieving Instrument (Magnetic)

The Golden Retriever is a metallic tube (4.2 mm OD) with a powerful miniature magnet in one end (Fig. 3-36). It functions with both applied suction forces and magnetic power. Its anodized gold color allows rapid visual identification in an environment of silver instruments.

The Golden Retriever will be effective only if the broken instrument fragment has magnetic properties. This is why metallic instruments and devices are necessary in arthroscopic surgery.

The force of flow created by suction will mobilize a fragment and draw it into a magnetic field. I have observed retrieval of metallic pieces located out of sight in the remote recesses of the joint with use of this instrument.

The suction tube applied to the end is purposely designed for a loose fit. If an adaptor is used to maximize suction, soft tissue often is drawn in between fragments and the magnet, interfering with attachment and retrieval. Thus the Golden Retriever by design cannot deliver suction as powerful as it would seem to be able to. In fact the suction should be removed the instant the metallic piece is close to the end of the tube to ensure good contact without interposition of tissue.

The final retrieval of the fragment is accomplished by direct visualization. A cannula is placed over the Golden Retriever. Under direct visualization, the fragment and Golden Retriever are removed through the cannula system. The cannula is removed last.

The surgeon should not attempt to pull a metallic fragment out through the tissues. A cannula must be used. The fragment could become loose outside the joint yet remain within the tissues. Such a situation seriously complicates the removal.

Cutting Instruments

Knife Blades. The knife blade has always been the traditional surgical means of tissue resection, which is also true in arthroscopic surgery. However, the small confines of the arthroscopic environment necessitated the development of special sizes and shapes of knife blades.

Originally, I used the available disposable knife blades. These particular blades had a high incidence of fracture, especially along the stress risers of the numbers stamped on the blade. The use of these blades resulted in the conception and development of the Golden Retriever.

The need for sharp knife blades specifically designed for arthroscopic surgery was urgent. Obtaining them was not an easy matter. The market demand was not great enough in 1977 to attract the interest of manufacturers. Thus it became necessary to develop and produce blades specifically for arthroscopic surgery outside of the existing industry. My serendipitous acquaintance with a precision grinder, Mr. Ted Hill, resulted in the production of a series of knife blades specifically designed for arthroscopic surgery. Virtually all manufacturers have copied these designs.

A

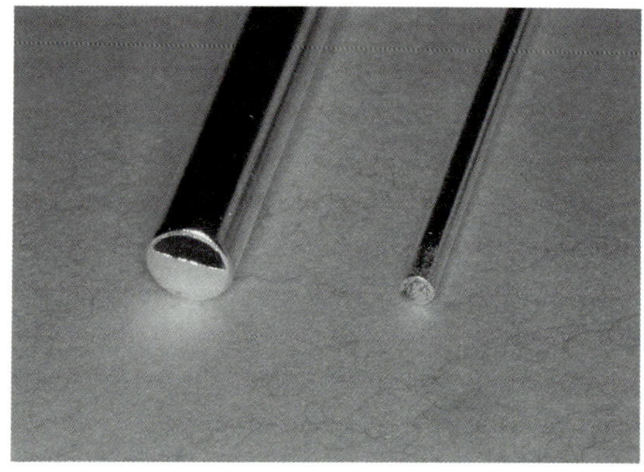

B

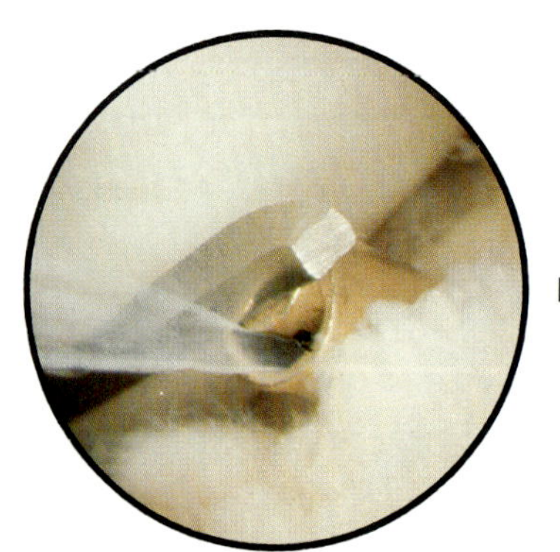

FIG. 3-36 Golden retriever.

A Regular and small sizes. The regular has magnet in end with small opening for suction. The small has only miniature magnet in the end.

B Arthroscopic view.

The first knife blades developed to meet arthroscopic specifications had the shapes of traditional blades (Fig. 3-37). They were designated Instrument Makar (IM) blades 771, 747, 764, and 767. The regular set blades are 3.4 mm in diameter and 23 mm long. The IM 711 blade is used for cutting of skin and subcutaneous tissue for various portals. It may also be used for sectioning fibrous bands. The IM 764 and 767 blades are used for cutting or dissection of labrum.

An arthroscopic knife blade must be sharp and breakage resistant and have magnetic properties. These do. The configuration of the cutting edge and shaft must be such that adjacent tissues are protected. The transition from cutting edge to shaft must be smooth to allow for gliding motion through capsular tissues. The knife must be deliverable by a cannula system; any knife blade placed blindly may cause tissue trauma. With separate passages, injury to the articular cartilage may occur. By use of a cannula, the blade is protected until it comes into view at the end of the cannula, the site of resection.

The retractable blade provides a similar safety factor, but the blade is breakable. The shaft-blade junction is abrupt, which results in bumping or catching on tissues.

Despite many requests for a retrograde blade set, I did not see a need for it. Eventually, after receiving a request from Dr. Richard Caspari of Richmond, Virginia, we designed five different retrograde blades of various sizes and shapes (Fig. 3-38). My associates and I also used the blades and were surprised at their value. The 710 blade led to the retrograde method of knee joint lateral release. The diameter of the retrograde blades is 4.1 mm, and they are 23 mm in length. The 707 is a reverse Smillie-type blade that permits retrograde cutting action yet has protective edges. The 708 is a retrograde right-handed blade that has the point facing left and concave surface up. It is used to shape firm tissue. The 709 is the mirror image of the 708 and has the same purpose. It has different cutting configurations for proper tissue beveling in a given situation.

The IM 761 blade is sharp on both sides and curved (Fig. 3-39). It is useful in cutting on an angle or following the curve of the glenoid in developing the interval for a pivot shift. Dr. Robert Hunter named the IM 761 blade the "banana blade." This name is used by all manufacturers.

The IM 747 blade is a miniature Smillie-type blade with a slight curve that follows the condylar curve to release tissue (Fig. 3-40). It has a protective guide on each side of the cutting edge.

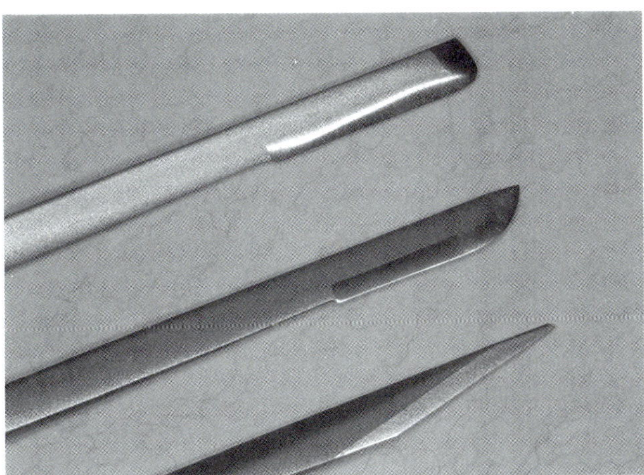

FIG. 3-37 Standard reusable knife blades: These shapes conform to No. 64, No. 67, and No. 11 and are labeled by Instrument Makar as 764, 767, and 711 from *top* to *bottom*.

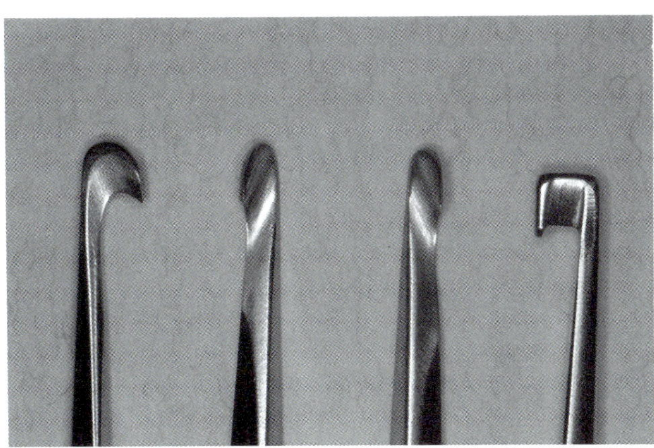

FIG. 3-38 Retrograde set: The retrograde set has several shapes; four are shown here. *Left* to *right*, One is straight hooked blade, two are opposite curved blades and the other is a shielded retrograde "Smillie-type" blade.

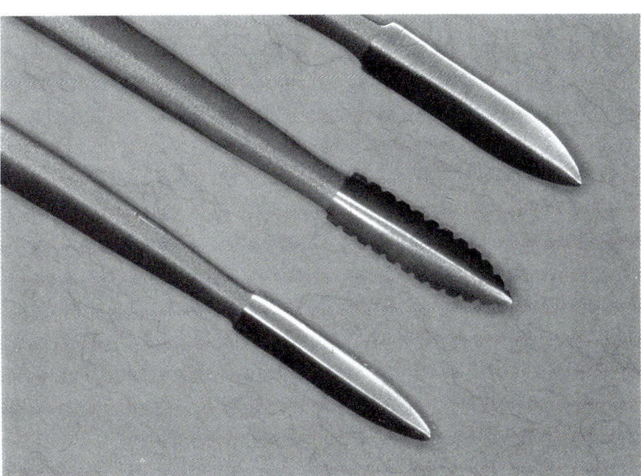

FIG. 3-39 The small curved blades (banana type) come in (*top* to *bottom*) regular, serrated, and miniature sizes.

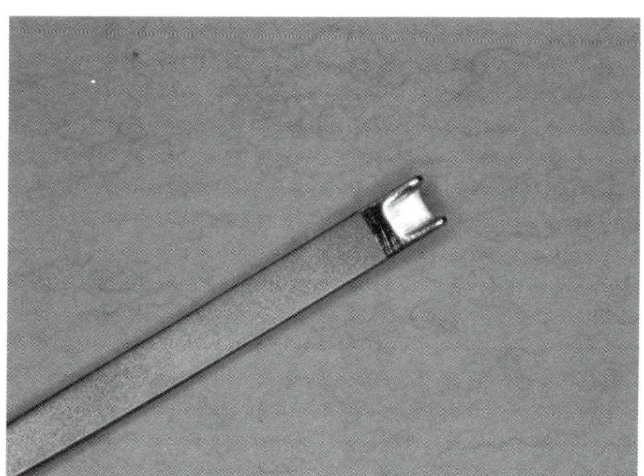

FIG. 3-40 The IM No. 707 blade is a miniature "Smillie-type."

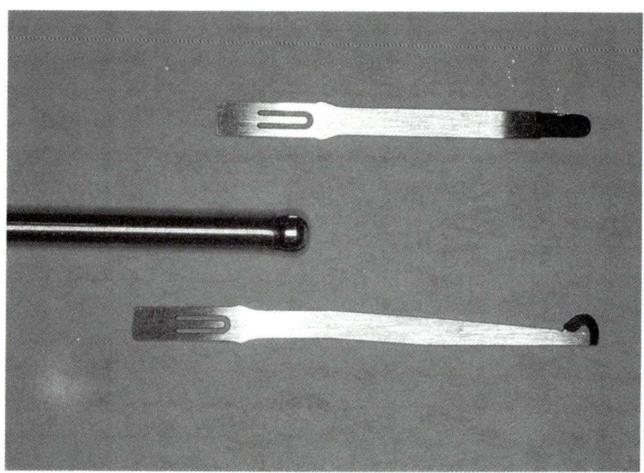

FIG. 3-41 Disposable blades.

Miniature Knife Blades. Because some joint spaces are so tight, rotational cutting was not possible with the regular 761 blade (see Fig. 3-39). I designed two smaller blades of similar configuration. The shaft is the same (3.4 mm OD), but the tips are small enough for any posterior cutting without injury to the articular surfaces. They are used with the miniature grasper and 2.7 mm basket forceps in the tightest environment.

Because these blades are reusable, care must be taken in their handling during and between cases. The commonly used 761 and 710 blades are part of the routine set-up. They are held in separate slots in the plastic knife holder for protection. They are disinfected by cold Cidex soaking methods between cases to reduce damage caused by jostling with other instruments in the autoclave. The less frequently used knives are individually wrapped and sterilized and held out of set-up. On request, they are unwrapped, used, and resterilized. With this method, sharpness and long blade life is ensured. Each reusable blade is good for about 30 uses. Single-case use is a result of abuse of the edges.

Disposable Blades. Since the original arthroscopic blades were designed, many have been adapted to disposable blades. The stress riser of the stamped number had been moved proximally. The objectionable abrupt junction between the handle and the blade itself was tapered with plastic. Occasional fracture of the plastic shafts has been reported, however, and retrieval of the fragments may be impeded by the nonmagnetic property of the plastic.

The main advantage of a disposable blade is its single-time use and sharpness. Per case, its actual cost is greater than the reusable blade (Fig. 3-41).

The disadvantages of the disposable blades are their flatness and flexibility, which do not allow tissue penetration and the rotation without deforming. These blades are limited to cutting similar to that done with other flat blade configurations. They do not offer any specific arthroscopic surgical advantages; this is especially so of the disposable "banana blade."

Basket Forceps. These were the initial cutting instrument, borrowed from other endoscopic disciplines, to be used for resection of labral flaps or fibrous bands. They have even been used in a rather primitive way for debridement of articular surfaces. Basket forceps have limited value in shoulder surgery (Fig. 3-42).

Because of its disadvantages the basket forceps has a lesser role in arthroscopy today. It must be passed without a cannula, and multiple passes injure the joint. Small fragments are left to obscure the view or to become free within the joint. The resection line is perpendicular, which fails to reproduce the normal triangular configuration of the labrum. A knife and motorized instruments will do most jobs better, cleaner, and faster than basket forceps. Nevertheless, they do have a place in selected instances.

Basket forceps designs have advanced to create stronger, smaller instruments. They come in a multitude of shapes, sizes, angles: up, down, and around. Recently Dr. Terry Whipple introduced a basket forceps that incorporates suction and is sold by Dyonics.

I believe most surgeons have complicated their surgical set-up enough with all the options available. To me, the basket forceps meet a perceived need rather than a real one. The following are the features of basket forceps I have found useful. They should be small in size. The edges must be smooth and have no protruding parts. They must be strong and durable so they will cut well. A few properly selected basket forceps will do all jobs.

Variable Axis System. The variable axis system provides various sizes and shapes of basket forceps and cutting instrumentation (Fig. 3-43). It allows cutting both right and left at various angles and with various sizes,

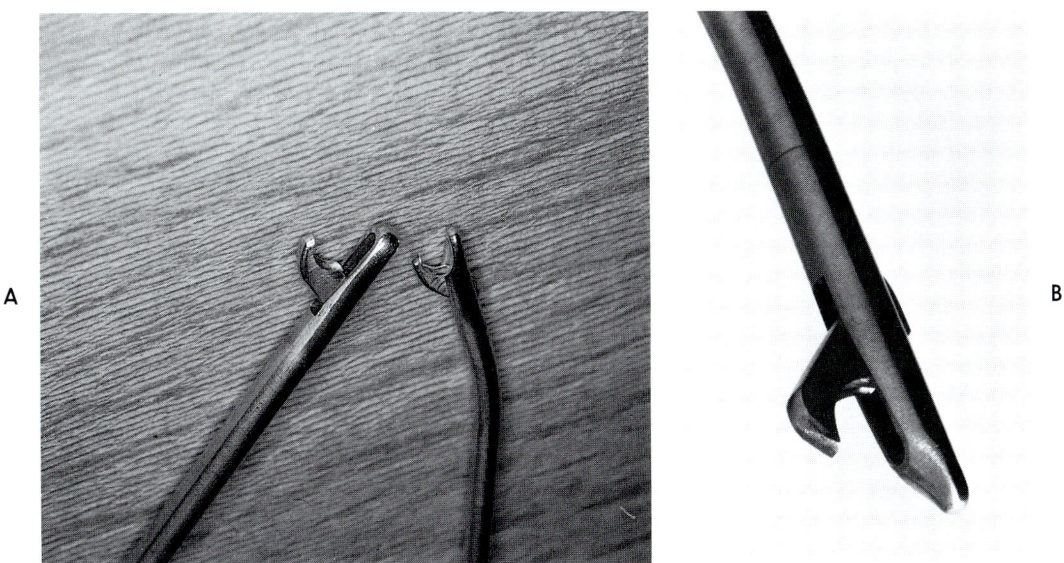

FIG. 3-42 Basket forceps.
A Curved and straight.
B Snowplow nose.

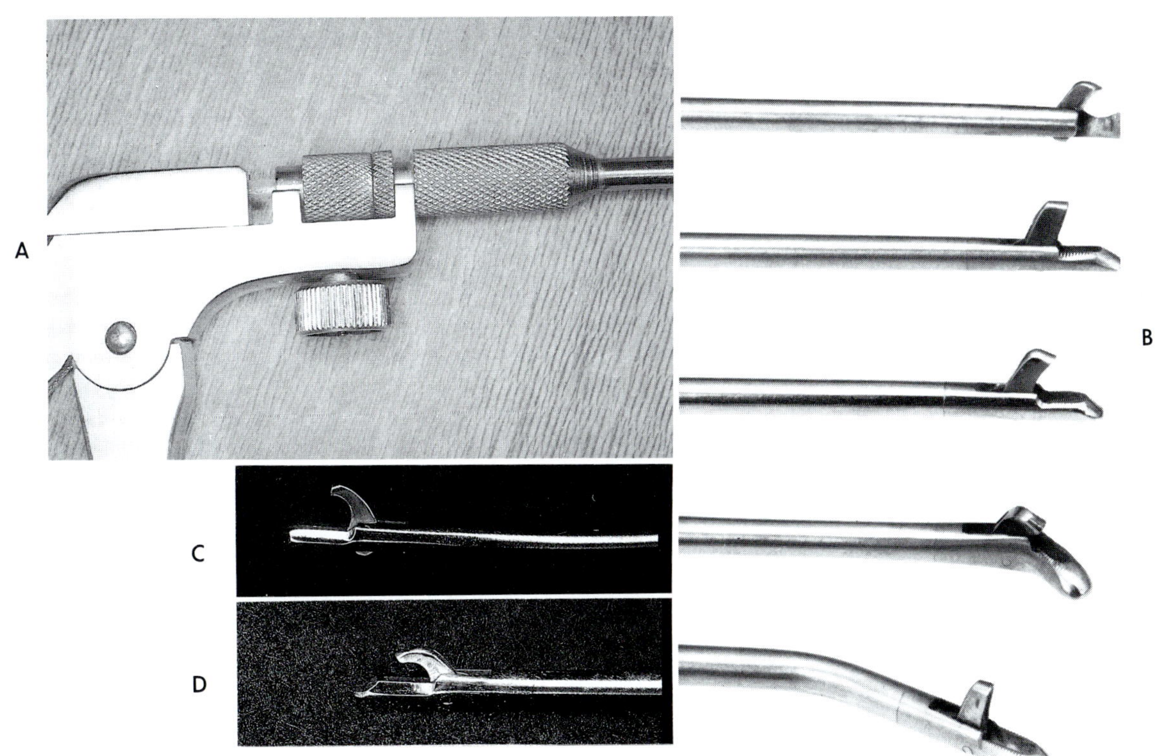

FIG. 3-43 Variable axis hand instrument system.
A Removable blade at handle.
B Various shapes, scissors, straight jaw, arc jaw, curve tip, curved shaft.
C Up-curved shaft, 2.7 mm, regular tip.
D Straight basket forceps, 2.7 mm, snowplow tip.

without the added expense of having multiple handles. Cutting devices are interchangeable. The variable axis system also facilitates resharpening, because only the cutting devices need to be sent for maintenance.

I use two handles, each with the most commonly used cutting shafts: the 2.7 mm angled and 3.5 mm with snowplow nose. Some may choose routinely to mount scissors; as a rule, I use basket forceps instead of scissors.

The 2.7 mm up-angle shaft, straight jaws forceps has a contour that conforms to femoral condyle. It reaches around the contour of the humeral head or margin of the glenoid.

The 3.5-mm straight shaft, straight jaws forceps is small enough to be used in the shoulder yet large enough to effect a meaningful bite. It is especially useful if designed with a scooped nose to elevate the edge of an elevated glenoid labrum.

I have found little use for a greater variety of angles and shapes. To have a shape and an angle for each and every bite is expensive and unnecessary. Surgical technique compensates for multiple-shaped tools, and a great variety of tools is not a substitute for good surgical technique.

Scissors. I have used a variety of scissors. Generally the durable scissors is too large and others are too fragile. A basket forceps is a better scissor for arthroscopy.

Curettes. Curettes are available in various sizes and shapes but most do not easily pass through cannulas (Fig. 3-44). They have limited use for shoulder arthroscopy.

POWER INSTRUMENTS

Cordless Instruments

Hand Drills. Hand drills have traditionally consisted of a simple brace-and-bit system. I presently favor the Dyonics battery-powered motorized system (Fig. 3-45). This system allows for Kirschner wire insertion and use of larger (5⁄16-inch) drill bits with good control and power. It is compact, lightweight, and easily maintained.

Oscillating Saws. Dyonics has an oscillating saw system for combined procedures, such as acromioplasty (Fig. 3-45, *B*).

Arthroscopic Motorized Instruments

Arthroscopic motorized instrumentation was introduced by Dyonics, Inc. of Andover, Massachusetts, in 1975 as the Intra-Articular Shaver (IAS). The IAS was a battery-powered, electric motor-driven, rotating-cutting-suction device. This patented device is the basic instrument used for modern day arthroscopic surgery.

The present Dyonics system is the PS3500 Arthroscopic Surgical System (Fig. 3-46). This system has diagnostic display panels that report whether the blade is engaged or if there are any system problems. This system accommodates the PS3500, mini, and universal motors.

Each blade has a computerized optimal rotational speed range, and an automatic blade speed recall with digital display. All blades have a forward, reverse, and oscillation mode of operation.

A

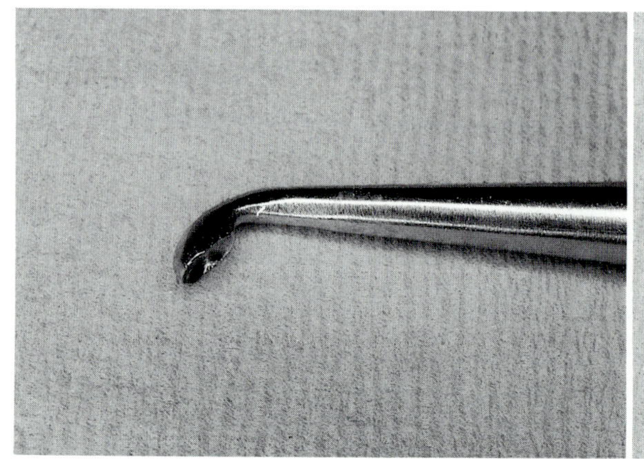

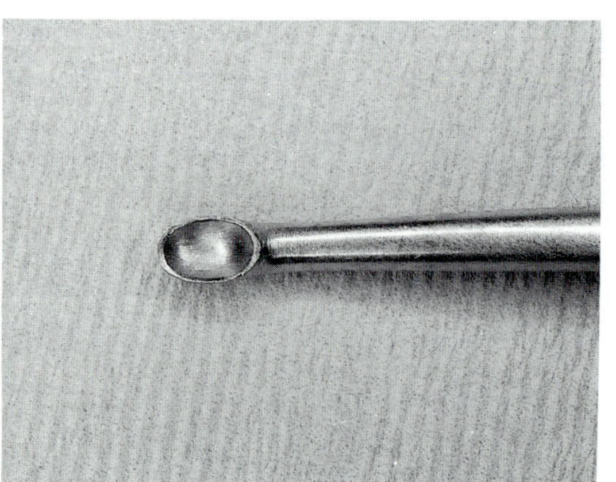

B

FIG. 3-44 Curettes.

A Angled curette.

B Regular curette.

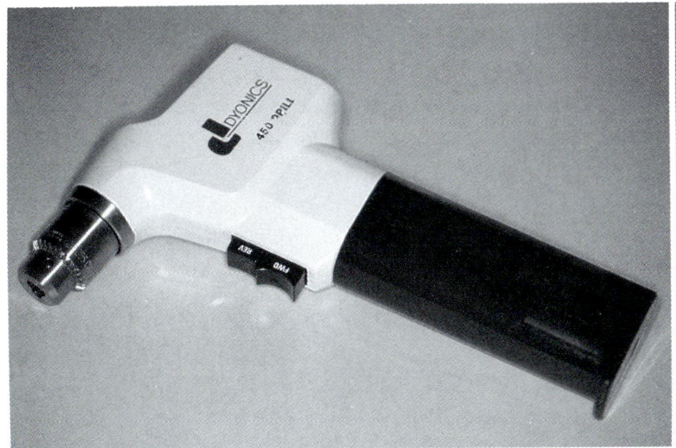

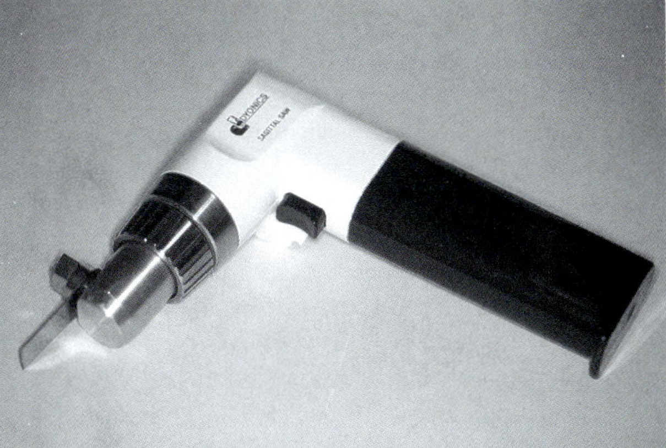

A B

FIG. 3-45 Dyonics Cordless Instrument System.

A Drill.

B Oscillating saw.

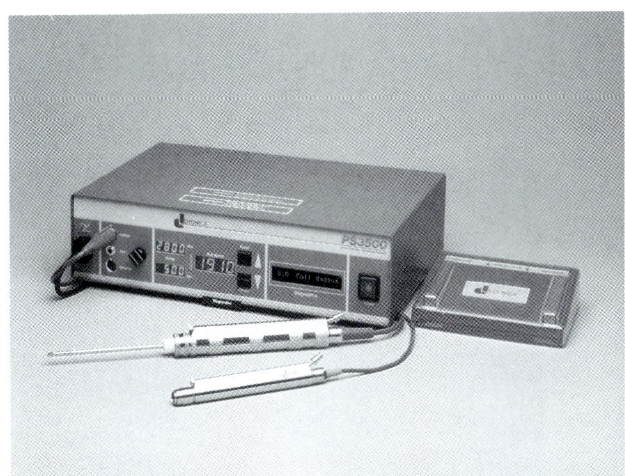

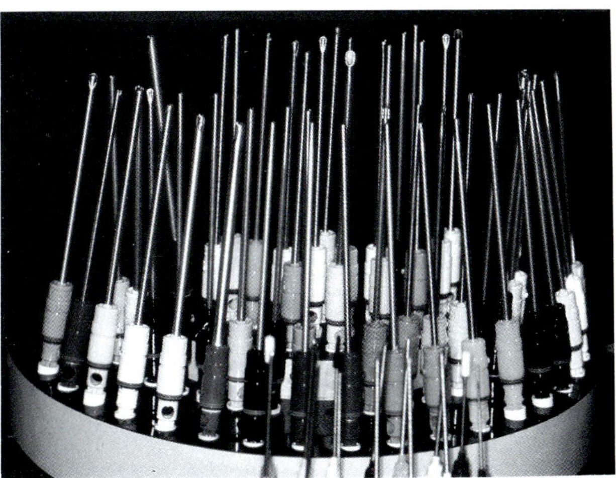

A B

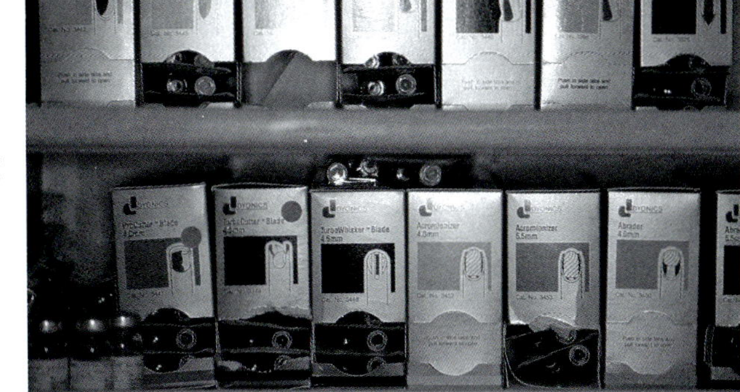

C

FIG. 3-46 Dyonics System 3500.

A Motor.

B Disposable blades.

C Disposable blades on shelf in operating room.

Cutting Attachments. Cutting attachments for the Dyonics Intra-articular System PS3500 are many and varied. Two basic groups of cutting heads exist: reusable and disposable. The reusable heads comprise the basic group of cutting attachment configurations. They are more expensive, are made of heavier steel, and last longer. They have closer cutting tolerances than the disposable blades. The disposable blade attachments have a broader selection of cutting heads. Disposable blades are popular because of the perceived need for a new sharp blade for each case.

The most commonly used attachments for arthroscopic surgery of the shoulder are cutters, full radius synovial resectors, burrs, and acromionizers. Sizes and shapes are too numerous to name, but the Dyonics catalog lists the original shapes and names that other companies have copied.

Shaver (3.0 and 4.5 mm). The bullet-nosed shaver head is commercially available but rarely used, because it is less effective at cutting than more recent configurations (Fig. 3-47).

Trimmer (3.5 and 4.5 mm). The trimmer was the first modification of the shaver head (Fig. 3-48). It placed the window closer to the end of the tube, which provided more effective cutting with tipping-in of the end into the lesion. The trimmer was designed for debridement of degenerative articular cartilage and was used for synovectomy before the Arthroplasty System was developed.

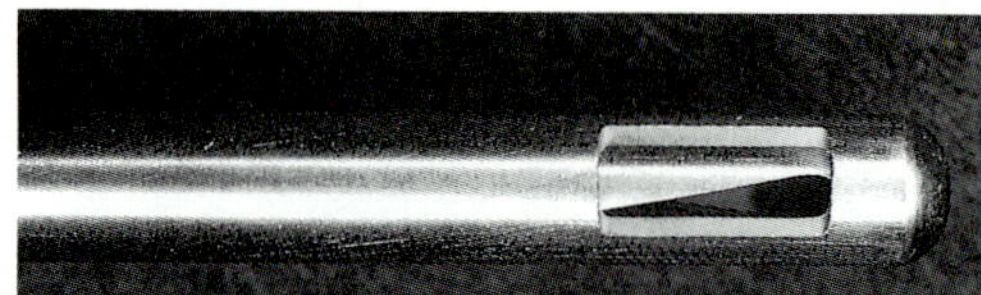

FIG. 3-47 Shaver, 4.45 mm.

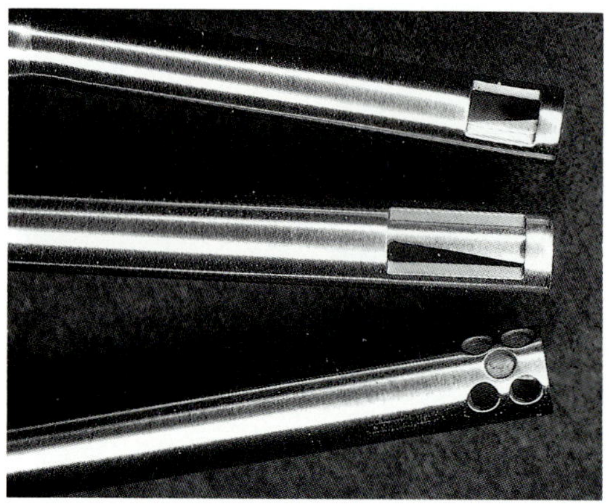

FIG. 3-48 Trimmers. *Top,* 3.5 and 4.5 mm. *Bottom,* whisker 4.5 mm.

Cutter (3.5, 4.5, and 5.5 mm). The keyhole-shaped cutter was developed in 1978 (Fig. 3-49). This unique design provides a means of end and side cutting. It is effective on the tough soft tissue like labrum. The cutter will cut bone but is not intended for that purpose; therefore, care must be taken not to injure normal articular cartilage.

Full-radius synovectomy blade (3.5, 4.5, and 5.5 mm). Dr. Thomas Rosenberg introduced this design to Dyonics (Fig. 3-50). This blade has greatly enhanced the efficiency and aggressiveness for synovectomy. The head configuration permits cutting on the end, as well as the side. It will cut normal articular cartilage, including cancellous bone. Therefore even an experienced arthroscopic surgeon must take care with its use.

Full-radius whisker blade (3.5 and 5.5 mm). This head design has multiple holes like a salt shaker (Fig. 3-51). It is not aggressive and provides a means of safely removing tissue without wide resection. It is effective in removing synovial villi while leaving the synovial base-

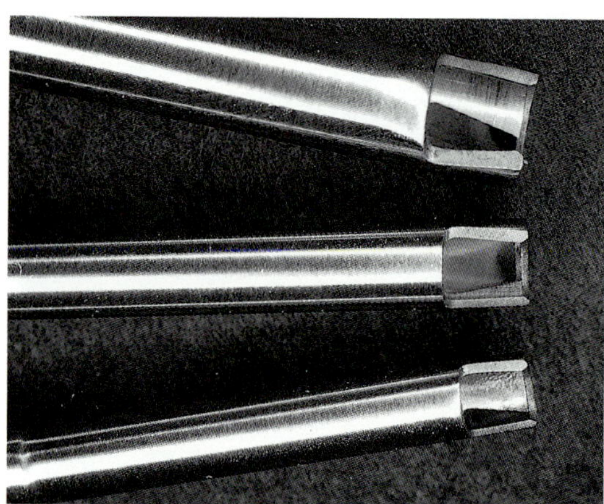

FIG. 3-49 Cutters, 3.5, 4.5, and 5.5 mm.

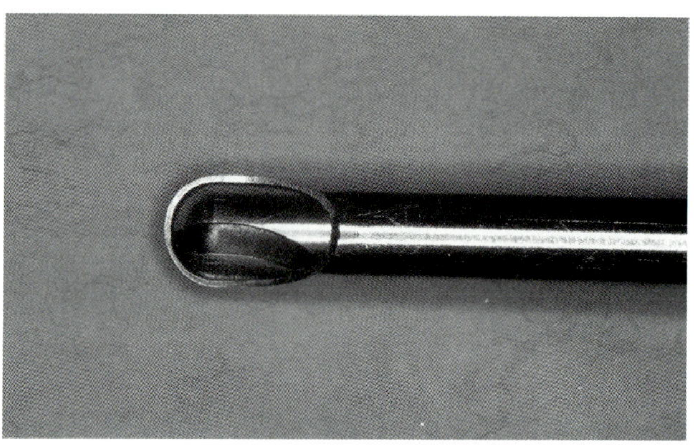

FIG. 3-50 Full-radius synovial resector.

ment membrane and capsule intact, and especially in removing furry areas of degenerative articular cartilage. This cutting head is best suited for faster speeds. The whisker facilitates the removal of small metallic debris from instrument or device fragments without cutting other tissue. This blade also serves well as a final clean-up instrument.

The 3.5 mm size is the instrument head of choice for small joint synovectomy. The smaller holes prevent decompression and joint collapse in a small reservoir. The head will not cut out of the capsule, thereby protecting adjacent neurovascular structures.

The Turbowhisker (4.5 mm) is a variation of the original whisker and moderately aggressive (Fig. 3-52).

Abrader (4.5 and 5.5 mm). This cutting head was designed to facilitate superficial debridement (1 to 2 mm) of exposed bony surfaces (Fig. 3-53). Both abraders have a retractable shaft on the cutting burr (for pistoning) to avoid inadvertent deep cutting if excessive pressure is applied.

The 4.5 mm abrader passes through the cannula system. It is most useful when portals of shoulder joints are interchanged, when a cannula approach is essential. This size is used to prepare the bone bed of anterior glenoid, before ligament reattachment, in acromioplasty and for resection of osteophytes.

The 5.5 mm abrader is more aggressive, but its size limits its use in the shoulder as no cannula is large enough to allow its passage. It may be passed transcutaneously for more aggressive acromioplasty.

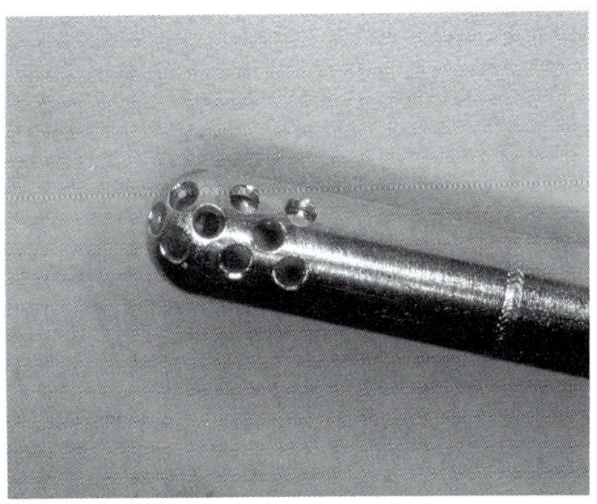

FIG. 3-51 Full-radius synovial whisker.

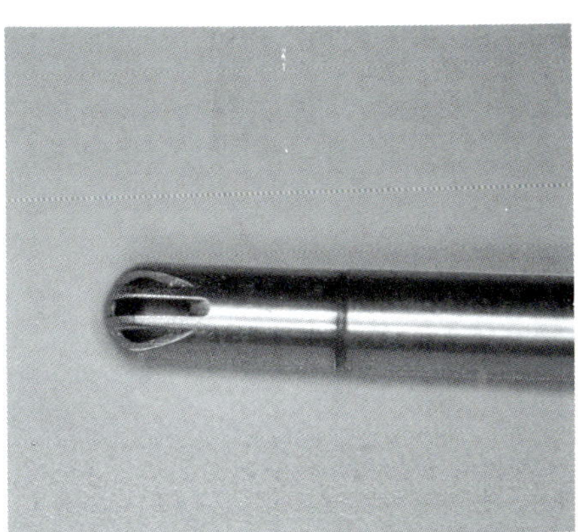

FIG. 3-52 Turbowhisker.

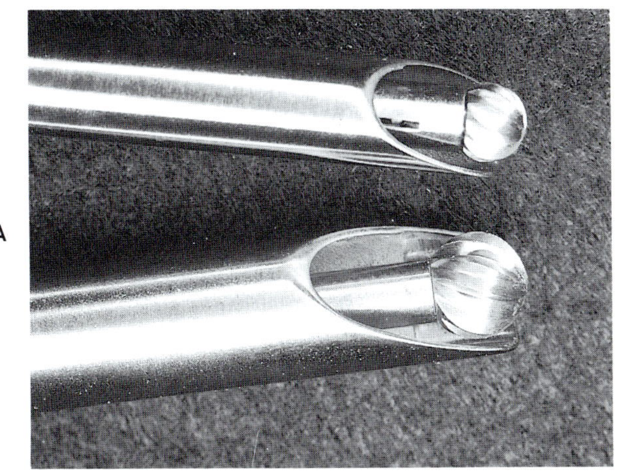

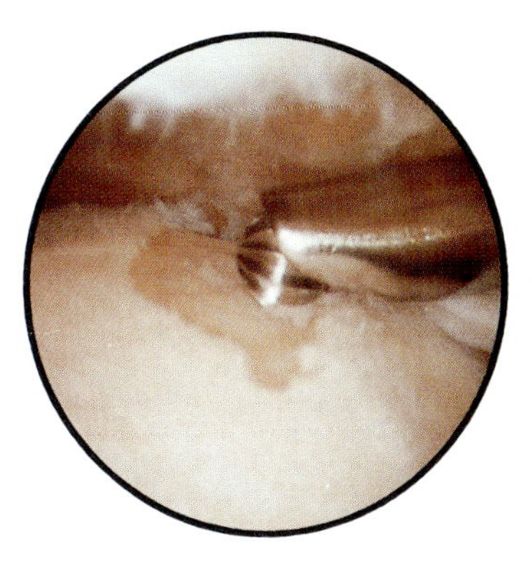

FIG. 3-53 Abraders.
A Regular.
B Larger.

Acromionizer (4.0 and 5.5 mm). Acromionizers are effective for acromioplasty. Their oblong length provides a means of cutting a flat surface on the underside of the acromion (Fig. 3-54).

Small Joint Instrument System. Dyonics has a smaller motor and various size cutting heads for small joint arthroscopic surgery (Fig. 3-55). This system may be useful in the acromioclavicular joint.

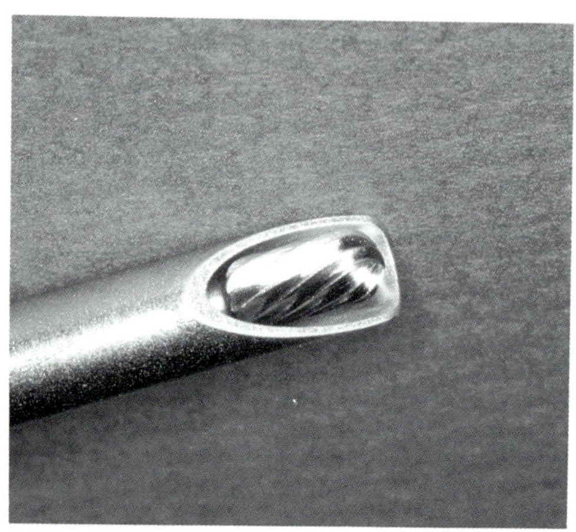

FIG. 3-54 Acromionizer. It comes in 4.0 mm. and 5.5 mm diameters.

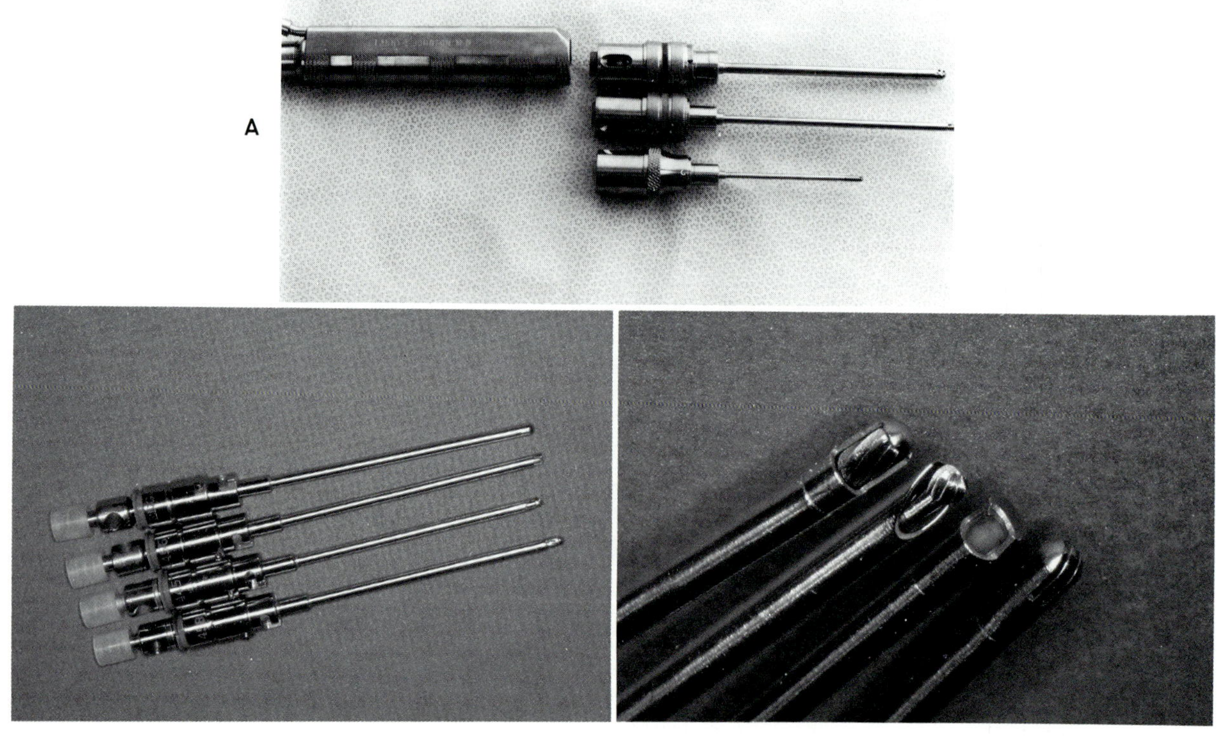

A

B

C

FIG. 3-55 Small instrument system.

A Motor.

B Various cutter heads.

C Close–up of cutter heads.

Cutting Effectiveness of Motorized Blades. The surgeon often perceives that cutting effectiveness is related to fast rpm and sharp edges. Both ideas are wrong. The common perception is that faster is better. Likewise, this is not always true. The surgeon's manipulation of the blades results in the most effective cutting (see Chapter 6 on Technique), and a variable-speed instrument is optimal.

The original IASS had a speed below 100 rpm in a liquid medium. Gradually, as improvements in metallurgy developed, speed was increased above 3500 rpm.

In general, the harder the tissue to be cut, the slower the rpm requirements; that is, the window must be open long enough for the material to enter. The reverse is true for soft pliable tissue, such as synovium. Over 1000 rpm is required to avoid deep, unregulated resections. Faster speeds are required to resect bone. Speed affects efficiency, but only when matched to cutting head and tissue type.

The Dyonics system has a built-in stall mechanism for safety purposes. The calibrated stall avoids unnecessarily deep resection and provides a mechanism of control for surgeons at all levels of experience. The Dyonics burred cutting heads have built-in retraction when too much pressure is applied. This design prevents stalling and cutting too deep.

The cutting edges of the shaver and trimmer are ragged on microscopic inspection, like conventional scissors. Another analogy to scissors is the tightness of the tolerance of opposing sides. If the screw is loose on scissors, the cutting is poor. If it is tight, the cutting is efficient. The surgeon should look for close tolerances on cutting heads. This is accomplished by looking at the head within the joint and with the suction on. If tissue goes between the two surfaces, then the tolerances are too great and the cutter will not be effective. Such a cutter should be replaced or repaired.

The cutter design has matched-angle sharp edges. Disposable cutting heads are a perceived need only; I used my last cutter for 6 months and 300 cases. Even an abused cutter will cut bone or the end of the arthroscope if the window is open long enough for entry.

It should be pointed out that faster speeds, greater power (torque), and sharp blades alone do not make a faster operation. The rpm, torque, flow, and cutting head selection must be suitable for the surgeon's manipulation skill. The hand that guides the instrument is the most important factor in cutting effectiveness.

RECONSTRUCTION INSTRUMENTS

The Ligamentous and Capsular Repair (LCR) System

The LCR system was originally designed for arthroscopic reattachment of the acutely torn anterior cruciate ligament (Fig. 3-56). It has been used in shoulder surgery to repair glenohumeral ligaments. Biceps (long head) tendon stabilization, labral reattachment, and rotator cuff re-

A

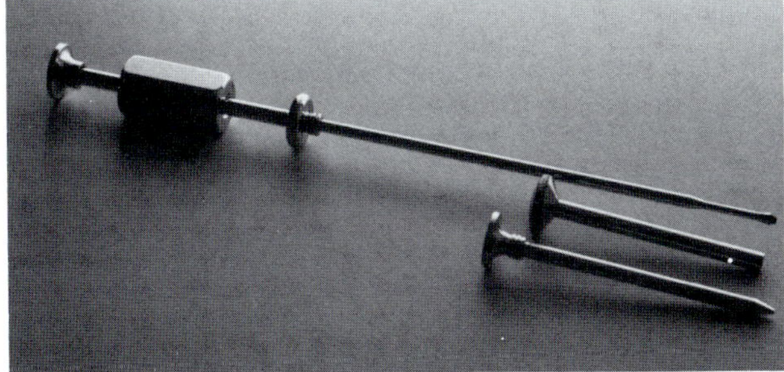

B

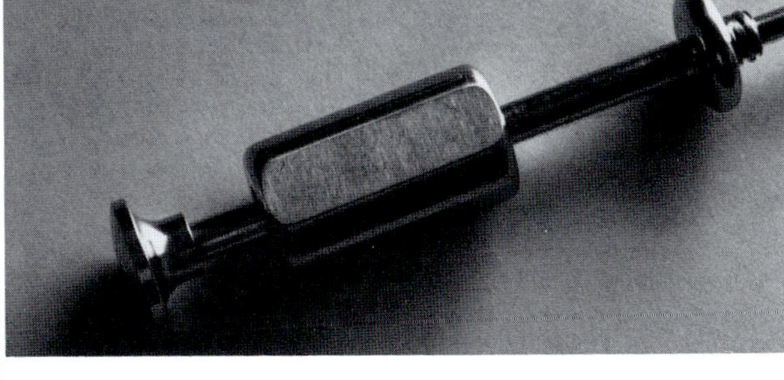

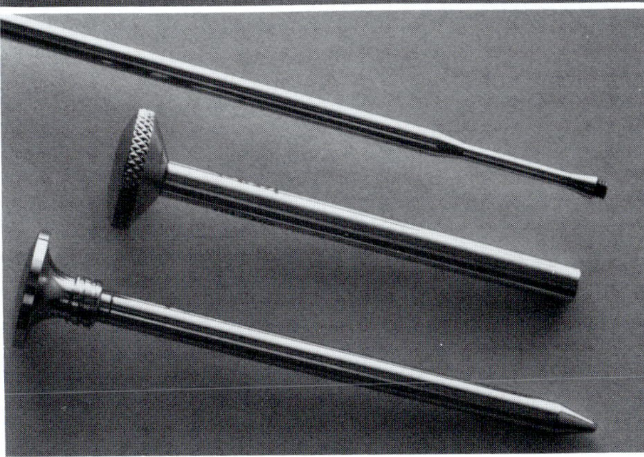

C

FIG. 3-56 Ligamentous and Capsular Repair System; Original.

A This photo shows the threaded driver, cannula, and obturator.

B The sliding hammer.

C Close-up of the driver, cannula and obturator.

pair have been performed arthroscopically using these staples (see Chapters 8 and 9).

The system consists of a cannula, an interlocking obturator, a driver-extractor and various sizes of staples. The cannula is large enough to deliver any of the staples. After the staple is placed intraarticularly, the cannula is withdrawn and secured to the driver-extractor by a rotation and locking-screw mechanism. This step avoids sliding of the cannula during impaction-extraction.

Cannula and Obturators. In 1990, a cannula was made larger to accommodate insertion of larger diameter biodegradable staples for the knee joint (Fig. 3-57). The new cannula has a tine to grasp ligament or tendon and secure it to the bone (Fig. 3-57, *D*). A staple tap is necessary to make a preliminary track in bone for the biodegradable staple (Fig. 3-57, *B*). A spiked insertion driver is used for the solid head, biodegradable staple (Fig. 3-57, *C*).

Driver/Extractor. The driver-extractor has a built-in sliding hammer (see Fig. 3-56, *B*) that permits the surgeon to watch the staple placement on the television screen instead of watching the end of the driver, as with a separate mallet. To better control force, the built-in hammer avoids side or missed hits. Extraction is immediately available by reversing the directional force of the sliding hammer. Threads are present at the distal end for staple attachment and they protrude so as to avoid cutting off ligament tissue against the bone (Fig. 3-58).

Staples. The staples are round for cannula insertion. They come in two styles and various lengths and diameters (Fig. 3-59). The smaller staples are used in children and small adults; the larger staples are more commonly placed. The limbs have reversed-angled teeth for securing to bone.

The original staples were too malleable, the crotch was sharp and the head too large, resulting in bending, cutting out, or joint irritation (Fig. 3-60). Subsequent modifications strengthened the metal, chamfered the crotch, and reduced the head size. In 1990, a tine was removed from the limb to make a longer and smoother crotch to the staple (Fig. 3-61). This Profile 90 staple is the current choice. The head and hips of the staples are shiny, and the legs are frosted (Fig. 3-62). These landmarks allow the surgeon to gauge depth of insertion so that the limbs of the staples are adequately embedded in bone with space remaining in the crotch of the staple to house tissue. Otherwise, the gaug-

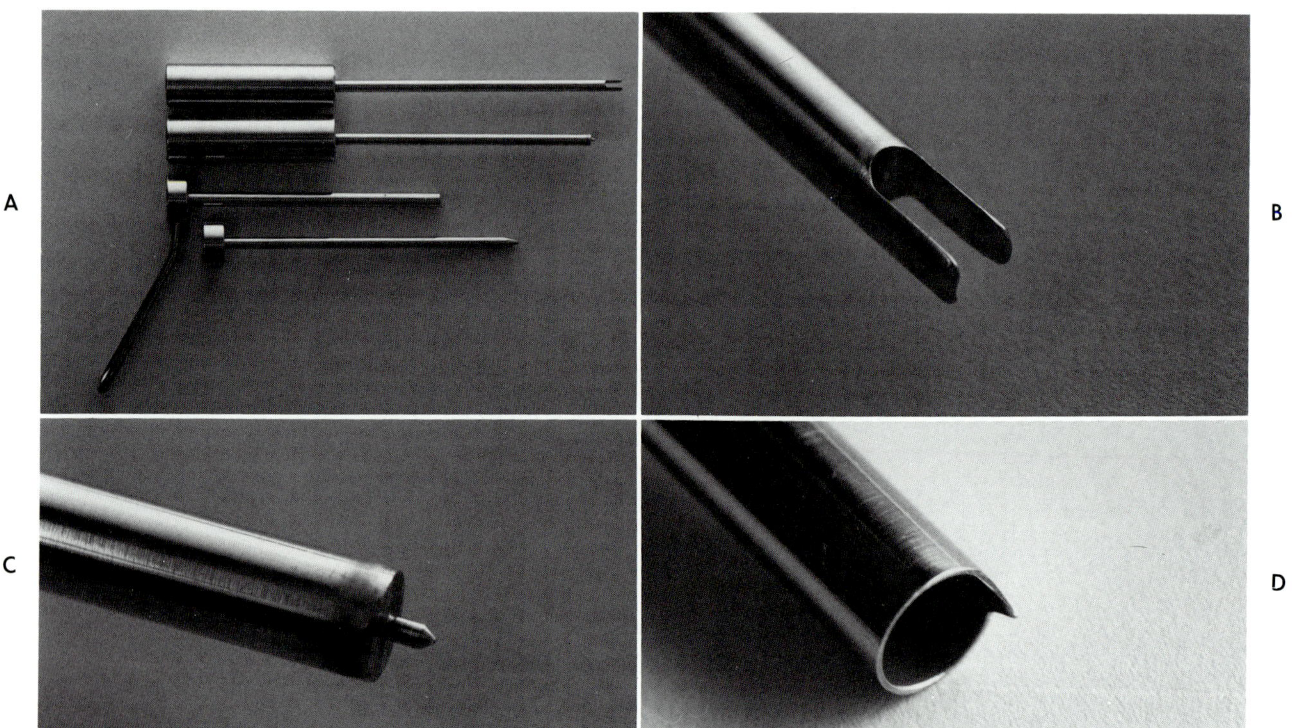

FIG. 3-57 LCR System 90's.

A **From *top* to *bottom,* the staple bone tap, the pinned driver, the spiked cannula, and the obturator.**

B **Close-up of the staple tap.**

C **Close-up of the pinned driver.**

D **Close-up of the spiked cannula.**

ing of depth would be inaccurate and complete insertion would cut through tissue held by the staple.

Major deformation, up to 90 degrees of angulation and 180 degrees of rotation of a limb of the staple, has not resulted in breakage. I am aware of two cases of fracture of the staple with more angulation and 180 degrees of rotation with continued impaction (hammering) and repeated angulation.

The metal of the IM staple has magnetic properties to facilitate retrieval if necessary, either broken or en toto. The metal is noncorrosive.

Biodegradable Staples. The Instrument Makar Biologic staple was approved by the Food and Drug Administration (FDA) for market labeling in 1991 for use in the knee joint (Fig. 3-63). Application for use in the shoulder is under way. The same type instrumentation used for the metal staple is used for the biodegradable staple.

Bullet-Nosed Staple Remover. Routine extraction is facilitated by a softer metal, bullet-nosed staple remover (Fig. 3-64). The shape allows the softer metal tip to enter and secure the staple to the extractor. The bullet-nosed staple remover is self-centering, even if the longitudinal axes of the extractor and staple are not aligned. Its gold color facilitates visualization. The remover was not intended for insertion or implantation.

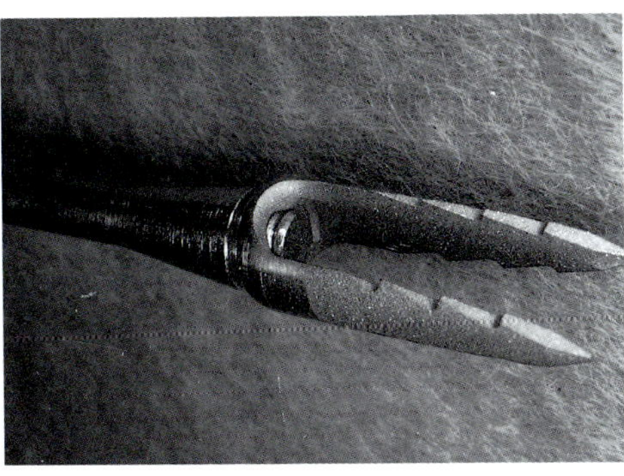

FIG. 3-58 Close-up of insertor/extractor in staple shows the protrusion of the threads into the staple crotch so as to prevent impacting staple against bone and amputating tendon or ligamentous tissue.

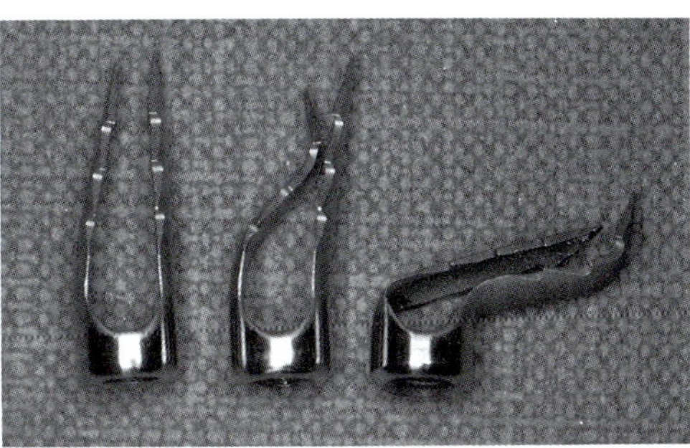

FIG. 3-60 The original staple in 1982 was intentionally malleable to avoid breakage, but bending was a problem. This problem has been corrected with a change in the tempering process.

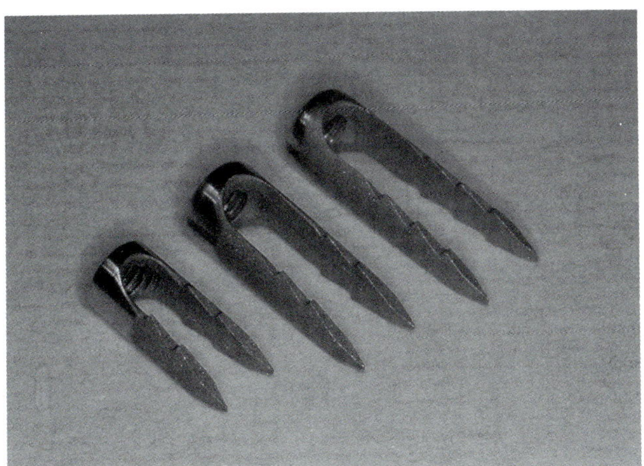

FIG. 3-59 Original style staple comes in three sizes. The crotches have been chamfered. Opposing sets of tines are visible.

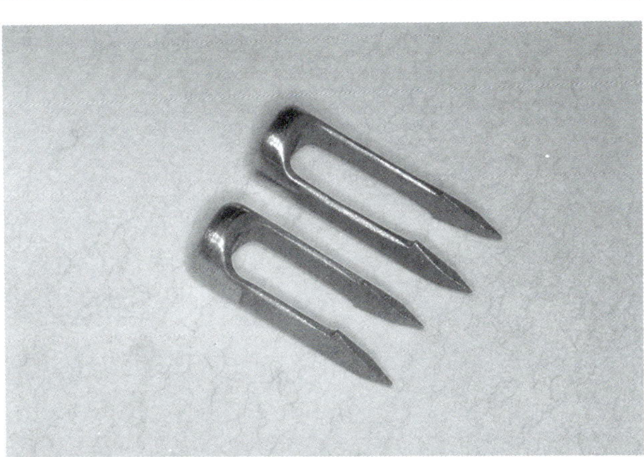

FIG. 3-61 The Profile 90 Staple comes in two sizes. Only one reverse tine exists, which allows smoother passage in tissue, thereby reducing cutting of soft tissues in the shoulder.

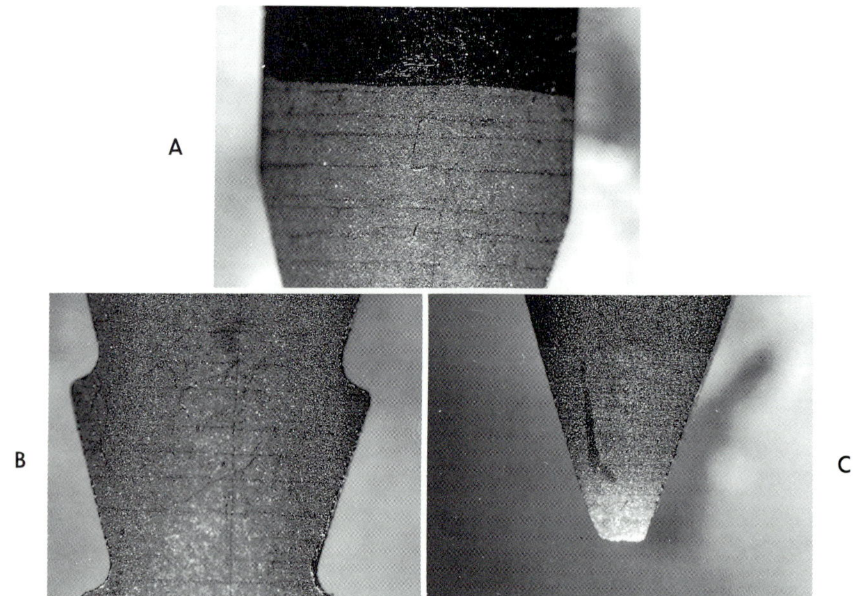

FIG. 3-62 Close-up of IM staple implanted over 1 year earlier. No corrosion.

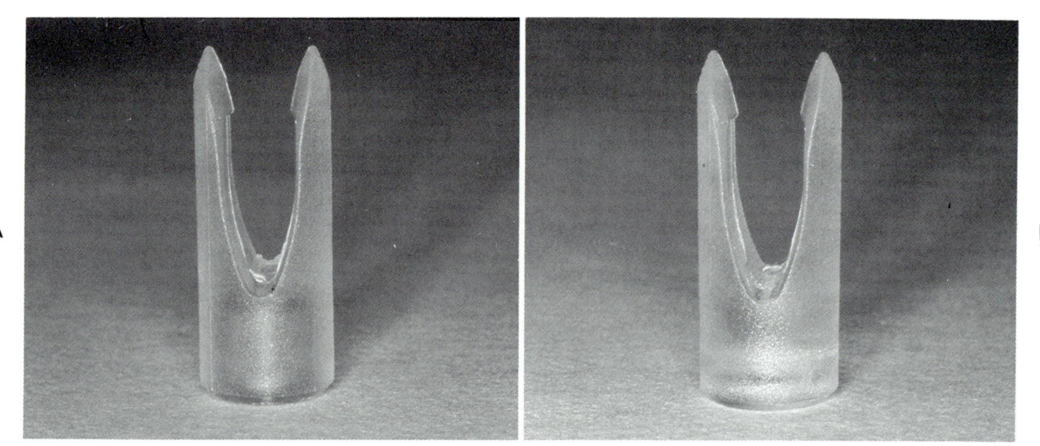

FIG. 3-63 Biodegradable staple.

A Threaded head.

B Solid head.

A 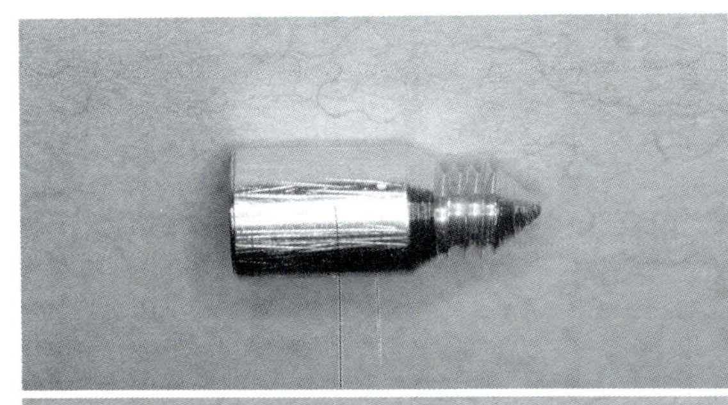

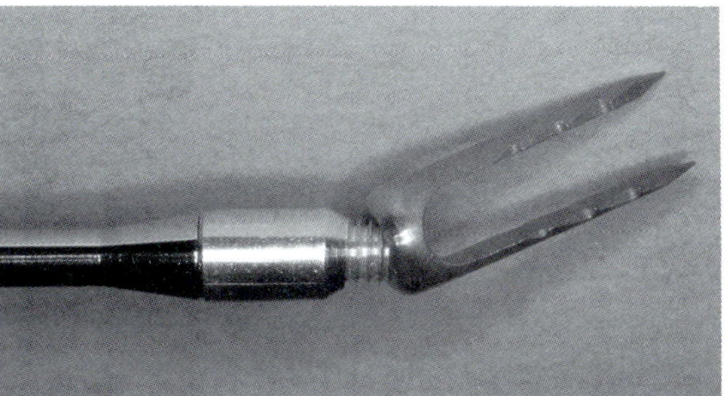 B

C 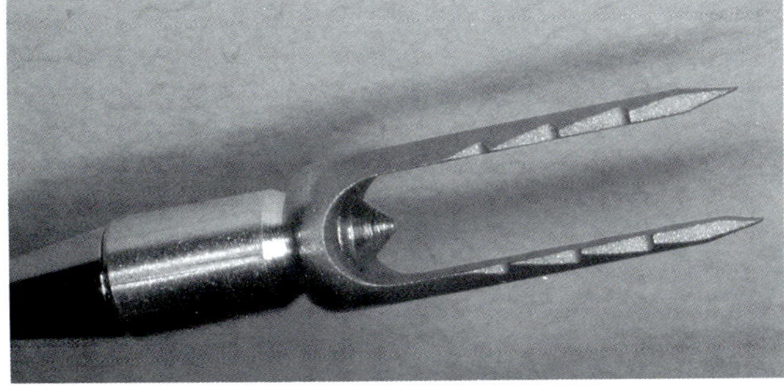

FIG. 3-64 Bullet-nosed extractor attachment.

A Gold-colored soft metal bullet acts as interface between extractor and staple for removal.

B Simulated benefit of bullet-nosed extractor attachment approaching the staple at an angle and self-seeking design.

C Extractor, bullet-nosed extractor, and staple engaged.

Cannulated Screw Sets

Transcutaneous, arthroscopically monitored, reduction-internal placement of bone fragments is technically challenging. A cannulated screw set facilitates this type of surgical procedure (Fig. 3-65). I have used screws to fix avulsion fracture of greater tuberostiy when it was pulled off with the supraspinatus tendon. The cannulation provides means of holding the bone reduced before drilling and subsequent screw placement (Fig. 3-66). After the reduction and fixation, the guide wire is removed.

Gradations in size and length are available: large, 40 to 130 mm in 5 mm gradations; and miniature, 10 to 30 mm in 2 mm gradations. Washers are available for a compression effect.

Bone Grafter

The bone grafter provides a means of procuring and delivering a cancellous bone graft by the transcutaneous method. Two sizes are available: 4 and 8 mm diameter (Fig. 3-67). Both the tube and the plunger are marked for 1 and 2 cm depths.

A 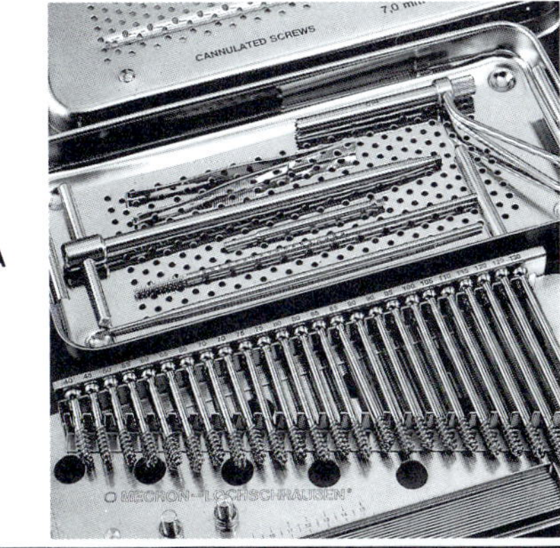

B 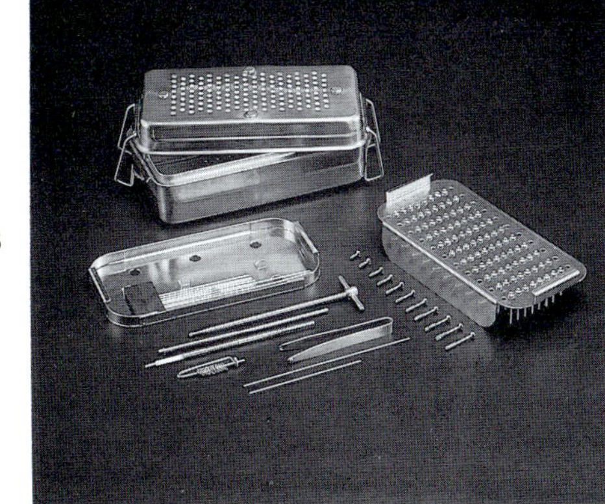

FIG. 3-65 Cannulated screw set.

A Large size for tibial plateau fractures.

B Small set for osteochondritis dessicans.

A

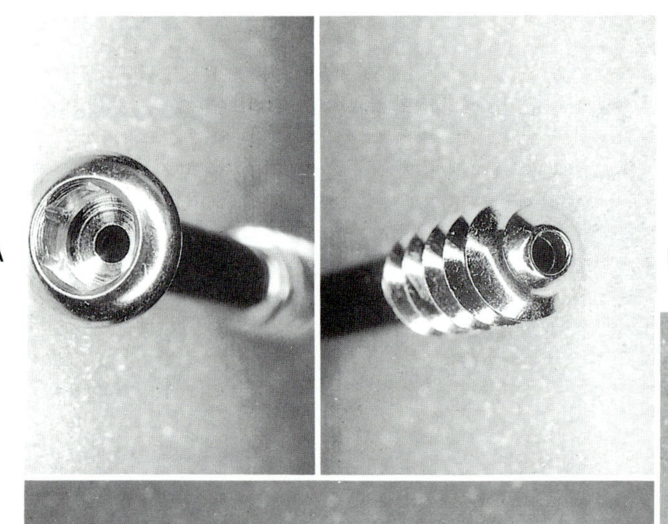

B

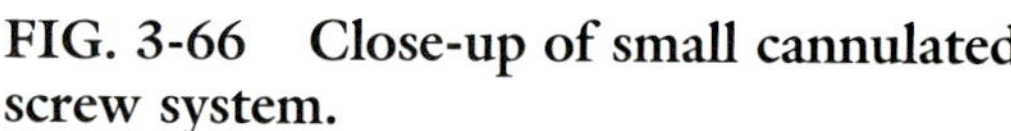

FIG. 3-66 Close-up of small cannulated screw system.

A Head of screw.

B End of screw with cancellous threads.

C *Left to right,* guide pin, countersink, drill, tap, screwdriver.

D Screw-on screwdriver over guide pin.

C

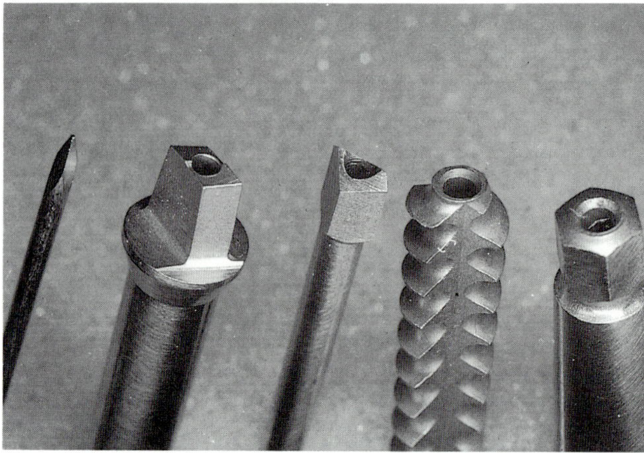

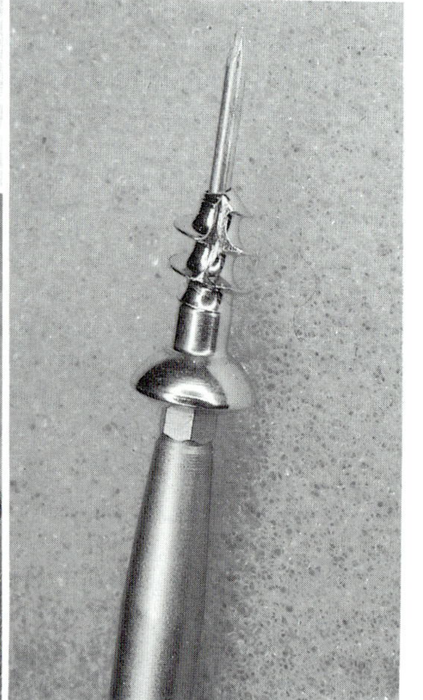

D

A

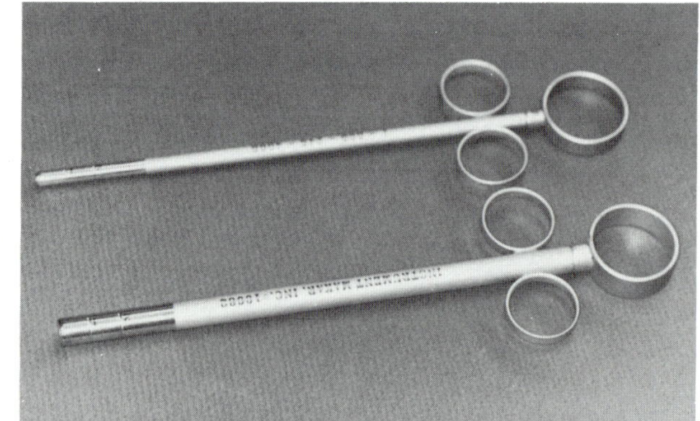

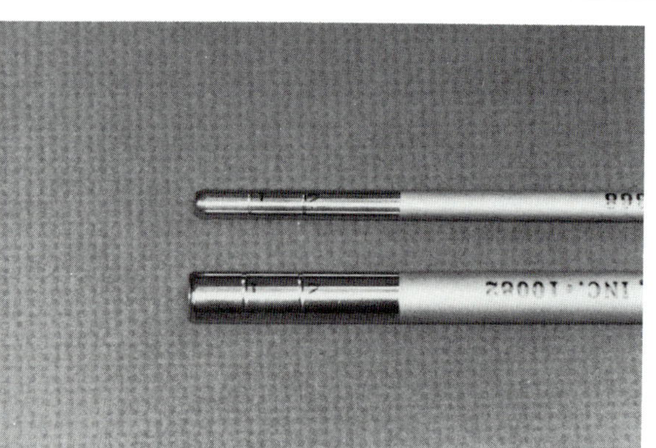

B

C

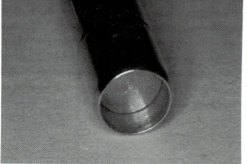

FIG. 3-67 Bone grafter.

A Two sizes; 4.0 mm and 8.0 mm diameter.

B Close-up of end shows depth markings.

C Close-up of end shows retracted plunger.

CARE OF INSTRUMENTS

Arthroscopic instruments are expensive, and they are more fragile than standard orthopedic instruments (Fig. 3-68). Proper care of instruments must be observed at all times. Besides obvious breakage related to dropping or excessive bending, injury can occur during clean-up, take-down, scrubbing, sorting, and packaging. Continuous educational efforts must be made to minimize breakage and maximize efficiency. The entire staff must take an interest, but the leadership must be by the surgeon's example.

It seems highly unlikely that a person who is not interested in arthroscopic surgery or a person on a rotational basis could take the kind of care of the arthroscopic surgical instruments, the video equipment, the suction and flow, and so on, that is necessary for this type of work. I therefore urge that one dedicated person be in charge of all a surgeon's instruments.

If no one person is assigned to this activity at an institution, the surgeon can anticipate the care of the instruments to be less than optimal. The cost of either repairing or replacing surgical instruments will be high and unnecessary. To have a team or an interested person to care for the instrumentation would be worth that dollar savings. I own my instruments, and only one person cares for them interoperatively and stores them between surgical dates.

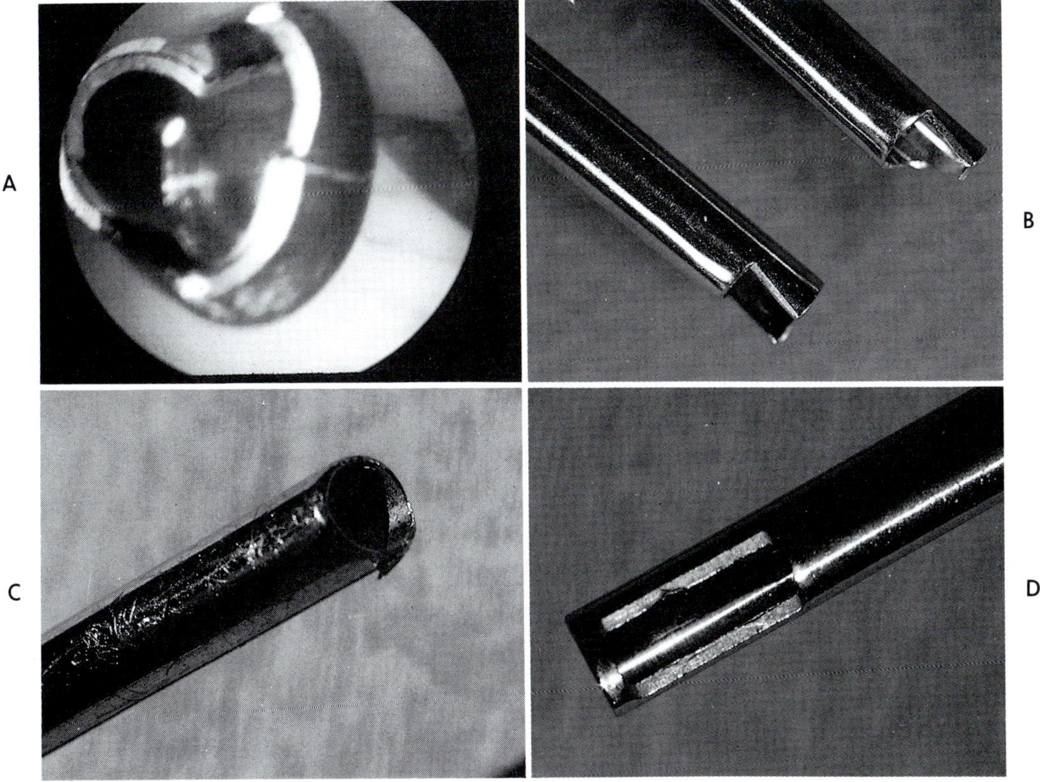

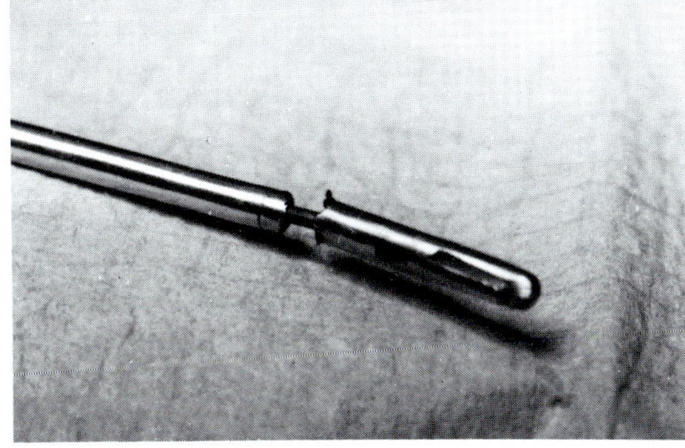

FIG. 3-68 Instrument breakage: Care of arthroscopic instruments.

A Broken cutter tip in early model.

B Fragment broken off inner rotating tube.

C Metal cut off tip of arthroscope cannula.

D Synovial resector with notch in edge after cutting cannula shown in *C*.

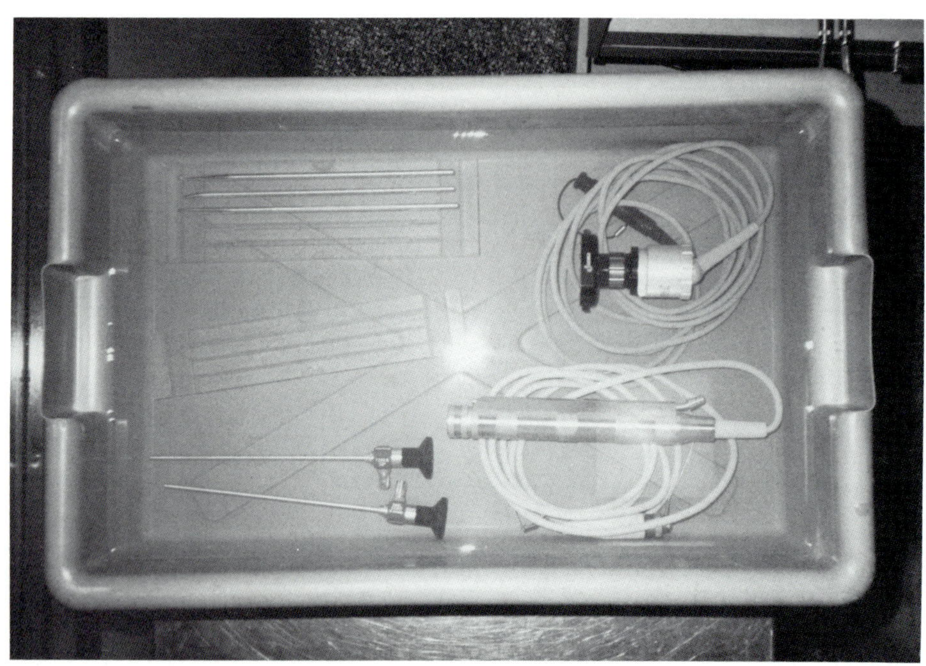

FIG. 3-69 Cidex soaking.

Sterilization and Disinfection

All metallic instrumentation may be steam autoclaved, as may most light guides. Arthroscopes deteriorate with steam autoclaving, even the ones that are advertised as being autoclavable. The life of the scope is shortened because of deterioration of the lens sealants. Ethylene oxide gas sterilization is preferred. As a practical matter, disinfection by cold soaking in activated glutaraldehyde (Cidex) is clinically safer (Fig. 3-69).[1,4,6,15]

Cold soaking is also used for motors to avoid the time necessary for the motor to cool down for comfortable handling after autoclaving. Hand-held television cameras are treated in the same manner or covered with sterile plastic. Knife blades are soaked in plastic containers to minimize handling injury, although they can be steam autoclaved.

VARIOUS ENERGY SOURCES

High-Speed Motors

The Midas Rex arthroscopic motorized instrumentation is a high-speed cutting device with a speed greater than 10,000 rpm. It was adapted from air-powered instrumentation for cement and bone resection. I have used it only in the laboratory. It is my opinion that the size, shape, contour, and concept were not, at the time of my observation, acceptable for the field of arthroscopic surgery.

I have also had an opportunity to watch videotapes of clinical cases performed with the Midas Rex. It is my opinion that the frequency of intraarticular cartilage injury depicted in those videotapes would not be acceptable in clinical practice. In its developmental state, I cannot recommend it for clinical use.

Acufex introduced a high-speed auger and cutting design in conjunction with Drs. Richard Caspari and Terry Whipple. This auger is also sold by Baxter Travenol and Biomet. The design and speed are aggressive in cutting firm, soft tissue. Clogging has been a problem, and turbulence may cause a momentary loss of visualization of the resection site. Control of resection requires a careful hand.

The introduction of these high-powered, aggressive resectors comes at a historical time in which emphasis in treatment has shifted from resection to preservation of tissue and repair.

Electrothermal Energy

Electrothermal instrumentation was developed to decrease post operative bleeding following knee joint lateral release.[2] The use of electrothermal cutting devices carries no advantage.

Electrocautery does have some benefit in shoulder arthroscopy, especially during acromionplasty. The least expensive yet effective method is the use of specially modified electrocautery probes called the Coagulators (Fig. 3-70). They come in various shapes and attach to existing generators in operating rooms, like the Bovie system. These probes are effective in sterile water or the room air environment. A more expensive system that provides electrocoagulation in electrolytic fluids is also available.

A

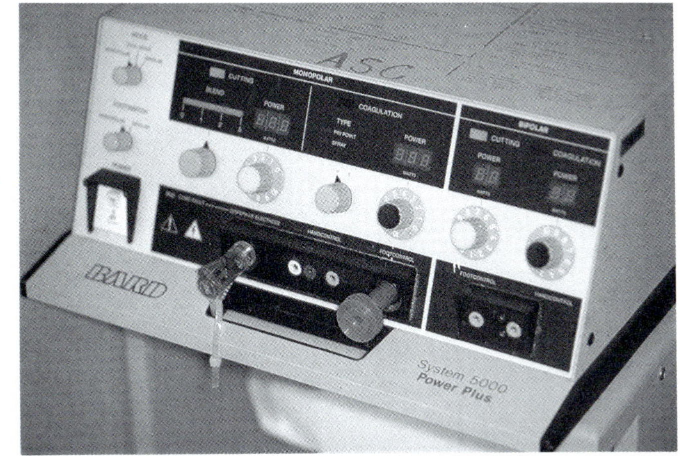

B

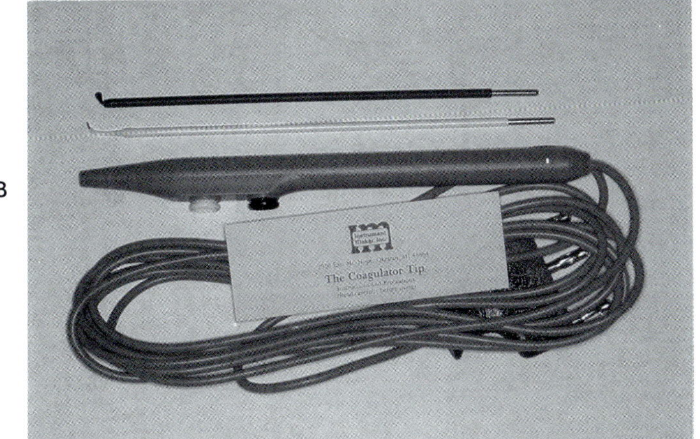

C

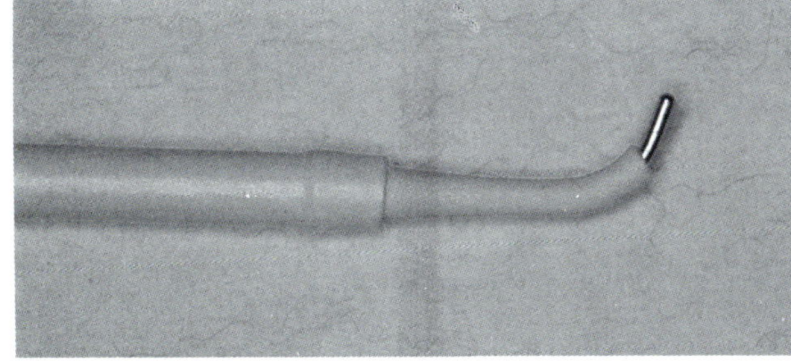

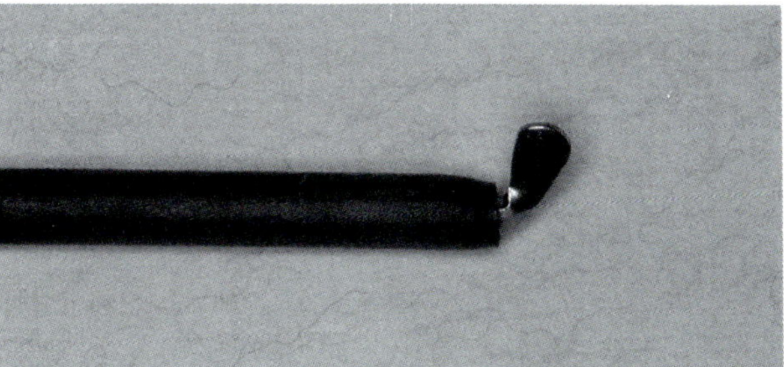

D

FIG. 3-70 Coagulators.

A A regular generator may be used with this system.

B The attachments are cost effective with this system.

C The small tip concentrates the energy.

D A paddle tip is used for outlining areas of anticipated acromioplasty.

Laser

I see no present benefit to laser energy in the shoulder.[7] It is expensive and slow. Its main advantage of hemostasis can be performed with less expense by electrocautery.

Early clinical trials in the shoulder by Dr. Chad Smith produced complications of subcutaneous emphysema of the neck and as far down as the scrotum with Helium gas.[12] In two other cases there was transient pneumothorax. Smith changed to carbon dioxide gas and reduced pressure to 1 psi.[12] Charring of tissue has been a problem following knee surgery with laser.[13,14,18]

Cryosurgery

Cryosurgery has not been of practical value in resecting tissue or effecting hemostasis.

REFERENCES

1. Crow S et al: Disinfection or sterilization? Four views on arthroscopes, *AORN J* 37:854-862, 1983.
2. Fox JM et al: Electrosurgery in orthopaedics, part 1, *Principles Contemp Orthop* 8:21, 1984.
3. Jackson RW, Dandy DJ: Arthroscopy of the knee, New York, 1980, Grune and Stratton.
4. Johnson LL et al: Two percent glutaraldehyde: a disinfectant in arthroscopy and arthroscopic surgery, *J Bone Joint Surg* 64A:237, 1982.
5. Johnson LL: Needlescope. In *American Academy of Orthopaedic Surgeons Symposium on arthroscopy and arthrography of the knee*, St Louis, 1978, Mosby–Year Book.
6. Johnson LL et al: Cold sterilization method for arthroscopes using activated dialdehyde, *Orthop Rev* 6:75, 1977.
7. Miller DV et al: The use of the contact Nd:YAG laser in arthroscopic surgery: Effects on articular cartilage and meniscal tissue, *Arthroscopy* 5(4):245-253, 1989.
8. O'Connor RL: *Arthroscopy*, Philadelphia, 1977, JB Lippincott.
9. O'Connor RL: Arthroscopy in the diagnosis and treatment of acute ligament injuries of the knee, *J Bone Joint Surg* 56A:33, 1974.
10. Prescott R: Optical design and care of the endoscope. In *American Academy of Orthopaedic Surgeons Symposium on Arthroscopy and Arthrography of the knee*, St Louis, 1978, Mosby–Year Book.
11. Prescott R: Optical principles of endoscopy, *J Med Primatol* 5:133, 1976.
12. Smith CF et al: The carbon dioxide laser: a potential tool for orthopedic surgery, *Clin Orthop* 242:43-50, 1989.
13. Smith JA: Personal communication, 1982.
14. Smith JB, Nance T: Laser energy in arthroscopic surgery. In Parisien JS, editor: *Arthroscopic surgery*, New York, 1988, McGraw-Hill.
15. Stearns CM: Preparation of arthroscopic instrumentation: the sterilization vs. disinfection controversy, *Orthop Nurs* 2:383, 1983.
16. Takagi K: The classic arthroscope, *Clin Orthop* 167:6, 1982 (from J Jap Orthop Assoc 1939).
17. Watanabe M, Takeda S, Ikeuchi H: *Atlas of arthroscopy*, ed 3, Toyko, 1979, Igaku Shoin.
18. Whipple TL, Caspari RB, Myers JF: Arthroscopic laser meniscectomy in a gas medium, *Arthroscopy* 1:2-7, 1985.
19. Wissinger HA: Personal communication, 1982.

CHAPTER

4 Documentation

Documentation is an important dimension of medical practice and must be integrated into the surgeon's daily activities.[1] Medical record information must be communicated to the patient for informed consent and to the insurance company/government agency for approval of recommended treatment and for billing purposes. Such information is also essential for medical malpractice risk management.

As of January 1, 1992, a new coding system was instituted for Medicare billing of office encounters. Under this system, the physician is to characterize the encounter based on complexity and time. The government has placed physicians on notice that spot checks will be made to determine if the billing reflected the intensity of the encounter. The medical record will be the measure used to support the magnitude of the billing. Reimbursement will be based on documentation.

In addition, the federal government has funded medical treatment outcome studies. This decision places a great emphasis on collection of patient demographic and treatment result data. Outcome studies are intended not only to evaluate various treatments, but also the doctors who render those treatments.

For these and other reasons I have developed over the past 11 years a computerized medical record.[4] I rely on this computerized system to store and generate reports on the patient's medical history, shoulder examination, x-ray results—even to the point of using the protocol to write the referral letters. The amount of time saved is tremendous, and in large part this system has replaced my former methods. This chapter details my experience with documentation methods, with an emphasis on the use of computers and video technology.

INITIAL DOCUMENTATION

Handwritten Chart Notes

Although the standard of practice in the past, handwritten notes now serve only an immediate purpose in documentation. They are not as suitable as a more legible, typed medical record.

Handwritten notes are valuable in an emergency situation and during hospitalization. They provide immediate postoperative documentation in the hospital flow chart while the permanent operative report is being prepared. Progress notes in the hospital and office provide timely documentation during the ongoing care of the patient and are necessary for communication between care givers. Handwritten notes may help reconstruct the patient's data base if dictation equipment fails.

Dictated Narrative

The dictated narrative medical record has been the standard of practice but has many limitations. These limitations include inconsistent order of recordings and deletion of essential information. Anyone who has ever performed retrospective clinical research would agree. A look back at some of my old medical records shows sketchy ramblings, apparently hurriedly constructed, perhaps even after the fact. Today, the best way of producing a dictated medical record is by a protocol at the time of the encounter so that the order of the report is consistent and deletions are avoided.

So many and varied events occur during postoperative, follow-up patient care that I have been unable to produce a practical protocol. Recognizing that a protocol would have to be long and complicated while the dictations were concise, I opted for dictation of these patient encounters. The information is not lost when material is subject to computerization. Software exists to search narratives for various subject material by words and even syllables. Recording progress notes related to the office hours still is an effective use of dictation.

Work Sheets/Diagrams

Work sheets and diagrams have been replaced by the computerized medical record. Drawings of unusual lesions can be helpful when placed in any part of the medical record. My computerized medical record includes a place for a drawing on the work sheet (see Appendix A, Form 4). Although computer software exists for drawings, at this time its use is impractical.

THE COMPUTERIZED MEDICAL RECORD

During my medical practice lifetime, the demands on the physician to collect, record, retrieve, and report information have grown enormously. Insurance company and governmental requirements have largely produced these ever-increasing demands. Also, medical malpractice risk management principles demand a comprehensive medical record. Documentation requirements are increasing in the face of increasing time constraints. With the multitude of reasons for documenting medical information, the value of such a record in patient care must not be overlooked.

As a result of these requirements and my interest in clinical research, I developed a proprietary computerized medical record for my practice. The software is called the Benevolent Dictator* and was written in C-language.[4] It runs on a personal computer as a stand alone or can be networked in multiterminal systems. This software functions on MS DOS or UNIX operating systems. The shoulder joint is one of many orthopedic modules in the program.

It is not the purpose of this text to provide all the details of this, or any, computerized medical record system. The following discussion is intended to explain the components and benefits of such systems.

Data Collection Forms

The common denominator of a computerized medical record is the data collection forms (see Appendix A, Forms 1A, 2A, 3A, and 4A). The multiple data points are best established over time and with daily use in clinical practice. Data must be collected for both billing and patient care purposes. Even if you do not anticipate computerizing your practice, you should construct or purchase forms that collect data in an organized manner. The best method is to collect data on forms that are used with existing computerized medical record software, so that if you later change to computers, the data can be placed retroactively into electronic files.

*Information Health Network, 2950 Mount Hope, Okemos, MI 48864

Surgeons have an inherent resistance to function by protocol. Most physicians believe that they are flexible and do not function by protocol. Furthermore, if they did, their protocol would be different than that of all other surgeons. In reality, all doctors work from some system, and the data points they use in their system are not unlike those used by their colleagues. The only differences in protocol are the number and order of the data points.

The use of a form arranges the data points into a protocol. The organization of the protocol can change over time to make the collection of data easy and practical. Input from physician users fine tunes the protocol. The "final protocol," if there ever is one, will not be that of any one doctor. The computerized medical record (CMR) illustrated here is not solely of my input, although I supervised its construction. Many surgeon users regularily contribute to enhancements.

Minimal Data Set

Because of the interest in outcome studies created by federal government funding, various organizations are addressing the minimal data set for various orthopedic conditions. Those investigations presently underway include total hip, fractured hip, total knee, and spine. The American Society of Shoulder and Elbow Surgeons is developing a minimal data set for patient encounters; the committee is headed by Louis Bigliani of New York. Ultimately, a minimal data set will be constructed in modular fashion. There will be a basic data set for demographics, a second for general medical history, a third for general orthopedics, and branching for each orthopedic subspecialty. At this time one has not been established for shoulder problems. The initial information collected will be correlated with subsequent follow-up data sets for outcome research.

The CMR shown here is modular in construction with software that provides for addition, deletion, and shifting of data points without loss of previous data.

THE PERFECT COMPUTERIZED MEDICAL RECORD

The following characteristics of the perfect medical record have been suggested at various committee meetings I have attended:

1. It would be simple and sophisticated.
2. It would be short and comprehensive.
3. Neither the patient nor the staff would have to do anything.
4. The physician would not have to change his or her ways.
5. No work would be involved.
6. It would be automatically available to everyone concerned with the proviso that confidentiality was protected.
7. It would be free.

This type of idealistic thinking only defers the day of computerization of one's medical practice.

THE BENEVOLENT DICTATOR SYSTEM

In the absence of the perfect computerized medical record, I started construction of forms in 1980. I was motivated by the desire to do clinical research without spreading and sorting charts all over my office floor. An added motivation was the medical malpractice–risk management aspect following an out of court settlement because of one of my records having inadequate documentation.

I wanted a system that collected data points for research and produced narrative record for hospital medical records. Forms were constructed for general orthopedic history, supplemental histories for anatomical regions like the knee and shoulder, and general orthopedics (see Appendix A, Form 1). A physical examination form was established for the knee and shoulder (see Appendix A, Form 2). An x-ray report was developed for both areas (see Appendix A, Form 3). An operative report was constructed for the knee and subsequently the shoulder (see Appendix A, Form 4). Modules now exist for the hand, spine, elbow, hip, foot and ankle.

Subsequently, software was constructed to meet the need for patient communication and referring physician letters (see Appendix A, Forms 5 to 7). Over time, while practicing, I identified all the factors involved in the initial patient encounter. These factors were placed on a form in an orderly and logical fashion for both collection and transmission of information regarding this encounter to the patient and referring physician. Although I "write" the letters by dictation while reading through the protocol, I have illustrated the forms and this method with a completed patient letter in writing (see Appendix A, Form 5A), plus the subsequent typed letter (see Appendix C, Form 5B). The data input for the patient letter is converted to the referring doctor letter with a single push of a key by the keyboard operator (see Appendix A, Form 6).

COLLECTION OF PATIENT MEDICAL HISTORY INFORMATION IN THE OFFICE

Three options are given to the new patient for means of collecting medical historical data. They may have printed forms to fill out by hand writing. A second method of input is by keyboard while reading routine questions on a computer screen. The other way is by interactive video.

Interactive Video (History Makar)

The Benevolent Dictator System serves my purposes well, but to date has not been a commercial success. One of the objections is the length of the forms; physicians are concerned that their patients will reject this system of data collection.

The application of interactive video technology to patient data collection has overcome this objection. I have combined interactive video technology to our medical record software to simplify the collection of patient historical data and instantaneously produce a type narrative (Fig. 4-1).

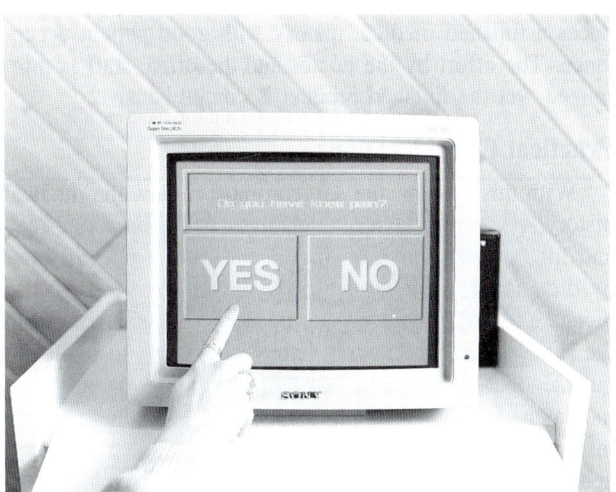

FIG. 4-1 Interactive video.

The new patient fills out the basic demographic and billing information form by hand so that the physical medical chart can be constructed while the patient is using the interactive video. Also, because billing information requires checking long insurance policy numbers, this approach gives the staff a head start.

The patient sits down in front of the television monitor and touches the screen to start the interaction. The doctor's image appears on the monitor to discuss the importance of this process. Next come instructions by illustration on the screen and voiceover instructions by the staff. The television screen then presents the first of a series of written questions with voiceover. There is a place on-screen with the proper response for the patient to touch. After the screen is touched, the next screen appears. When the patient answers "yes," branching automatically occurs within the software to ask more specific questions to define the problem. When the patient answers "no" the software automatically skips to the next category (Fig. 4-1). When completed, a narrative report is generated on a laser printer. The patient removes the rough draft from the printer. He or she reviews the history, makes corrections by hand, and signs this draft.

Patient acceptance of this method is good. Although this process takes an average of 40 minutes, questioning after the visit shows the patient believes the interactive video experience lasts only 20 minutes.

The medical history draft is taken to the surgeon at the time of the patient interview. The draft has space for the surgeon to make further notations (see Appendix A, Form 8).

After the interview and examination, the paperwork is given to the staff. The rough copy generated by the patient is brought up on the monitor, corrections and additions are made, and a final report is stored electronically and generated (see Appendix A, Form 1C).

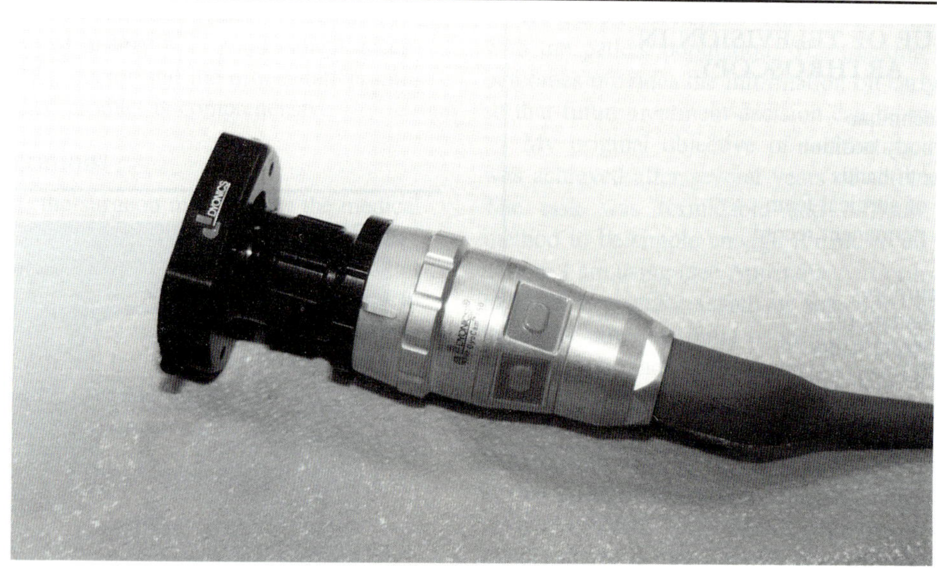

FIG. 4-3 Hand-held television camera.

Hand-Held Video Camera

The hand-held miniaturized television cameras have antiquated other systems of projecting an image (Fig. 4-3). These cameras are coupled with a light source that varies the intensity with the needs of the camera to produce an image. The electronic output is projected on a monitor, recorded on videotape, and available for slide and print photography. The most common system used at our institution is the Dyonics model Dyocam 750.

Video-Generated Slides/Prints

This system of slide and print production is simple (Fig. 4-4). The video image is captured electronically without interruption of the surgical procedure. However, the video-generated slides are not as sharp as those made by conventional photography. They are grainy and lack color balance. Nonetheless, this type of slide may be suitable for lecture presentation slide projection. The prints are acceptable for the patient's chart. Some surgeons give printouts to the patient as a marketing tool.

We have a Polaroid system for making slides and prints depending on the film used (Fig. 4-4). This system does not produce instant development of slides or prints. This method requires that each surgeon have his or her own camera, so that photos taken by one surgeon are not confused with those of another. More expensive and higher quality producing electronic camera systems are available.

Recently, Dr. David Shnieder in our institution adapted a retail Sony printer for our video systems. This adaptation makes prints of functional quality. It is model #CVP-G500 and retails for $1000. Prices of higher quality systems are over $5000.

35 mm. Slide Photography

The best quality 35 mm slide photographs are made with a single-lens reflex camera attached via an adaptor directly to the arthroscope with Ektachrome ASA 400 color film. Procurement of these photos requires detaching the television camera, re-gloving, and changing the arthroscope to maintain sterility. These photographs are of publication quality.

I use an older model Olympus OM 1 camera and an adaptor (Fig. 4-5). A good quality image requires a matching color balance between the film and the light source. Our Dyonics 510 light source generates illumination in the 550 K range. Unfortunately, the present day light sources are balanced for television and do not produce a good color image on 35 mm slides.

I use Kodak Ektachrome ASA 400 film which is fast enough to take photos with available light at $1/30$ to $1/8$ seconds. The lesser time is used for bright reflecting articular cartilage and the longer time for cavities like the subacromial space. Faster films up to ASA 1000 have not proven any better. Black and white prints do not illustrate the arthroscopic image as well as color photos. Also, the conversion of color slides to black and white for publication do not have the detail of the original.

A

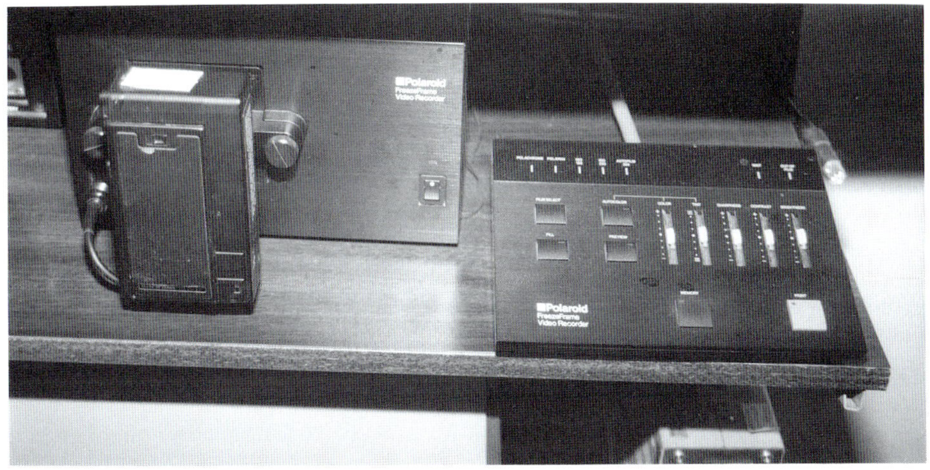

FIG. 4-4 Polaroid generated slides.

A Polaroid slide generator.

B Sample slide from electronic image.

C Sony Video Printer CVP-G500.

B

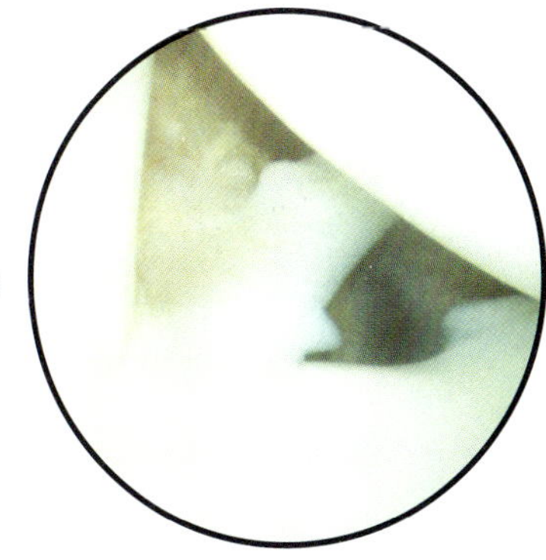

C

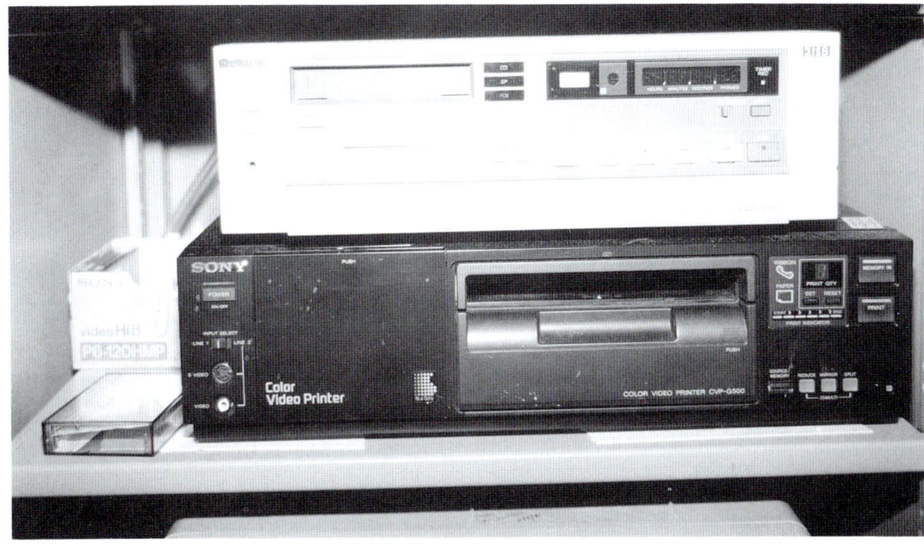

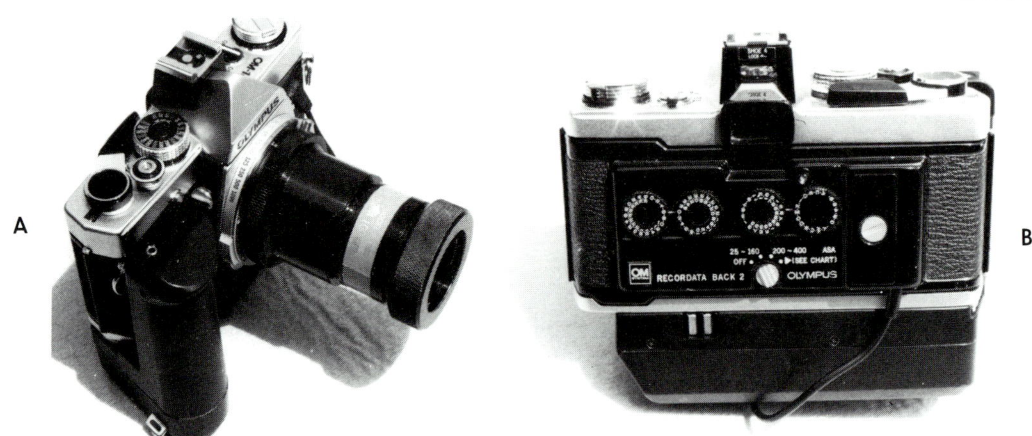

FIG. 4-5 35 mm slide photographic camera.

A Motor drive and direct scope attachment with single lens.

B Databack 2 for Olympus system.

Movie Photography

As the quality of intraarticular video has improved the need for movie photography has become obsolete. Some presentations are made with outside movie photography to be combined with inside film after conversion of the video to this format.

REFERENCES

1. Haralson RH III: Computerized information retrieval and medical education for orthopedists, *JBJS* 70A(4):624-629, 1988.
2. Jackson DW, Ovadia DN: Video arthroscopy: present and future developments, *Arthroscopy*, 2:108, 1985.
3. Jackson DW: Video arthroscopy: a permanent medical record, *Am J Sports Med* 6:213, 1978.
4. Johnson LL: A rationale for systematized record keeping and improved documentation, *Arthroscopy* 3(4):258-264, 1987.
5. McGinty JB: Closed circuit television in arthroscopy, *Int Rev Rheumatid* 35:45-49, 1976, (special edition devoted to arthroscopy).

CHAPTER

5 Arthroscopic Surgical Principles

The principles of arthroscopic surgery of the shoulder are adaptations of known basic surgical principles practiced for years during conventional open surgery. The adaptation of the open surgical principles to arthroscopy occurred during the development of arthroscopic surgery of the knee.[15-17,19,21] These basic surgical principles must be appreciated and implemented for successful arthroscopic shoulder surgery.[45]

TRANSFERRED GENERAL SURGICAL PRINCIPLES

Knowledge

Basic knowledge of the shoulder structure, function, injury, and disease is a prerequisite. Knowledge gained in care of patients with shoulder problems and open surgery can form a foundation for arthroscopy.[28,34,35] Anatomical dissections and cadaver surgical exploration should precede any arthroscopic procedure (see Chapter 6). The subsequent shoulder arthroscopy techniques developed will enhance or build on the previous experience of any orthopedic surgeon who cares for patients with shoulder joint problems.

Arthroscopy widens the surgeon's perspective of anatomical structure, function, and relationships. The arthroscope allows access to areas of shoulder joints not before appreciated by open methods.[6] More specifically, the arthroscope offers an inside-out view rather than the conventional outside-in perspective.[13] The anatomical structures remain in situ, providing enhanced appreciation of the intraarticular structures.

Surgical Plan

Planning of the arthroscopic surgery is necessary so that you do not paint yourself into a corner (Fig. 5-1). Lack of planning may be manifest by prolonging the arthroscopic attempt at surgery such that resultant extravasation of fluids or lack of anesthesia time precludes shifting to an open procedure.

Asepsis

Infection is a rare complication of arthroscopy, although it does occur, especially when direct viewing immediately precedes open surgery.[22,23] A complete skin preparation and sterile draping should precede open surgery if direct viewing is performed. The system outlined in this textbook gives arthroscopic surgical sterile technique the same respect as in open procedures.

Hemostasis

Hemostasis is provided during the shoulder arthroscopy with fluid distention, adrenalin solutions, and electrocautery. Also, air instillation can have a drying effect on tissues and promote hemostasis (see Fig. 5-4, *A*). This later technique is especially useful in arthroscopic acromionectomy. Postoperative hemostasis is enhanced with a compression dressing.

Gentleness

The restrictions of space, size of instruments, and delicacy of the articular cartilage require maximum gentleness in arthroscopic surgery. Any lack of gentleness is magnified by the lens systems and projected on television for all to see. The arthroscopist has a minimal margin for error.

Working From Known to Unknown

The general surgical principle of working from known to unknown is absolutely necessary in arthroscopy. The arthroscopic view is small; if the view is up close to a structure, no adjacent landmark for orientation is identifiable (Fig. 5-2). During arthroscopy, the view should be as wide as possible to show relative anatomical relationships. If a close-up view is necessary, the scope can be moved in and

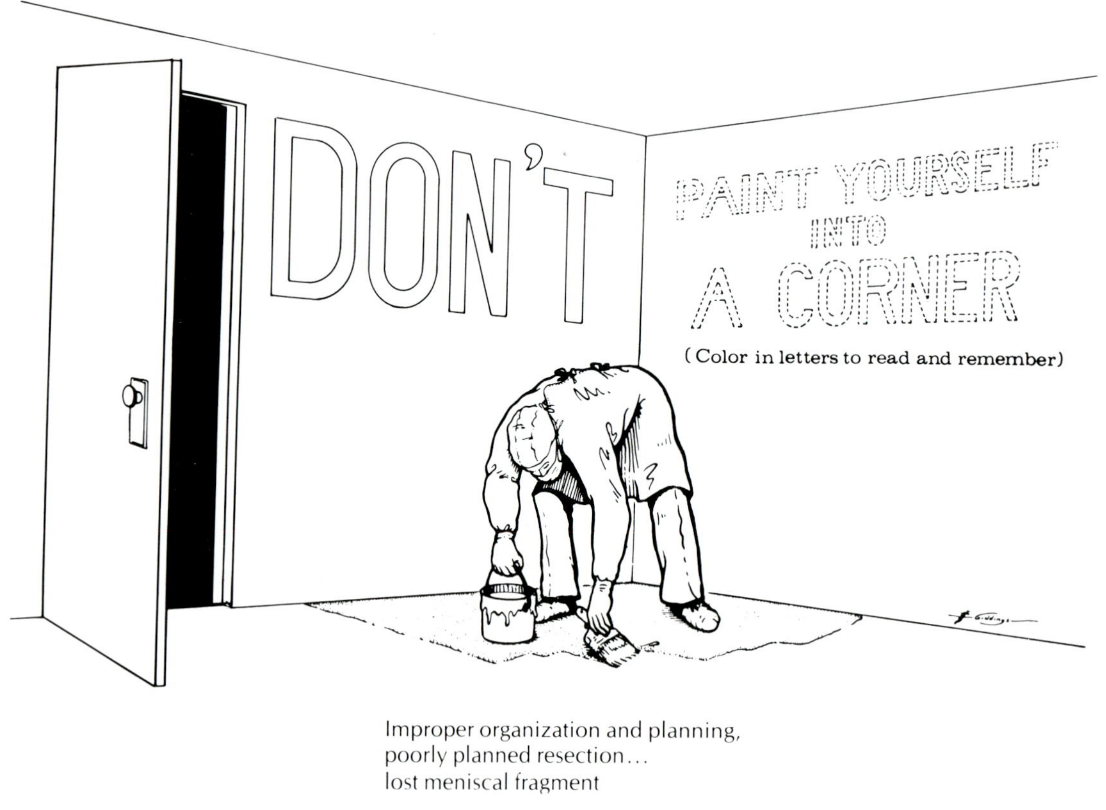
DON'T
PAINT YOURSELF
INTO
A CORNER
(Color in letters to read and remember)
Improper organization and planning,
poorly planned resection...
lost meniscal fragment

FIG. 5-1 Don't paint yourself into a corner.

out for perspective (pistoning) (see Fig. 5-45). In the shoulder joint, the biceps tendon is the initial landmark and the humeral head surface serves as a horizontal reference point (Fig. 5-3).

Orientation in the glenohumeral joint is achieved by knowledge of the biceps tendon position of attachment to the superior glenoid (Fig. 5-4). If lost, the surgeon should go back to the last known area. The scope may scan back and forth from a known landmark like the humeral horizon to the less distinct homogenous areas (i.e., articular cartilage) to maintain orientation.

Orientation in the subacromial space may be difficult not only because of the patient's reclined position, but also because anatomical structures are not well defined. This problem may be overcome by preliminary placement of transcutaneous needles into the space to gain perspective (Fig. 5-5).

Retracing of steps may be necessary to regain position. The surgeon should walk himself or herself through the joint as with a flashlight in a darkened room (Fig. 5-6). The surgeon's head should be looking in the same direction as the light is shining. In case of arthroscopy, this maneuver is performed by rotating the 30 degrees–inclined arthroscope.

"Getting lost" is a common problem for the beginning arthroscopist. The classic "whiteout" and "redout" pictures confirm you are lost (Fig. 5-7). The surgeon should stop at this point and retrace his or her steps or return to an area of identifiable anatomy.

Attention to Detail

Many details involve surgical judgment, technique, and result. These details are not unique to arthroscopy, although arthroscopy seems to demand a higher level of attention to detail and surgical technique than the more familiar open surgical methods.

Momentum

Maintaining momentum throughout all operative procedures is essential. The concept of momentum means

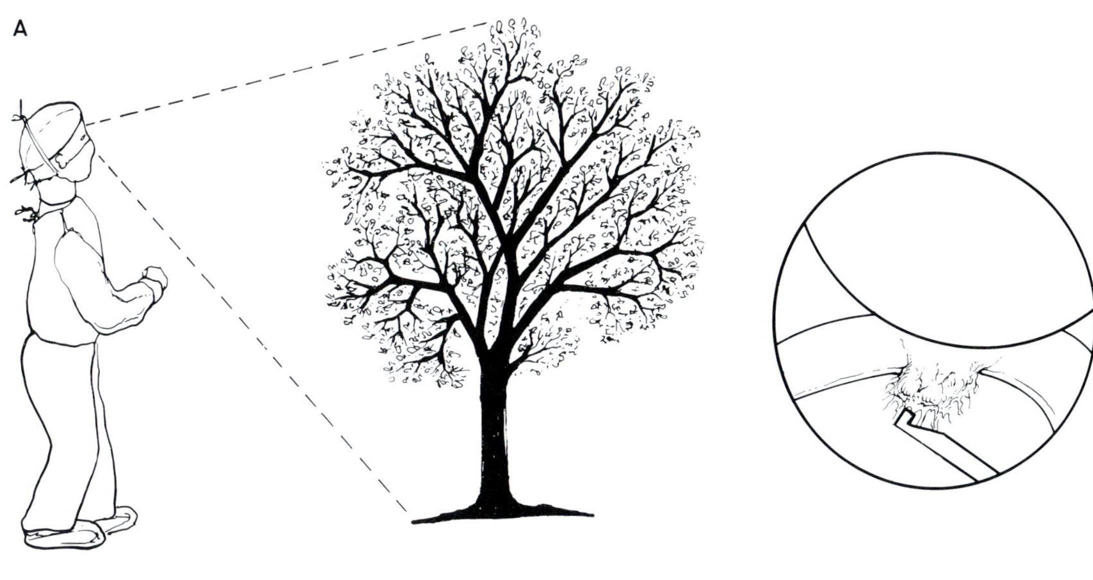

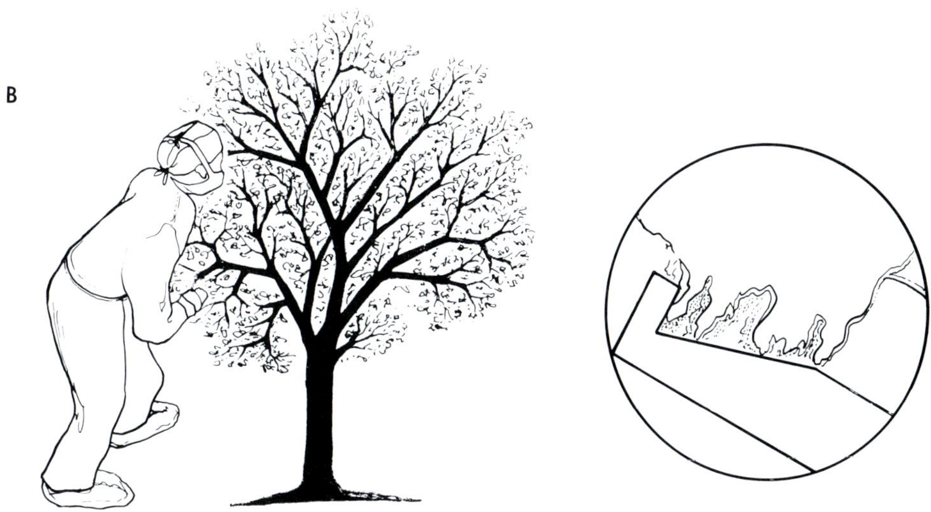

FIG. 5-2 Optimal position of arthroscope.

A Scope retracted to give overview.

B Surgeon and scope too close to lesion for comfort or instrumentation.

there is a continuous flow of sequential events that result in a steady progression toward completion of the task at hand. Many potentially distracting events in surgery can interrupt the flow of the procedure. Intraoperative complications such as a broken instrument, excessive bleeding, inattention of the assistants, or surgeon fatigue interferes with momentum. Once the momentum is lost, every effort must be made to regain the smooth functioning teamwork and progress throughout the procedure. Such an effort may even require stopping and regrouping. The many details involved in arthroscopy create an even greater risk of loss of momentum. If the surgeon is not aware of this principle, he or she will achieve momentum but be left to wander to and fro without a steady progression.

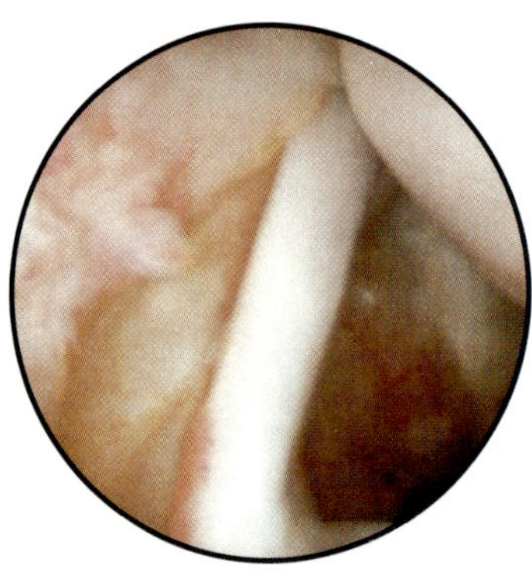

FIG. 5-3 Arthroscopic view of biceps tendon provides the best initial landmark for orientation.

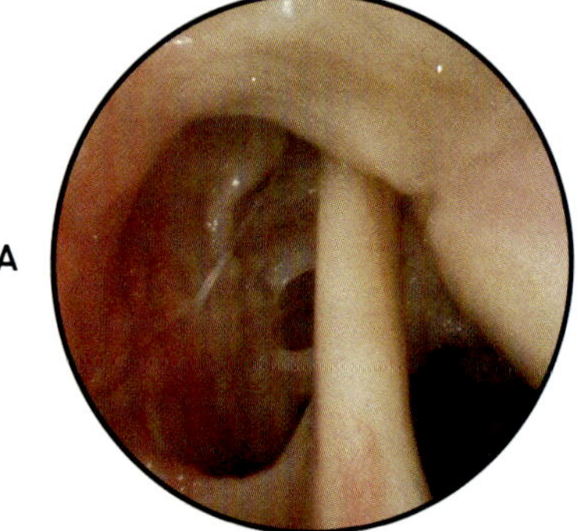

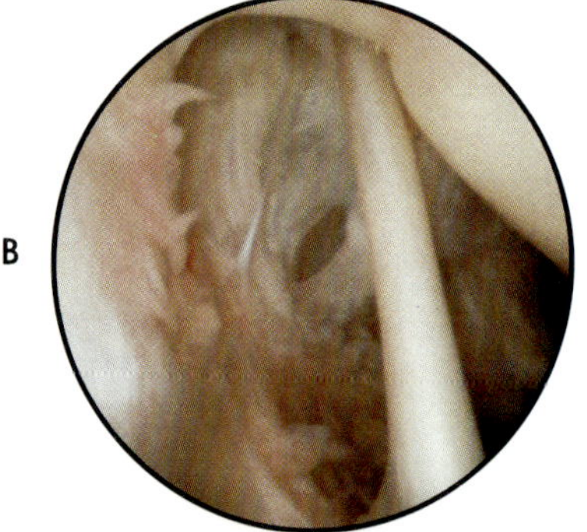

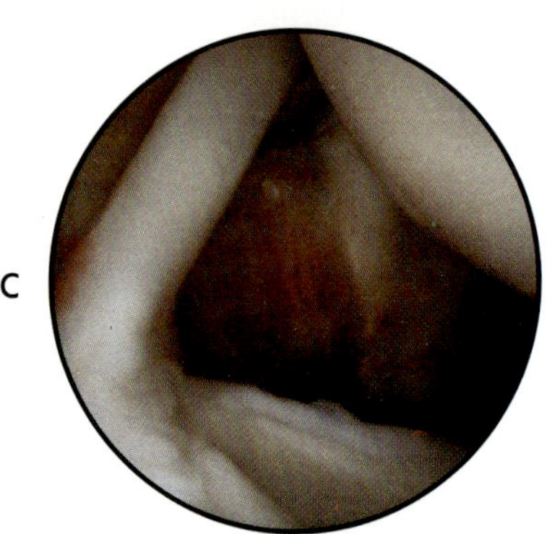

FIG. 5-4 Initial arthroscopic views in air and fluid.

A Air distention. Note biceps tendon, optical clarity, and vascularity.

B Adrenaline fluid distention. Note blanching of tissue due to adrenaline effect.

C Arthroscopic view of biceps tendon, glenoid, and superior humeral head. This triangular area is orientation position for penetration of the arthroscope to anterior in the glenohumeral joint.

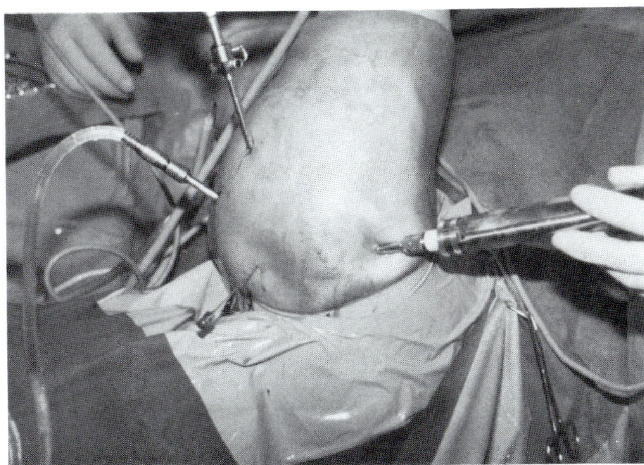

FIG. 5-5 Orientation in the subacromial space is assisted by transcutaneous placement of needles. The position of the needle is known and penetration into the subacromial space gives landmark for orientation of arthroscope and instruments.

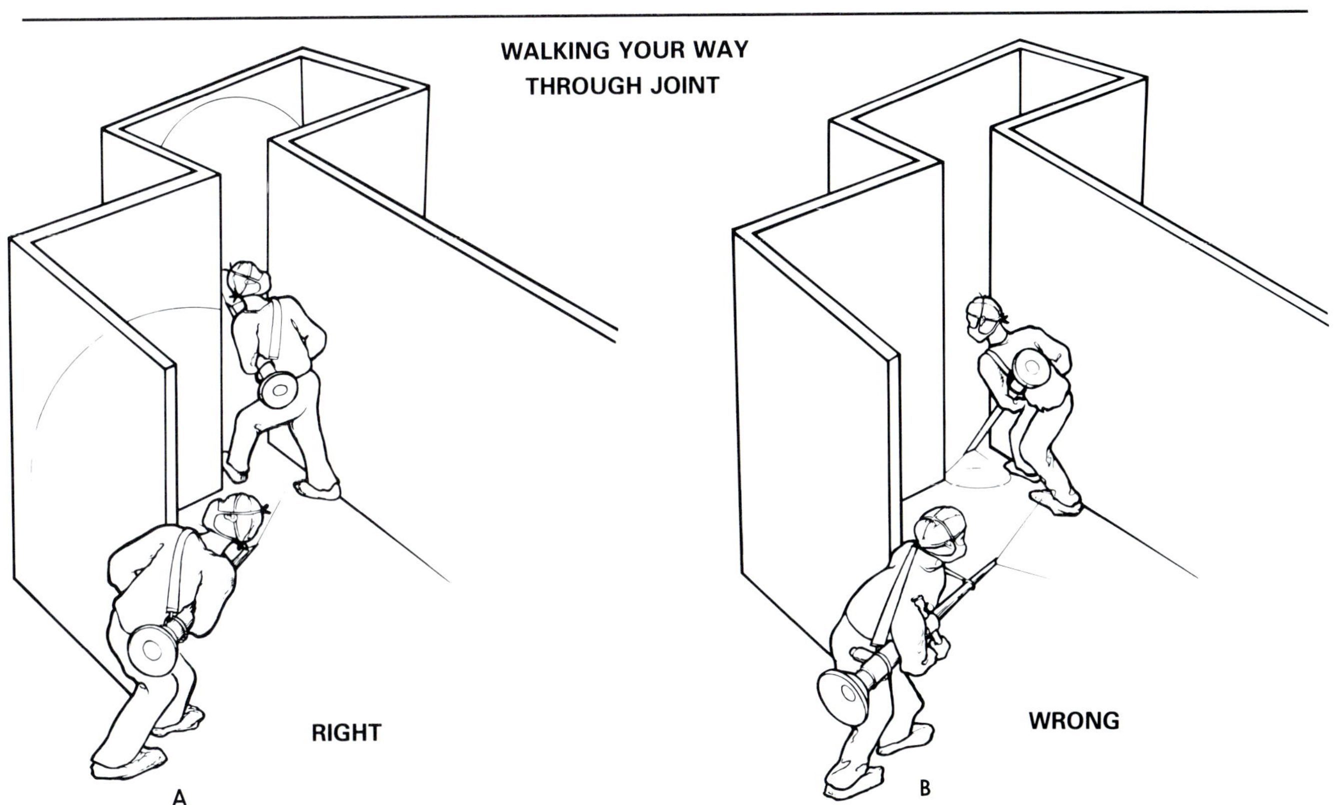

FIG. 5-6 Following light around corners.

A Right.

B Wrong.

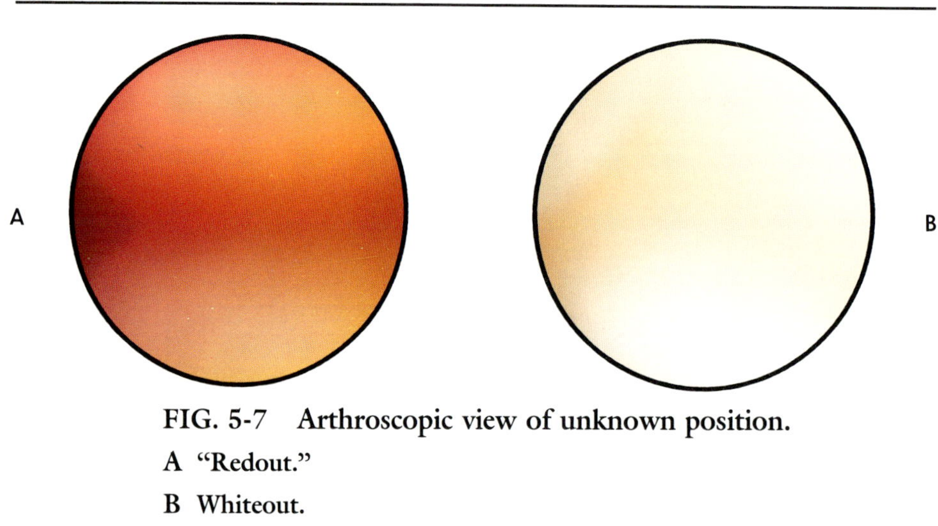

FIG. 5-7 Arthroscopic view of unknown position.
A "Redout."
B Whiteout.

SPECIALIZED ARTHROSCOPIC KNOWLEDGE

It can not go without saying that an understanding of arthroscopy's unique environment and principles is crucial. No matter what or how vast the orthopedic surgeon's experience or number of years in open or arthroscopic surgery, he or she still will require specialized knowledge and training before approaching the shoulder joint with an arthroscope.

The unique arthroscopic surgical environment must be appreciated. Arthroscopy is usually performed in a fluid medium instead of room air. Proper patient position, arthroscope placement, fluid distention, and external manipulation are principles utilized in arthroscopic surgery to create surgical exposure.

The monocular arthroscope produces only a two-dimensional image. The surgeon must compensate for this loss of depth perception by scope movement, knowledge of anatomy and pathology, appreciation of relative sizes, and instrument palpation.

The surgeon is remote from the anatomical structures. To compensate, the surgeon mentally projects himself or herself into the joint (Fig. 5-8).

Problems can occur in shoulder arthroscopy because the patient is in a reclined unanatomical-oriented position. The surgeon must choose to orientate the scope to the operating room floor or to the anatomical position of the shoulder. If the surgeon chooses to correct the anatomical position of the shoulder, the arthroscope is rotated 90 degrees. The picture on the television monitor will appear as if the patient is in vertical position. If the surgeon accepts the patient's surgical position, then the arthroscope must be orientated to the room horizonal position on the television monitor. I prefer to accept the real position in space and compensate for the anatomical relationships with adjustment in my mind. This approach provides for no other spatial relationship correction while passing surgical instruments (Fig. 5-9).

In either case, the surgeon should ignore his or her body and hand outside positions. Repeated glances to outside positions distract and confuse orientation (Fig. 5-10). The hands should be felt, not inspected. Only when the surgeon is completely lost should he or she look at the hands or the instrument. External viewing may be helpful to get perspective of triangulation during placement of a second instrument. Otherwise, the surgeon must focus only on the view on the television monitor. All other placements and surgical maneuvers are made in relation to the initial choice of orientation.

The distortion produced by arthroscope inclination may require removing the television camera and direct viewing to gain orientation. After the direction of the arthroscope is determined, the motion of pistoning or rotation is viewed in relationship to the original perspective. When the surgeon is reoriented, video monitoring can be resumed.

The inability to directly touch the anatomical structures is compensated for by developing skill with instrument probing (Fig. 5-11).

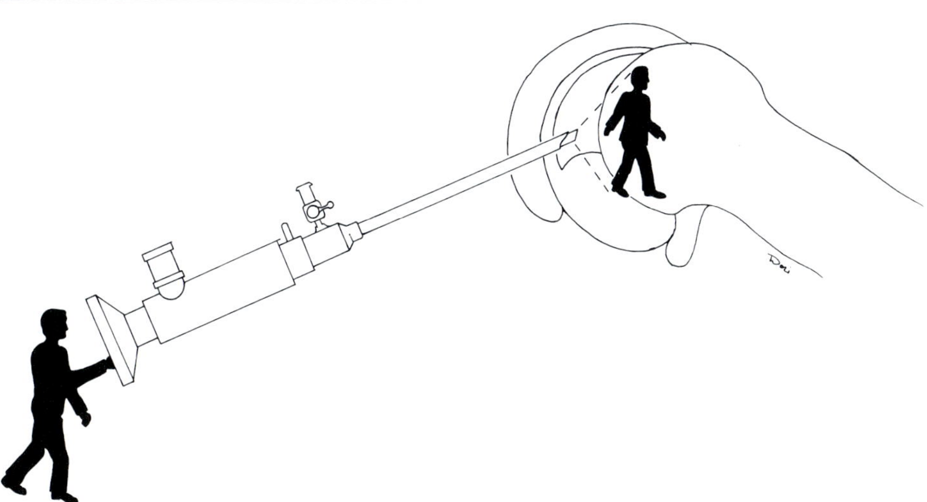

FIG. 5-8 Mental projection into joint.

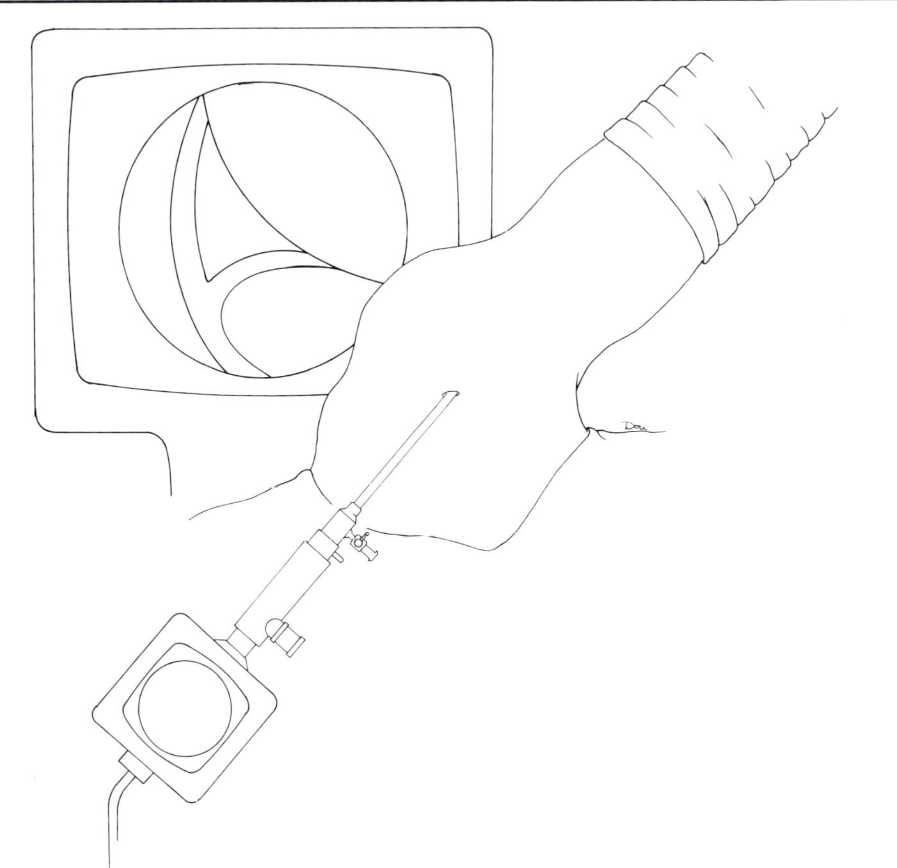

FIG. 5-9 Horizontal orientation of television image, without regard to body or scope position, is necessary to accomplish maneuver.

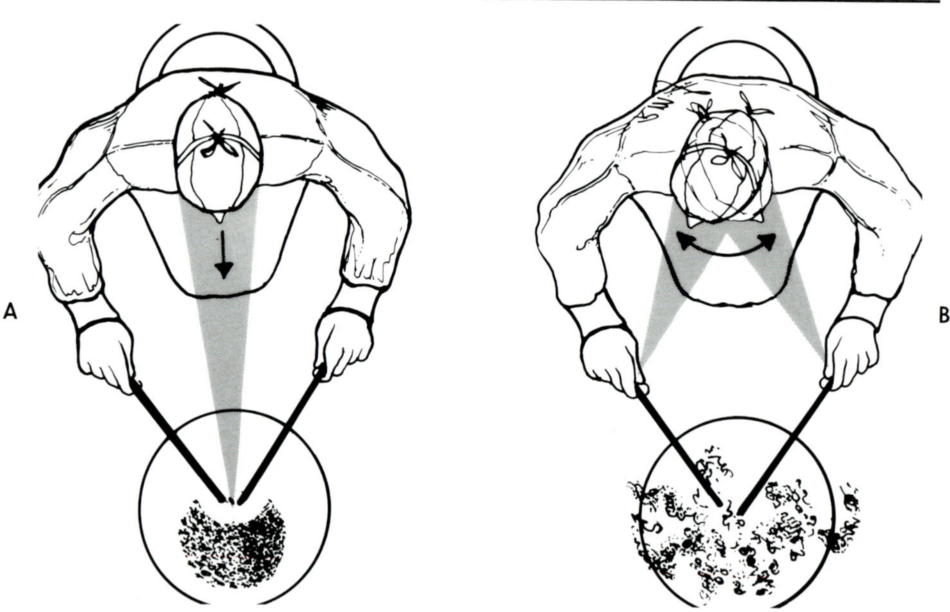

FIG. 5-10 Surgeon's focus on inside of shoulder.
A Inside focus gives best control.
B Outside look causes loss of control and position.

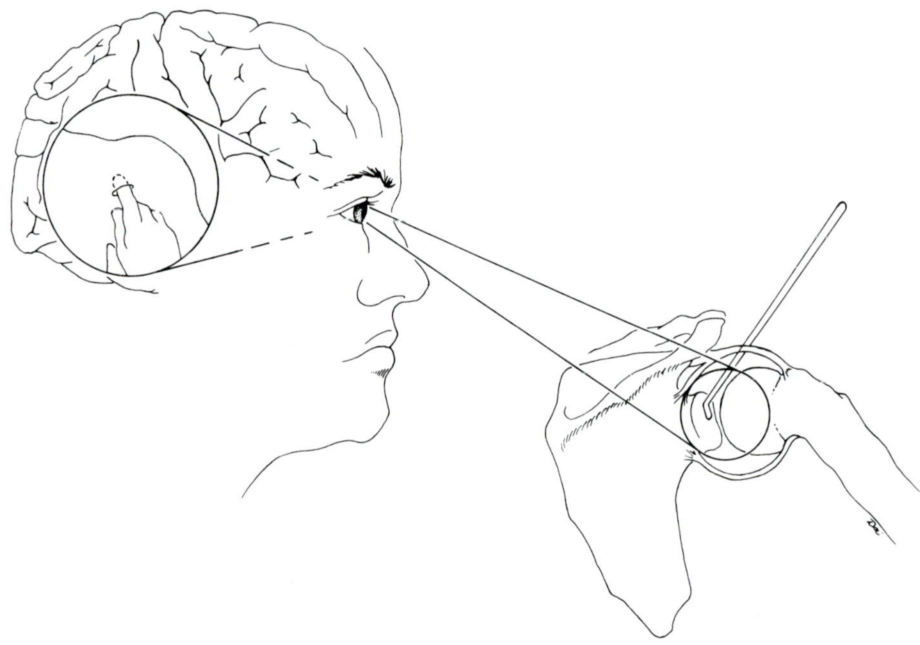

FIG. 5-11 Palpation inside of joint with a probe requires mental concept of finger palpation.

THE SURGEON'S PERSONAL PREPARATION

Staged Experience

A staged experience within the discipline of arthroscopic shoulder surgery is necessary to be successful.[33] During the development of arthroscopy in the 1970s, pioneering surgeons like myself enjoyed the luxury of performing thousands of diagnostic arthroscopies before any surgical arthroscopy. The standard of practice in those days was to perform a diagnostic arthroscopy before every knee arthrotomy. We were able to develop basic arthroscopic skills over time and without any peer or socioeconomic pressures.

In addition, we enjoyed the slow and measured introduction of surgical procedures with simple procedures preceding the more difficult. A surgeon would start with loose body removal, then meniscectomy, followed by anterior cruciate reconstruction.

Another benefit was the gradual development of instrumentation from hand to motorized over several years. I was intimately associated with the development of new instrumentation and the introduction of new techniques. I learned about this sophisticated equipment over a period of time. On the other hand, sophisticated instrumentation will not alone do the job. Golf clubs do not play golf. Also, the surgical assistants (in the golf analogy, the caddie) cannot do it for you.

Unfortunately, the circumstances are different today. Today's surgeon has professional and socioeconomic pressures to perform complicated and technically difficult arthroscopic shoulder procedures with a vast assortment of instrumentation.[33]

A continuing education course is only the lecture one attends before the laboratory experiment of surgery. What another surgeon can do may be different from what you do. You will have to play your own game.

Although learning from the experiences of predecessors is possible, there is no substitute for the surgeon's own measured progression from diagnostic arthroscopy to simple procedures before attempting the more technically challenging operations.

The inexperienced surgeon, resident, or fellow often has factual knowledge that exceeds his or her technical ability. Untempered by experience, one's excitement with the instrumentation and adventure into the unknown may result in a less than desirable surgical outcome.

The surgeon entering the field of arthroscopic shoulder surgery today is confronted with thousands of dollars' worth of equipment (new toys), a new environment (a new field), and new personnel (new players). Somehow, this surgeon expects to be an expert in arthroscopic surgery (a new ballgame). This expectation is unreasonable, unrealistic, and frankly, impossible. The present dilemma results from consumer demand and intraprofessional competition. Even though this is a whole new ballgame, all the standards of surgery, patient care, and professional integrity can not be abandoned. The surgeon must accept staged development in arthroscopic surgery. Case experience over time will be necessary to achieve proficiency; a few successes are often followed by a frustration or two. This is to be expected in any growth pattern.

Often the old adage "pride precedes the fall" becomes operational. If one exalts oneself, one will be humbled; if one chooses to humble oneself, then one has a chance of being exalted. In arthroscopic surgery, the surgeon will be humbled in one way or another. The best choice would be to be humble going into the operating room rather than humbled coming out.

Environment

The surgeon must learn about the unique environment necessary for successful arthroscopic surgery (see Chapter 2). He or she must inspect the environment in his or her institution and assist in correcting any deficiencies.

Instrumentation

The surgeon must become familiar with arthroscopic instrumentation, its assemblage, and function (see Chapter 3). The fragility of the arthroscopic instruments must be appreciated and respected.

Motor Skill Development

Arthroscopy has always been and still is technically challenging. Arthroscopy requires a high level of eye-hand coordination. The surgeon must prepare himself for the unique motor skills requirements of arthroscopy in a motor skills laboratory or on a cadaver before initial arthroscopic experience.[44] Unfortunately, few avail themselves of this experience. Arthroscopic shoulder techniques and procedures are still developing. All orthopedic surgeons are learning new technical skills and use of instrumentation. In spite of the requirement of "good hands" technical skill will not compensate for the lack of sound surgical principles.

Team Leadership

Arthroscopic surgery requires a team effort (see Chapter 2). The surgeon is the logical team leader. The characteristics necessary to be a team leader include an attitude and presence not often required for most open surgical procedures. Beyond the surgeon's technical preparation is his or her emotional demeanor. A disciplined, systematic, deliberate approach must be tempered with exact execution and patience. Therefore the surgeon must prepare himself or herself as team leader, not just as surgeon-technician.

Team Effort

Training of the team should occur under the leadership of the surgeon—it is not the responsibility of the hospital administration, the operating room nurses, or the instrument company representative. All of these individuals may make a contribution to the learning process, but the surgeon must not shift his or her responsibility. Not only is the surgeon "playing" many instruments and thinking, but he or she is responsible for directing or "conducting" the surgical team (see Chapter 2).

Team members are encouraged by recognition of their meaningful contributions.[2] The surgeon should share in the satisfaction of the team approach.

Realistic Expectations

Most surgeons expect too much when they start arthroscopy. One must be realistic because shoulder arthroscopy is a new discipline. The experienced surgeon has confidence in his or her abilities, but this confidence can be challenged in arthroscopic surgery. Arthroscopy may bring frustration and discouragement. The orthopedic surgeon who has performed well for many years in general orthopedics, or even specialized in the shoulder joint, will find a challenge in arthroscopic procedures. Visualization may be difficult, the perspective is not the same, cutting proceeds slowly, and the operating room floor is wet from fluid spillage. The beginning arthroscopic surgeon is uncomfortable and knows the procedure would have gone much faster and better by opening the joint.

Time and experience are required to develop new skills. With patience and diligence, the surgeon will be well satisfied and his or her patients well treated.

PATIENT CONSIDERATIONS

Once the surgeon prepares himself or herself, creates the proper environment, knows the instruments, and gathers and trains an arthroscopic shoulder surgical team, the focus turns to the patient.

Preoperative Evaluation

Arthroscopy is NOT the first tool to use in making a diagnosis. It is NOT the only tool for making a diagnosis. In fact, arthroscopy may NOT reveal the patient's diagnosis. Therefore, arthroscopy must be proceeded by a comprehensive evaluation, including a physical examination of the neck and chest (see Chapter 1). The source of the problem could be in anatomical structures juxtaposed to the shoulder joint (e.g., pain of cervical spine origin or a Pancoast tumor in the apex of the lung). Arthroscopic inspection is limited to the intraarticular structures.

Patient Selection

The inexperienced arthroscopic shoulder surgeon should select patients for whom an open conventional surgery is planned. A diagnostic arthroscopy would be reasonable before conventional open surgery and would provide a patient benefit. This approach will permit a staged experience for the surgeon.

When choosing a patient for operative arthroscopy only, the case should be well documented preoperatively, with a single, simple preoperative diagnosis. For example, a loose body or a labrum tear without glenohumeral instability is a reasonable first case. A degenerative joint may be chosen because articular disruption already exists. This situation allows the surgeon to operate well within his or her developing abilities. More difficult cases like reconstructions or acromioplasty should be deferred until the surgeon gains experience.

Avoiding a Trap

The patient approaches arthroscopic surgery with high expectations. I have had patients ask at the conclusion of the office evaluation, "Are you going to fix it now? Here in the office?" In the patient's imagination, fostered by the lay press, one may think he or she is having "laser" surgery. The patient expects not only to be healed, but also restored to normal. The patient might think he or she will be younger following the procedure. He or she may also believe that the recovery period will end when he leaves the operating table. The patient may be surprised that anesthesia is required or that a skin blemish results. In my experience arthroscopic surgery requires more explanation and "deprogramming" of patients than any other type of orthopedic surgery. Ignoring this problem will only result in subsequent prolonged discussions with the patient and/or family concerning their disappointments.

In addition, patients should be prepared to understand there are alternate methods and other physicians from whom they might seek either treatment or a second opinion. The patients may be disappointed to learn from you, the arthroscopic surgeon, that their case requires an open operation or a combined arthroscopic and open procedure. Another concern might be that the arthroscopy will be the first of several operations in a patient's life, especially when degenerative arthritis exists.

The convalescence period and eventual return to work are important to the patient, but the desire to return to recreational and competitive sports is usually stronger. The patient often assumes that "if the shoulder is opened," the convalescence will be longer. The convalesence may not be any different for open or arthroscopic surgery. The result may *not* be better just because the surgery was performed by arthroscopy.

What does all this discussion have to do with arthroscopic technique? Considerable! I will illustrate a worst possible scenario. Consider that you are operating on a patient who expects the surgery will be performed without opening the shoulder. You identify the preoperative anterior labrum tear, but a previously unrecognized partial thickness articular cartilage loss in the area of the Hill-Sachs lesion changes the diagnosis to traumatic anterior instability. The glenohumeral ligaments are attenuated and contracted. If this condition was recognized preoperatively, you would have proposed an open procedure. You have not performed this type of case before arthroscopically, though you could perform an open reconstruction. The patient chose the surgeon and surgery because you said it could be performed arthroscopically. The patient's expectations close the open procedure option, so you try an arthroscopic Bankart procedure.

The extracapsular edema increases along with the operative time. You are unable to visualize the operative area. The patient's preoperative expectations have restricted the intraoperative alternatives. The pressure on the surgeon increases, and his or her technical performance is impeded in the face of frustration. The choices are to open the shoulder or abort the procedure. The extravasation of fluid would complicate the open procedure. What do you do? In this case, stop and proceed on another day.

A better solution would have been to avoid the circumstance. Anticipate potential problems and do not promise that the operation will be performed only by arthroscopy. Arthroscopic procedures, let alone mastery of technique, is difficult enough without the added pressures of patient expectation on the surgeon. Avoid painting yourself into a corner (see Fig. 5-1). A reconstructive procedure solely by arthroscopy is not a good selection for the beginner surgeon.

The surgeon should know his or her limitations. Cases should be chosen by diagnosis, inherent joint mobility, and the patient's physical size to ensure technical simplicity. You might consider accepting one difficult preexisting factor, like an obese patient, but not one with a series of potential problems, such as an obese patient with a stiff shoulder and scar of previous surgery.

The surgeon should have complete candor about his or her level of arthroscopic development with the patient. What is the chance of success by arthroscopy in your hands? What is your experience with the anticipated diagnosis or operation? Have you performed similar operations? Do you have permission to abort the arthroscopic procedure? More importantly, would you be willing to abort the arthroscopic procedure? Would you perform the procedure by open methods with good outcome?

A disappointing result can occur when the surgeon's or the patient's expectations are unrealistic. Both circumstances can be avoided.

OPERATING ROOM PLANS OF ACTION

Preoperative Plan

After the previous conditions have been fulfilled, the scene shifts to the operating room. Based on the preoperative impression and the differential diagnosis, an operative plan is formulated. The surgeon should avoid "painting himself into a corner". This occurs with improper organization and planning such as a poorly planned resection or a lost fragment in the joint (Table 5-1).

The patient's expectations and the surgeon's ability influence the surgical approach. The operating room staff must have proper set-up for anticipated open procedures to avoid delays and unnecessarily prolonged anesthesia time.

Table 5-1 Operative Plan

Diagnostic arthroscopy	Operative arthroscopy	Combined procedure	Conventional open surgery
Now	Later	Later	Later
	Now	Later	Later
		Now	Later
			Now

The routines of the diagnostic and operative system presented in this text accommodate every technical eventuality of diagnosis and operation or intraoperative problem. These routines are discussed at the end of this chapter.

All anatomical compartments can be entered with instrumentation from primary and secondary portals. Multiple perspectives and multiple portals are necessary for successful diagnostic and operative arthroscopy. Most pathological conditions are treatable, usually by arthroscopic or combined techniques.

Alternative (Contingency) Plans

No matter how sure the surgeon is of the diagnosis and his or her ability, a contingency plan is necessary. The surgeon, patient, and the surgical team must be prepared for an alternate plan. These plans include initiating, deferring, aborting, or referring based on the surgeon's ability and the patient's expectations and preparation (Table 5-1):

1. The surgical procedure may be initiated and concluded with diagnostic arthroscopy.
2. The operative arthroscopy may be modified, completed, deferred, aborted, or referred.
3. The open surgery may be modified, completed, deferred, aborted, or referred.

If the surgeon is failing to make progress in any phase of arthroscopy, to modify or conclude the operation is reasonable. If the surgeon cannot see or make a diagnosis, the procedure should stop. If an arthroscopic diagnosis is made and the operative procedure is not within the skill level of the surgeon, then the procedure should be aborted. If the lesion is visible, but not approachable in a tight shoulder, then you will have to accept that it is not possible to proceed. Simultaneous television monitoring resolves this question of meaningful progress, clearly demonstrating the situation to all who are viewing or who might subsequently view the videotape.

Operative Time

As an operative procedure approaches 1 hour, the surgeon should formulate a plan to conclude. This may mean finishing the arthroscopy and leaving open surgery for another time. If acromioplasty cannot be accomplished arthroscopically, the shoulder should be opened early in the procedure.

These opinions on time restrictions are intended as guidelines. Time is a measure of preparation, not just execution (Fig 5-12). When the surgeon has both, the operative times decline. Judgment precedes experience in the production of reasonable operative times.

As a rule, if diagnostic arthroscopy exceeds 30 minutes, no arthroscopic operative work should be initiated. Diagnostic arthroscopy exceeding 1 hour is unnecessary when other surgeons are available to perform this type of surgery with greater dispatch. Complicated operative work should not be initiated when a reasonable amount of time is not available for completion.

Arthroscopic debridement procedures should not exceed 1 hour. Surgeons with operative times that regularly exceed 1 hour for diagnostic and 1½ hours for operative work should limit their case selection to conform to reasonable operative times. Some orthopedic surgeons should choose another interest within their specialty.

In spite of this discussion of operative time, I am an advocate of "how well," not "how fast," the procedures are performed. However, prolonged operative times often are a reflection of "how well" the procedure has progressed or been accomplished.

Modified Procedure

In some cases one may have to "change horses in midstream." For instance, extraarticular extravasation of fluid is common during arthroscopic surgery of the shoulder. You may have performed much of an anterior glenohumeral ligamentous reconstruction procedure, only to lose your visualization before final securing of the tissues. You may have to abort the procedure and open the shoulder for the reconstruction. Be prepared. Extravasation of fluid may require stopping an arthroscopic acromioplasty because of failure to visualize or poor instrument approaches. An intraoperative complication of major bleeding or instrument breakage is a reason to change to an open method.

Aborted Procedure

Any operative procedure can and should be aborted when it is in the patient's best interest. The usual reason to stop a procedure is when it exceeds a reasonable operative time. Arthroscopic procedures should not exceed 2 hours. It is reasonable to perform diagnostic and complicated operative shoulder arthroscopy, including most combined open procedures, well within this time. If not, then staging or deferment of the open operative dimension should be considered. Prolonged arthroscopic operative times result in increased fluid extravasation, frequency of instrument passage, tissue damage, surgeon fatigue, surgical team inefficiency and anesthesia risk.

AN ABORTED PROCEDURE REFLECTS GOOD JUDGEMENT, NOT FAILURE

Every attempt should be made to retrieve a broken arthroscopic instrument, including the use of x-ray imaging. Retrieval is usually easier by arthroscopy than by opening a swollen joint. Even if the instrument is not retrieved, the operation should be aborted in the patient's best interest rather than use excessive time or create further tissue damage. A second procedure, usually by arthroscopy on another day, is sound judgment.

In summary, if for any reason the surgeon is unable to complete the surgery safely for the patient, the operation

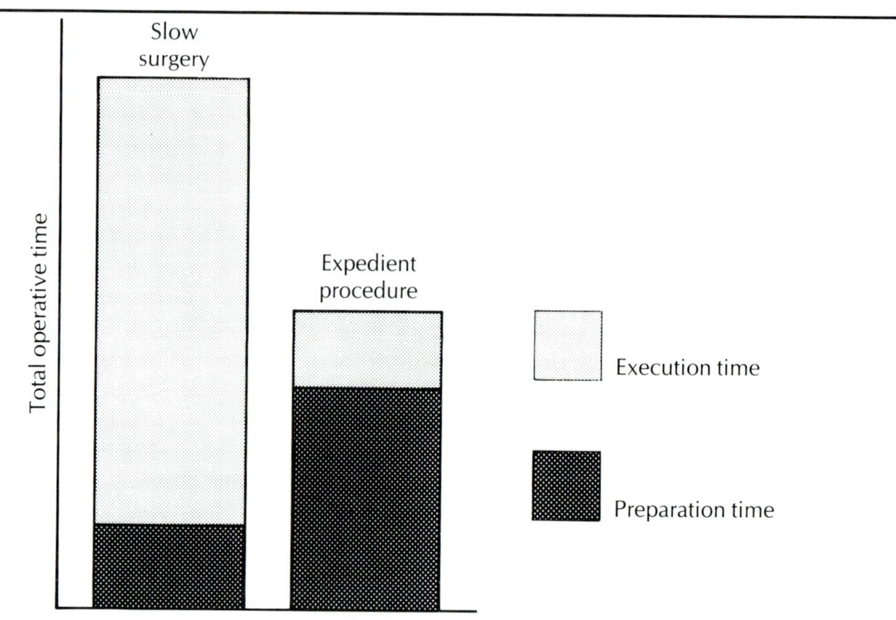

FIG. 5-12 Relationship of operative time to organization and planning.

should be aborted. This includes mishaps to the surgeon and any of the just-mentioned factors or anesthetic problems. There is always another day or another way. The case can be deferred or referred. Dogged determination to complete arthroscopic surgery without regard to time is not only unfortunate but also unreasonable and unnecessary.

Fatigue and Frustration

Fatigue and frustration are a dimension of arthroscopic surgery, no matter what the surgeon's experience or skill level. These problems can result in inexact instrument manipulation and tissue damage. Failure to make progress and the factor of fatigue may lead the surgeon to lose his or her composure, self-control, or surgical imagination. Resultant strife among the operating room team may have to be resolved.

One approach is to stop for even 5 minutes early in the procedure to allow regrouping and subsequent progress. If the operative progress continues to be hampered by fatigue and/or frustration, then sound judgement dictates concluding the procedure.

Combined Procedures

Another plan of action is to combine arthroscopic techniques with conventional open surgery. The patient should recognize ahead of time that a combination procedure is being considered. This scenario is the most common in cases of glenohumeral instability and rotator cuff tears. In anterior instability cases the patient may have to be repositioned (see Chapter 8). In rotator cuff disease the lateral decubitus position lends itself well to open surgical reconstruction (see Chapter 9). Intraarticular surgical debridement and preparation is performed arthroscopically, thereby minimizing the surgical exposure for cuff repair.

SHOULDER ARTHROSCOPIC TECHNIQUES

Patient Positioning

Lateral Decubitus Position. The surgical principle of a secured extremity is very important in arthroscopy. I prefer the lateral decubitus position with a suspended upper extremity (Fig. 5-13). This position eliminates the need for an assistant to hold the upper extremity. The arthroscope enters the shoulder from the horizonal position, avoiding fluid flow by gravity on the video, which can obscure the im-

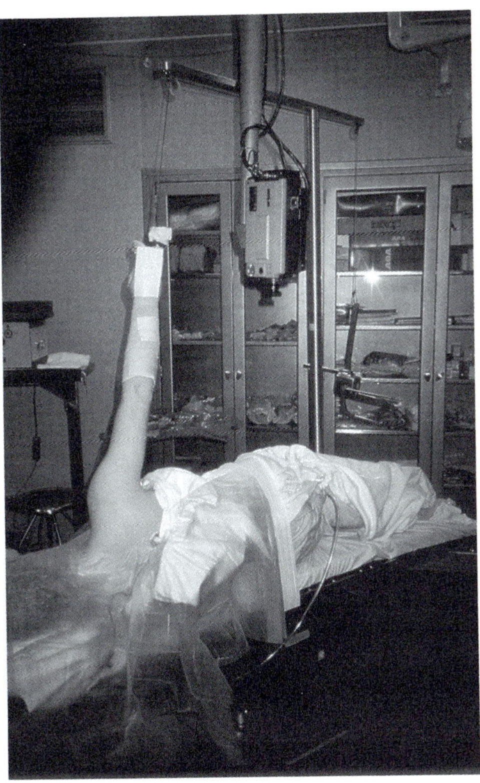

FIG. 5-13 The patient is placed in the opposite lateral decubitus position. The patient is held with an Olympic Vac Pac and tape secures both to the table. The arm is suspended with skin traction by two pullies attached to a mechanical T-shaped bar attached to the table by a C-clamp device.

age. Orientation in space is obtained by holding the scope parallel to the floor. The lateral decubitus position need not be changed for combined open rotator cuff surgery.

The patient is secured on the table with an Olympic Vac Pac. The involved upper extremity is suspended.[25,31] The forearm is secured to a suspension apparatus (Fig. 5-14). In this position, although the patient's thorax and pelvis are secured to the table, the scapula is not anatomically secured to the thorax. Therefore, often the scapula must be stabilized by manual counter pressure during operative arthroscopy.

The patient's position is easily changed from lateral decubitus for anterior surgery by releasing the suspension apparatus, and covering the unsterile hand and wrist with sterile stockinette and wrapping with sterile Coban (Fig. 5-15). The vacuum is removed from the Olympic Vac Pac until the patient's position is shifted toward supine until satisfactory to the surgeon. Vacuum is re-created and the patient is secured in the new position for open surgery (Fig. 5-16, *A*). The shoulder surgical field is again prepared with skin antiseptic. The posterior puncture wound remains within the sterile field (Fig. 5-16, *B*). The change to any position for the open surgery is easily obtainable.

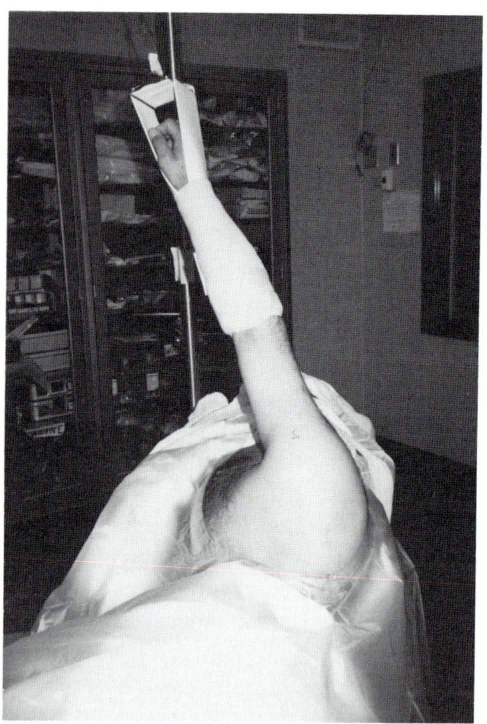

FIG. 5-14 The upper extremity is suspended by skin traction. A perforated latex foam strip is placed on the skin and secured with an Ace wrap. The Ace wrap is secured with strip of tape. A metal frame connects to the suspension cable.

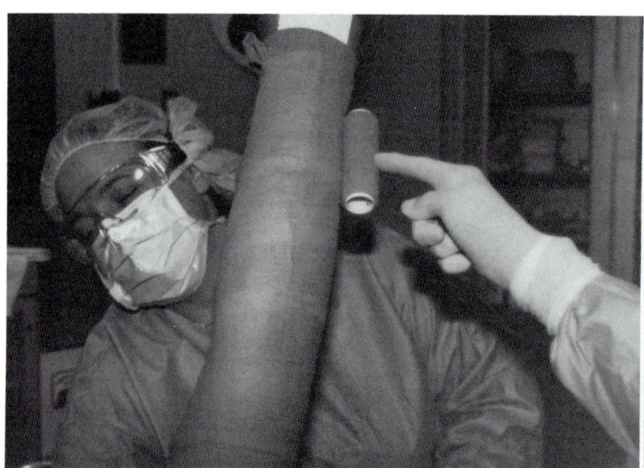

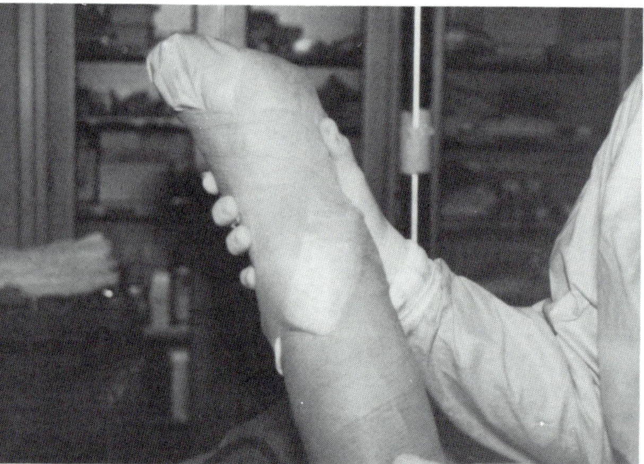

A B

FIG. 5-15 Change in patient position.

A The suspended forearm is covered with sterile toweling and wrapped with sterile Coban. The roll of Coban remains on arm for subsequent use to cover hand when suspension is removed.

B Suspension was removed. The unsterile hand was covered with sterile draping and wrapped with remainder of Coban.

Beach Chair Position. Some surgeons prefer the beach chair position, especially when open anterior surgery is anticipated.[37] This position requires the arthroscope to be placed in a dependent position from posterior. The posterior dependent positioning results in increased soft tissue depth to the area of arthroscope placement. After the scope is placed, the dependent position results in fluids running onto the scope and obscuring the view from time to time. One or more assistants are required to "pull" on the arm for distraction. Orientation of the arthroscope is more difficult, because the scope approaches the patient from a different angle than the surgeon's eyes view the screen.

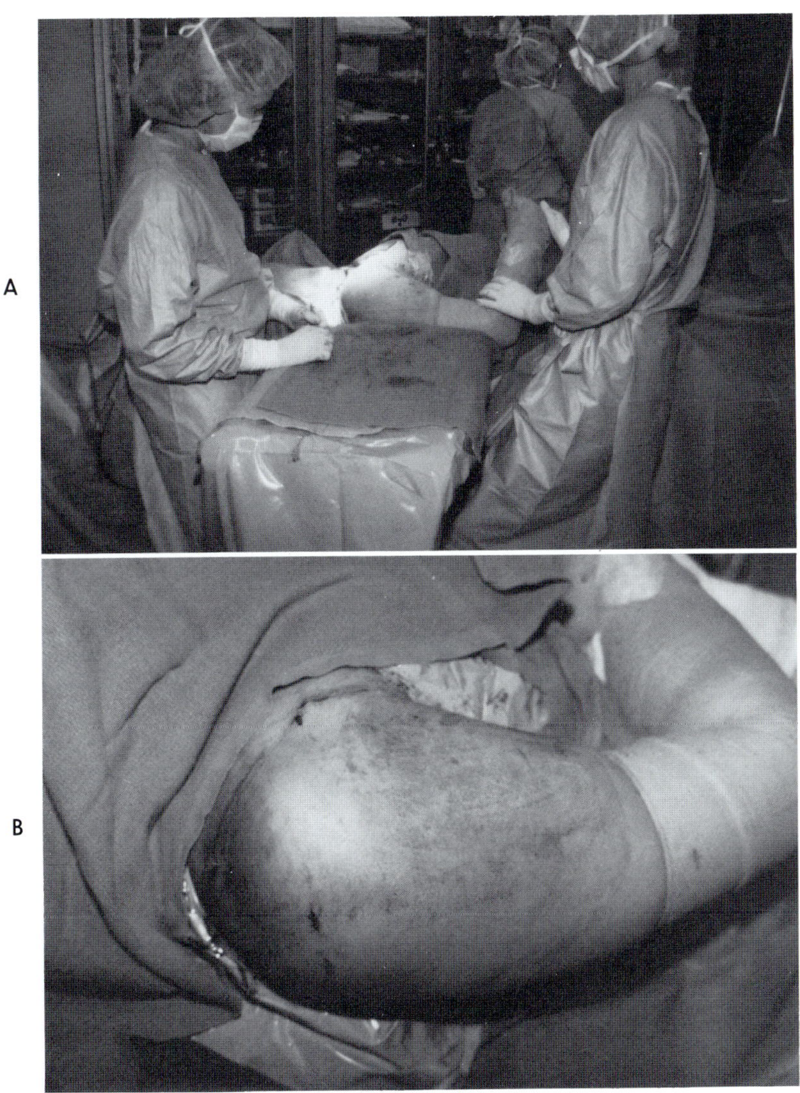

FIG. 5-16 Open surgical position.

A The patient is rolled to new position for open surgery. In this illustration, the position is supine, with slight elevation of the head. The full beach chair position would also be possible.

B The new position retains the previous draping. The arthroscopic wounds are within the sterile field. A repeat skin antiseptic has been applied.

Surgical Set-Up

For details on the ideal operating environment, see Chapter 2. The surgical preparation includes a Betadine skin preparation. The draping is accomplished with a sterile water impervious draping (Fig 5-17). The Johnson & Johnson Arthroscopy Shoulder Pack has special loops to hold various tubes and cords (Fig. 5-18). The drape is folded and secured behind the shoulder to catch and deflect fluid out of the operative field to a container on the floor (Fig. 5-19, *A* and *B*). The draping is gathered and taped over the patient's pelvis to provide pockets to hold surgical instruments (Fig. 5-19, *C*).

The arm is covered with a sterile towel and secured with 3M Coban wrap (see Fig. 5-15). The wrap starts proximal and proceeds distal to cover the hand. The reason for this direction of application is to facilitate removal at the end of the case. Unwrapping from distal to proximal is performed with little movement of the arm.

Also, if open surgery is anticipated and the arm is to be draped free, I leave the remaining tube of Coban attached to the arm so that it can be used to secure the subsequently placed sterile tube sockenette (see Fig. 5-15, *B*).

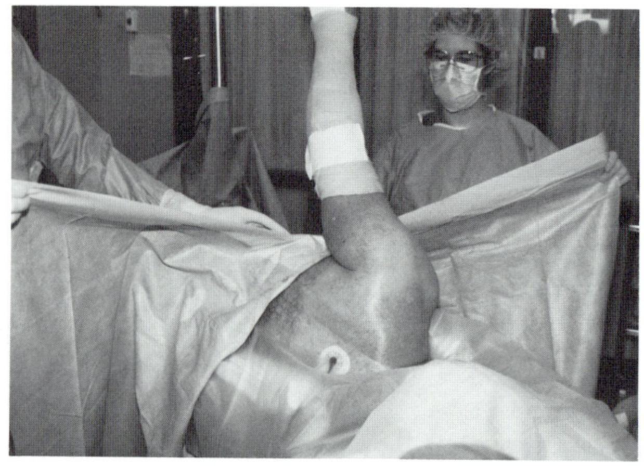

FIG. 5-17 **A Johnson & Johnson paper draping system was devised to form a fluid-impervious barrier. Note the unsterile plastic drape covering the towel over the patient's head.**

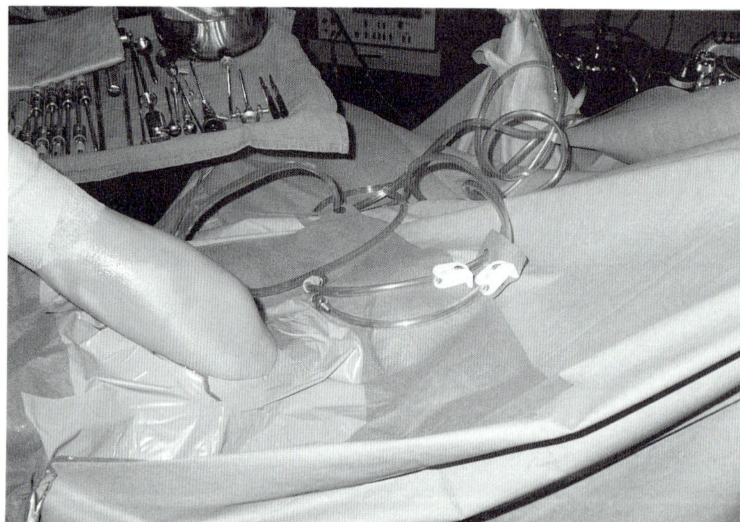

FIG. 5-18 **The draping system has tabs that provide means of securing tubing and cords to the operative field. This prevents falling of the field to the unsterile floor.**

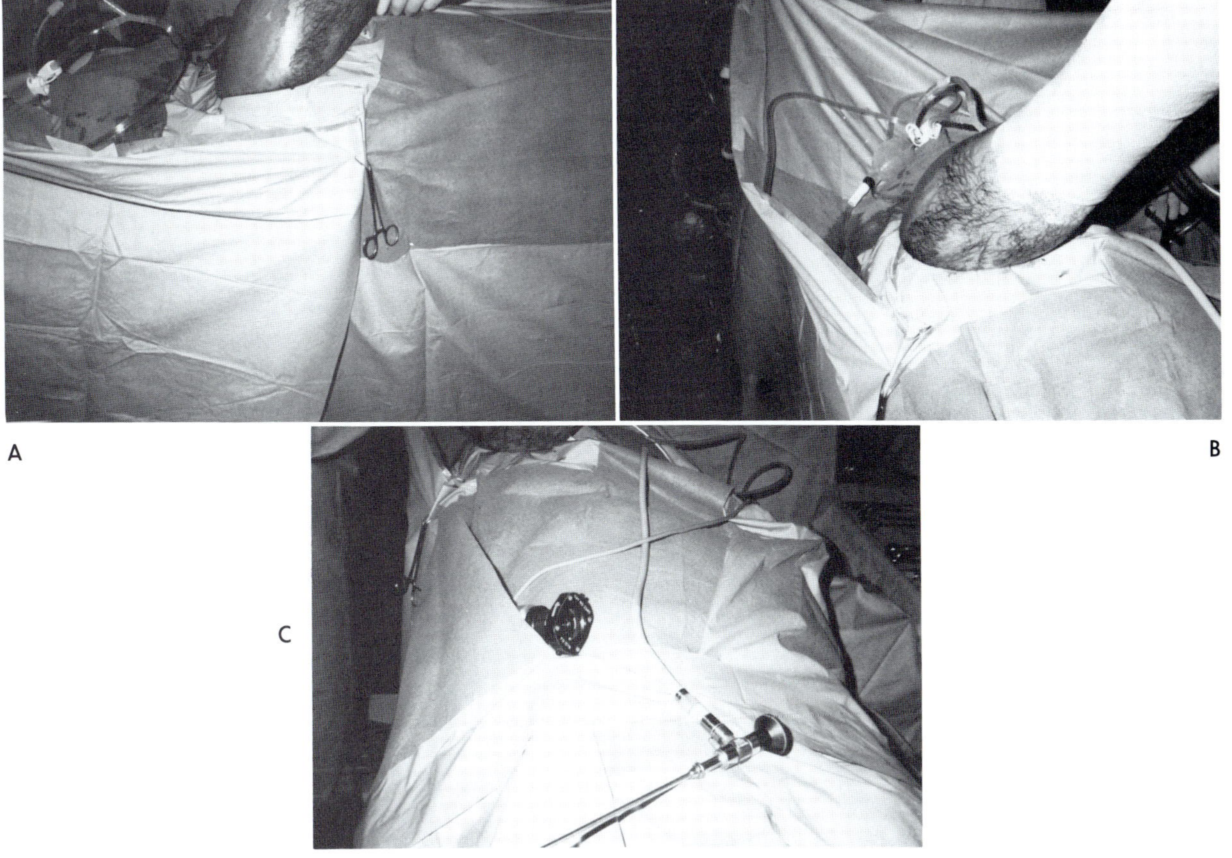

FIG. 5-19 The draping is modified to contain and direct fluid flow. Folds are made to hold instruments on the operative field.

A A fold is made on the surgeon's side of the table to catch fluids and direct them to the opposite side into a floor bucket.

B Another angle of this fold shows the "pocket" with fluid and inflow system.

C The folds in the draping over the patient's pelvis provides a place to secure arthroscope, camera, and instruments.

Joint Distention

Gaseous Medium. The joint can be distended by room air or CO_2 delivery systems (Fig. 5-4, *A*).[8] For diagnostic purposes, the field of view is optically wider in air than in a liquid medium. CO_2 must be used for a CO_2 laser.[40,41,42] The air medium has some advantage over sterile water for use with electrocautery, but no other advantages. I have used room air for joint distention to enhance a slide photograph with a wider angle of view. The practical value of intermittent distention with room air will also control bleeding, as the drying effects of air cause a clot to form. This effect is often used in subacromial bursa surgery.

Room air is delivered with a 60-ml syringe via a K-52 catheter attached to the arthroscope spigot or with the Gravity Assist hand pump. Air quickly dissipates, and a repeat volume is delivered. I have seen no complications of infection, air embolism, or troublesome subcutaneous emphysema. The concern over injecting nonsterile room air is no more hazardous than the same air coming into contact with the wound at open surgery. Gas infusion under continuous mechanical pressure could result in subcutaneous or tissue emphysema, however.[36,40]

One disadvantage of air distention is the absence of liquid circulation for mobilization of loose fragments. Also, operative motorized instruments are designed for fluid medium and fragment removal by suction. Nonetheless, room air is inexpensive, readily available, and a safe gaseous medium for joint distention.

Fluid Medium. Ringer's lactate is the preferred fluid because articular cartilage metabolism is not altered by its physiologic nature.[29,32] Normal saline is used in degenerative arthritis because of its effect to decrease cartilage metabolic activity and its greater propensity for attachment of blood clot to surgical surfaces.[12]

Adrenalin Solution. Adrenalin may be used for hemostasis. An adrenalin solution is used only with the knowledge and approval of the anesthesiologist and only when the patient has no mitigating circumstances. The adrenalin solution is mixed in a sterile basin as 1 vial of 1:1000 (1 mg) in 1000 cc fluid. I use the solution during the diagnostic phase, with repeated injections with a syringe and catheter attached to the arthroscope spigot. If bleeding becomes a problem during operative arthroscopy, I prefer to use electrocoagulation.

If additional adrenalin solution is to be given, I prefer repeated controlled injection over continuous infusion. The continuous infusion method may result in lack of control and/or recognition of the amount of adrenalin that may have extravasated into the patient's tissues. Later absorption may have deleterious cardiac effects.

I do not use adrenalin in the operative fluid reservoirs.

Preliminary Distention with Needle. The synovial joint is normally in a decompressed state unless pathological effusion is present. Distention is necessary for access and visualization.

The arthroscopist may choose to distend the joint with a needle and syringe to facilitate entry of the arthroscope cannula and obturator. If successful, the maneuver provides maximal distention that enlarges the target for the arthroscopic cannula. Fluid backflow through the needle cannula confirms entry. Originally, I delivered fluid into the shoulder joint with a No. 18 spinal needle. This method often resulted in extraarticular extravasation of fluid when injection was made without confirmation of being inside the joint. The extravasation of fluids complicated subsequent arthroscopic penetration due to extrasynovial fluid compression of the joint from without.

I no longer use this method.

Placement of the Arthroscope

Direct Entry with Arthroscope Cannula. Subsequently, I found it is easier to determine intraarticular penetration with the larger arthroscope cannula and obturator than with a small needle. I enter the glenohumeral joint with the cannula and obturator (Fig. 5-20). Palpating unvisualized tissues and recognizing joint penetration is easier with the larger instrument. This method also provides an opportunity for a visual confirmation of entry with obturator removal and placement of the arthroscope. A small amount of fluid (<5 ml) is instilled via the syringe system through the arthroscope to clarify the view before further instillation of fluids. If misplaced, then large amounts of fluid have not been injected.

Arthroscope Cannula/Obturator Penetration. Safe penetration of the joint capsule is facilitated by internal rotation of the suspended arm and measured rotatory motion on the scope cannula with the obturator (Fig. 5-20). The surgeon should avoid plunging with the arthroscope (Fig. 5-21). Entry is confirmed when the obturator is removed and a rush of air is heard with a change of negative joint pressure.

Cleaning and Vacuuming. Confirmation of entry may be obscured by bloody or cloudy joint fluid. The liquid medium used in arthroscopy lends itself well to clearing up the joint by dilution of joint effusion, plus mobilization and removal of loose fragments. Surgical exposure and visualization are enhanced by preliminary cleansing and vacuuming cloudy joint fluid and fragments. This is accomplished by first filling the joint with clear irrigating fluid injected via a K-52 catheter from a 60-ml syringe (see Fig. 5-24). Even massive hemarthrosis can be cleansed with proper technique and washing with saline solution.

Joint cleansing is enhanced by large-volume inflow from a separate cannula (Fig. 5-22). Suction vacuuming on the arthroscope draws fragments to the scope for removal. Small, soft pieces fold up and are removed along the scope. Medium-sized pieces come out of the cannula with momentary scope removal. Suction can be applied directly to the end of the scope cannula to help with removal (Fig. 5-23). Large pieces may require forceps or motorized instrument removal.

Ballottement from exterior of a joint creates turbulence within. This activity mobilizes fragments from joint recesses toward the force of suction on the arthroscope. This effect can be created during shoulder arthroscopy by gently wiggling or rotating the arm back and forth on the glenoid.

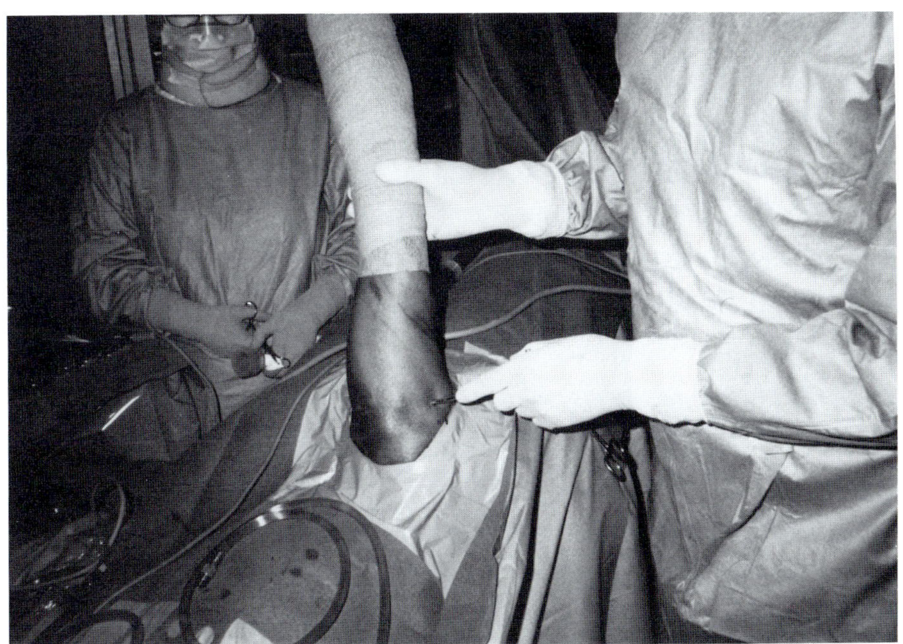

FIG. 5-20 Internal rotation of the humeral shaft facilitates joint penetration.

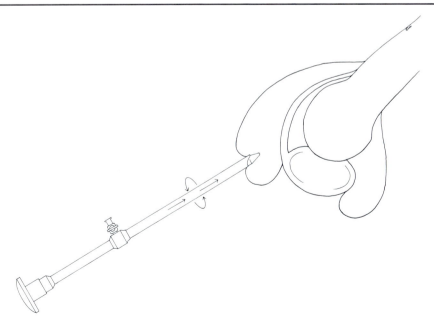

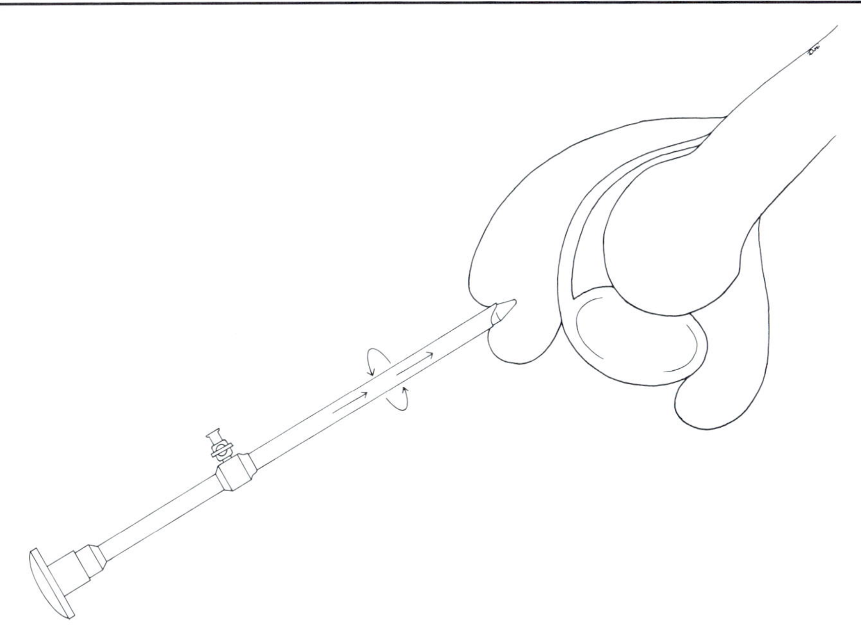

FIG. 5-21 Manipulation of the cannula/obturator for safe penetration requires a rotation motion to avoid plunging.

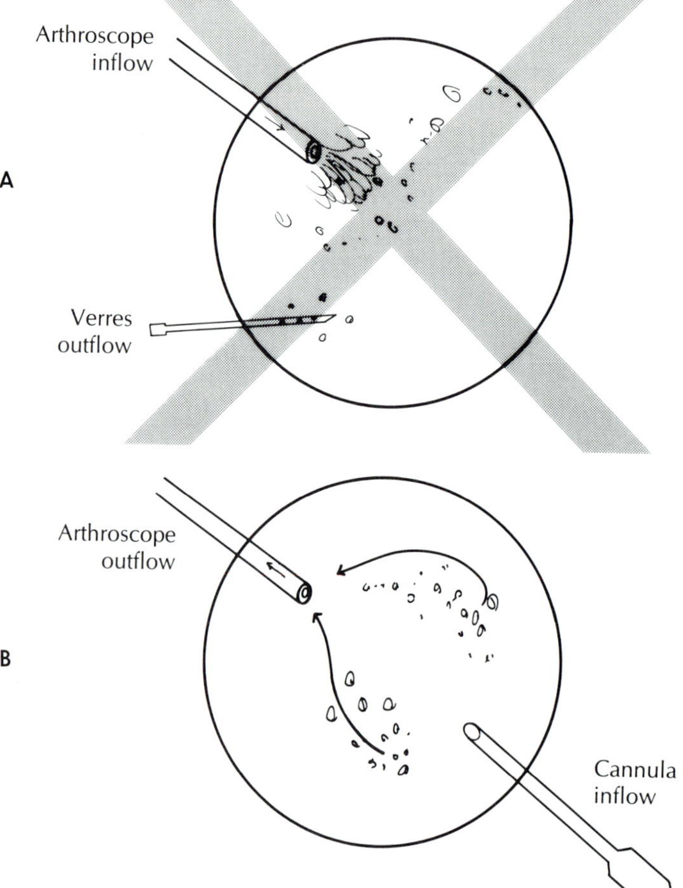

FIG. 5-22 Flow systems.

A Impractical inflow on arthroscopic and outflow via needle.

B Large cannula inflow and intermittent outflow on arthroscope during diagnostic phase.

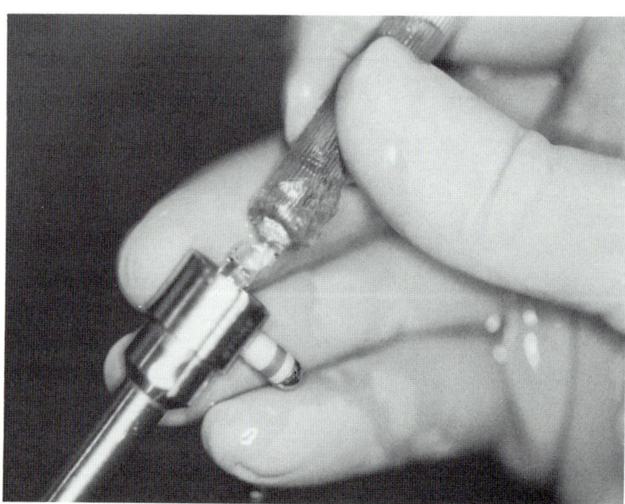

FIG. 5-23 Suction is applied directly to the end of the arthroscope cannula to expedite joint cleansing and remove larger loose bodies.

FLUID MANAGEMENT SYSTEMS

Original System

Originally, the fluid flow system for diagnostic arthroscopy was inflow on the arthroscope (Fig. 5-24). Inflow via the arthroscope has the one advantage of not requiring a second joint puncture for an infusion cannula. The disadvantages are several. The amount of fluid delivered along the arthroscope is limited by the small spigot openings on the arthroscope cannula (approximately 1 to 2 mm in diameter). This cross-sectional area is far less than that of a 4.2 mm inside diameter of a separate cannula. Thus the amount of fluid delivered though these small spigots would not be comparable to flow or volume through a larger diameter cannula.

The arthroscope sheath must be enlarged to provide space for fluid flow along the scope to the joint. If this method is used, a greater pressure is required to deliver the fluid, as with a K-52 catheter and 60-ml syringe or arthroscopic pump.

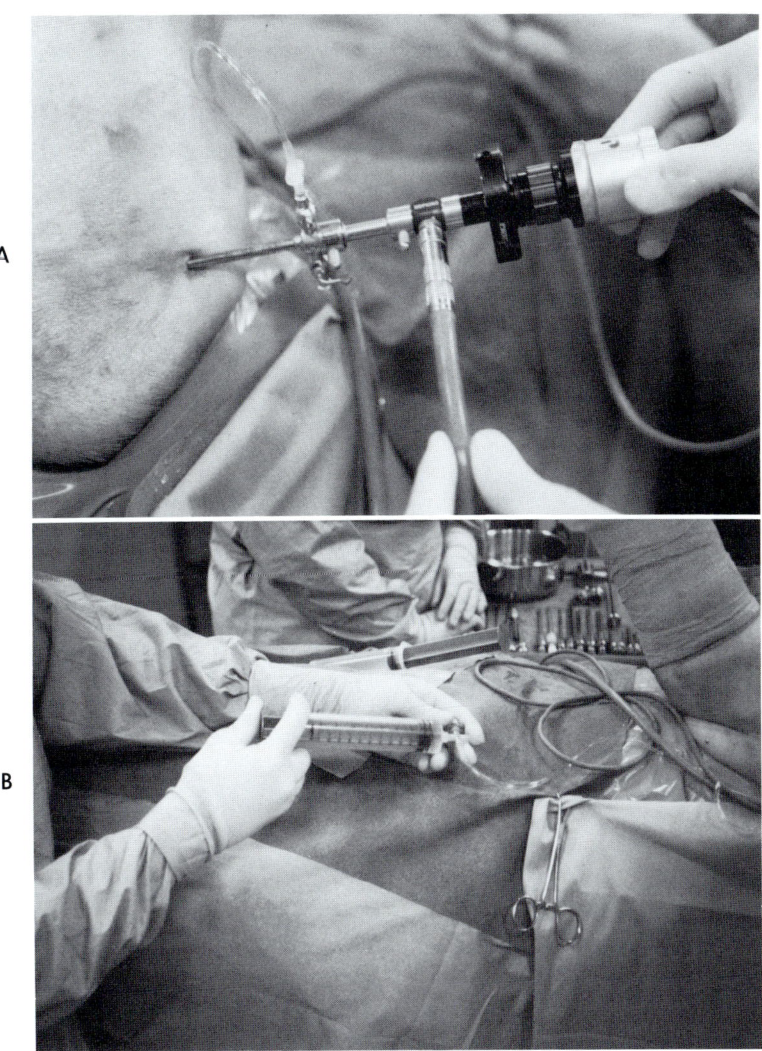

FIG. 5-24 Original system of inflow is used for diagnostic phase.

A A K-52 catheter is attached to the arthroscope spigot.

B Fluid is delivered from a 60-ml syringe with manual pressure by the first assistant. Intermittent bolus is delivered. Two syringes, alternately filled facilitate this method.

Previous Misconceptions About Irrigation Systems

Traditionally the infusion system for diagnostic arthroscopy was brought through the arthroscope via one of the side spigots of the cannula system. This technique was adopted from urology. In the past, some surgeons simultaneously opened both inflow spigots on the arthroscopic cannula. They insisted the fluid would flow in along the arthroscope, into the joint, back out the joint, and into the opposite spigot. Of course, fluid flows to the area of least pressure; in this case, that was directly across the cannula. No fluid flowed into the joint! This system provided a nonexistent irrigation system.

In addition, the traditionalists used what was called a Verres needle for drainage. They insisted that small particles were blown from in front of the scope and moved 2 to 3 inches, where they flowed out of the joint from one of the many tiny holes in the Verres needle. I have not seen this happen.

Their previous proponents have now abandoned these ideas.

Mechanical Fluid Infusion Pump

In 1975, during the development of the Intra-articular Shaver System with Dyonics, Inc., a heart-lung machine was used as an infusion pump to measure flows and pressures as well as record volumes. This was the first mechanical pump used in arthroscopy.

Today arthroscopists commonly use mechanical infusion pumps to overcome flow problems (see Fig. 3-18). I do not use an expensive arthroscopic infusion pump. My main objection to infusion pumping of fluids via the arthroscope is the turbulence produced in the visual field of view. The fluids flowing rapidly around the scope shake the tissues in the visual field. My concentration is disrupted by this constant motion of synovium. In addition, inflow on the arthroscope does not facilitate removal of potential loose bodies. The inflow on the arthroscope moves free fragments away from the end of the scope but out of sight into remote recesses of the joint and is therapeutically counterproductive. Other disadvantages of the mechanical pumps are expense, time in set up, and unrecognized continuous pumping that results in extravasation of fluids.[30]

Arthroscopy pumps have the benefit of electronically controlling pressure and flow, although intraarticular pressures are not always reflected in machine readouts. I have tested two of the most popular arthroscopy pumps against my gravity flow system, using the sensors in the mechanical system to make the comparison. The gravity flow system was comparable to the mechanical pumps in every category of evaluation.

A

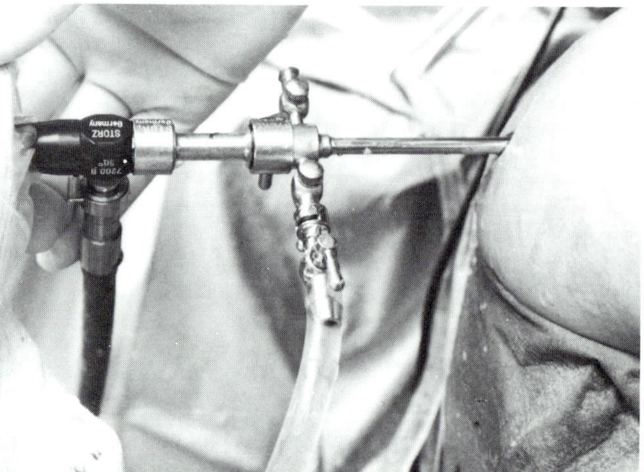

B

FIG. 5-25 Inflow fluid control.

A Inflow fluids are contained in a reservoir. Suspension of two 3 L bags, at least 1 m above the patient creates enough of a pressure head for most procedures. The plastic bags allow additional manual compression to increase flow when needed.

B Inflow adaptor on arthroscope permits direct attachment to arthroscope via Y-tubing.

Gravity Flow. A less expensive alternative method to the original heart lung machine was established with a suspended fluid reservoir (Fig. 5-25). We settled on this irrigation method as being simple, safe, and effective. The gravity flow method is just as effective as the most sophisticated arthroscopic pump. In fact, my testing showed this gravity flow system superior to existing commercially available mechanical pumps in replenishing the decompressed joint (see also Chapter 2).

Gravity Assist Hand Pump

For short periods during shoulder arthroscopy additional flow or pressure is required. This need may occur at the end of a capsular ligament reattachment case or during arthroscopic acromioplasty. I devised a unidirectional hand-bulb pump that places a fluid reservoir near the joint and provides a simple and inexpensive means of assisting gravity during those short periods of need in surgery (Fig. 5-26). This method prevents the unrecognized continuous high pressure of mechanical pumps that causes extravasation of fluid. It is installed in line with the gravity flow tubing, and gravity flow is unobstructed by its presence. The hand pump is activated by the second assistant applying manual pressure and controlling outflow (Fig. 5-27).

Outflow Suction Pressure

Gravity outflow is not adequate to mobilize intraarticular fragments or maximize efficiency of motorized instruments. Suction is required. In 1975, during the development of the Intra-articular Shaver System, we tested all the various pressure suction apparatus. The wall vacuum system in our operating room was measured at 14 to 16 inches of mercury (40 cm Hg) (see Fig. 3-26). This measurement should be in-line and not end-on. End-on measurements will tend to falsely elevate the value of the suction over the in-line test. We have learned most operating rooms suction systems measure between 14 and 16 inches of mercury. The surgeon should measure and calibrate the suction pressures in the operating room for optimal function of motorized instrumentation.

The Dyonics Intra-articular Shaver System (window size, and diameter and rotator speeds) were calibrated for this in-line amount of suction pressure. I am not familiar with calibration of replica systems.

Since maximal distention distracts the humerus from the glenoid and distorts normal anatomical relationships, suction is valuable to partially decompress the glenohumeral joint. Natural relationships of the anatomical structures are less distorted when the joint is decompressed.

Monitoring Fluid Flow

Both the glenohumeral joint and the subacromial space have a small potential fluid volume. The acromioclavicular (AC) joint is even smaller. The lack of volume may compromise adequate exposure or effective use of motorized instrumentation. Maintenance of volume depends on monitored balance of inflow and outflow systems.

In my system, manual means are utilized to increase flow. On the inflow side, pressure may be applied to the reservoir bags. The circulating nurse manually clamps off one bag and squeezes the other (see Fig. 3-27). A more effective and inexpensive way to do the same thing is the

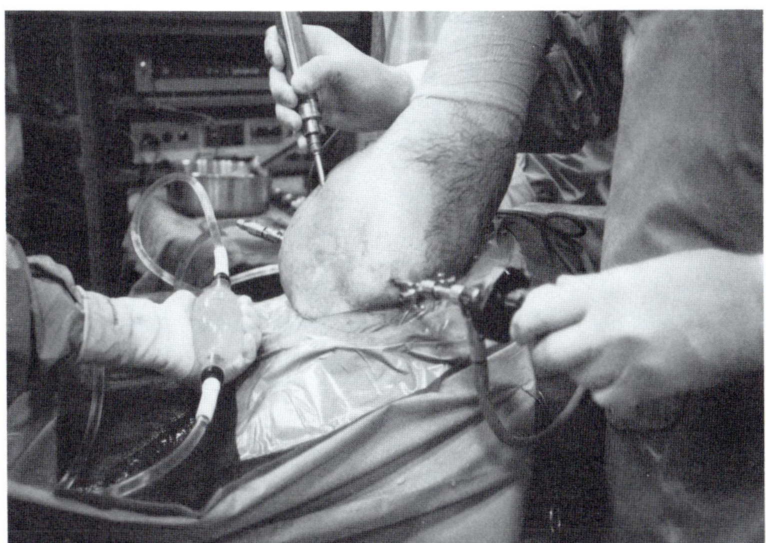

FIG. 5-26 Gravity Assist Hand Pump. This device is a simple, inexpensive, and effective means of increasing flow during critical times in the procedure. It is most often used in arthroscopic acromioplasty.

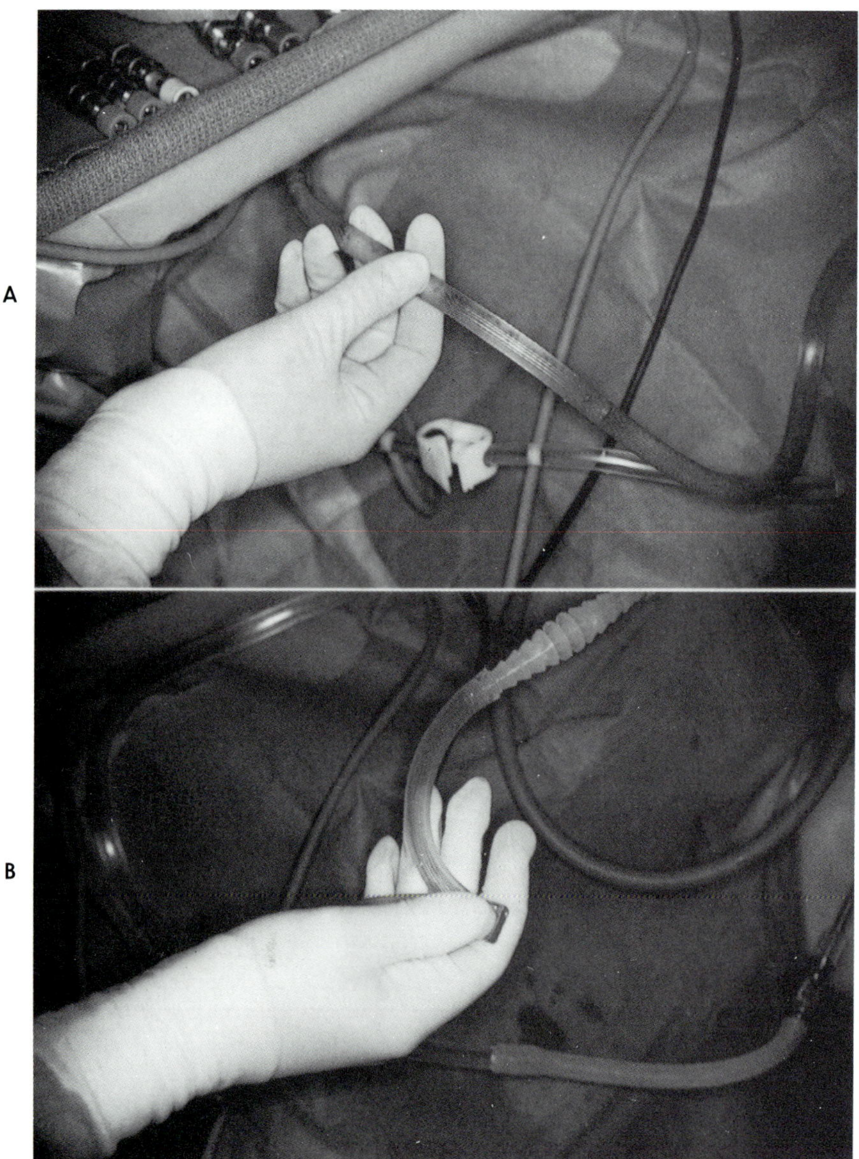

FIG. 5-27 Outflow fluid control.

A Outflow control affected by carefully restricting the outflow tubing. The second assistant partially bends the tubing.

B Outflow is shut off with complete fold in the tubing.

use of the Gravity Assist Hand Pump. A more expensive and no more effective way is to use a commercial arthroscopic pump.

Because the AC joint has such a small intraarticular volume, I routinely use a 60-ml syringe via a K-52 catheter to create maximum flow and pressure (see Fig. 5-24, *B*).

The outflow may not be in perfect balance with the inflow. The joint may be over vacuumed. The arthroscopic view will be obliterated by the rush of air bubbles and by joint lining encroachment. This problem is avoided by preoperative calibration of the suction pressure in the operating room and vigilant monitoring of the outflow by the second assistant during surgery. He or she can partially restrict outflow by bending the outflow tubing (see Fig. 5-27, *A* and *B*). The experienced assistant can perfectly coordinate (fine-tune) the flow by watching the surgical field on the television monitor.

In some cases, both increased inflow pressure and restriction of outflow are necessary.

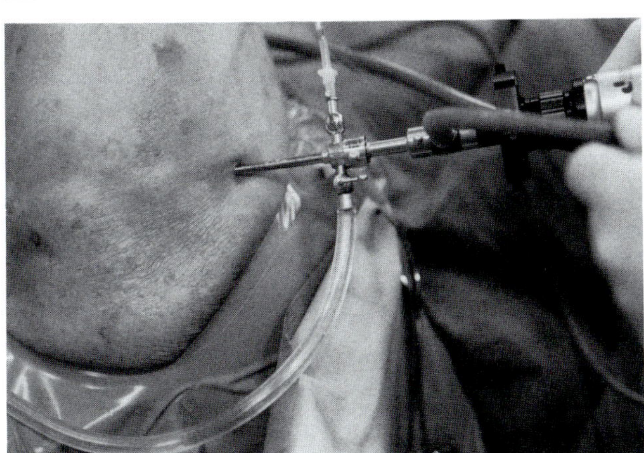

FIG. 5-28 This set-up provides inflow on one spigot and outflow suction on the other. In this instance the inflow spigot is open, and the outflow spigot is shut off. The joint is maximally distended.

Fluid Management System for Diagnostic Arthroscopy

My fluid infusion system for the diagnostic phase of shoulder arthroscopy is a closed system. Fluids are delivered from a 60-ml syringe, via a K-52 plastic catheter, along the arthroscope into the joint.[18] The fluid usually contains adrenaline. Pressure is applied by the first assistant (see Fig. 5-24, *B*) This method provides sufficient flow and pressure. To provide increased flow at specific times during shoulder arthroscopy, the second assistant squeezes the Gravity Assist Hand Pump (Fig. 5-26).

During the diagnostic phase with a closed irrigation system, intermittent joint distention and cleansing is performed for optimal visualization.

The inflow is on one spigot and the suction tubing is attached to the other (Fig. 5-28). When distention is desired, the outflow spigot is off. When suction is desired, the inflow valve is turned off. If large loose bodies exist, then intermittent distention is followed by removing the arthroscope from the cannula; both fluid and fragments flow out of the joint because of the pressure differential. Cleansing is more efficient when suction tubing is attached to the open end of the empty cannula (see Fig. 5-23). A simple joint lavage procedure can be performed with this system.

Fluid Management System for Operative Arthroscopy

During operative arthroscopy a fluid reservoir is established with two 3-liter bags of fluid. These are suspended at least 1 m above the patient (see Fig. 5-25, *A*). They connect to the operative field via sterile Y-tubing. Joint distention is created by the hydrostatic pressure and gravity flow. A balancing of inflow and outflow is necessary to provide optimal visualization and function of motorized instrumentation (see Fig. 5-27, *A* and *B*) If suction exceeds inflow, the joint is decompressed (Fig. 5-29). The outflow spigot may be closed to maximize distention (see Fig. 5-28).

This method has several advantages. Particles are drawn into view and out of the joint rather than being blown away. Fragments or loose pieces are drawn toward the arthroscope for identification and removal. If the pieces are very small and supple, they can be removed by the suction alone. If large, they may cover the end of the arthroscope and block visualization. Simply removing the arthroscope from the cannula and letting the fluid rush out removes the fragment. With only a momentary delay, inspection can proceed by replacing the arthroscope.

A piece too large to exit by this suction system should be delivered by suction to a site for easy removal by another instrument. For instance, a loose body from the depths of the subscapular bursa can be delivered to rest on the glenoid surface for visualization and removal. Using suction of the arthroscope allows recessed areas to be vacuumed, such as under an elevated labrum or in the subscapularis bursa.

One disadvantage of this system occurs when suction draws synovium over the end of the arthroscope, obscuring the view. Simply turning off the suction and moving the arthroscope will release the synovium and allow visualization.

Additional Portals for Glenohumeral Joint. A second arthroscopic portal is reserved until the diagnosis is made and a surgical plan is formulated. If a simple and short debridement procedure is indicated, I use only one additional portal, that being anterior for the surgical instruments. I continue with the inflow on the arthroscope and repeated bolus of fluid delivered with syringe and catheter. The system is sufficient for short cases.

Separate Superior (Supraspinatus) Inflow Portal. This portal is routinely used for the inflow of fluids. It is established when a longer operative procedure is anticipated. The standard separate inflow cannula in shoulder arthroscopic surgery comes through the superior supraspinatus portal, described by Neviaser and popularized by Caspari (Fig. 5-30). The inflow portal may be interchanged with the anterior or posterior portal to facilitate operative arthroscopy from the superior portal (Fig. 5-30, *F*).

Auxiliary Inflow. Additional cannulas or attachments to the arthroscope are sometimes used as auxiliary sources of inflow to tight or small reservoir spaces like the subacromial space or acromioclavicular joint. The inflow system can be attached to the arthroscope with the use of an adapter (see Fig. 5-25, *B*).

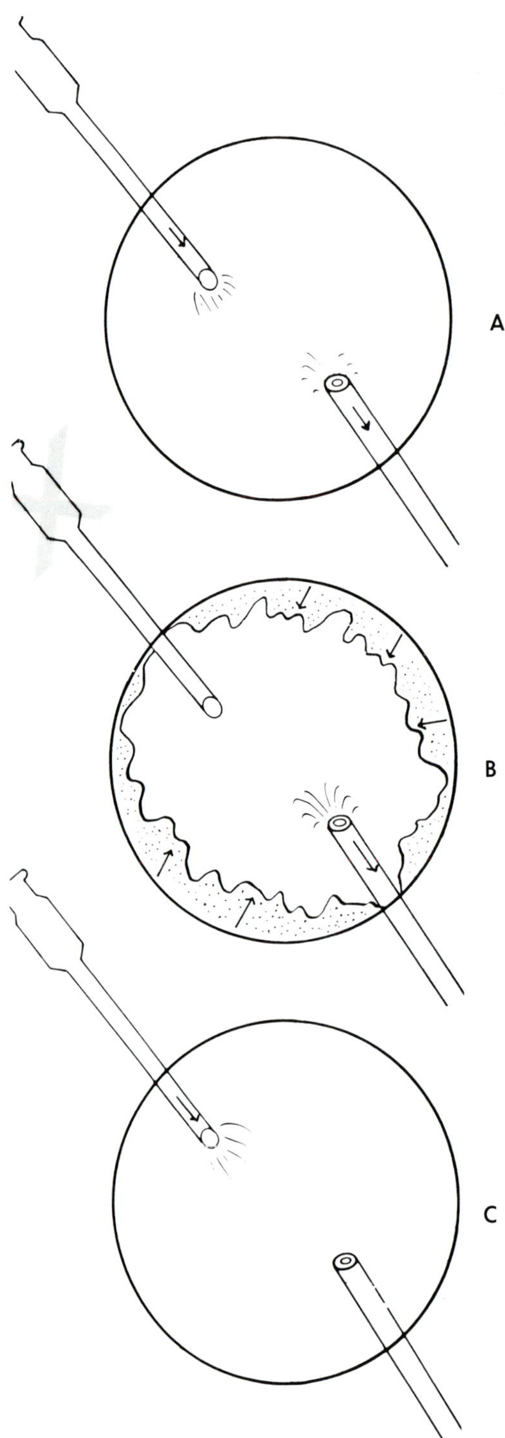

FIG. 5-29 **The various combinations of inflow and outflow create maximal distention and visualization.**

A **Inflow should exceed outflow at all times for optimal viewing.**

B **When outflow exceeds inflow there is joint collapse.**

C **Inflow without outflow creates maximal distention.**

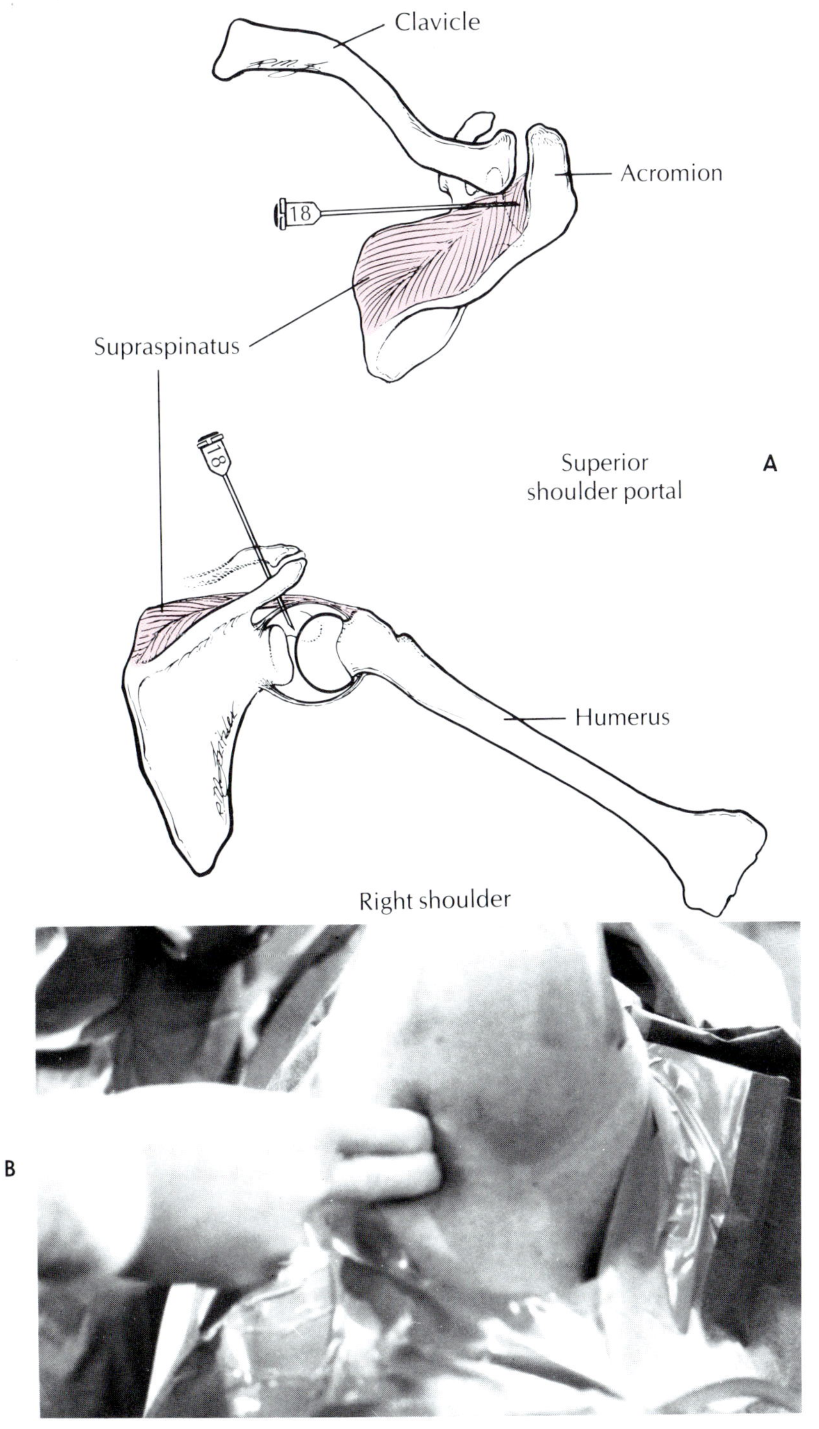

FIG. 5-30 Superior inflow portal.

A Drawing of landmark of entry at apex of clavicle and scapula and through musculature of supraspinatus.

B Sulcus is palpated with fingers.

Continued.

C

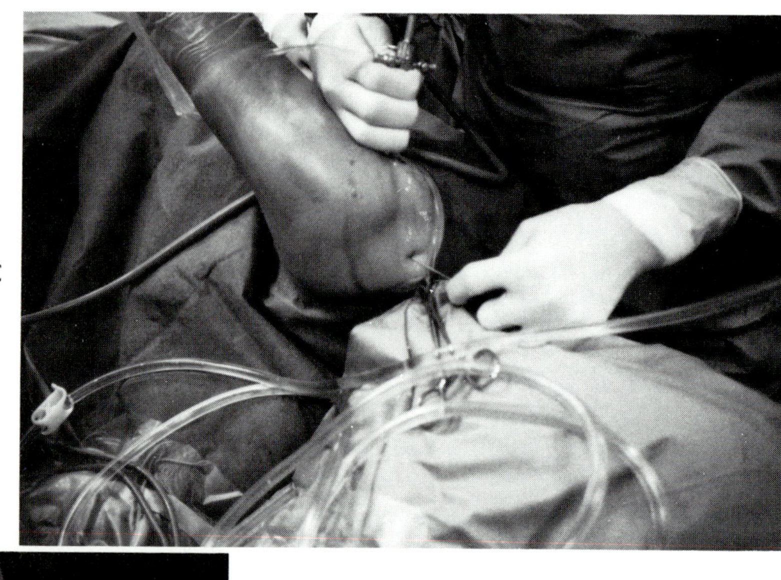

D

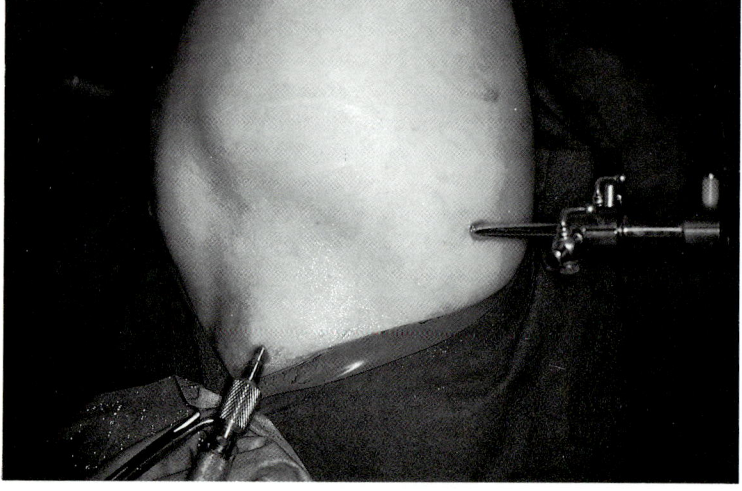

E

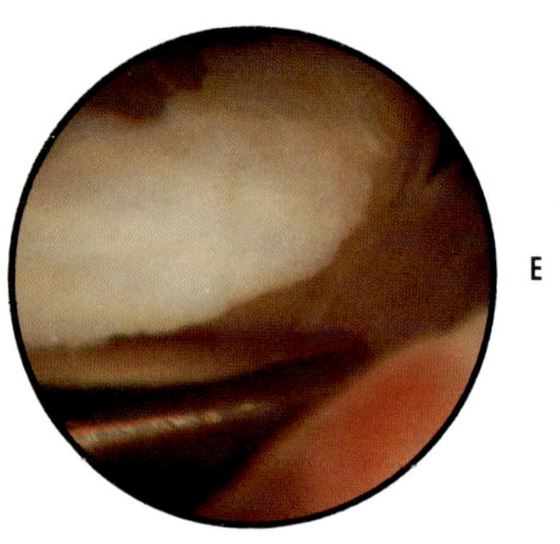

FIG. 5-30 ***cont'd*** **Superior inflow portal.**

C No. 18 spinal needle approach safely secures entry tract before cannula insertion.

D Superior inflow cannula through supraspinatus muscle and arthroscope placed from posterior.

E Arthroscopic view of inflow cannula resting below posterior glenoid labrum.

Continued.

Control of Joint Leakage. If an incision made for portal placement exceeds the diameter of the cannula, leakage occurs. Leakage out of the joint may cause decompression. Extravasation into the capsule and skin is even worse, lengthening the distance from the skin to the joint, resulting in a longer fulcrum that interferes with scope manipulation. Cannula systems decrease fluid leakage by creating a single hole of entry. When the portal is not in use, the obturator placed in the cannula preserves the portal for subsequent use and controls the leakage. When hand instrumentation is passed through the cannula, the cannula is removed over the instrument if possible and returned to the Mayo stand. When instrumentation is complete, the cannula is placed back over the probe or knife for interchange to another instrument. Passage without cannulas is necessary with the use of forceps, but the small incisions still reduce leakage. Motorized instrumentation is also passed through cannulas.

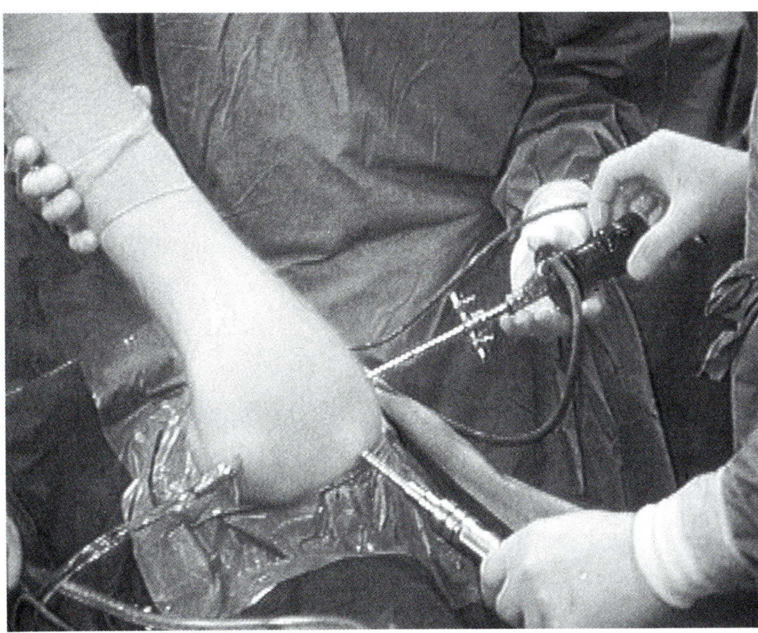

FIG. 5-30 *cont'd* **Superior inflow portal.**

F The inflow portal may be interchanged with the anterior or posterior portal to facilitate operative arthroscopy from the superior portal.

Potential Problems with Inflow

Joint Position. Joint position may affect fluid flow. Both humeral rotation and displacement has the potential to decrease joint space volume or obstruct an inflow cannula.

Empty Fluid Reservoir. The most common problem is an unrecognized empty fluid reservoir. This is solved by diligent monitoring by the circulating nurse. Careful attention is necessary to avoid an empty fluid reservoir. The two bags rarely empty in unison. When emptying is unequal, the empty bag is clamped off and another is suspended. Pressure is applied to the other bag until it is empty. The first bag is unclamped to maintain flow during change of the second bag. This alternating emptying system is very functional.

Unopened Tubing. It may seem obvious, but troubleshooting a lack of fluid often uncovers a failure to unclamp the inflow tubing. Attention to details avoids this problem.

Inflow Cannula Obstruction. Malposition of the cannula is another potential problem to compromise fluid inflow. The cannula may not have been placed in the joint. The cannula may be placed at an acute angle or pushed in so far that the opening may be occluded by the opposite joint wall. Cannulas with side openings were intended to overcome this problem in knee arthroscopy, but are not recommended for shoulder inflow because retraction of the cannula in the smaller spaces around the shoulder may cause extraarticular extravasation through these small openings. Inflow disruption may occur during shoulder joint manipulation, especially rotation or posterior displacement of the humerus. The opening of the cannula may be occluded by compression of the joint wall against the humerus. Sometimes the inflow cannula may be blocked with a loose body or a large blood clot.

Potential Problems With Outflow

The common intraoperative causes are a clamped tube, debris clogging the tubing at the junction with an adaptor, and loose connections. An unmeasured suction system of below 14 inches of mercury will be ineffective for Dyonics motorized instrumentation.

No-Flow Viewing

After the glenohumeral joint has been cleansed and examined, the outflow spigot is closed. The inflow remains open via superior cannula for optimal distention. No flow is needed during most hand instrumentation.

After hand instrumentation resection, small fragments are removed by gravity flow or use of motorized instrumentation like a vacuum cleaner.

Operative Out-Flow

The effectiveness of motorized instruments is based on the surgical principle of cutting tissue under tension. The tissue tension is created by force of suction that draws the tissue into the cutting orifice of the tool. Flow moves the material through the instrument and out of the joint. If for some reason flow can not be established for motorized instruments, then resection with hand instruments is substituted.

Postoperative Inspection

At the conclusion of a procedure, the space is redistended and a postoperative inspection is accompanied by reapplication of vacuum suction to the arthroscope to remove any remaining surgical debris.

ARTHROSCOPE MANIPULATIVE TECHNIQUES

Placement and Direction

Proper placement of the arthroscope is essential to successful shoulder arthroscopy (Fig. 5-31). It constitutes the surgical approach. If the surgeon is unable to enter the shoulder joint, any further discussion about arthroscopy becomes academic.

Arthroscopic portals are initiated with superficial laceration of the skin. A No. 11 blade is utilized (Fig. 5-31, *A*) to minimize cutting cutaneous nerves. The surgeon must be careful not to penetrate into the joint with the knife blade. The skin puncture should be only wide enough to accommodate the cannula. Otherwise, fluid leaks out and causes joint decompression, wet feet, and a wet floor.

An arthroscope cannula with a sharp trocar pierces the skin and the deltoid muscle (Fig. 5-32). The trocar is replaced with a blunt obturator for joint capsular penetration. The commercially available cannula systems have trocars that are too sharp and obturators that are often too blunt for this task. I have smoothed the end of a commercially available sharp trocar, and it serves both functions to allow a single obturator for joint entry (Fig. 5-32, *D*).

Accurate placement and direction is necessary for proper entry. If the arthroscope cannula is angled too superior, it enters the subacromial bursa. If the cannula is angled too low, it enters the inferior aspect of the glenohumeral joint (Fig. 5-33). If angled lower, the axillary nerve is at risk. If angled too medially, the suprascapular nerve, which is only 2 cm away, is at risk.[3,7] A portal or direction that is too lateral may create an injury in the posterior humeral head (Fig. 5-34).

In arthroscopic surgery, a separate puncture or redirection is required to correct a misplaced portal of entry. This is unlike open surgery, in which if a skin incision is misplaced a correction is possible by sliding the wound.

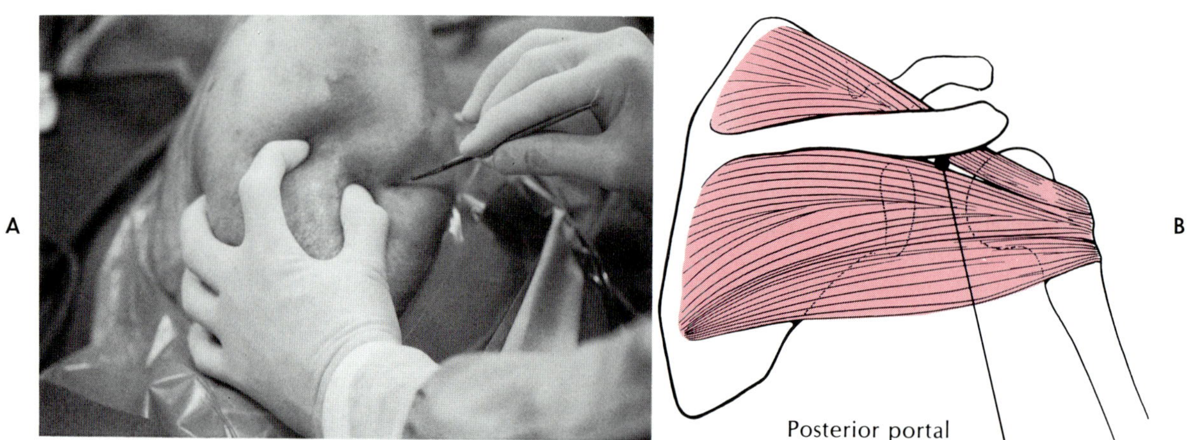

FIG. 5-31 Posterior skin incision and topographical landmarks.

A The posterior angle of the acromion is "captured" with the surgeon's thumb and index finger. The skin incision is made on the tangential surface of the skin in a place that will allow passage of the arthroscope 1 cm below the undersurface of the acromion and 1 cm medial to the posterior tip.

B Graphic illustration of plane of passage of the arthroscope to the glenohumeral joint.

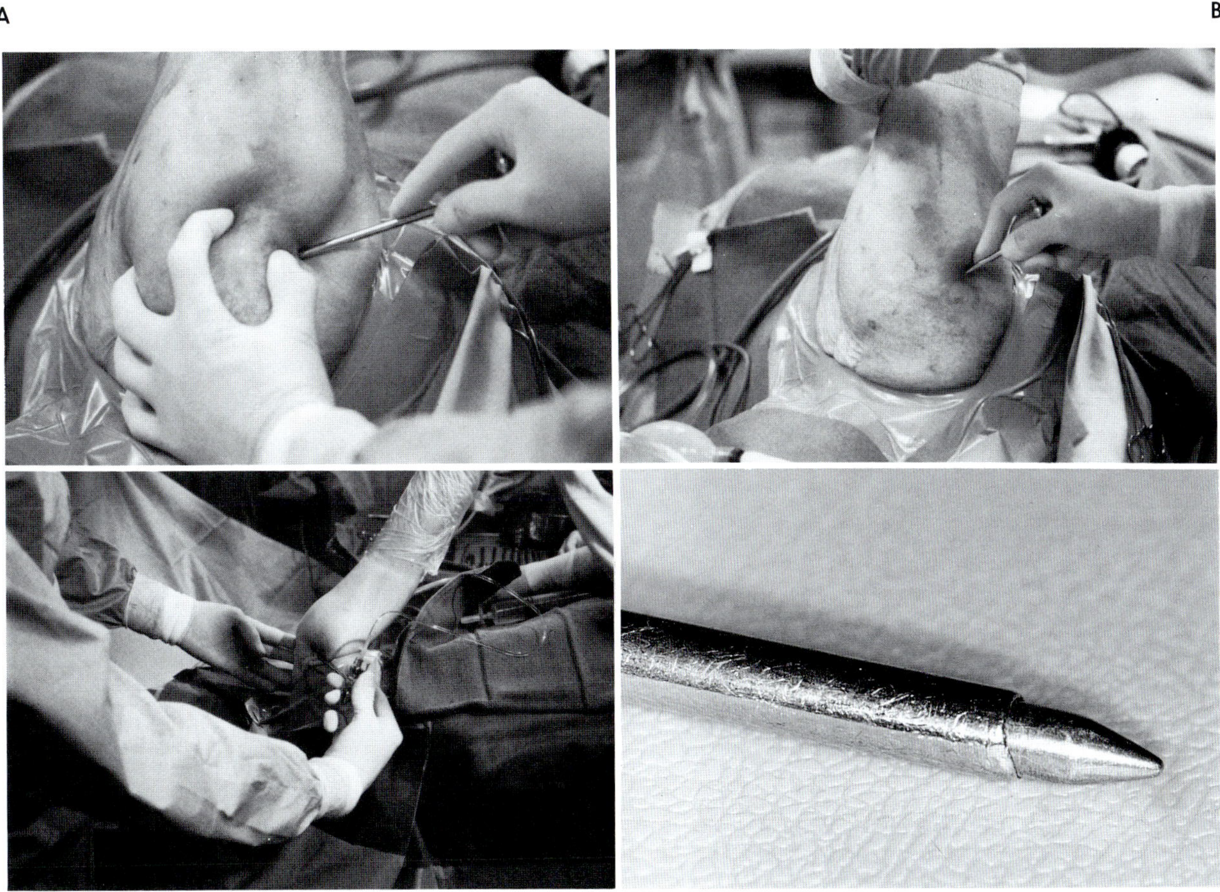

FIG. 5-32 Arthroscope placement.

A The surgeon's free hand captures the posterior angle of the acromion. The arthroscope cannula/obturator is passed with firm pressure and rotation motion to avoid plunging.

B The surgeon's free hand internally rotates the humeral shaft and the arthroscope cannula/obturator angles toward the glenohumeral joint.

C Palpation of the coracoid process with the free hand will give general direction for the cannula/obturator to approach the glenohumeral joint.

D Close-up view shows modified obturator, neither sharp nor totally blunted, and evidence of use.

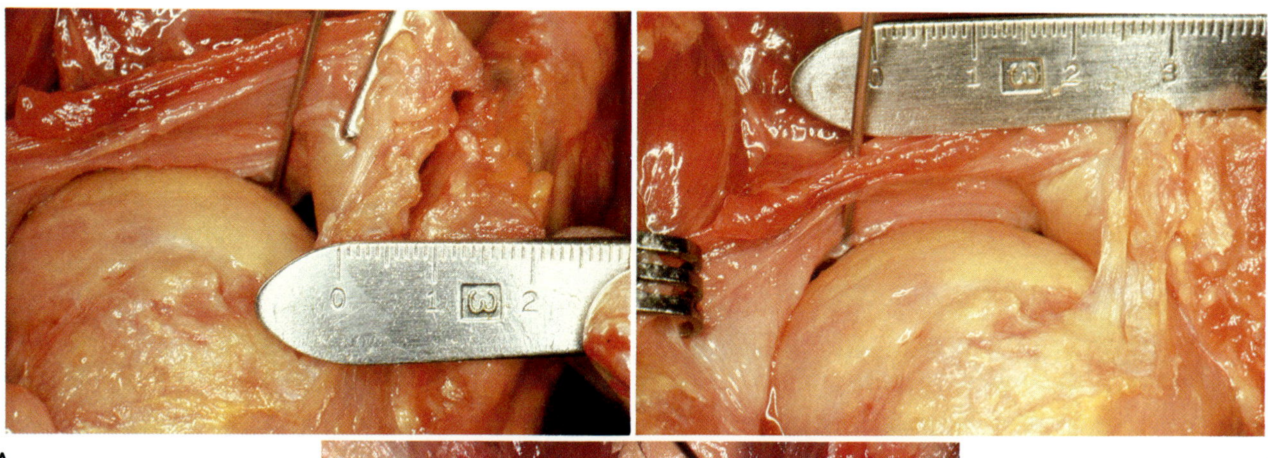

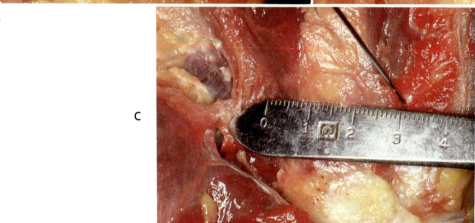

FIG. 5-33 Arthroscope placement in relation to the anatomical structures.

A The proper placement is 1 cm below the acromion. This delivers the arthroscope to the superior aspect of the joint.

B A placement 3 cm below the acromion places the arthroscope in the inferior aspect of the joint and compromises both manipulation and visualization.

C If the arthroscope is placed lower, then the axillary nerve is at risk of injury.

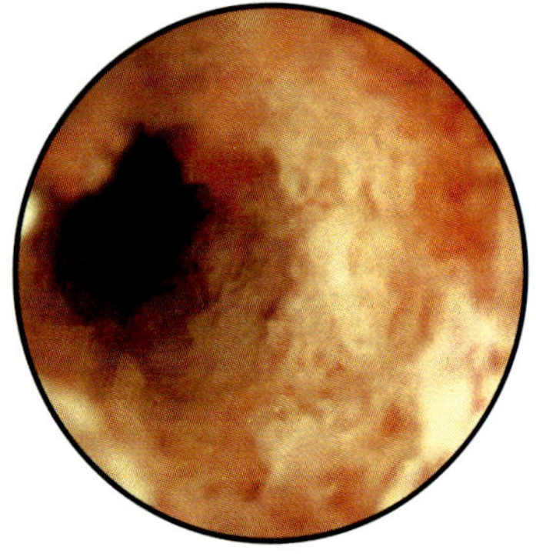

FIG. 5-34 Arthroscopic view of inadvertent penetration of the humeral head. Notice the disruption of the articular surface and the exposed cancellous bone where the obturator penetrated the posterior humeral head.

Fulcrum Principle

All instrumentation placed arthroscopically operates off a fulcrum principle. The skin, subcutaneous and capsular tissues, make up this long fulcrum, which limits side to side and angulatory motions. Because of the fulcum, a force applied to the scope on the outside by the surgeon results in opposite direction movement of the end of the scope within the joint. A move to the right moves the scope or instrumentation on the inside of the left and vice versa. Recognition of this principle allows the surgeon to adjust to the perspective.

The depth (or width) of the fulcrum is greater in shoulder arthroscopy than in the knee. The increased depth of shoulder tissue decreases mobility of the scope and instruments during glenohumeral or subacromial bursa arthroscopy as compared to the knee.

Tissue Resistance Provides Control to Instrumentation

Intentional creation of small puncture wounds provides a tight grip around the arthroscope and instruments. The instruments are secured in the tissue, thereby resisting sudden movement. This results in more controlled and exacting motions. A large portal incision allows the instrument to slide not only side to side, but in and out, thus losing manipulative exactness.

Control of Fluid Leakage

Troublesome leakage may also occur around a large opening. If the hole is large, hand pressure or even suturing may be necessary at the skin to stop the leak and keep the instrument from inadvertently pistoning. A sponge may be draped over an instrument to divert a leak from spraying out of the joint (Fig. 5-35).

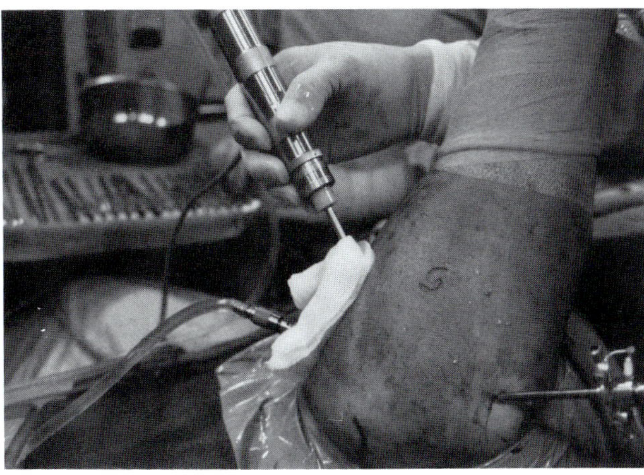

FIG. 5-35 A sponge is draped over the instrument portal to divert fluid leakage.

Glenohumeral Joint Entry

A posterior portal is routinely used for initial arthroscope entry into the glenohumeral joint. Passive internal rotation of the suspended humerus facilitates entry into the glenohumeral joint (see Fig. 5-20).

The posterior angle of the acromion serves as an anatomical landmark for arthroscope passage. I capture the posterior angle of the acromion with my index finger and thumb to establish the topographical landmark (see Fig. 5-31).

The scope should pass 1 cm inferior and 1 cm medial to the acromion (see Fig. 5-33, *A*). The size and shape of the patient determines the site of the skin incision. In a muscular or obese patient, the actual skin incision will be far removed from the posterior angle of the acromion in order to parallel its undersurface while approaching the glenohumeral joint.

After initial soft tissue penetration, the surgeon may place his or her opposite hand on the coracoid process as an external landmark for scope cannula/obturator direction (see Fig. 5-32, *C*). Palpation, not visualization, is the method used for placement. Since palpation is so important, I often look away from the shoulder, so as to eliminate any false attempt at visualization and provide maximum sensory input for palpation. The cannula and obturator serve as extensions of the surgeon's hand.

Rotation must be simultaneously combined with advancement of the scope cannula and obturator. Penetration is accomplished with firm forward rotational pressure (Fig. 5-36). This combined motion will place the cannula and obturator safely into the joint. This technique avoids "plunging," mishap, and joint surface injury (see Fig. 5-34).

If entry is not immediate, the location of the cannula tip may be ascertained by the following observations. If the resistance is soft, then you are in muscle or fat. If the resistance is hard you are against bone. To determine which bone you are against, rotate the humerus. If no force is transmitted to the cannula, then you probably are against the glenoid. If the tip of the cannula moves with passive motion of the humerus, you know your location (Fig. 5-36). If you are against the humerus, use this location to check whether you are too high or too low. Gently push with the obturator against the humeral head. If internal rotation results, you are located superior. If external rotation occurs, you are inferior. If only anterior humeral displacement occurs, then you are centered on the humerus. Confirm this position with another maneuver. Use passive humeral shaft rotation while monitoring movement with the arthroscope cannula.

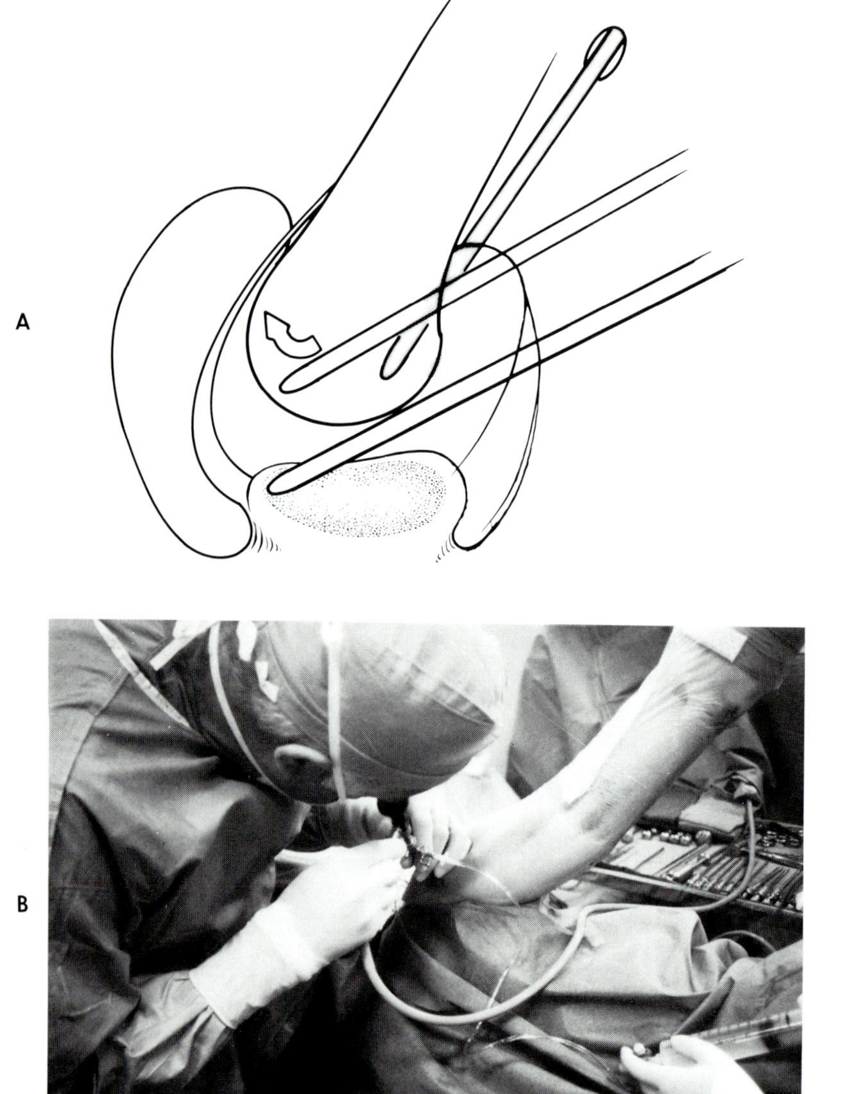

FIG. 5-36 Palpation skills necessary for shoulder entry.
A Rotation of humerus indicates position of cannula to joint.
B Direct viewing confirms joint entry.

Penetration into the glenohumeral joint is preceded by the sensation of passing through the distinct posterior capsule. Before removing the obturator, the surgeon should gently advance the cannula and obturator deeper into the joint. Slow retraction without rotation hangs up the synovium and capsule on the instrument shaft. This avoids accidental exit and covering of the end of the scope with tissue, obscuring the view (Fig. 5-37). Entry is confirmed by placing the arthroscope in the cannula for direct viewing. The synovial lining with small vessels is easily contrasted with muscle or adventitia. A small amount of fluid distention (5 ml) along the scope will improve the view without massive extravasation of fluids.

Glenohumeral operative portals will be discussed in Chapter 8.

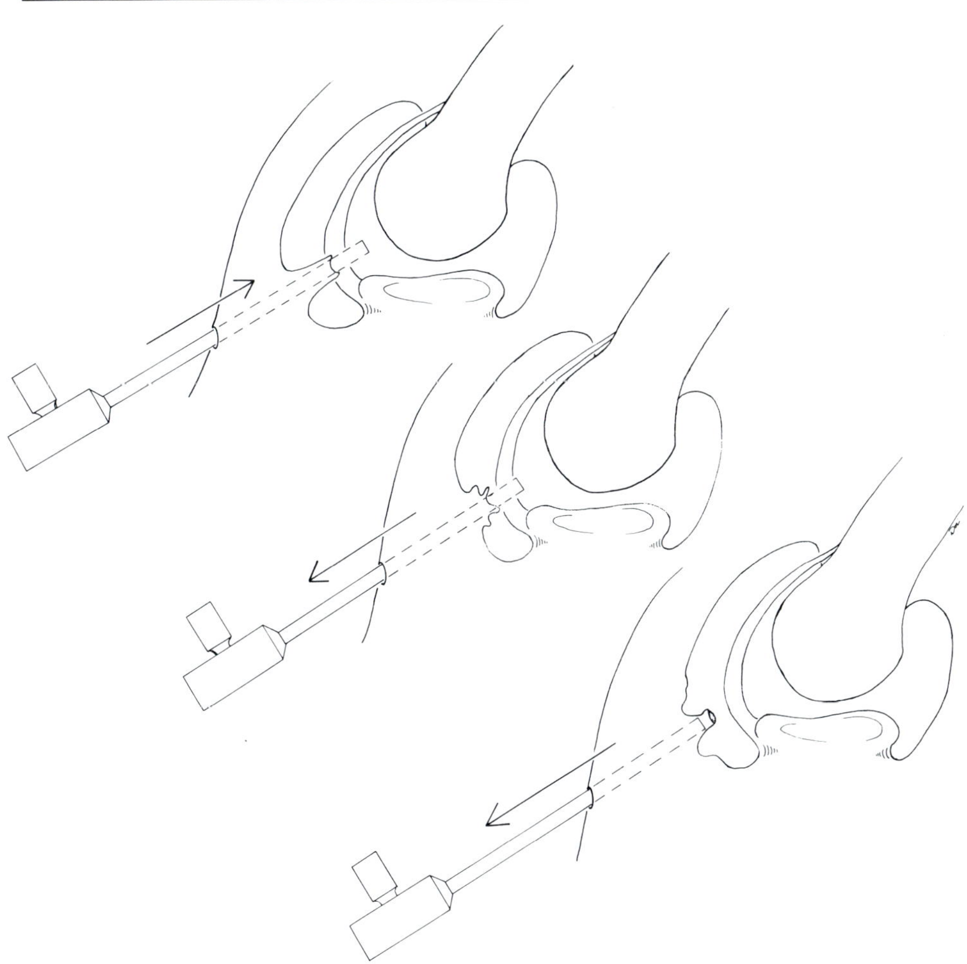

FIG. 5-37 Secured entry of scope. The arthroscope cannula penetrates into the joint with authority. Retraction is a slow movement so that tissues "hang" on cannula and remain retracted from end of scope.

Subacromial Space Entry

The subacromial space is also approached from posterior through the same skin incision used for the glenohumeral joint. In some cases of an obese patient or intervening massive fluid extravasation, another skin incision may be necessary to gain a proper angle of approach to the subacromial space.

Measurement of the distance from the posterior skin incision to the anterior acromion with the arthroscope cannula is a safety precaution (Fig. 5-38). This imaginary mark provides one measure of position after penetration. The surgeon's free hand is used as a guide by palpation of the acromion. This hand can be moved over to the tip of the coracoid process for another topographical landmark. The arthroscope cannula/obturator enters the skin incision but is redirected superior under the acromion. Palpation of the undersurface of the acromion with the cannula/obturator is helpful for locating the bursa. Entry is simple when a large bursa exists. Entry is difficult in normal patients as the bursa is small. The normal subacromial bursa is immediately under the free span of the coracoacromial ligament. When the arthroscope cannula has been inserted, the tip of the obturator can be palpated under the free portion of the coracoacromial ligament. Repeated obturator removal and scope insertion may be required if the bursa is small or the view is obstructed by synovitis and fibrous bands.

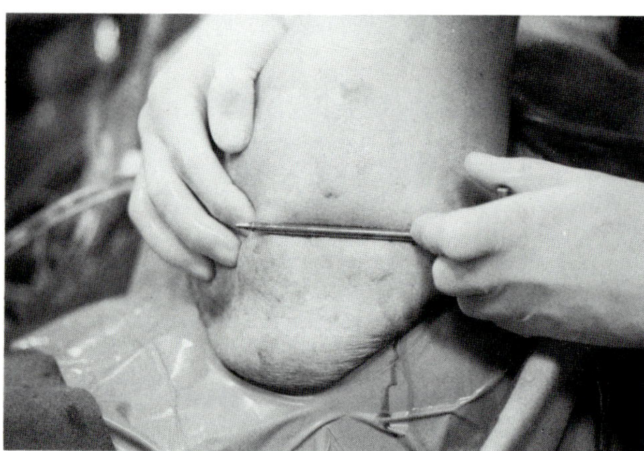

FIG. 5-38 Subacromial space entry. A preliminary measurement is made with the arthroscope cannula to estimate the depth necessary to reach the undersurface of the coracoacromial ligament. The surgeon's finger remains on the scope cannula so penetration does not exceed this distance.

Preliminary distention may be required to confirm location, just as for the glenohumeral joint. As a last resort the cannula/obturator may be moved side to side to expand the bursa. This maneuver will enlarge the potential space, but if too vigorous the walls of the bursa will be torn and subsequently contained fluid will be lost. This spillage makes subsequent surgery difficult.

Repeated attempts at entry into the subacromial space are justified. If clinical symptoms of impingement or a rotator cuff tear are present, entry into bursa is possible for even the inexperienced. In normal patients with a small bursae and no subacromial symptoms, the surgeon should abandon attempts if entry is not accomplished after three well-placed attempts. Further tissue damage may occur.

Blind debridement of the subacromial space area should not be a substitute for failure of exposure. Surgical debridement should follow only a confirmed bursal entry. Optimal surgical exposure of the subacromial space may come only following debridement of the bursal bands with motorized instrumentation.

Subacromial operative portals will be discussed in Chapter 9.

Acromioclavicular Joint Entry

Two surgical approaches to this joint exist: one is superior and transcutaneous; the other is inferior and from the subacromial space.

The transcutaneous approach requires preliminary needle penetration and distention. The subacromial approach is facilitated by transcutaneous placement of a No. 18 spinal needle through the skin and joint from superior to inferior as a locator medial to the subacromial bursa. Using a combination of approaches may be advantageous, with the arthroscope inferior to the joint after acromionectomy and the motorized instrumentation placed transcutaneously from superior to enter the exact plane of the AC joint. The arthroscope placement and surgery of the AC joint will be discussed in Chapter 10.

EXTRAARTICULAR ARTHROSCOPIC TECHNIQUES

Replacement

The inexperienced arthroscopist focuses so intensely on difficulties of viewing that he or she fails to recognize that the original portal placement may be less than optimal. Perhaps another site should have been selected. It is considered good technique to either replace and/or redirect an arthroscope. This maneuver avoids struggling with poor exposure throughout the entire case.

Poor placement sites are commonly seen in patients seeking second opinions after failed arthroscopic surgery. I have seen some sites placed as much as 3 inches away from the optimal position. No amount of manipulation could produce proper surgical exposure from this position. Reoperation usually shows unrecognized lesions and iatrogenic articular cartilage damage (traumatic arthritis) or even penetration fracture of the posterior humeral head (Figs. 5-39 and 5-40).

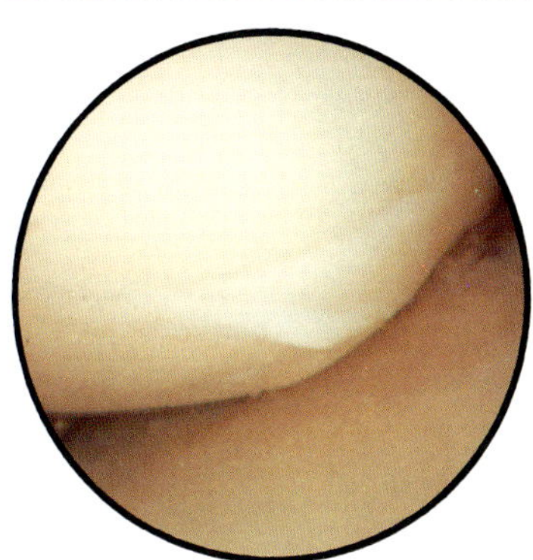

FIG. 5-39 Scrape of the articular surface as made with the arthroscope.

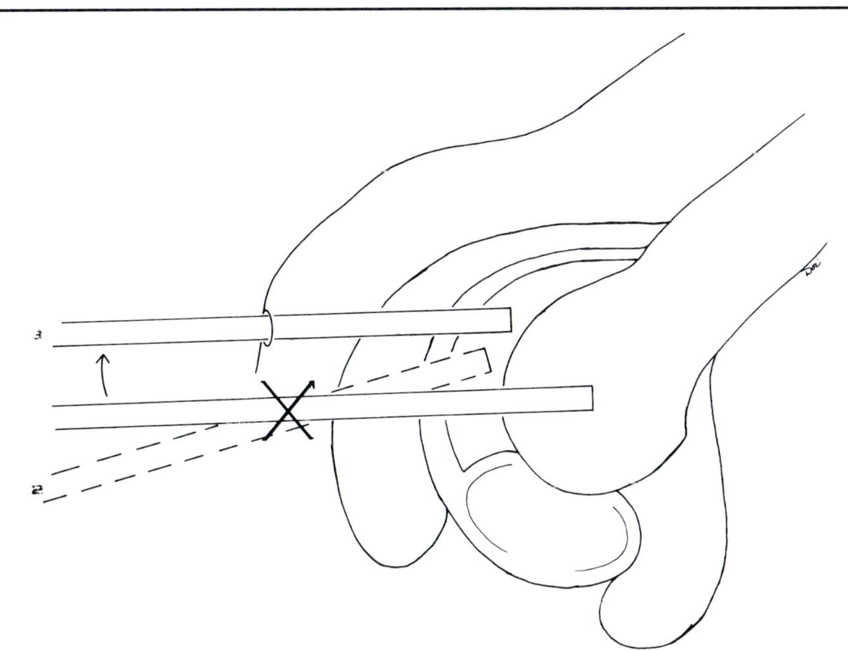

FIG. 5-40 Replacement. The scope is removed and replaced at a different position in the tissue, up, down, or side to side.

If surgical exposure is not optimal, the scope should be removed and replaced to another site (Fig. 5-40). Attention to proper portal sites is discussed under specific techniques in later chapters. If the site appears close to optimal, then the same skin incision could be used if the skin is moved sideways up or down, and another capsular penetration is accomplished via the same incision.

Replacement is chosen if either scar tissue or depth of tissue decreases instrument mobility. If visualization of a certain area is compromised, an alternate portal is chosen.

Direction

The scope or instrument is directed toward a known anatomical target. Viewing the surface anatomy with bony landmarks is helpful. However, the internal structures are still not seen as in open surgery, with layer by layer exposure. Palpation is the sense that is of greatest value in proper direction. To enhance palpation, it is helpful to look away; this removes the useless temptation to visualize. This same technique is valuable for placement of instrumentation. Specific operative portals are discussed in later chapters.

Redirection

If the position is acceptable yet visualization is inadequate, the problem may be misdirection (Fig. 5-41). Redirection should be tried before portal position is changed. The instrument is withdrawn through the capsule, not the skin, and reinserted by palpation in another direction. Redirection may be used in patients who are obese or have a scar from previous surgery or injury. Forcing the arthroscope through a wide fulcrum or through tough tissue can only result in injury to the arthroscope and/or the patient's articular tissue. In some patients with a very tight or scarred joint, redirecting as many as three times may be necessary to gain adequate view. This should be considered good technique, not failure of the initial placement.

Redirection is routine when switching from the glenohumeral joint to the subacromial space. Redirection is less effort than struggling and produces less tissue injury than does forceful angulation. Furthermore, redirection facilitates complete inspection of all the areas of the joint.

If redirection fails, then a minor change of portal position will be necessary. In some cases, an alternate portal at another area of the joint will be necessary.

Lower Body Control

The arthroscopist may appear as a one-man-band with all body parts being involved. The feet must be firmly planted on the floor or the surgeon firmly seated on a stable stool. This is the platform from which various surgical maneuvers take place. One foot secures balance as the other operates the foot pedal of motorized instruments or electrocautery. Some surgeons prefer to have an assistant activate the surgical controls because this decreases the number of things they must do. I refrain from this technique, prefering all control in the surgeon's hands (or feet).

Upper Body Control

Although a firm grip on the arthroscope is needed, the rest of the body must remain relaxed. The intensity of the procedure may cause unconscious tenseness and fatigue. The combined and coordinated action of the surgeon's wrist, elbow, and shoulder make up a "universal joint" to position the surgeon's hand.

A firm grip allows precise movements and prevents any slippage or inadvertent joint injury. Dexterity is provided by the wrist, elbow, and shoulder. Lack of precision in handling the arthroscope, cannula and/or trocar could result in quick motion and potential abrasions to the intraarticular structures, especially the articular cartilage. Damage to the arthroscope is also possible.

Hand Control

With direct viewing the scope is handled firmly, like a pencil, between the thumb and fingers (Fig. 5-42). When using video projection, the hand is cupped around the scope and the television camera is balanced. The scope is controlled with very slow, deliberate motions to allow time for assimilation of the image. Quick motions lead to disorientation or even joint damage. The motion can be likened to that used to smooth frosting in cake decoration. The pressure is firm, but gentle and rhythmical.

Free Hand Activity

The most common use of the surgeon's free hand is for rotation of the humerus (Fig. 5-43). The free hand is also used to palpate the acromion and the CA ligament. Humeral positioning may be accomplished by the assistants.

With the patient under local anesthesia, the patient's tightness or anxiety can be monitored by noting spontaneous tightening of the musculature. Such tenseness can alert the surgeon to any quick motion by the patient and thus avoid damage to the joint or the arthroscope.

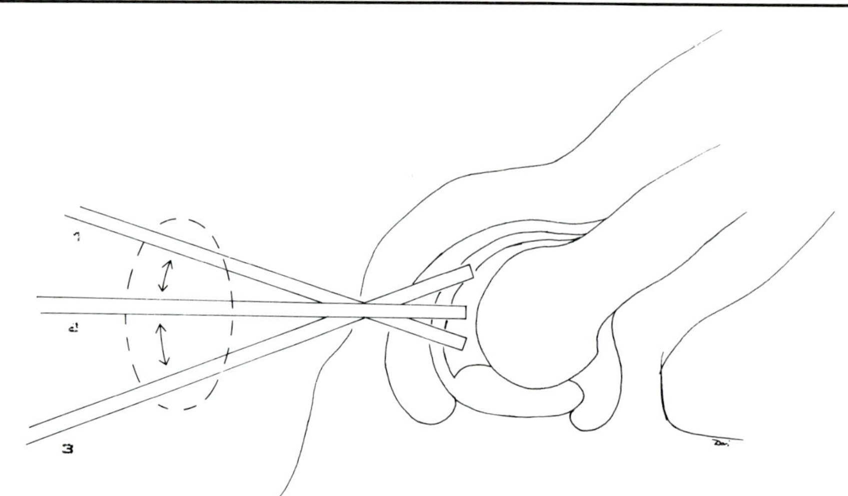

FIG. 5-41 Redirection. The placement position remains the same, but the direction of the scope cannula insertion differs.

A

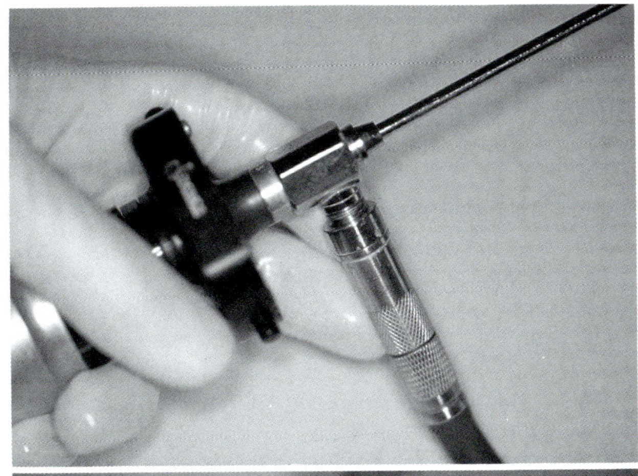

B

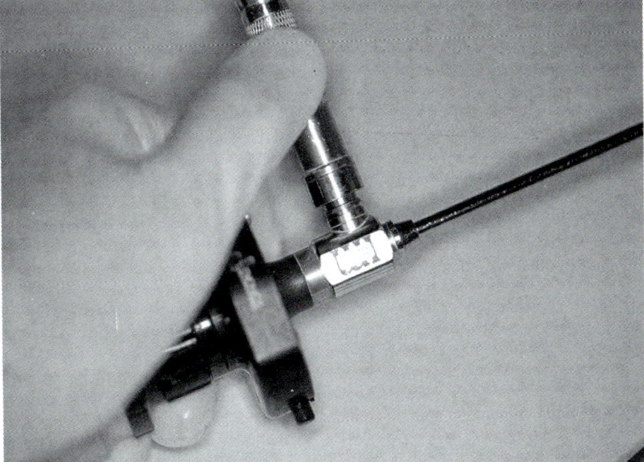

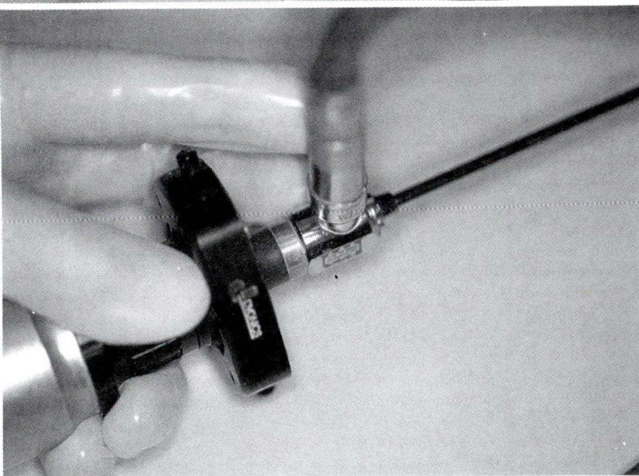

C

FIG. 5-42 Hand control.

A The hand-held television camera is held in palm of the hand and the scope is rotated with pressure on the arm of the light cable.

B The scope is rotated 90 degrees and the arm of the light cable is now controlled with the surgeon's thumb.

C Further rotation is provided with pressure from the surgeon's index finger.

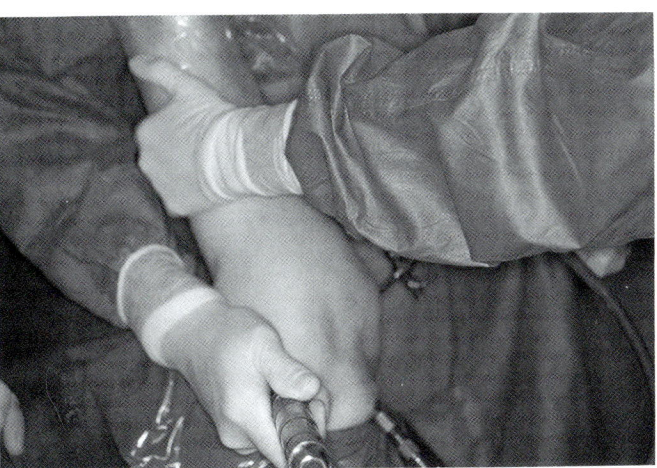

FIG. 5-43 External manipulation of the joint. Manipulation of the humerus will provide another method of gaining optimal visualization or instrument access.

External Manipulation of the Joint

Too much emphasis has been placed on scope manipulation and too little on manipulation of the extremity to gain arthroscopic composition (Fig. 5-43). The surgical exposure is facilitated by application of various forces to open or distract the joint. The glenohumeral joint is exposed by suspension, distention, rotation, and flexion and abduction. The composition is affected by external manipulation.

Rotational force can be applied to the humerus with coordinated motion of the arthroscope to gain access to an otherwise inaccessible area of the shoulder. Another technique is to hold the arthroscope fixed within the joint and move the humerus to create the view in front of the arthroscope. The humerus may be rotated, providing a panoramic view of the posterior surface without moving the arthroscope. This maneuver is a common method of observing the humeral surface: from anteror to posterior and from superior to inferior surface.

Arthroscope positioning becomes quite complex when various combinations of forces are applied to the scope and the extremity. Exact awareness of individual manipulation factors is not possible during surgery, but becomes second nature to the experienced arthroscopist.

Increased distention will move the humerus away from the glenoid (Fig. 5-44). The pressure is applied with syringe and K-52 catheter attached to the arthroscope. This method is more effective than external traction on the arm, even at forces of great magnitude. Distention is also safer than traction.[1]

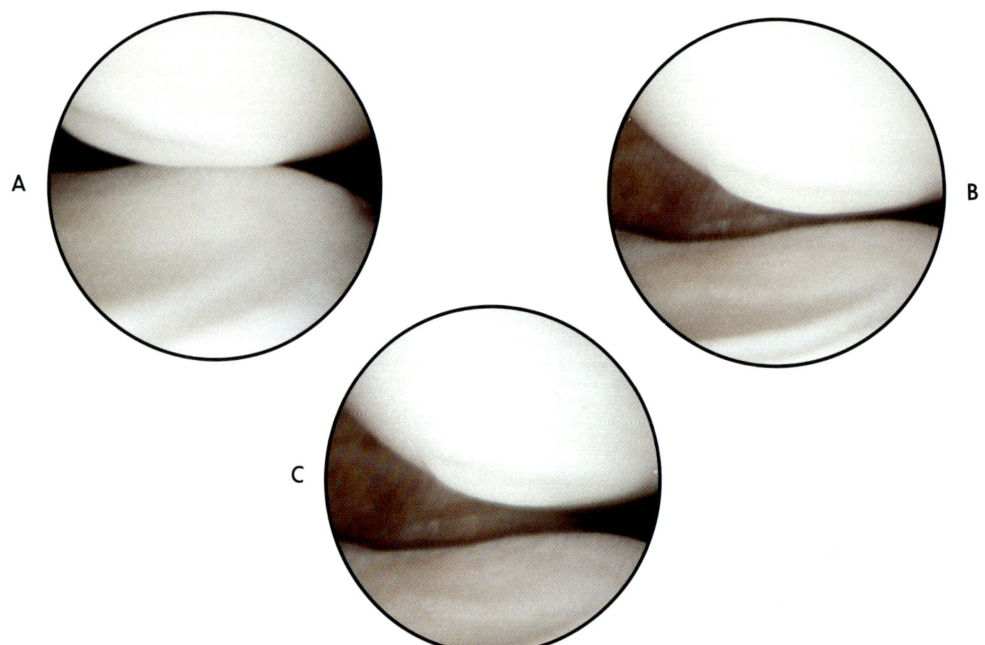

FIG. 5-44 Exposure is facilitated by intraarticular pressure that distracts the humeral head from the glenoid.

A Minimal distention shows the humerus resting on the glenoid.

B Increase in distention lifts the humerus off the glenoid.

C With maximal distention supplied during the diagnostic phase with syringe and K-52 catheter, the anterior joint is seen through the space between humerus and glenoid.

INTRAARTICULAR ARTHROSCOPIC TECHNIQUES

Palpation

Although arthroscopy draws attention to visualization, palpation skill is as important. Visualization follows that placement or sense of placement. As one's technical skills improve, so does the ability to sense by palpation the proper location within the shoulder joint. For instance, one learns to sense by drag and palpation the different layers of fat, capsule, and synovium during joint penetration. Palpation is used to determine the position of the arthroscope in relation to the various intraarticular parts, whether the humerus, biceps tendon, or acromion. After some experience, one can even palpate soft tissue structures such as the biceps tendon in the shoulder without looking. The skill of palpation is essential as one advances to arthroscopic shoulder surgery.

A well-placed arthroscope, with the surgeon keeping an awareness of the sense of palpation and not emphasizing or attempting just the visualization, will facilitate the arthroscopic examination with a high level of eye-hand coordination.

Pistoning

The most primitive motions applied to the arthroscope are push and pull. The pistoning motion moves the scope forward and then it is retracted backward (Fig. 5-45).

Pistoning should be a controlled, gentle motion. Pistoning will provide information concerning relative size and shape in relation to other intraarticular objects.

The beginning arthroscopist generally makes very gross in and out movements. Brisk withdrawal of cannula or scope will slide the instrument out of the joint cavity, obscuring the view or causing the surgeon to lose the location of a cutting instrument.

Scanning

A second basic manipulative procedure involves moving the scope from side to side (Fig. 5-46). This motion is valuable in identifying the horizon of an articular surface,

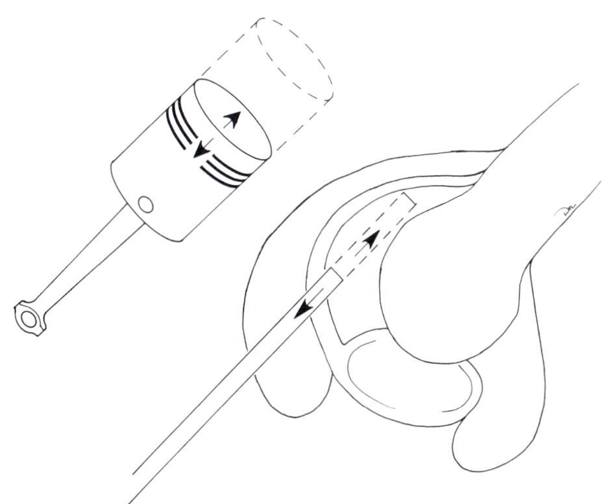

FIG. 5-45 Pistoning in joint.

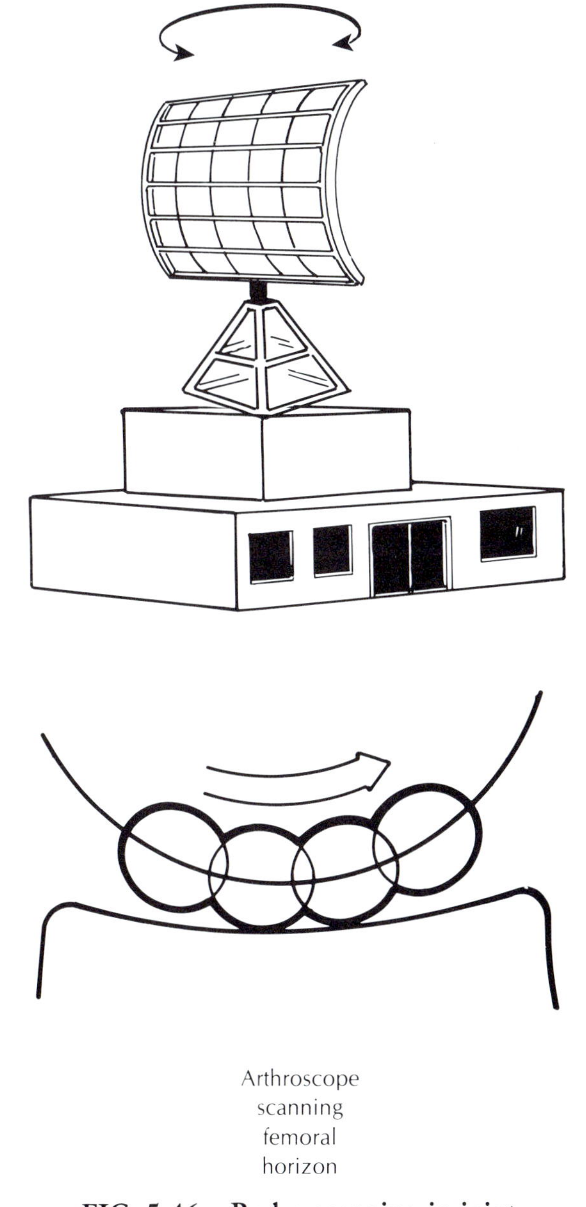

FIG. 5-46 Radar scanning in joint.

the tangential portion of the joint, and then the joint space and adjacent structures. The edge of the humeral condylar horizon should be kept in the edge of the image for orientation (Fig. 5-47).

Scanning is helpful in working from known to unknown. The arthroscopist identifies a known structure like biceps tendon or the horizon of the humeral head opposite the glenoid fossa (see Figs. 5-3 and 5-4). Finding these important landmarks arthroscopically, even if they are not the focus of the inspection, restores confidence to the surgeon concerning orientation. He or she can then move to the various structures from that point. If the surgeon becomes lost or disoriented, he or she can move back to a known horizon and to the area in question, thereby reestablishing position in the joint.

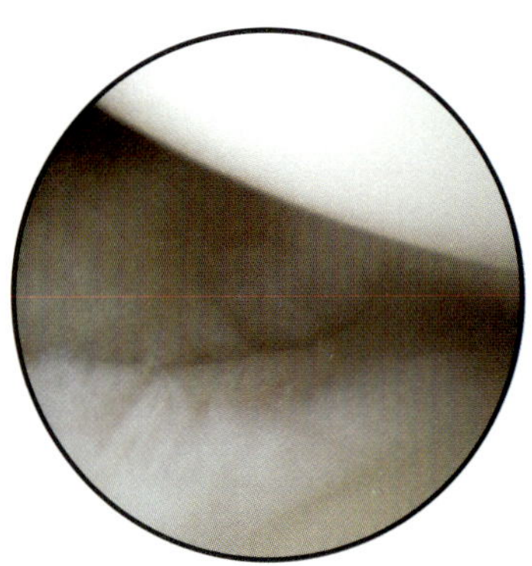

FIG. 5-47 Horizon of the humeral head is landmark for scanning.

Rotation

Scope rotation is the most valuable of the manipulative techniques. I prefer, as many arthroscopists do, an arthroscope with a 30-degree fore-oblique field of view. In a direct-viewing arthroscope, rotation will not change the view. Without any motion except rotation, a 30-degree inclined arthroscope produces a much wider view of the entire area to be inspected (Fig. 5-48). It does not necessitate any motions of the joint and/or the arthroscope to view areas to one side or the other, above, or below. This can be a distinct advantage in a circumstance in which one does not want to or cannot change position. Scope rotation can accomplish what otherwise would not be achievable by either pistoning or scanning.

Although this technique was clearly illustrated in my first textbook on arthroscopy, rotation continues to be overlooked even by experienced arthroscopists. The effective use of scope rotation is the mark of an expert arthroscopist.

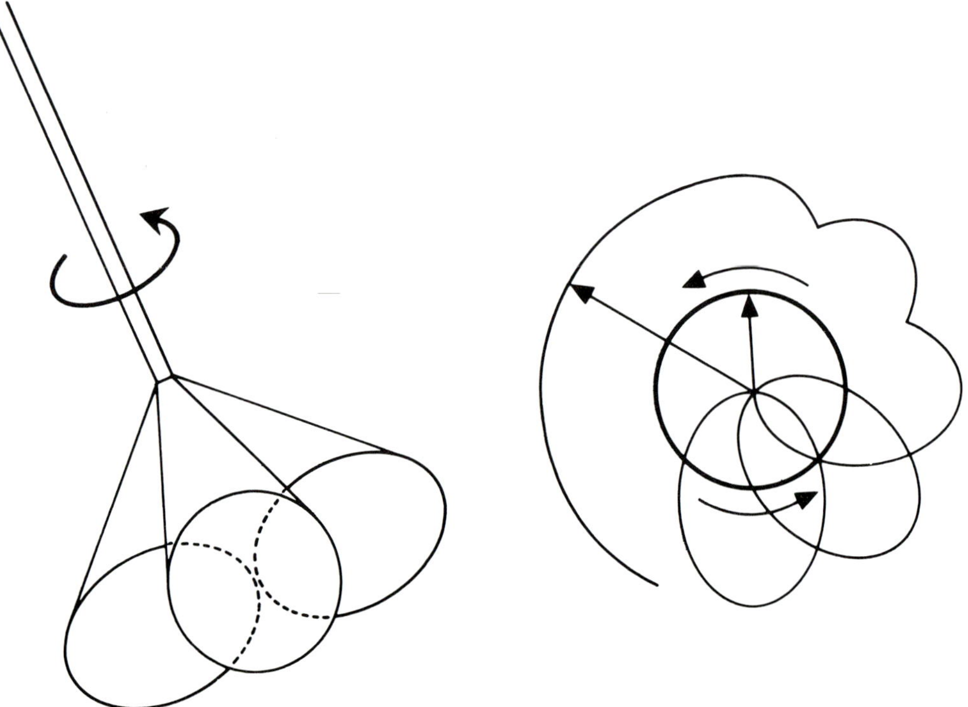

FIG. 5-48 Rotation of the arthroscope provides widest possible view without changing position of the scope.

Scope Sweeping

Scope sweeping should be a controlled motion of combined angulation and rotation (Fig. 5-49). One can visualize a pencil pushed through a cardboard square, which is the tissue fulcrum in shoulder arthroscopy. When the pencil is moved to the right, the portion of the pencil on the other side of the cardboard moves in the opposite direction. Similarly, angulation of the arthroscope on the outside of the joint produces movement in the opposite direction inside the joint.

Sweeping from side to side with very rapid motions may injure the joint and certainly blurs visualization. Gross movements of the scope should be avoided. The observations made during quick movements are useless. When the scope is moved very slowly, the surgeon can observe and comprehend the actual sequence of images.

Composition

At open surgery, the doctor has the luxury of scanning the entire wound directly with the eyes in three dimensions. This is not possible in arthroscopy. The surgeon must use many arthroscopic maneuvers to collect the data. Only one image is captured at a time. Depth perception is lacking because the arthroscope is a monocular instrument. Slow, deliberate movements combine with manipulative procedures to enable the surgeon to fully comprehend and create sequentially organized images for storage in his or her brain (Fig. 5-50). The collection and simulation of these observations construct what I call an arthroscopic composition.

The single arthroscopic view cannot visualize a joint in its entirety. A single view encompasses part of a compartment or anatomical structure. Appreciation for the entire joint is accomplished intellectually after proper techniques are mechanically executed. This is similar to the construction of photographs taken from outer space, in which individual electronically produced dots are printed in an orderly manner, line after line. The printout of these various bits of information illustrates the entire image.

Many mechanical factors contribute to composition. They include the arthroscope position, light, nature of the patient's anatomy, adherence to surgical principles, and performance of arthroscopic techniques. In addition, the proper combination of these factors influences the resultant arthroscopic picture. For example, the proper light up close to the condyle blanches out any detail. This could be corrected by retracting the scope away from the object or by dimming the light. Another surgical approach would provide a tangential view of the same area. Rotation, abduction, and adduction of the humerus show various different contact areas. Palpation with a probe determines the texture of tissue. All of these experiences are performed in concert to visualize one area of the joint.

The summation of all visual, position, and palpation experiences is recorded on television. The television records, but it cannot conceptualize. The imagery is simulated and constructed in the surgeon's mind (see below). The quality of the composition is affected by the surgeon's ability, capacity, discipline, and willingness to follow strict protocol yet allow for surgical imagination.

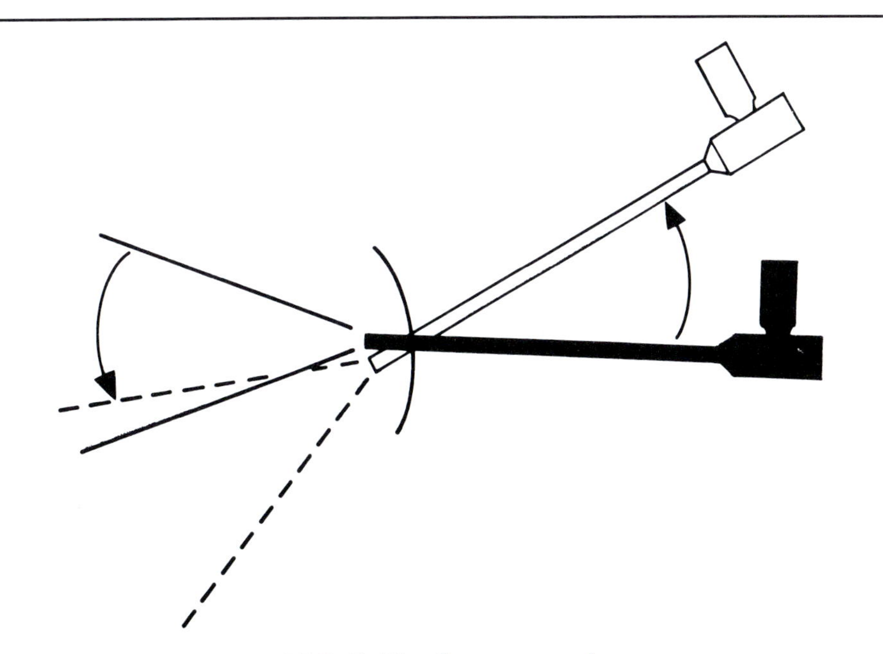

FIG. 5-49 Scope sweeping.

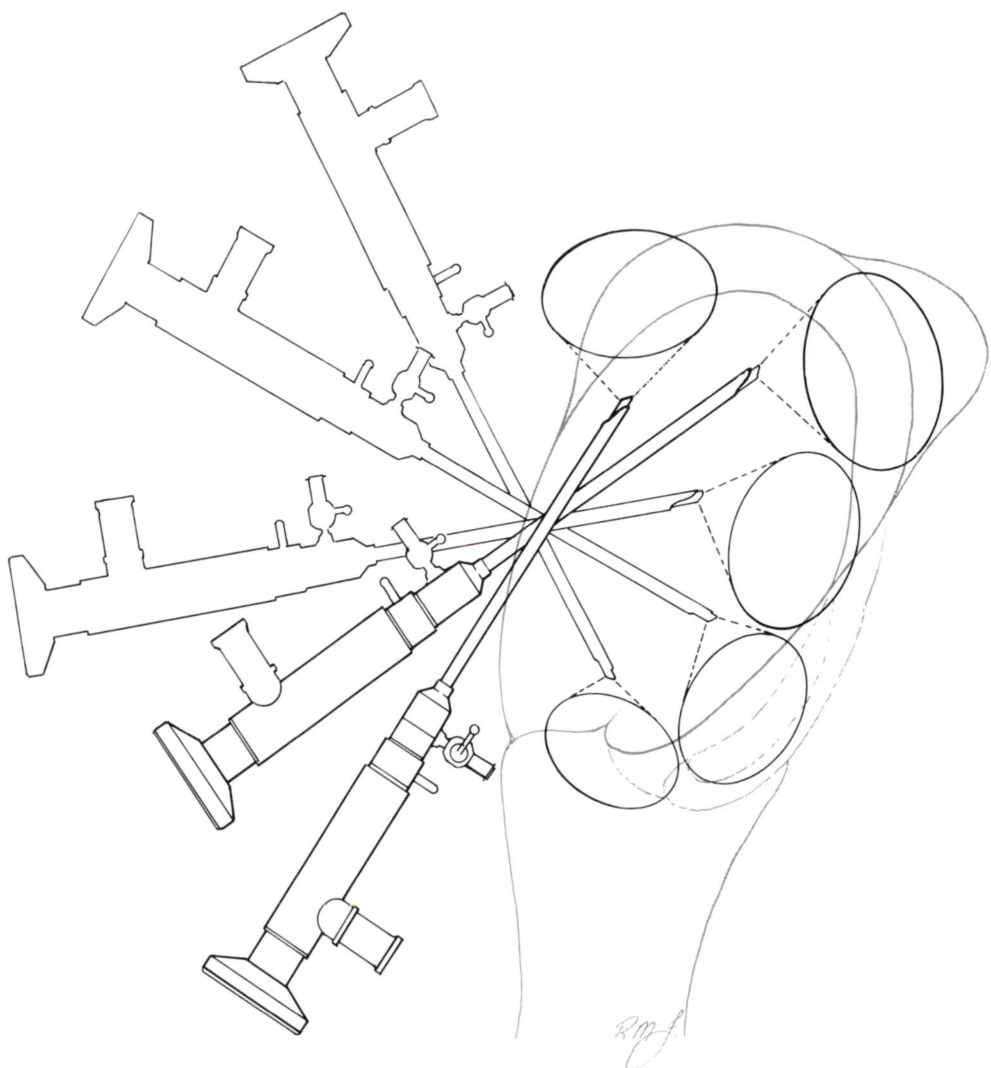

FIG. 5-50 Composition: sequence of images constructed in surgeon's mind.

Arthroscopic composition is a matter of penetration, rotation, scope sweeping side to side, or any variety of these techniques. The beginning arthroscopist generally uses a lot of scope sweeping, jumping from side to side with very rapid motions. The observations made during that quick movement is virtually useless in collecting data and is potentially damaging to the joint or scope.

When the scope is moved very slowly and the surgeon comprehends the sequence of images, slow movements combined with manipulative procedures make it possible to fully comprehend or make composition arthroscopically.

The sign of an expert arthroscopist is the ability to make comprehensive compositions.

Motor Skills

Arthroscopic technical ability is not solely dependent on intellect. It is a motor skill. Certain skills can be improved by education and motor skills training. No direct correlation exists between athletic skills and the intellect—you either run fast or you don't. Techniques and training will maximize natural abilities. Some limitations do exist, however. Lack of innate abilities for arthroscopy should not reflect poorly on a surgeon. A certain natural endowment makes arthroscopy easier for one surgeon than another.

In addition to physical skills, the surgeon must have an emotional capacity for arthroscopic surgery. The qualities of patience, gentleness, and self-control are needed, and the surgeon must have a willingness to discipline himself or herself and the staff. The delicate tools, small spaces, and remote control of manipulations are demanding. Repeated practice will cause the discipline to become natural and satisfying. The surgeon's disposition affects the motor skills.

A

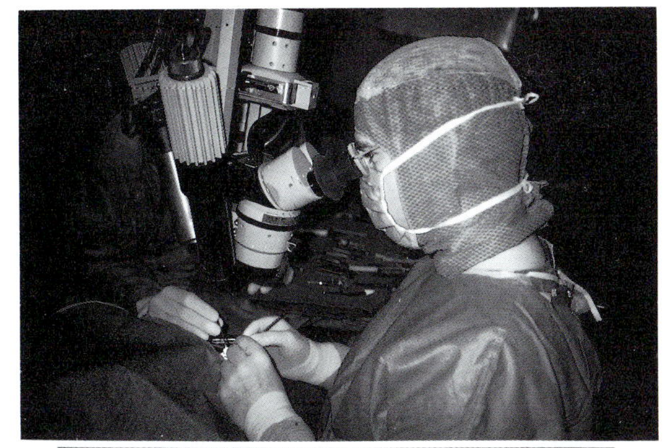

B

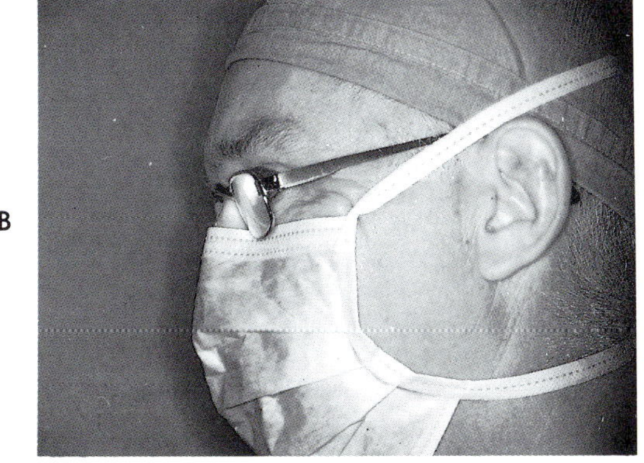

FIG. 5-51 Multiple lens systems of surgery.
A Operating microscope.
B Surgeon's eye and eyeglasses.

VISUAL INTERPRETATION

Surgical Imagination

Surgical imagination is the key ingredient of any surgery. Some surgeons are more gifted than others at conceptualizing or applying imagination in problem solving. One's innate skill will be developed with experience. The small confines of the arthroscopic exposure, the lack of three-dimensional image, the inability to directly touch the structures, the use of television, the hand positions in one direction, and the gaze away from the operative field—all these factors require considerable imagination. The physician's surgical imagination is the intangible ingredient that aids in overcoming the unexpected and even the unknown. This is the design, the dance, the excitement, and the sound that is recognized in other art forms.

Arthroscopic Imaging

Image enhancement is used in most surgery, but none so magnified as during arthroscopy. The operating microscope is an example of a surgical lens system (Fig. 5-51, *A*). Several lens systems are used in arthroscopy. The intraarticular image is transmitted via glass lens within the arthroscope. The small television camera has a lens that requires focusing. The image is transmitted to the electronic chip and onto the television monitor. The image passes through the surgeon's glasses and lens system of his or her eye to the brain (Fig. 5-51, *B*) (see also Chapter 2).

The arthroscopic lens also magnifies. Further magnification occurs with an electronic image on a television monitor with minimal loss of optical clarity. Projection during presentations or demonstrations creates great magnification on the silver screen.

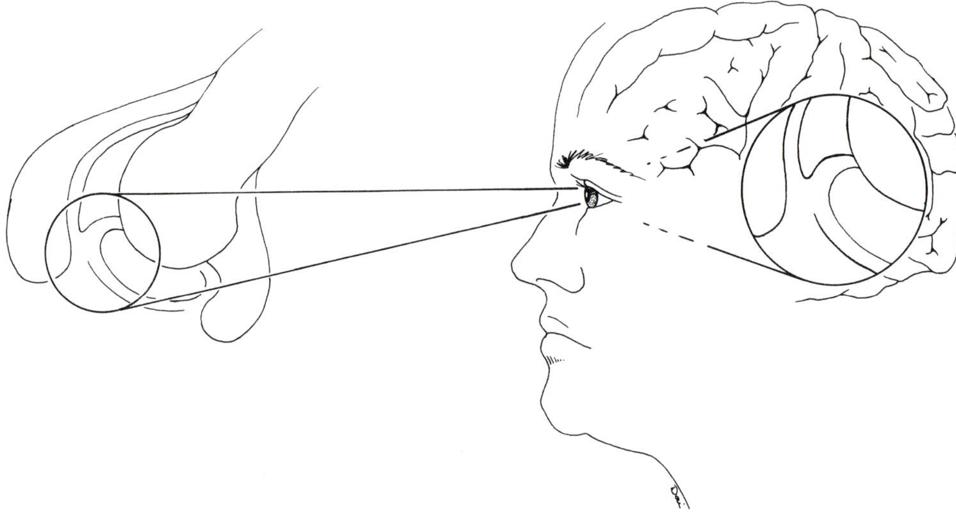

FIG. 5-52 Arthroscopy is restricted to a two-dimensional image. The instrument and scope motions of scanning, pistoning, plus rotation create a continuous video recording, but the composition is created in the surgeon's mind.

Two-Dimensional Image

The arthroscopic lens system provides only a two-dimensional image, compared to the binocular vision at open surgery. The spatial relationships of exposure are gained by appreciation of shadowing, relative size, and position, and these are assisted by probing and palpation (Fig. 5-52). The surgeon makes the final composition within his or her mind.

Illumination

Most surgical procedures are performed with supplemental light. The requirements of open surgery are met with suspended lamps or head-mounted lights. In arthroscopy, the intraarticular spaces are dark, requiring a powerful light supplement for surgical exposure.

Varying illumination is necessary with television viewing. If the camera does not have automatic gain control, some areas will be too bright and others too dark. Manual control of light source intensity may be necessary. Articular cartilage requires less light than the cavernous subacromial space. A decrease in light is necessary to properly evaluate subtle changes in articular surfaces.

The color balance of a television camera may require attention to maintain realistic colors of tissue. Most system manuals outline the procedure for correction. Our Dyonics model has built-in color bars and an external button for ease of light balance correction (see Fig. 3-9, *A*).

Orientation

Orientation is easiest when the surgeon's body and eyes are behind and in line with the arthroscope (Fig.

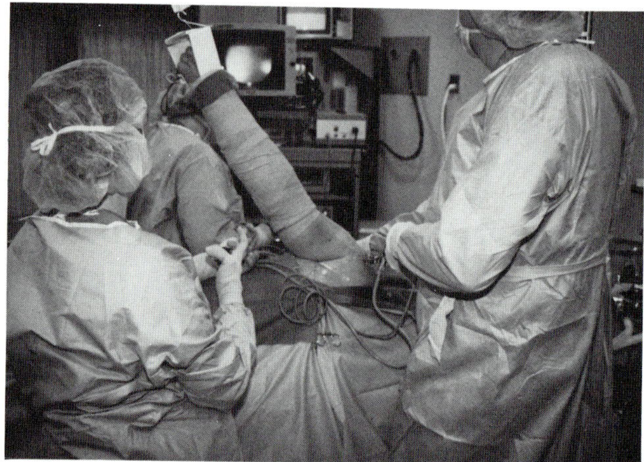

FIG. 5-53 Orientation. The surgeon's body and eyes are positioned behind the arthroscope for orientation.

5-53). The television monitor should be perpendicular to the axis of the scope. The angle of the arthroscope's inclined view is oriented with the side arm of the light guide attachment for orientation of direction of the intraarticular view. The arthroscopist should note that some scopes angle toward from the light guide attachment and others angle away. The angle of scope incline in relation to the light guide attachment is a necessary reference point for scope manipulation. The direction of scope viewing inside the

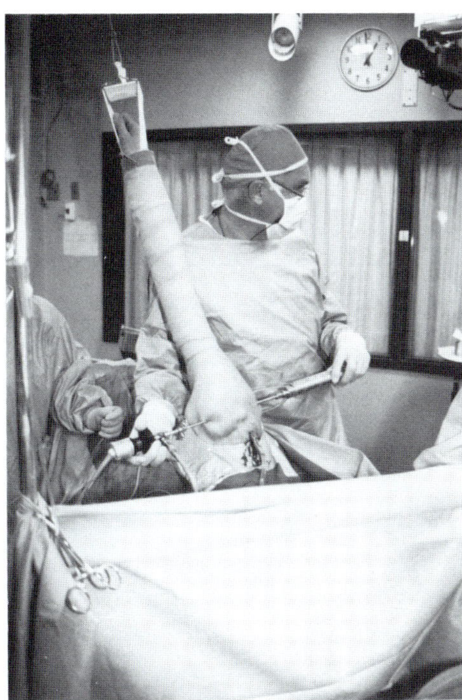

FIG. 5-54 Reorientation. Time must be taken for orientation. When the arthroscope is switched to the side away from the surgeon and the instruments are placed from his or her side of the table, the surgeon must reorient to this change of position. This is best accomplished if the surgeon will rotate his or her body and eyes to look at video camera behind him or her. This places the surgeon in line with the view of the arthroscope even though he or she is not behind it. This maneuver removes the mirror image on the video monitor and makes subsequent manipulation easier.

joint is oriented with observation of the light guide attachment outside the joint.

Orientation is more difficult when the surgeon is behind the arthroscope, but the instrumentation enters from the opposite side of the joint. This is the usual case in shoulder arthroscopy. Instrumentation is more difficult than when both arthroscope and instruments enter from the same side of the joint. Instrumentation movements appear as a mirror image of what is expected. When the instrument enters opposite the arthroscope portal, the surgeon moves the instrument to the right to produce an intraarticular move to the left on the television monitor. Orientation is enhanced by moving the instruments slowly back and forth, testing resultant angulation, before commencing with surgery. Rotational direction must also be figured out.

Reorientation With Repositioning

The most difficult orientation problem occurs when the scope enters from the side opposite the surgeon yet the television monitor remains behind rather than in front of the scope (Fig. 5-54). When instrumentation is placed on the surgeon's side, the matter is further complicated. With some approaches, the surgeon cannot change position of his or her body along the axis of the arthroscope. In this case the monitor should be rotated 90 degrees to a position perpendicular to the scope. The surgeon enhances orientation by viewing the monitor with his or her head rotated. This maneuver reduces the disorientation that accompanies the malposition. It may be necessary to face in another direction, looking at the monitor, although the body cannot gain complete reorientation.

Another compensatory maneuver is for the surgeon to remain behind the patient and do an about-face and view a monitor that was previously behind him or her. The scope still enters from anterior. The instruments are on the same side as the surgeon, but orientation is maintained because viewing is in the same direction as the scope. The surgeon is manipulating the instruments behind his or her back. A slow approach and testing of the movements of instruments are necessary.

If this explanation is not clear, imagine the difficulty in orientation during actual arthroscopy. These techniques may not suffice. The surgeon may have to go to the other side of the table.

Disorientation and Vertigo

On rare occasions during arthroscopy, I have experienced momentary disorientation and even vertigo. Such occurrences have happened during complex cases with multiple portal interchanges in which I was operating from all possible perspectives. Fatigue usually preceded the vertigo experience. Vertigo is most likely to happen while viewing in the subacromial space, where anatomical landmarks are not distinctive. I once mistook the bare humeral head for the acromion and started resecting bone, only to become confused with my orientation and instrument movement. I stopped, waited, relaxed, rested, reoriented, and completed the procedure without incident. No further problems developed on that day or subsequent days. Disorientation and vertigo problems can be minimized by systematic approaches and proper position of the surgeon, arthroscope, television monitor, instrumentation, and avoidance of fatique.

Contrast Dye

In some cases a contrast dye may assist in highlighting intraarticular structures.[10] The determination of the amount of roughening or fragmentation or of fissure depth may be enhanced. I have used dilute solution of methylene blue (1 ml in 500 ml fluid) injected along the scope to the desired area of observation. The dye clears easily from the joint for further arthroscopy. It selectively stains fibroid exudate or loose bodies (Fig. 5-55). I have seen no complications with the use of methylene blue in hundreds of arthroscopy cases.

This same method is helpful in identifying small rotator cuff tears. A needle is placed in the glenohumeral joint under direct observation. The arthroscope is removed and placed in the subacromial space, viewing the top of the rotator cuff. The dye is injected via the previously placed No. 18 spinal needle into the glenohumeral space. The subacromial space is monitored for flow of the blue dye through the rotator cuff tear (Fig. 5-56).

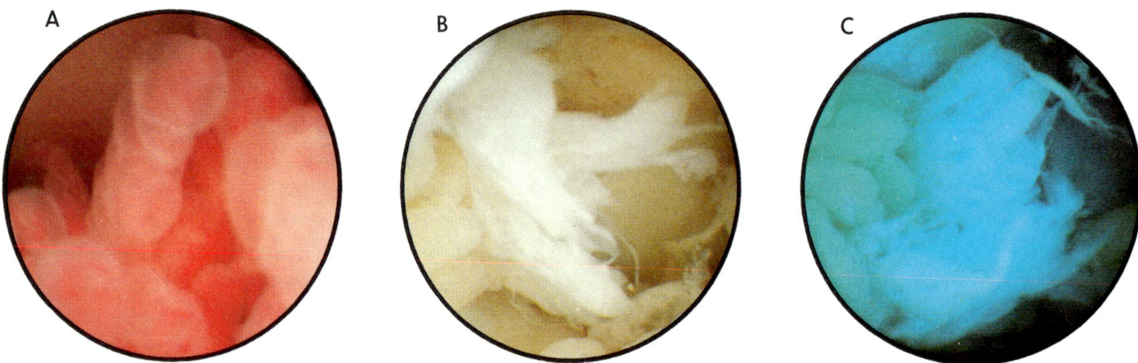

FIG. 5-55 Contrast dye. The fibroid exudate on rheumatoid arthritis synovium is selectively stained with methylene blue.

A Rheumatoid arthritis with a marked inflammatory component.

B Rheumatoid arthritis with villous fibrinoid exudate.

C Methylene blue injected into joint defines villi.

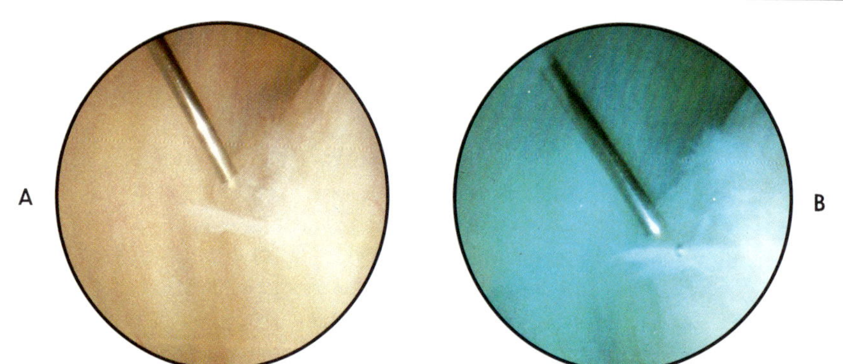

FIG. 5-56 Contrast dye injected into the glenohumeral joint will identify small, rotator cuff, full-thickness tears with leakage into subacromial space.

A Arthroscopic view of subacromial space before placing dye in glenohumeral joint. Only a small roughened area of superior rotator cuff is identified with No. 18 spinal needle.

B Methylene blue dye leaks through the small tear in rotator cuff and causes subacromial space to demonstrate dye.

THE ROUTINE OF DIAGNOSTIC ARTHROSCOPY
With General Anesthesia

The patient is placed on a regular operating room table in the supine position. The patient marks the surgical extremity with the letter "S" with ink pen in the presence of the preoperative nurse (Fig. 5-57). An anesthetic is administered, and a physical examination is performed with the patient under anesthesia. Passive range of motion is determined with comparison to preoperative motions. Joint stability is assessed (Fig. 5-58). The patient is turned into the opposite lateral decubitus position. The patient is held with an Olympus vacuum bean bag (Fig. 5-59, *A*) and secured to the table with 3-inch wide adhesive tape placed over the pelvis (Fig. 5-59, *B*). The patient is positioned with 15-degree posterior rotation to the body. Michael Gross pointed out the advantage of this positioning to compensate for the 15-degree anteversion of the glenoid. The joint space is now positioned in the same plane as the floor.

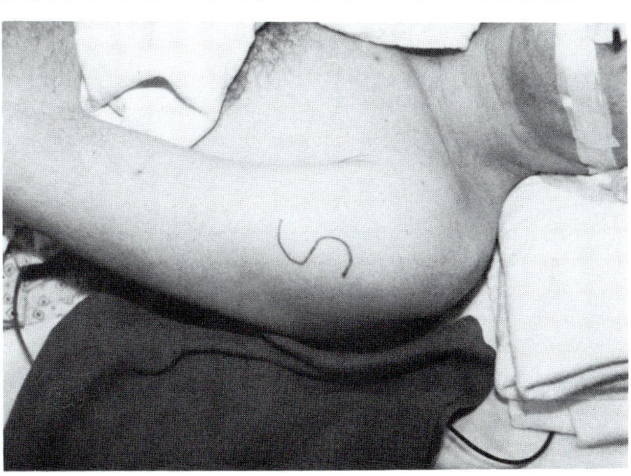

FIG. 5-57 The patient marks the operative region with ink with the letter "S."

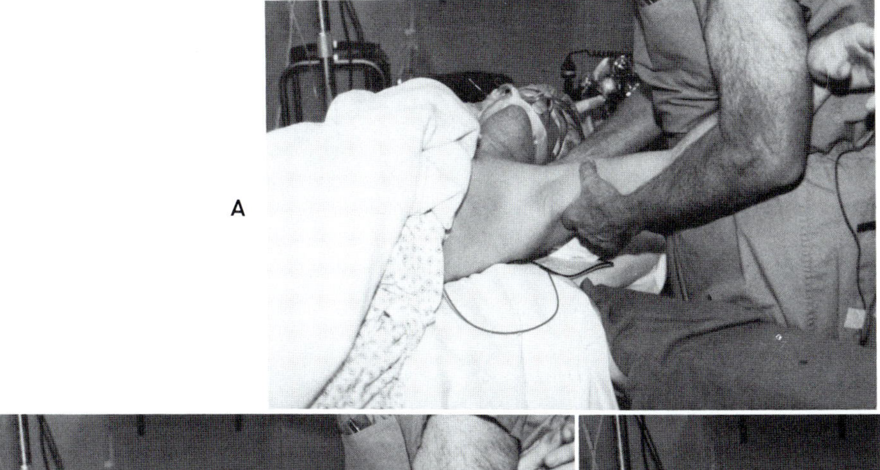

A

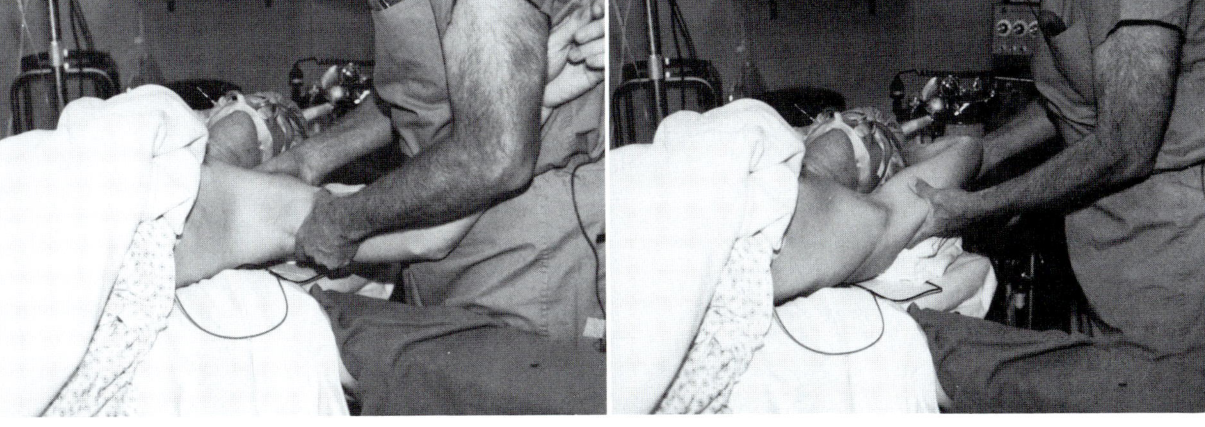

B

C

FIG. 5-58 Examination under anesthesia provides yet another opportunity to evaluate the patient's shoulder.

A The arm is held at 90 degrees abduction and an anterior force is applied.

B The arm is held at 90 degrees abduction and a posterior force is applied.

C The arm is taken into elevated position and the stability is retested.

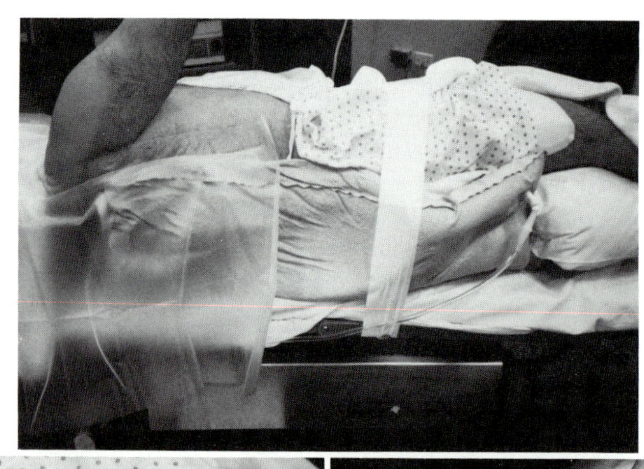

A

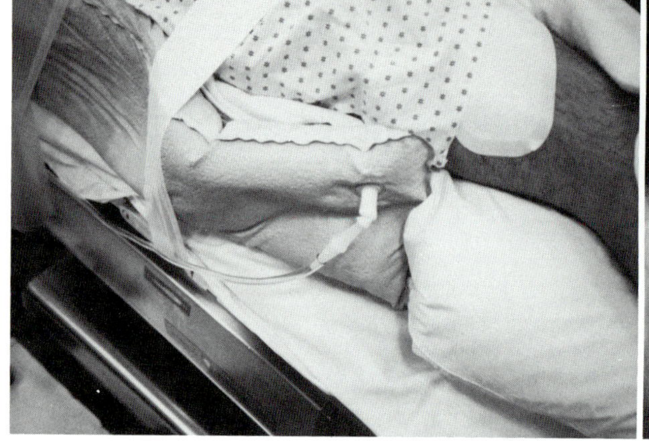

B

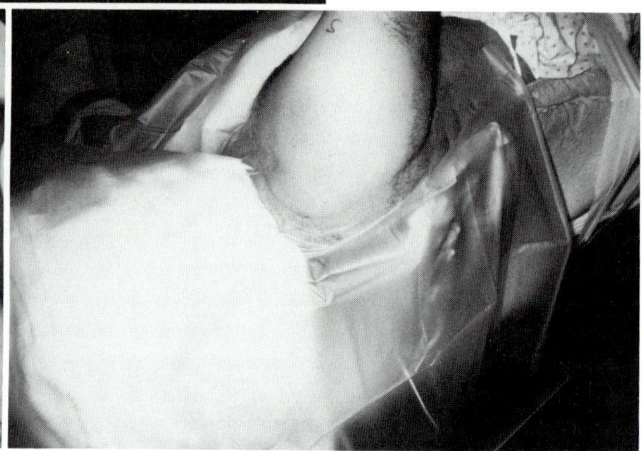

C

FIG. 5-59 Patient positioning.

A The patient is placed in the opposite lateral decubitus position with an Olympic Vac Pac. Tape is placed over the patient's pelvis to secure the patient to the table.

B Suction remains attached in case a small leak occurs in the Vac Pac.

C A 3M plastic drape is placed over the patient's head to keep fluid leakage off the patient. Notice the posterior tilt of the patient's body, which compensates for the normal anterior slope of the glenoid, so that the glenohumeral joint is parallel to the floor.

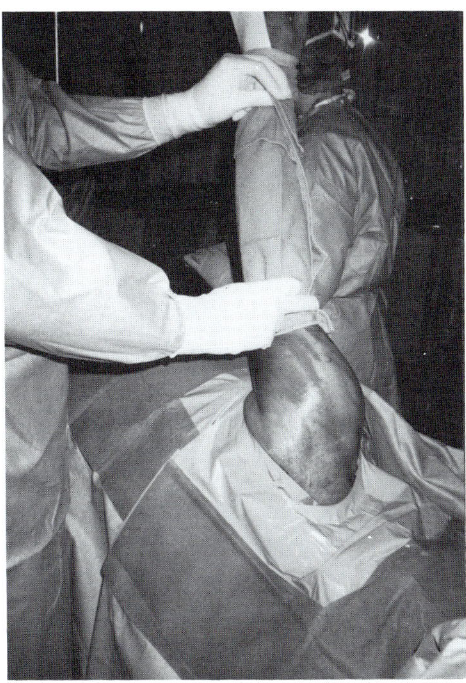

FIG. 5-60 A Johnson & Johnson drape is placed over the patient, and a sterile drape is placed over the forearm.

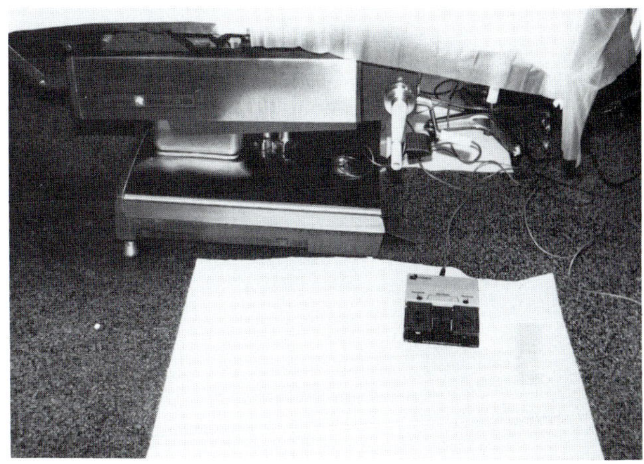

FIG. 5-61 A disposable paper drape is used to absorb not only fluids, but also debris.

A shoulder suspension apparatus is attached to the operating room table by a C-clamp holder (see Fig. 3-15).

The arm is secured to the suspension system with foam tape and ace bandage wrap. The technique of application of the suspension device is outlined in Chapter 2. The foot of the operating table is lowered or elevated to adjust the proper angle of the upright that creates the angle of the patient's suspended arm. Lowering the foot of the table lowers the angle of the arm to the side. Elevating the foot of the table raises the arm away from the side.

An unsterile towel is placed over the patient's head. This area is covered with a 3M company plastic U-drape with adhesive margins to seal off the patient from intraoperative fluid drainage (Fig. 5-60). An antiseptic is applied to the skin about the shoulder girdle and arm.

The Johnson & Johnson arthroscopic shoulder disposable drape creates a sterile, water-impervious barrier (Fig. 5-60). The excess drape hanging down on the floor is swept under the table to clear this area for placement of disposable absorbable paper matting (Cloud-9) (Fig. 5-61). The foot pedals of the motorized instrumentation and electrocoagulator are placed on the mat. The surgeon and first assistant stand in this area.

The disposable drape is folded behind the shoulder and attached to the anesthesia pole to create a trough for directing fluids away from the surgeon and into a bucket on the opposite side of the operating field (Fig. 5-62). Folds are also made in the drape over the patient's pelvis to hold instruments between usage (see Fig. 5-19, *C*).

A simultaneous, coordinated effort of the team brings the instrumentation tables into place (Fig. 5-63). The Mayo stand with the surgical instrumentation is on the opposite side of the patient from the surgeon. The second assistant stands in that area. The cabinet holding the television monitor and power supplies is moved adjacent to the operative field beyond the Mayo stand. The light cables, television camera, and powered surgical instrumentation are extended from the sterile field to the power sources for attachment. All instrumentation is tested for function before initiation of the surgical procedure.

The electrical cords and inflow-outflow tubes approach the operative field from the side opposite the surgeon. The electrical cords and fluid tubing are placed through the loops in the arthroscopy drapes so they do not slip off the operative field.

The team members have assigned positions in the operative field and designated assignments (Fig. 5-64), as detailed in Chapter 2.

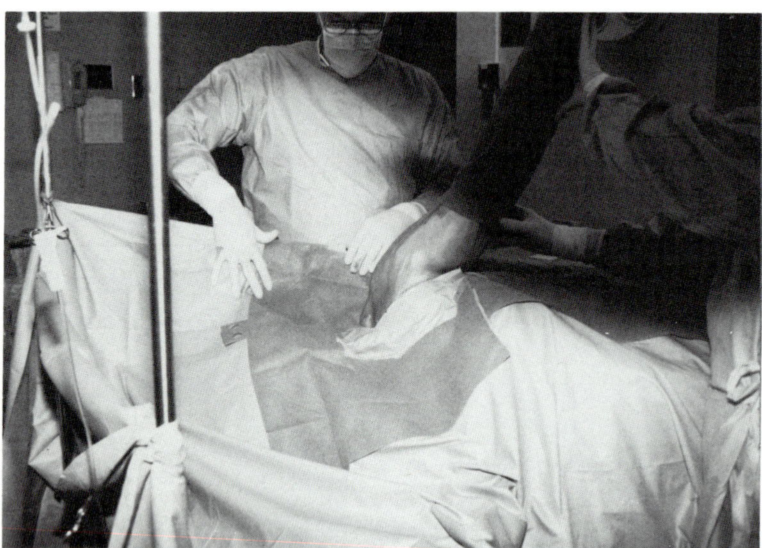

FIG. 5-62 Folds in the sterile draping direct fluids away from the operative field.

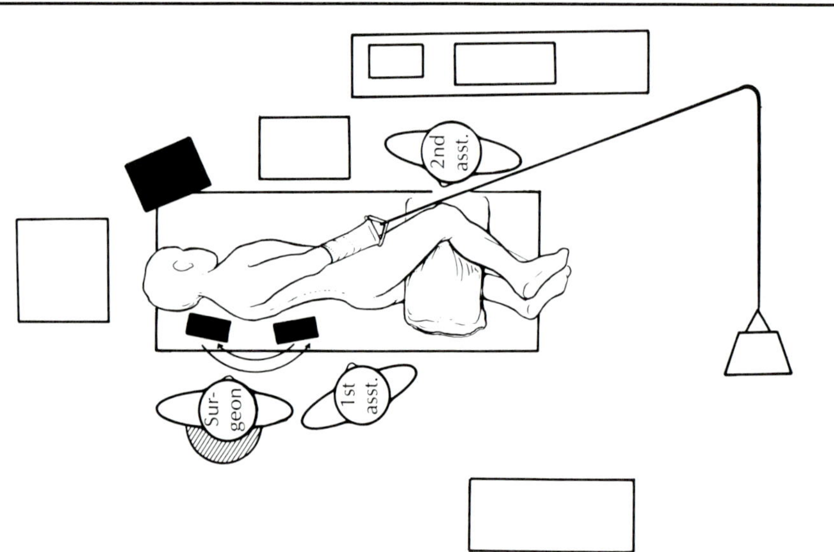

FIG. 5-63 Diagram of the arthroscopic room set up for shoulder surgery.

Fluid Irrigation System. When prolonged use of motorized instrumentation is anticipated, an infusion system is established to a fluid reservoir as previously discussed. Two different fluid reservoirs are used when electrocoagulation is anticipated as in acromioplasty. One is for sterile water (nonelectrolytic for electrocoagulation), while the other is for Lactated Ringer's solution.

The circulating nurse suspends the two 3 L bags of sterile fluids (Fig. 5-65). The sterile Y-tube is handed to the circulating nurse, who connects it to the suspended fluid reservoir. When two fluids are used the separate systems are marked with sterile pen and ink for identification. The gravity assist hand pump is placed in the system (Fig. 5-66); see Chapter 3 on Instrumentation for details.

While fluids are being set up, the first assistant prepares the television system.

Arthroscope placement is accomplished from posterior as previously described.

Intraarticular viewing is from television monitor with simultaneous videotape recording.

Routine for Intraarticular Viewing. The surgeon and the team members must develop a routine for intraar-

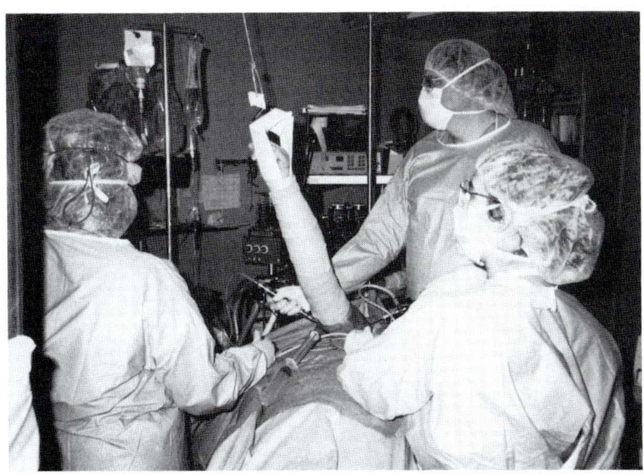

FIG. 5-64 Each team member has the same position for each procedure. Notice the attentiveness of not only the surgeon, but the other two team members in the photo.

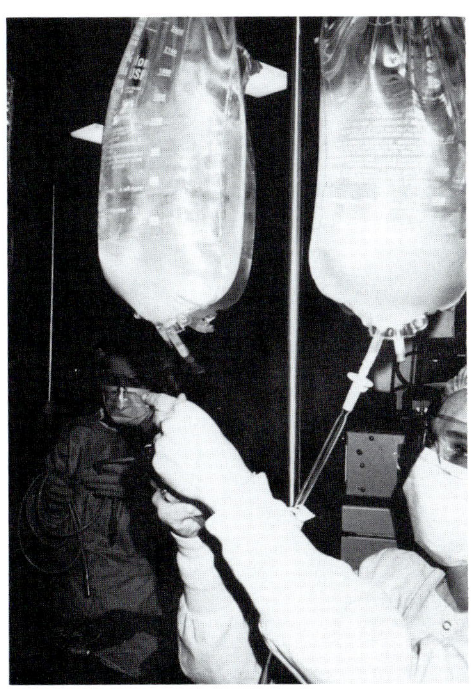

FIG. 5-65 The circulating nurse watches for emptying of fluid reservoir bags and makes the necessary changes.

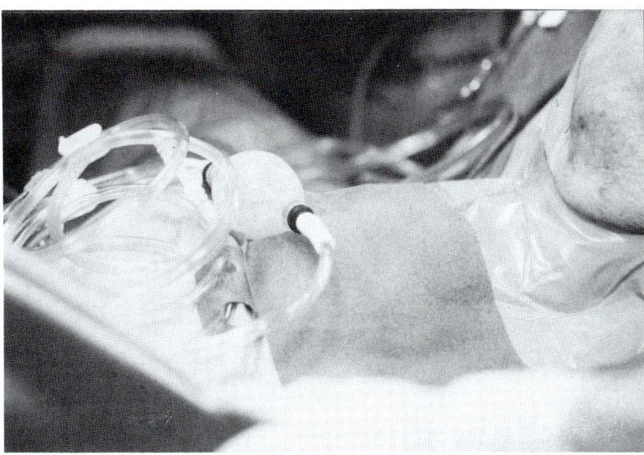

FIG. 5-66 The Gravity Assist Hand Pump is placed in line with the infusion tubing and rests in the operative field.

ticular viewing. Adhering to the same routine ensures completeness and avoids overlooking any area.

I first inspect the glenohumeral joint. The biceps tendon is identified. My routine starts with superior, moves to posterior, anterior inferior, and then anterior superior and anterior. The posterior aspect of the joint is best inspected from anterior. This step may be deferred until the placement of the anterior operative portal. Cannulas may be interchanged with switching sticks, with the arthroscope ending up in the anterior portal. (See Chapter 5 on anatomy for visualization of the routine.)

The subacromial joint is inspected next in most cases. The AC joint is reserved for last and inspected only when diseased and surgery is anticipated. An anterior and lateral arthroscopic portal is used during the operative phase, but is not routine for diagnosis.

Positional Testing. Penetration of the joint decompresses the intraarticular pressure, resulting in minimal anterior inferior humeral subluxation. This result is normal under these circumstances. Intraarticular increases in pressure further accentuate the subluxation. Increases in intraarticular pressure distract the humeral head off the glenoid fossa (see Fig. 5-44).

Abnormalities in glenohumeral position may be evaluated under arthroscopic control with external manipulation of the upper extremity. Instability is assessed in the same manner. Removing the suspension apparatus may be necessary to accomplish this task. The humerus may also be repositioned to show the kissing lesion of impingement in the subacromial space.

Wissinger Rod Technique. The Wissinger rod technique is a simple method to establish an anterior portal (Fig. 5-67). This method was suggested by Dr. H. Andrew Wissinger of Pittsburgh, Pennsylvania, while watching me struggle with an anterior transcutaneous needle to establish

FIG. 5-67 Use of Wissinger rod to establish anterior operative portal.

A Diagnostic arthroscopy with joint distention supplied through syringe via K-52 catheter.

B Scope removed and rod placed. Knife lacerates skin over rod tip.

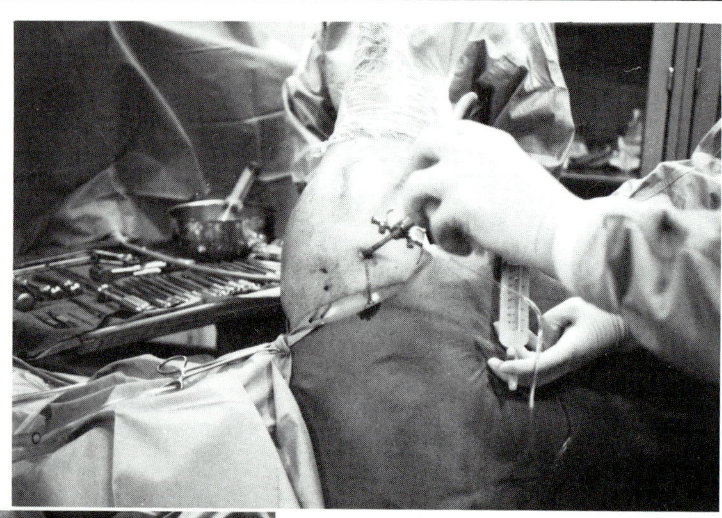

A

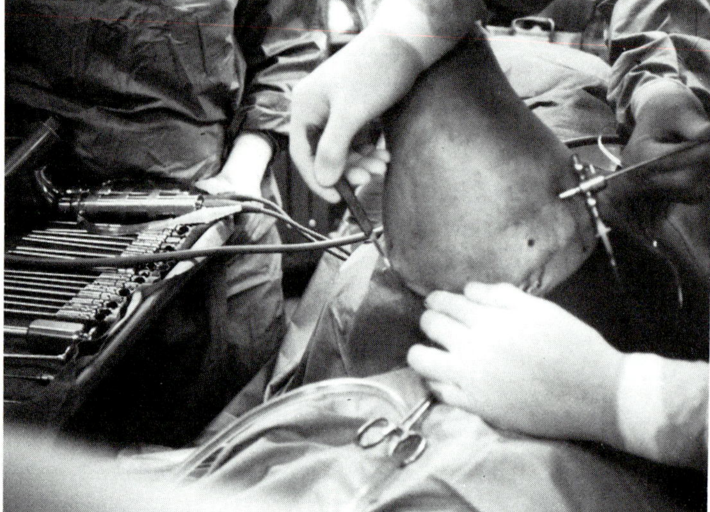

B

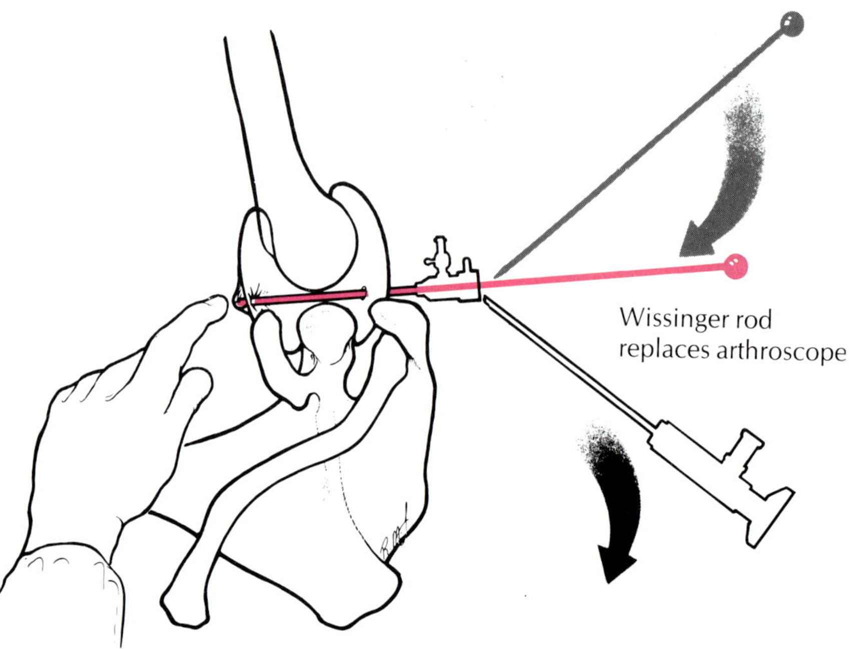

Continued.

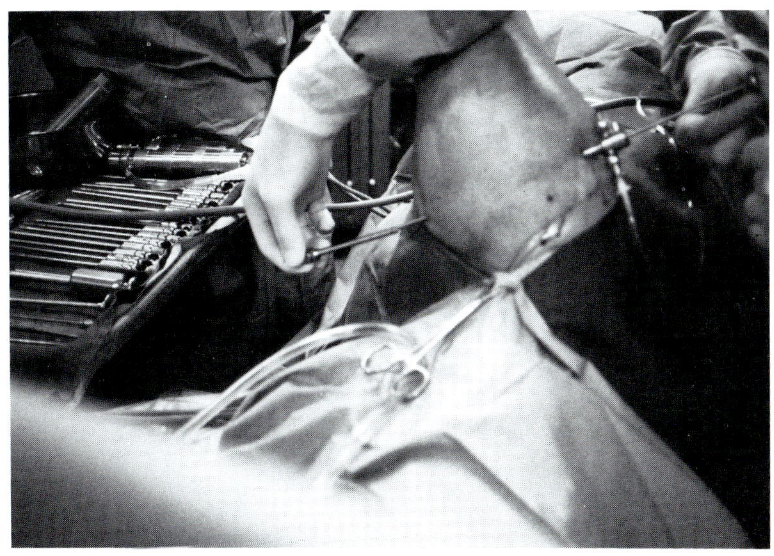

Wissinger rod
through anterior wall
and fitted with
retrograde cannula

FIG. 5-67 ***cont'd*** **Use of Wissinger rod to establish anterior operative portal.**

C Cannula retrograded over rod.

Continued.

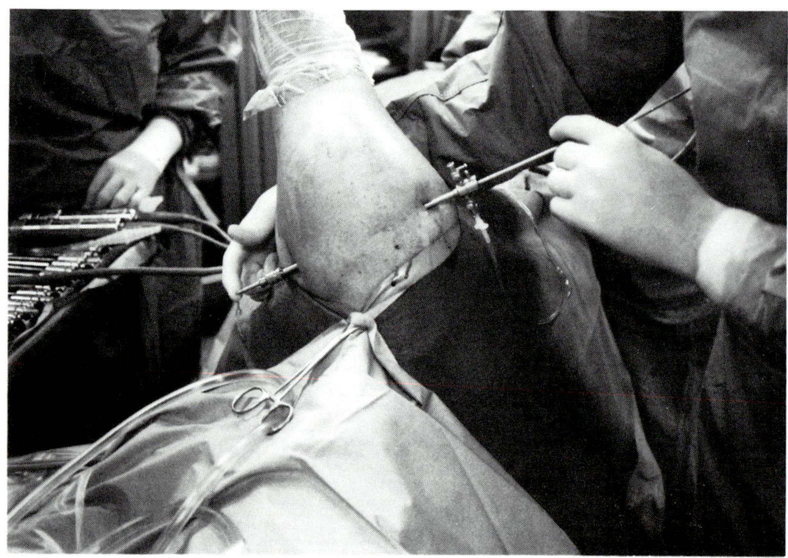

D

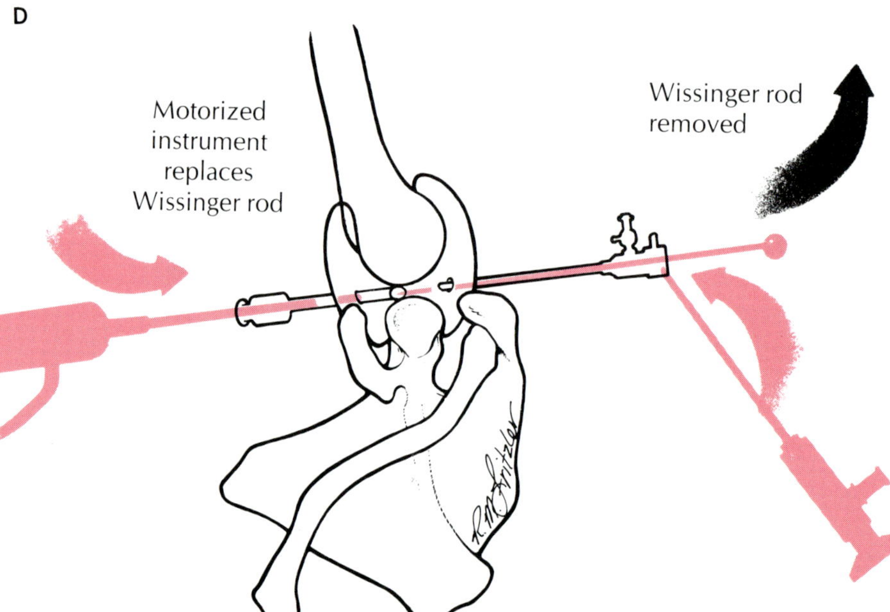

FIG. 5-67 ***cont'd*** **Use of Wissinger rod to establish anterior operative portal.**

D Both cannulas in joint over rod. Rod is removed and scope and instruments placed.

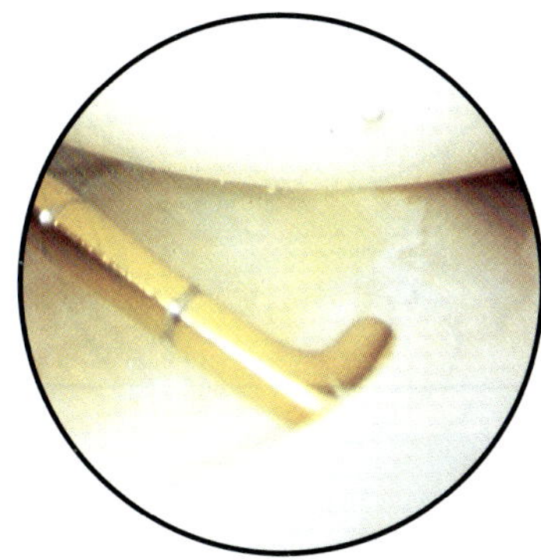

FIG. 5-68 Probing is an important aspect of arthroscopic diagnosis. Probe touches posterior inferior labrum tear from anterior portal.

this portal.[46] Wissinger's suggestion, which is now standard practice, was to pass the arthroscope from posterior to anterior to the desired internal position immediately superior to the subscapularis tendon. This is performed with direct visualization. The scope is pushed against the anterior capsule, which obliterates the view. The cannula is held in place while the arthroscope is removed. The Wissinger rod is placed down the cannula and forced against the anterior capsule. The capsule is penetrated from inside to just under the anterior skin. A knife blade cuts the skin to expose the tip of the rod. The arthroscope cannula is retracted 1 or 2 centimeters. An operative cannula is passed from anterior in a retrograde fashion over the Wissinger rod and into the joint. Joint penetration is determined by palpation. In some cases extravasation of fluid confirms the entry. The Wissinger rod is removed and the arthroscope reinserted to confirm the entry.

This technique is used in the glenohumeral joint, but is also helpful in the subacromial space and the AC joint.

Probing. Visualization will give only a portion of the information that one hopes to gain, and palpation is essential with a probe. The probe, although it is not considered a surgical "instrument," is an integral tool of the arthroscopic procedure (Fig. 5-68).

I place the probe into the glenohumeral joint from the anterior portal that was established with the use of the Wissinger rod technique. With the cannula in the joint, the probe is placed in the cannula. After the tip of the probe is seen in the joint, the cannula is removed and placed back on the Mayo stand. No leakage occurs around the probe or cannula, and free palpation is allowed within the joint. The tip, as well as the knuckle, of the probe can be used to palpate any interstitial tears or disruptions.

The probe can be used to elevate the labrum or pull the biceps tendon further into the joint. The integrity of the glenohumeral ligaments is tested by probing.

In some cases it is necessary to initiate the operative phase to improve visualization for diagnosis. Intraarticular fluid, especially blood and blood clots, may require placement of motorized instruments to cleanse the joint. Loose bodies may need to be removed. In some instances, the synovitis is very proliferative and obstructs the view. A localized synovectomy will clear the area. In fact, the diagnostic observations continue throughout the subsequent operative phase as well.

With Local Anesthesia

The technique is identical to that outlined previously, except for the instillation of local anesthetic agent.[11,20,24] Preoperative sedation is optional. The suspension apparatus is surprisingly comfortable if the procedure is less than 15 minutes.

1% plain lidocaine is injected into the area of the posterior portal along all layers including synovium. Adrenaline and intraarticular anesthetic is optional. Other portal sites will require the same type of infiltrative local anesthetic.

With the use of local anesthesia, the surgeon must be sensitive to the patient's potential discomfort or sudden movements. This response can be monitored with talking to the patient and by having the free hand on the patient's body to sense muscle tightening or motion.

D

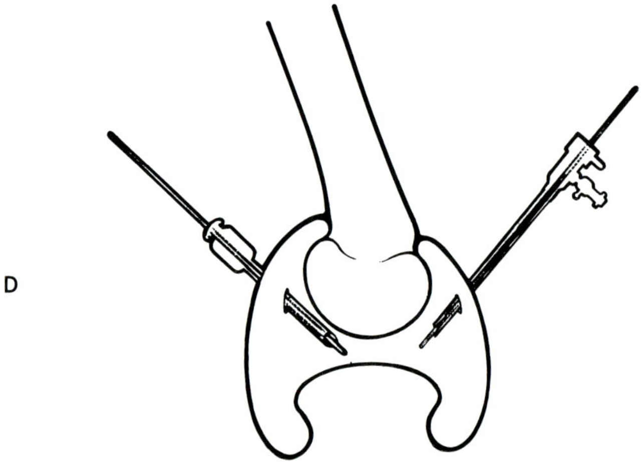

Switching sticks in place,
ready for cannula "switch" (swap)

E

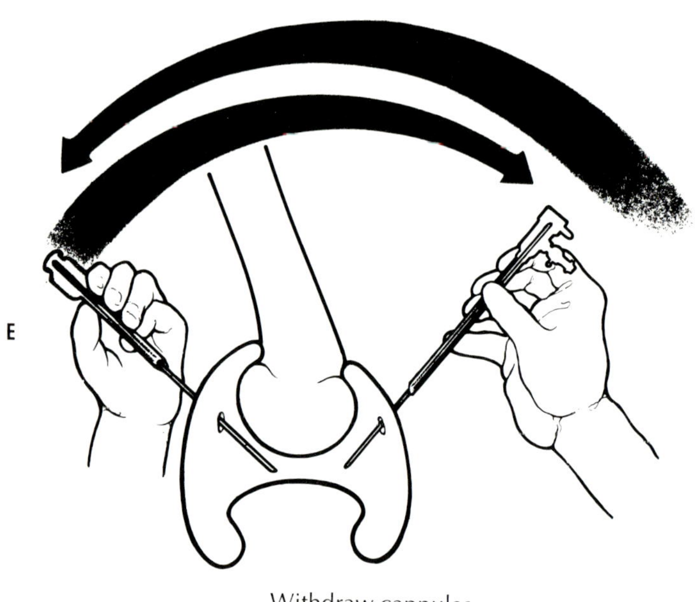

Withdraw cannulas
over switching sticks

FIG. 5-70 cont'd Interchanging instrument portals with switching sticks.

D Switching sticks in place.

E Cannulas removed off sticks and interchanged.

Continued.

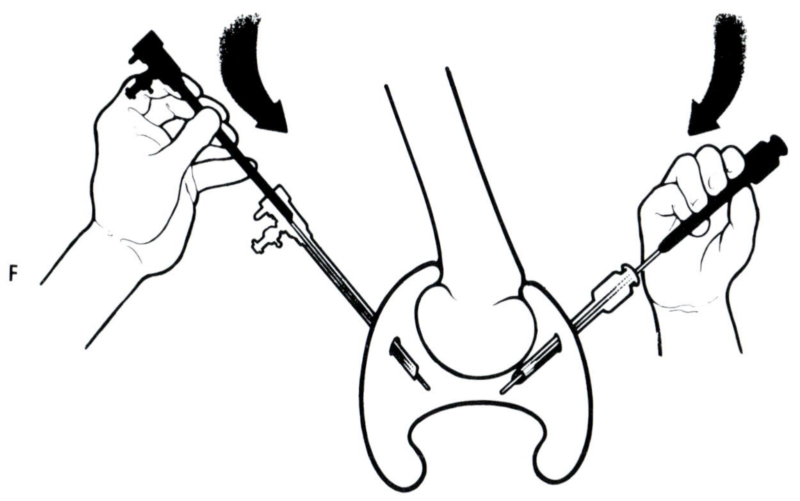
F
Slip cannulas over switching
stick ends into work positions

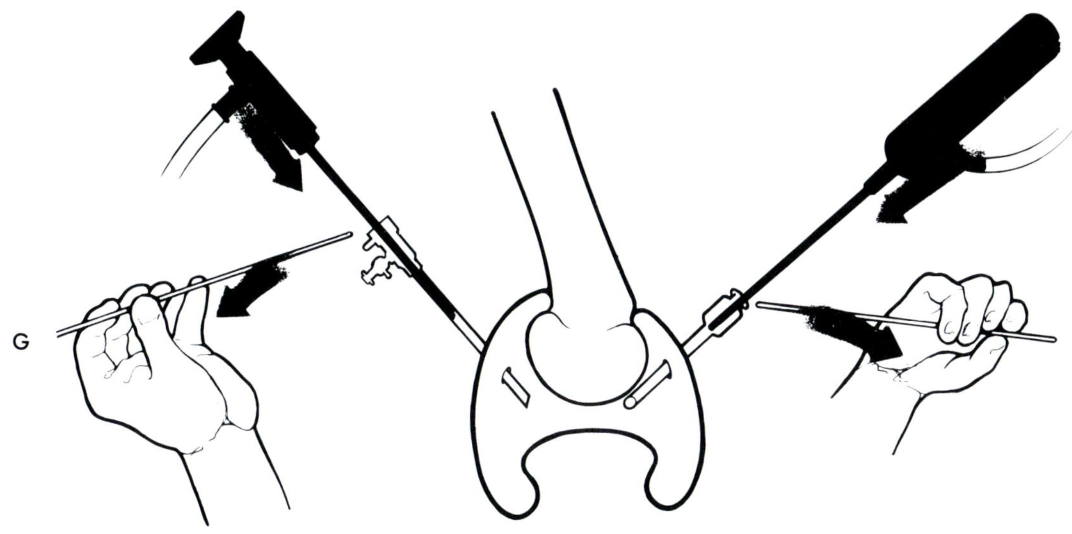
G
Remove switching sticks
and replace instruments

FIG. 5-70 cont'd Interchanging instrument portals with switching sticks.

F Cannula over switching sticks.

G Cannulas in, sticks out. Arthroscope and instruments are now interchanged.

THE ROUTINE OF OPERATIVE ARTHROSCOPY

Upon completion of the diagnostic phase, the indicated operative arthroscopy may commence. If the inflow cannula system has not been previously placed and is required, it is placed at this time. The inflow is established with preliminary placement of a No. 18 spinal needle along the anticipated course. The needle is identified within the joint, with rotation of the scope to superior and angulation to posterior. The cannula follows in the same plane, first with a sharp trochar and then exchanging it for a blunt obturator to penetrate the joint. The inflow cannula is placed behind the glenoid in the posterior sulcus. The cannula is attached to the inflow system.

The anterior portal, if not already established, is secured with use of the Wissinger rod technique. The anterior portal will serve as the initial operative portal. Most areas of the glenohumeral joint can be reached from the anterior portal. Care must be taken when penetrating from anterior to posterior with the instruments to observe the cannula tip to avoid scuffing the joint with the protruding margin. Throughout the procedure the surgeon must concentrate on the cutting tip of the instrument.

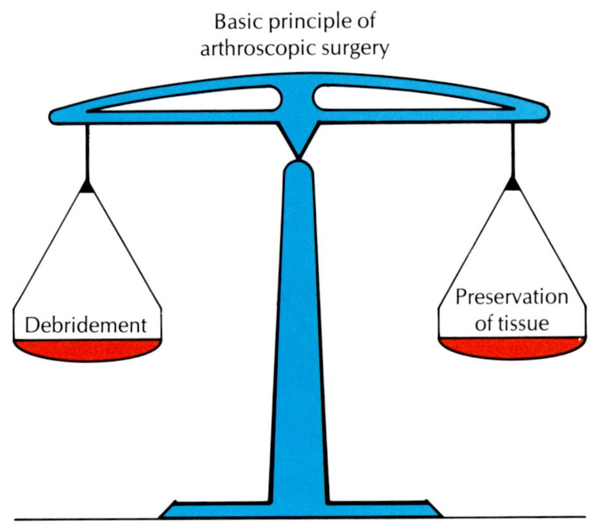

FIG. 5-71 Debridement must be balanced with preservation of tissue.

Arthroscopic Operative Principles

Surgical Skin Incision Sites. In arthroscopy the small incision sites are called portals and are used to pass the arthroscope and instrumentation into the joint.

Cannula System. A cannula system is essential to operative arthroscopy (see Fig. 3-21). This system is the same as that used in diagnostic arthroscopy. The use of cannulas provides a simple means of interchanging position of the arthroscope, inflow, and instruments.

Surgical Exposure. Exposure is developed in the same way that is mentioned in the previous section on diagnostic arthroscopy and composition. Adequate joint distention is a primary factor in optimal surgical exposure.

Incision Principles. Hard material requires sharp incision. Rather than cut entirely through the tissue, like a separated labrum, it is best to first inscribe with the knife blade, leaving a small area intact. The inscription in the labrum will clearly outline the pattern to be resected. Either basket forceps or motorized instruments can go up to the line of inscription, which is perhaps two thirds to three fourths of the way through the labrum. This approach prevents the piece becoming loose in the joint. The fragment can be grasped and removed with an avulsion of the attached tag.

Clean-up can be performed with a motorized system.

Resection Principles. Debridement is a common denominator of all arthroscopic surgery. It is balanced by tissue preservation (Fig. 5-71). The surgeon must use discernment concerning the limitations of the resection in order to remove torn or degenerative tissue while preserving the viable tissue. Determining the acceptable extent of debridement is difficult. The general principle is to debride less rather than more.

Tissue must be placed under tension to perform a clean cutting. Tissue tension is created in arthroscopy by fluid flow and suction pressure for motorized instruments. The firm or larger pieces of tissue have tension within themselves and are amenable to cutting with hand instruments.

The order of resection in arthroscopic surgery is first to remove the soft parts. This is best performed with motorized instrumentation with a nonaggressive cutting head like a small diameter synovial resector. Resecting the soft parts improves visualization, and the extent of further resection can be assessed.

The remaining firmer tissue requires a more aggressive cutting head, such as a cutter or hand instruments.

Plan of Attack. The surgeon should plan out every step concerning the debridement or resection. Experience, planning, and surgical imagination can prevent "painting yourself into a corner" (see Fig. 5-1).

Surgical Techniques: Visualization and Instrumentation of Various Compartments

Location

Anterior glenohumeral. Usually the 30-degree inclined scope is from posterior. This may be changed to a 90-degree inclined scope to see over the top of the glenoid into the subacromial bursa or the anterior inferior glenoid. The instrumentation is placed anterior. In some cases both the arthroscope and the instrument portals may be placed anterior.

Superior glenohumeral. The viewing may be from anterior or posterior with interchange of instrument portal.

Posterior glenohumeral. The view may be from posterior and the instrument portal may be from anterior or superior portal. A better view is obtained from anterior portal with a shift of instruments to the superior or posterior portal.

Inferior glenohumeral. The inferior aspect of the glenohumeral joint is easily visualized from the posterior portal. The scope is directed inferior. The view follows the labrum to inferior with the scope looking down. Once the scope is anterior and inferior, it is rotated to look up at the anterior joint. Another maneuver is to start anterior and superior. Rotate the scope to look inferior. A simultaneous posterior traction on the humerus displaces the head on the glenoid, creating more space for viewing. The same type of maneuvers can be made from an anterior portal. The instrumentation is placed from the opposite side.

Anterior humeral head. Both the arthroscope and the instruments are from anterior.

Posterior humeral head. The arthroscope is from the posterior portal and the instruments are from the superior portal. These two portals may be interchanged. Rotation of the humeral head is also required.

Subacromial space. I start with the arthroscope from posterior and the inflow from anterior. My initial operative portal is anterior and lateral. An interchange of arthroscope and instrument portals from anterior, anterolateral, and posterior may be required. I finish with the arthroscope lateral and the instrumentation from either or both anterior and posterior to create a flat surface resection to the acromion (see Chapter 9).

AC joint. From the inferior approach I start with the arthroscope posterior and instrumentation anterior. The scope is shifted lateral if swelling occurs. The instrumentation may be shifted to superior to adequately resect the superior osteophytes (see Chapter 10).

From a superior approach the arthroscope is placed posterior and the instruments anterior. They are interchanged to complete the resection.

Depth

Superficial. The superficial lesion is best resected with a limited-opening, motorized instrumentation, such as a whisker. A 3.5 full-radius resector is also useful.

Deep. This type of lesion requires an instrument of a large opening like a 5.5 cutter or full-radius synovial resector. A burr might also be used (see Chapter 3).

Tissue Type

Articular cartilage. The articular cartilage must be preserved. It is soft and easily incised or resected. Injury to articular cartilage is permanent. For this reason the less aggressive cutting heads, such as a whisker, are indicated to both initiate and complete debridement of this tissue. The more aggressive cutter or full-radius synovial resector may be used to remove large detached flaps. Using a well-housed cutting shape is safer when resecting hard tissue adjacent to intact articular cartilage. The depth of the cut may be controlled by rotating the cutter opening away from the tissue surface to minimize the amount of tissue that can enter the mouth of the cutting head.

Synovium. The nonaggressive synovial whisker is best for resecting synovial villi. A full-thickness synovectomy might be desirable in rheumatoid arthritis or pigmented villinodular synovitis. The 5.5 cutter or synovial resector are the instruments of choice for this procedure.

Tendon. The small-diameter, full-radius synovial resector is the best choice for resecting a portion of tendon when the remainder is to be preserved. This occurs with frayed biceps, rotator cuff, and superior supraspinatus tendons. A more aggressive resection is performed with the 5.5 cutter head. In some cases resection with knife blade and forceps removal might be most effective for a bicipital tendon stump.

Bone. The Abrader and the Acromionizer are choices for bone. These are used for resection of osteophytes, preparation of the anterior glenoid and during acromioplasty. The full-radius synovial resector, although not intended to do so, will cut bone.

Shape of the Lesion. If the lesion is well circumscribed with film articular adjacent to the edges, the surgeon might use a knife blade or a curette. For a lesion that is spread out and has a gradation of softness at the center to a gradual healing or fissuring at the margins, the small full-radius synovial resector or whisker head is more appropriate than a knife blade. Only the degenerative articular tissue can enter into these resectors, however, and the resection is limited to reshaping into the contour of a saucer.

Instrument Selection

Although instruments have been designed for specific purposes, a surgeon through experience may effectively use a tool for another purpose.

Hand Instruments

No. 18 spinal needle. This instrument is used to locate portals, palpate and elevate structures, and hold lesions in place for resection.

Cannula. The cannula with an obturator can be used to probe articular surfaces or labral tears. It will give a sense of palpation of softness or firmness of any given tissue.

Probe. The probe is used for probing under or above the labrum or to catch an articular piece. It can also be used as a retractor; the labrum can be elevated to look for loose bodies.The probe can also be used to determine the mobility of labrum or the suitability of the glenohumeral ligaments for repair.

Knife blade. The knife blade is used most to cut the firm tissue like biceps tendon or labrum. Knife blades are passed through cannula systems to minimize trauma to soft tissues of the capsule and to protect articular cartilage. The blade is observed closely as it enters the joint from the cannula. The cannula is then removed and placed on the Mayo stand. The knife is held with a fingertip grip for precision.

Basket forceps. The basket forceps are not commonly used in the shoulder. They are not placed through a cannula system, which is a disadvantage in the shoulder. Basket forceps are placed transcutaneously. They are most useful in resecting labral tissue if the surgical approach can be direct. If angulation is necessary, then a motorized instrument or a knife blade is indicated. The basket forceps can be used as a scissors. It removes pieces along the line of the incision to allow for better visualization along the cut. The remaining fragments do not overlap as with scissor cutting.

The disadvantage of using a basket forceps is that it requires multiple passes and leaves multiple pieces. If space restrictions are such that the forceps cannot be opened, resection is impossible. The basket forceps are best used with the flow system turned off. The pieces will stay in place for removal with cannula suction or motorized instrumentation.

Scissors. There are few indications for the use of scissors when other instruments perform the same task.

Graspers. The graspers are used either with or without a ratchet. I favor using the graspers without a ratchet for quick release. Although the ratchet holds well, it does not release easily. The graspers can be used to advance the glenohumeral ligaments or rotator cuff tendon as an assessment tool.

The Jaws type of grasper is beneficial for removal of loose bodies. The smaller Jaws grasper is good in the shoulder because it fits through the cannula.

Switching sticks. Switching sticks are useful for interchanging cannulas of various lengths and diameters (see Fig. 5-69). These simple straight rods, which are blunt on the end, provide for change of portals without loss of position. The technique is simple and effective.

Golden retriever. The Golden Retriever is used to retrieve loose, metallic fragments with magnetic properties (Fig. 5-72). The gold-colored retriever is easily identifiable in a surgical pan of silver-colored instruments.

When an incident of breakage occurs, the surgeon should pause and collect his or her thoughts. The device is inserted via the cannula system. The fragment is manipulated end-on to the magnet for removal through the cannula. With the cannula in the joint, the Golden Retriever and fragment are removed. The fragment should not be removed transcutaneously because it may be lost in tissues.

Suction will aid in retrieval, but suction that is too strong will bring soft tissue in between the magnet and fragment. This is why a tight suction connection is not possible while using the Golden Retriever.

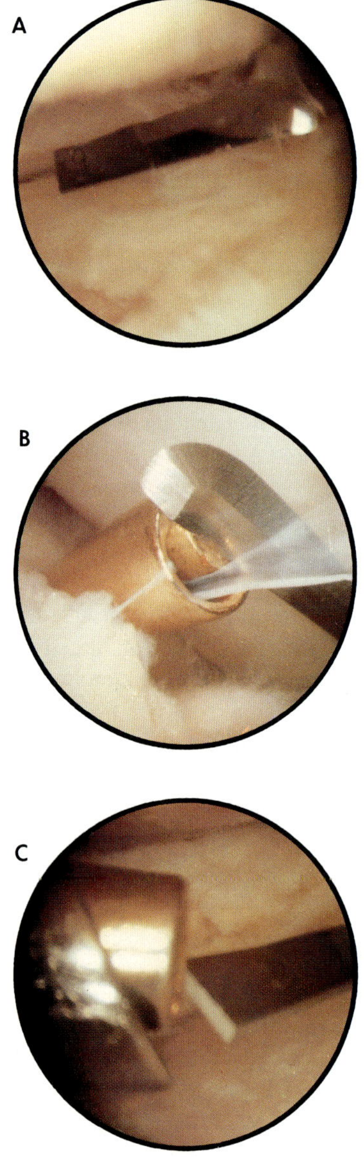

FIG. 5-72 Golden Retriever.

A Fragment broken off in joint.

B Golden Retriever passed via cannula. Magnet attracts fragment on side. Notice effect of suction on tissues.

C Cannula pushed over Golden Retriever into view.

Continued.

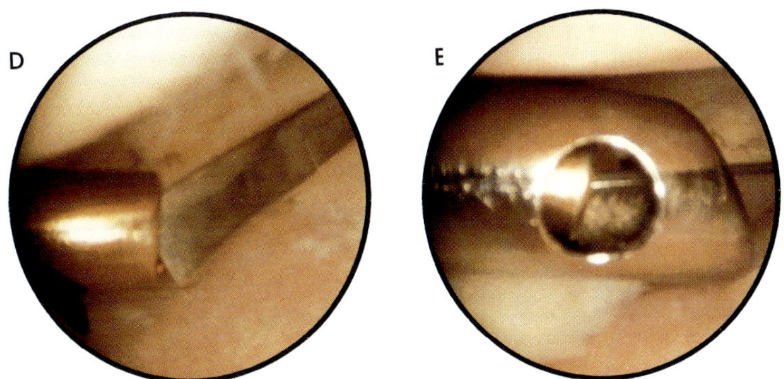

FIG. 5-72 *cont'd* **Golden Retriever.**

D Fragment end on magnet to facilitate cannula removal.

E Fragment seen in cannula opening.

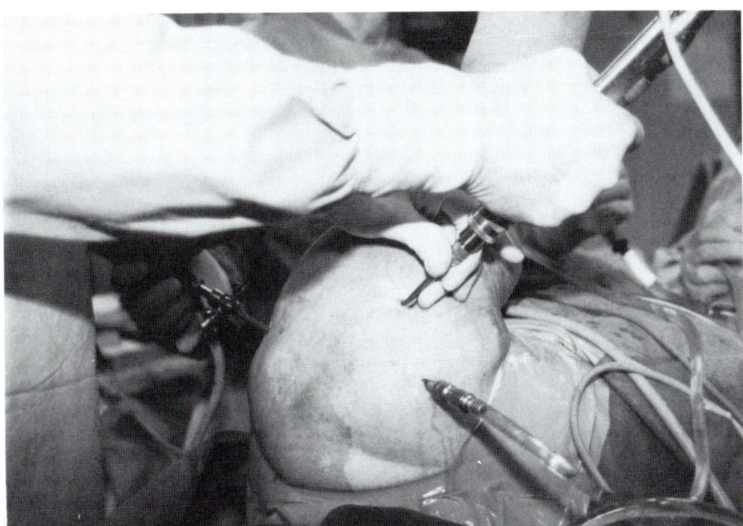

FIG. 5-73 Two-handed control on the motorized instrumentation will give better control, especially if the nondominant hand is required for the control.

Motorized Instruments. Motorized instrumentation facilitates simultaneous resection and removal, and it reduces the number of entries necessary into the joint. The risk of articular cartilage injury or scuffing is less. Motorization decreases the amount of hand activity necessary by the surgeon, and minimizes his or her fatigue. It is especially effective in articular cartilage debridement and synovectomy, which could not be as easily accomplished in any other way.

A motorized instrument is handled much like a pencil. To use one that has a "gun" or pistol grip, the surgeon has to supply rotation with the forearm rather than motion with the hand. Some systems rotate by manipulation of the barrel with the second hand. The axial alignment of the Dyonics system allows for greater ease of handling and encourages precision gripping. Using one's second hand may be necessary for control (Fig. 5-73).

Manipulative techniques for motorized instruments

Shaving. Shaving is the technique that started the development of motorized instrumentation (Fig. 5-74). The shaver or cutter head is moved back and forth across a surface very much as an electric razor is guided across a beard. The tissue comes into the instrumentation by suction. The rotating-cutting device removes the soft articular parts. The shaving technique is basic, and instrument head changes are made based on tissue type.

Dabbing. Dabbing is an oscillating action that can be likened to blotting spilled fluid with a towel (Fig. 5-75). The towel is placed on the fluid repeatedly until the water is drawn up into it. As the towel approaches, the fluid will seem to jump up into it. This is actually the case with arthroscopic dabbing; the instrument is held away from ei-

SHAVING

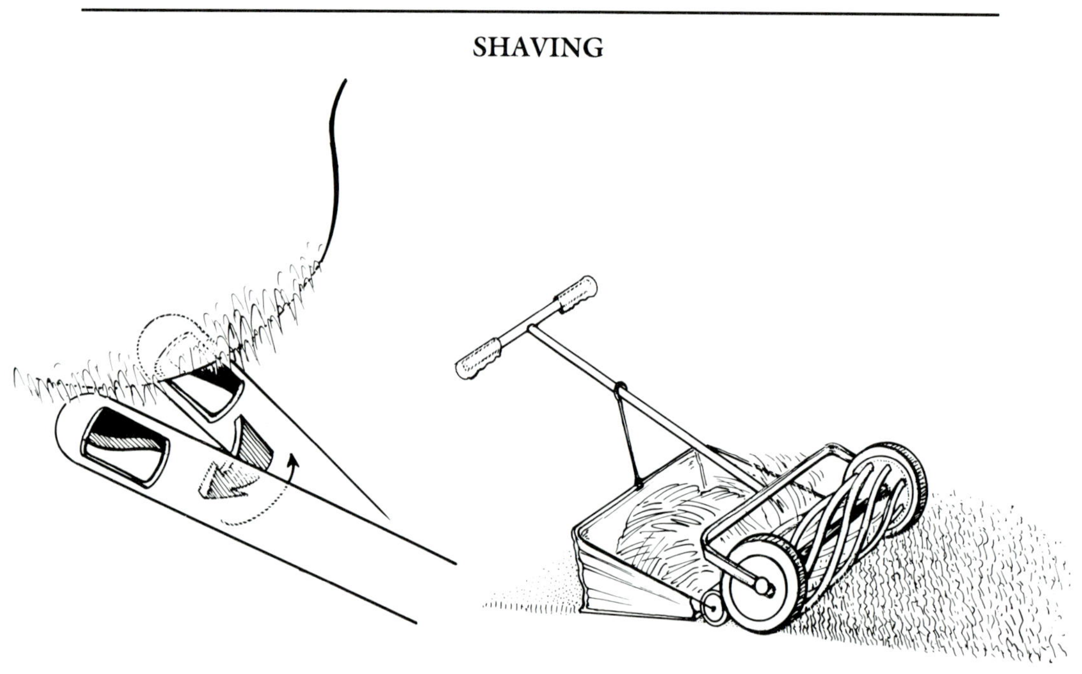

FIG. 5-74 Shaver head.

DABBING

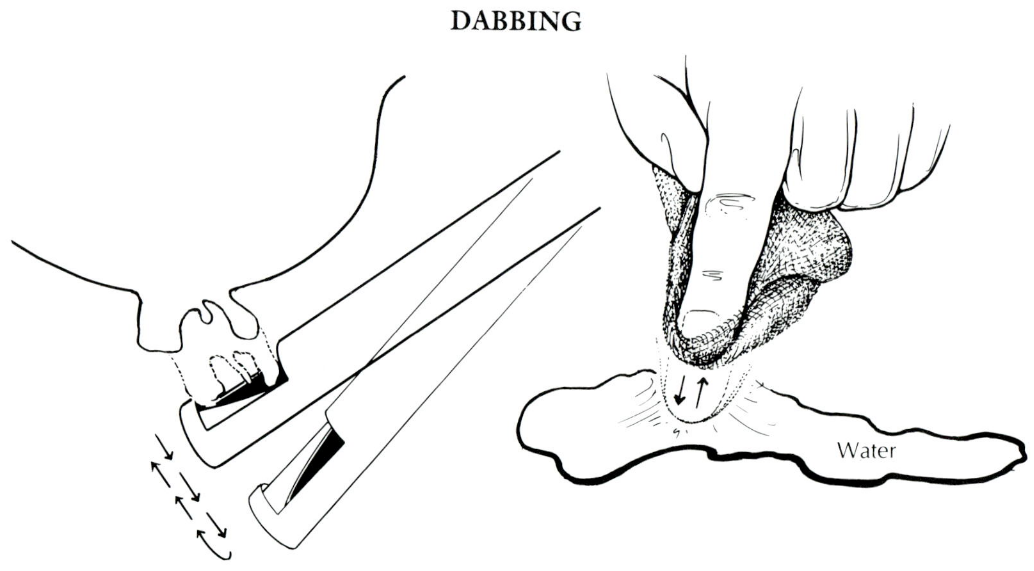

FIG. 5-75 Dabbing motion.

ther synovium or the soft part. The suction is open on the instrument. As the instrument moves toward the object, the material is moved under tension into the instrumentation. This suction tension permits sharp cutting action.

Pawing. Another technique is pawing (Fig. 5-76). Pawing is used in the Intra-articular Shaver System, with a trimmer head for use on articular cartilage or the cutter head on meniscus. The motion is as if one were pawing or scratching in the dirt. It is a very slow motion, and the surgeon can pull down toward his or her body, go back, and pull toward the body again several times. Repeated pawing and pulling goes over the same area. This approach is used on labral and articular cartilage flaps.

Whittling. Whittling is accomplished by using the oscillating mode of the foot pedal (Fig. 5-77). This advanced control system is better than moving one's foot back and forth; reverse and then forward. This technique is likened to whittling wood. Whittling on one side of a green stick

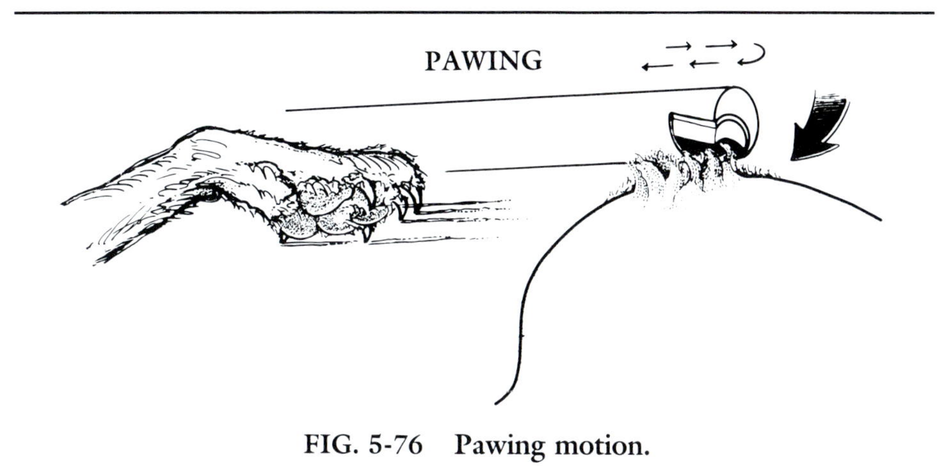

FIG. 5-76 Pawing motion.

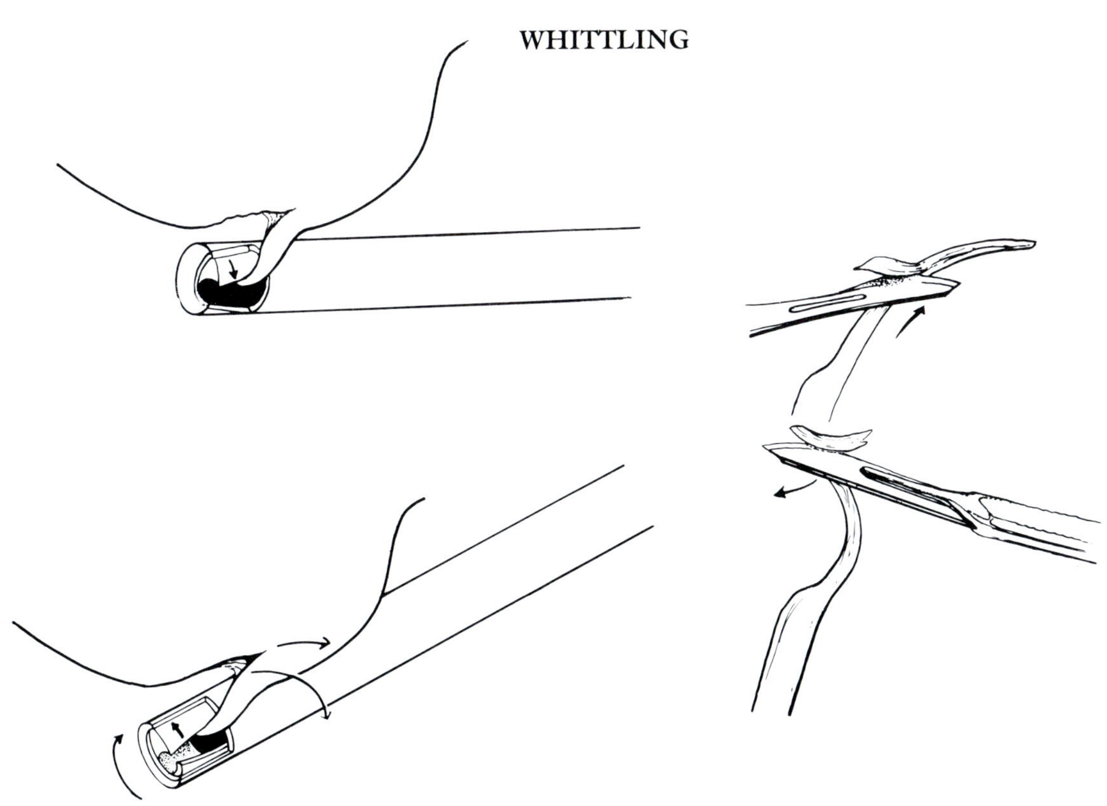

FIG. 5-77 Whittling motion.

bends it over without further resection; reversing the twig provides an angle for cutting. A more effective method of resection is to alternate whittling from one side of the stick and then from the other side. The foot pedal is used in the same way, alternating forward and reverse on any given fragment, to produce the whittling effect.

Scooping. The scooping action is like that used in scooping ice cream (Fig. 5-78). The open portion of the cutter head rests along the edge of tissue to be resected. The motor is activated, and cutting is initiated. The instrument is rotated to lift material with a scooping motion as it is resected. This motion is used on irregularly shaped tissue of hard consistency.

Joint manipulation. In another approach, the surgical instrument can remain stationary in the shoulder joint. For instance it can rest over the glenoid and the humerus can be rotated, bringing remote areas of the humeral head in front of the cutting instrument (see Fig. 5-30, *F*).

Technique by motorized cutting head type

Shaver. The shaver is used with a side-to-side motion; this is analogous to mowing the lawn. The bullet-nose prevents an effective pawing motion, but dabbing is possible (see Fig. 5-74).

Cutter. With a cutter head, both pawing on hard parts and dabbing on soft free edges is used on the labrum (Fig. 5-79). If a cutter is used on undermined edges of articular cartilage, scooping is the proper technique. Whittling is a function of all these motions. Scooping is used when working under the labrum edge, at the junction of a tear and normal labral tissue. This manipulation is useful for resecting the intact extension of the CA ligament under the acromion.

Trimmer. The shaving motion is the most common for the trimmer head (Fig. 5-80). A combination of pawing and scooping facilitate resection of tissues.

Whisker and turbowhisker. This head has small openings (Fig. 5-81). It is less aggressive. The whittling, side-to-side motion clears small holes of tissue. When this cutting head is held away from synovial villa, its draws in only the villi. A dabbing motion may be required.

Abrader. With the abrader the hand action is that of shaving, with an even pressure to progressively resect bone (Fig. 5-82). The reverse mode is less aggressive than the forward mode, in that the cutting edges are angled for the forward movement. A combination shaving and scooping or pawing action gives even control to resection. The whittling action cleans the burr of bony debris. A curetting

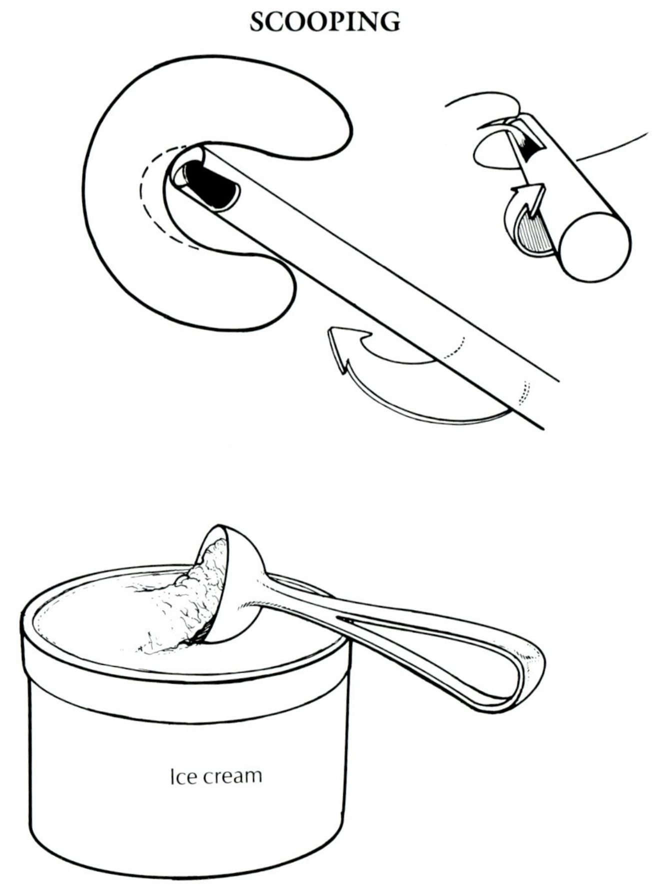

FIG. 5-78 Scooping motion.

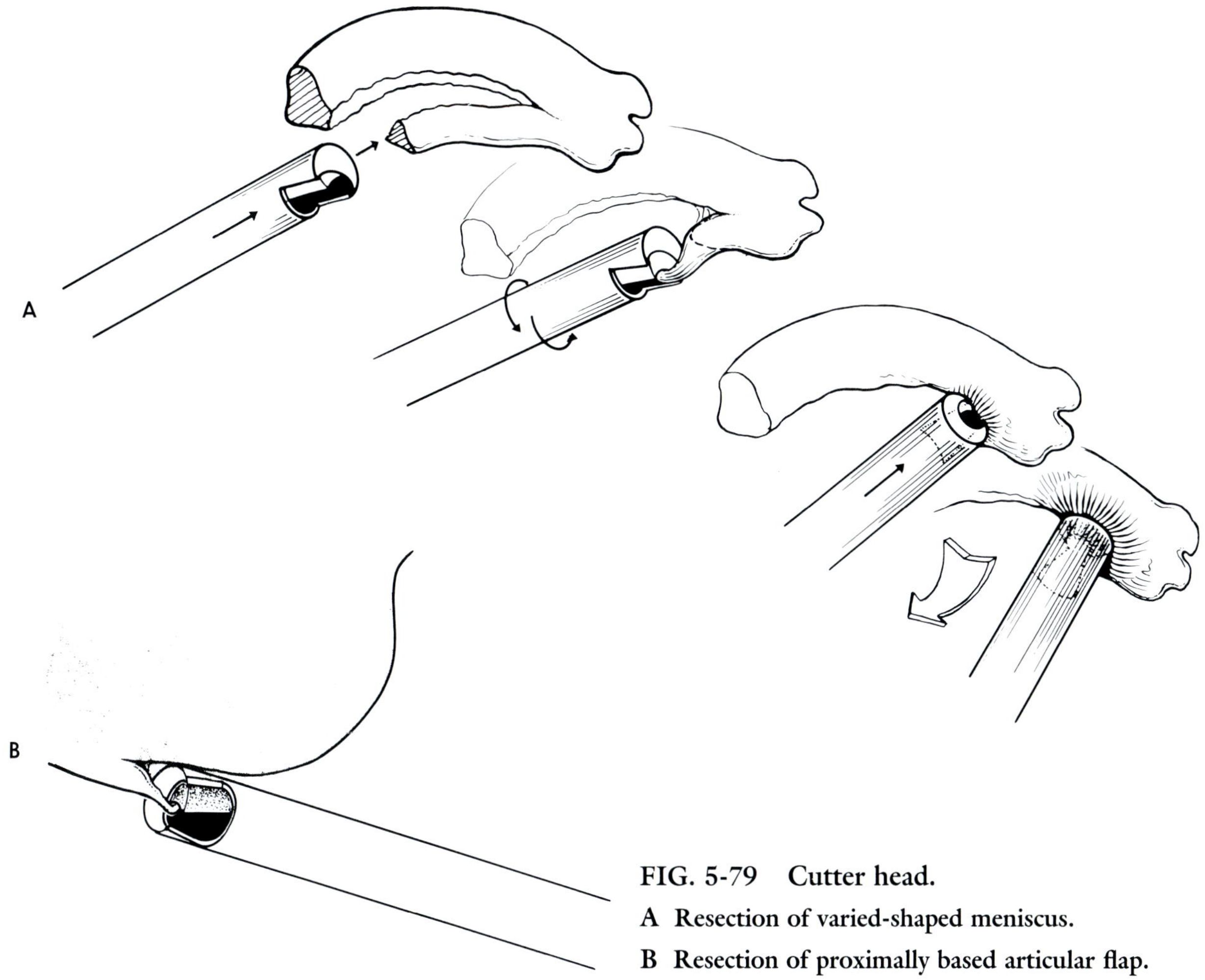

FIG. 5-79 Cutter head.

A Resection of varied-shaped meniscus.

B Resection of proximally based articular flap.

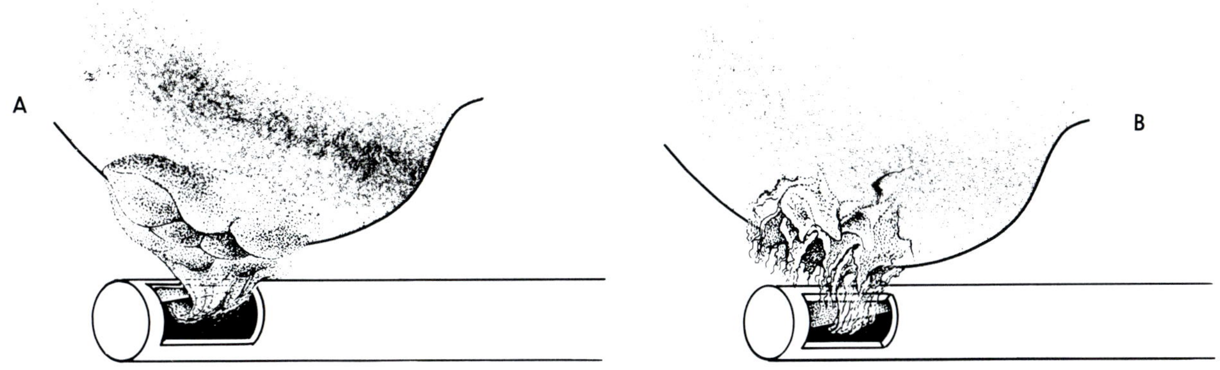

FIG. 5-80 Trimmer head.

A Removal of long, loose fragment.

B Resection of proximal-based articular flap.

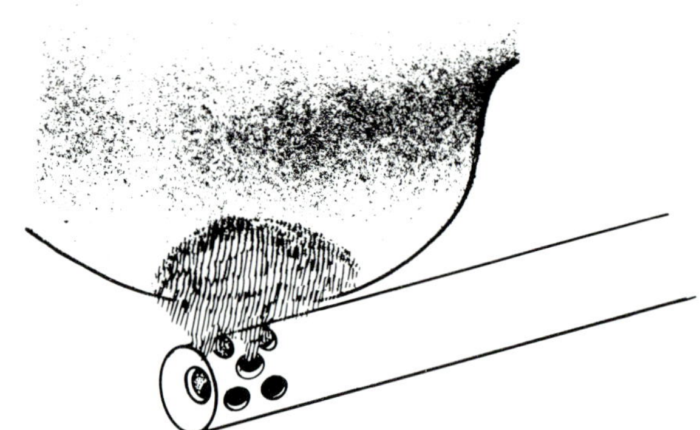

FIG. 5-81 Whisker and turbowhisker head.

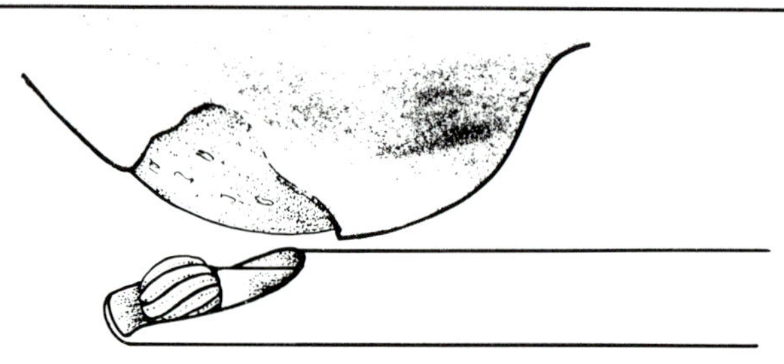

FIG. 5-82 Abrader head.

motion is used on deep holes. The scooping motion elevates and resects the edges of osteophytes. It is beneficial for resection inside the AC joint.

Acromionizer. The action is the same as the abrader, but a sweeping motion is effective for creating a flat, smooth undersurface of the acromion.

Synovial resector. The nature of the cut by the synovial resector is affected by shaving and dabbing. The distance from the synovium determines the depth of the resection. When held off the villi and slowly moved by dabbing, the resector cuts only the villi. A closer position removes synovial basement membrane. A pawing action with pressure will resect the capsule. Care must be taken not to resect the underlying muscle.

Final Operative Steps

The final step of any arthroscopic technique is to repeat the diagnostic arthroscopy. This review of the joint inspects the overall result of the surgical procedure. The areas of resection or the debridement are reprobed to see that all the remaining tissue is firm and of the proper shape. A motorized instrument is used to vacuum or debride and clean up the area to leave behind the cleanest possible wound. The final clean-up reduces the amount of work that the joint itself has to do in cleaning up.

Host Tissue Response

One factor that surgeons tend to ignore is that the body responds not only to disease or injury, but also to surgical intervention. Any debridement and/or repair has to be thought of in terms of the opportunity for the tissue to respond. For instance, a replaced glenohumeral ligament or rotator cuff tendon rapidly repairs to the bone.

Following surgery, bleeding occurs.[12] The incised areas are covered with clot. Synovial and vascular covering surrounds the injury site. Areas of resection heal on the intraarticular free span of the biceps tendon.

Careful debridement of a partial-thickness lesion removes potential fragments from the joint. Often, fibrous repair is seen on the surface without drilling to the bone.

If sclerotic exposed bone is debrided, hemorrhage occurs and is followed by spindle cell formation.[14] If the area is properly protected, reparative fibrocartilage will develop.

During any operative procedure, the diagnostic phase continues until the resection or repair is complete. Although the body has a great potential for repair, the resection of tissue should be adequate but not excessive or unnecessary.

INTRAOPERATIVE COMPLICATIONS

The shoulder joint has the highest complication rate in arthroscopy.[5,38,39] Part of this is due to the time in history when the surveys were collected. Those surveyed were experienced for years in knee arthroscopy, but new to the shoulder joint. They were new to shoulder reconstruction and arthroscopic metallic staples. This procedure was technically difficult and the complications easily identified by x-ray films.

The only way to avoid surgical complications is to avoid surgery. The issue then becomes recognizing the potential for complication and minimizing its occurrence. Knowing this potential, proper preparation for complications with backup instruments, retrieval tools, and alternate or additional procedures is mandatory. Recognition of complications is based on knowledge of their potential. The exercise of sound judgment in management is based on the surgeon's previous experience or that of others.

Instruments

All optical, electrical or mechanical devices are subject to breakage or failure of function. Therefore backup devices or methods must be available to substitute or compensate for the problem.

An arthroscope can fracture when it is dropped before or during the procedure. The arthroscope can also be fractured during intraarticular manipulations. The arthroscope is not a crowbar; it is a fine surgical optical instrument and should be handled as such. The surgeon should recognize that the scope is bending if an elliptical picture is seen ei-

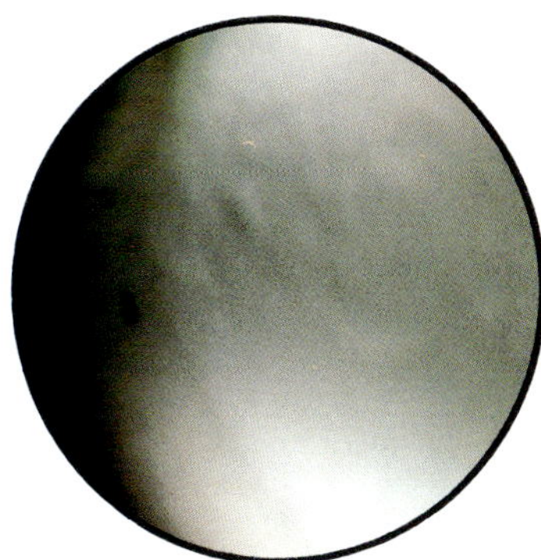

FIG. 5-83 Elliptical shape to arthroscopic view with bending of the scope.

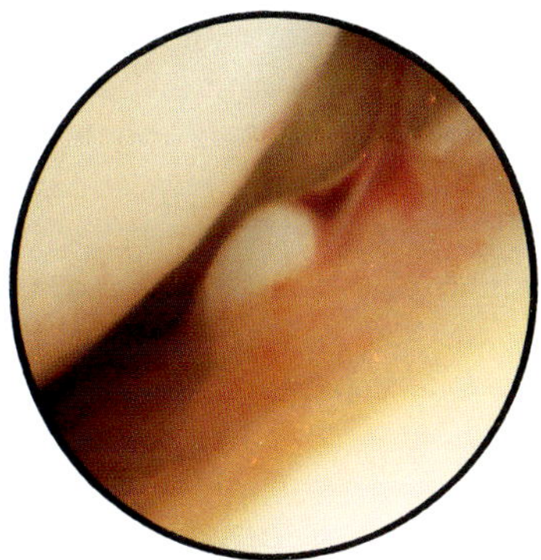

FIG. 5-84 Arthroscopic view of a lost piece of tissue caught in the capsule.

ther on direct visualization or on the video screen (Fig. 5-83). With all the distractions of the operation, the elliptical deformation of the arthroscope will often go unnoticed by the surgeon. Assistants are trained for observation and they will bring it to the surgeon's attention.

The arthroscope coverplate is subject to fracture or scratching. Also, a piece of glass could drop into the joint. From a visual standpoint, the scope maintains its integrity, but optimal visualization is lost. A change of arthroscope is necessary in this instance.

You must have a backup arthroscope.

Fractured Instruments. It is imperative that all instruments placed within the joint have magnetic properties. This property allows retrieval by a magnetic-suction device (see Fig. 5-72). Such a device must be in the arthroscopic surgical setup. The major problems occur when too great a rotational or angulatory stress is placed on the instrument. With small arthroscopic instruments, breakage can occur with a powerful grip on the handles. The surgeon must have a sense of the magnitude of pressure these instruments can tolerate.

Virtually all instruments made for arthroscopic surgery are breakable. They need not be broken if the surgeon is familiar with the instrument's proper use and tolerance.

Technical Problems

Scuffing. The most common interoperative complication is injury to the articular surface, so-called scuffing (see Fig. 5-39). These articular cartilage injuries can happen accidentally, unknowingly, or inadvertently. Although they seal with fibrous tissue and smooth away, scuffs are permanent. The hyaline cartilage is not replaced. Every effort should be made to avoid scuffing. This can be done by minimizing the number of passes of instrumentation and also by exercising gentleness, "treading light," and conceptually placing yourself on the end of the instrument (see Fig. 5-8).

Ligament Injury. The capsular ligaments could be inadvertently cut or resected during removal of adjacent tissue. For instance, the anterior capsular ligaments may be "wrapped up" with the motorized burr while the surgeon is roughening the anterior glenoid before anterior capsulorrhaphy.

Vascular Injury. Transcutaneous surgical approaches cannot identify vessels. The cannula system establishes a portal to the side of these veins by pushing them aside during entry. Care must be taken during placement to avoid cutting the cutaneous veins. The cephalic vein courses over the deltopectoral groove. Preoperative identification and marking with a skin scratch locates the vein during the surgical approach.

During glenohumeral surgery, the axillary and circumflex humeral vessels are at greatest risk, but injury is uncommon. Laceration would occur only with extraarticular instrument penetration. Having cutting tips in view at all times avoids this mishap. Knife blade cutting should be careful, slow, and measured. Fingertip control avoids "plunging." Control of the surgical hand may be provided by assisting with the other hand. Another method of control for the cutting hand is to rest the wrist or base of the hand against the patient. The acromial branch of the CA ligament is often lacerated during arthroscopic acromioplasty.

If major vessel injury occurs, its recognition is followed by repair, even with vascular surgical consultation. If laceration of the saphenous or cephalic vein occurs, suture ligation is sufficient. The acromial branch of the CA artery is controlled with electrocautery.

Lost Tissue in Joint. A frustrating intraoperative complication is sudden loss of a tissue fragment (Fig. 5-84). The surgical technique of inflow on the scope draws pieces toward the view, not away from it. The use of motorized instruments with suction assists in controlled removal; knife blade inscription, not resection, techniques keep the piece in place. Infrequent use of the basket forceps reduces the potential for multiple fragments.

When a tissue piece is lost, it may be in the joint, part of the way out into the tissues, or even out of the joint. I look at the easiest place first. Inspection of the drapes, gowns, floor, graspers, and Mayo stand eliminates these places. Inspection of instrument exit portals from the inside may show the "tail" of the fragment. If so, the piece should be placed back into the joint before removal. Attempts to remove the piece from its position in the capsule may lose it altogether. If a fragment is completely lost in the capsule of subcutaneous tissue, a motorized instrument is pistoned in and out, widening the hole and freeing the fragment from its attachments. The force of fluid flow may push it out of the joint. In another case, the fragment may be caught in the window of the cutter head and then moved into or out of the joint. Finally, after the portal is widened, an open forceps pushes through the portal to dislodge fragments back into the joint. I have not yet had a fragment lost in the capsule or subcutaneous tissue that was not retrievable by this method.

However, before extensive enlargement of the portal, a search should be made throughout the joint. The enlarged portal causes leakage that decompresses the joint.

If the fragment is believed to be in the joint, the inflow cannula is opened and suction is applied to the arthroscope. All recesses of the joint are vacuumed. Ballottement is helpful to mobilize the pieces.

Intermittent clamping of the inflow tubing will decompress the joint, creating movement of fluids and hopefully of the fragment to the arthroscope. Finally, a small full-radius head on the motorized instrumentation is placed into the joint and used as a vacuum cleaner, probing every recess. When the fragment is identified, it is brought on to the glenoid surface for removal.

Fluid Leakage. Leakage from various puncture wounds has two disadvantages: it decompresses the joint, compromising visualization and it is a nuisance to have fluid flowing over the surgeon and on the floor. Fluid leakage interferes with concentration.

Leakage is prevented by making small puncture wounds and using a cannula system. The large puncture wounds made for transcutaneous placement of instruments result in leakage. When multiple punctures are used, the cannulas can be left in place with their obturators, reducing the leakage from any given portal.

Leakage that does not come completely out of the joint can be an even worse problem.[26] If it enters the space between the synovium and the skin, the depth of tissue that the instruments must pass increases. Swelling can increase the length of the instrument fulcrum and make manipulation impossible. The angle of approach may be altered by this swelling, so that replacement is necessary.

Extravasation is one of the main disadvantages of having the inflow on the arthroscope. If the arthroscope is retracted out of the joint, the extravasation causes tissue edema and visualization is compromised.

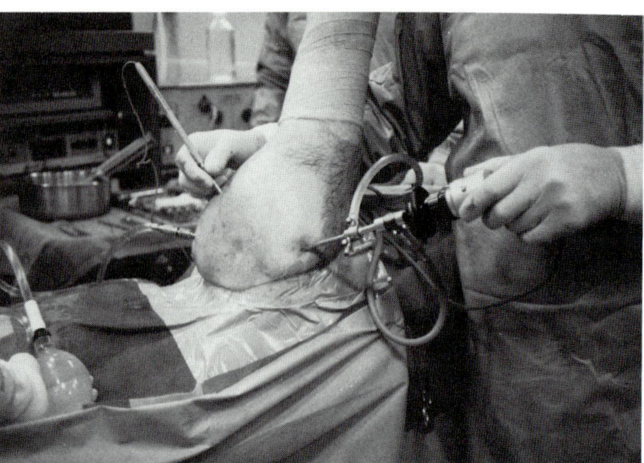

FIG. 5-85 Electrocautery is effective method of controlling hemostasis. A water (non-electrolyte) medium is required in this system.

If leakage occurs around an instrument and the operation is to continue, a suture ligature may be placed adjacent to the scope or instrument to control the leak. A small leak that is spouting fluid can be controlled by gauze around the instrument to dampen or redirect the flow (see Fig. 5-35).

Extrasynovial extravasation of fluid may cause temporary (a few minutes) blanching of the skin adjacent to the shoulder.[30] This problem resolves within a few minutes when absorption takes place.

Intraarticular bleeding

Adrenaline. Epinephrine solution (a vial of 1:1000 or 1 mg is placed in 1000 ml of saline) is used in the shoulders during the diagnostic phase only. A continuous infusion of adrenaline solution could cause extravasation and delay absorption, resulting in cardiovascular problems. This may occur especially in elderly patients or those with existing medical problems.

Distention. Maximal distention will control intraarticular bleeding when intravascular pressure is exceeded.

Electrocautery. Electrocautery is the most effective means of hemostasis (Fig. 5-85).[9] A "Coagulator" is used. A change to sterile water is necessary to create a conductive medium. Air and glycerol have also been used.

Injection of Air. Injection or distention with room air controls bleeding through its drying effect (see Fig. 5-4, *A*).

Extraarticular bleeding

Laceration of the cutaneous vein may require ligation. I have not had a case with major vascular injury.

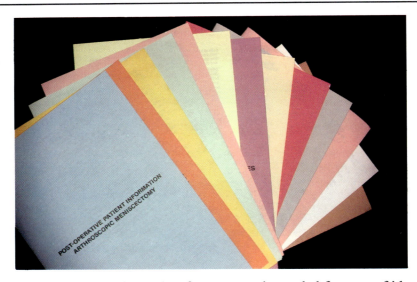

FIG. 5-86 Patient information forms are color coded for ease of identification for various arthroscopic procedures on any joint.

POSTOPERATIVE CARE

The success of surgical technique does not end at the operating room or recovery room door. Preoperatively, the patient is instructed on what to anticipate. Postoperatively, he or she is given both verbal and written instructions (see under specific operations).

I do not use suture material in routine puncture wounds. The larger wounds of loose body retrieval are sutured. I use a soft dressing with foam tape. This dressing is easily removed by the patient or by me without scissors. Band-Aids are applied the next day.

I give patients color-coded instruction sheets that are operation specific (Fig. 5-86). For further details on postoperative care, see Chapter 1.

REFERENCES

1. Andrews JR, Carson WG Jr, Ortega K: Arthroscopy of the shoulder: techniques and normal anatomy, *Am J Sports Med* 12:1-7, 1984.
2. Becker RL, Johnson LL: Role of the assistant in arthroscopy. In American Academy of Orthopaedic Surgeons Symposium on arthroscopy and arthrography of the knee, St Louis, 1978, Mosby–Year Book.
3. Bigliani LU et al: An anatomical study of the suprascapular nerve, *Arthroscopy* 6(4):301-305, 1990.
4. Caspari RA: Personal communication (with credit to Jules Neviaser), 1984.
5. DeLee JC: Complications of arthroscopy and arthroscopic surgery: results of a national survey, *Arthroscopy* 1:214, 1985.
6. Detrisac DA, Johnson LL: *Arthroscopic shoulder anatomy: pathological and surgical implications*, Thoroughfare, NJ, 1986, Slack.
7. Drez D, Proffer D: *Suprascapular nerve anatomy and relationship to the glenoid*. Presented at American Academy of Orthopedic Surgeons in Anaheim, CA, March 1991.
8. Eriksson E, Sebik A: Arthroscopy and arthroscopic surgeon in a gas versus a fluid medium, *Orthop Clin North Am* 13:293, 1982.
9. Fox JM et al: Electrosurgery in orthopaedics. Part 1: Principles, *Contemp Orthop* 8:21, 1984.
10. Guten GS: Methylene blue staining of articular cartilage during arthroscopy, *Orthop Rev* 6:59, 1977.
11. Ivey M et al: Serum bupivicaine concentrations following intra-articular injection for pain relief after knee arthroscopy, Scientific Presentation AANA annual meeting, San Diego, CA, 1991.
12. Johnson LL: Characteristics of the immediate post arthroscopic blood clot formation in the knee joint, *Arthroscopy* 7(1):14-23, 1991.
13. Johnson LL: The shoulder joint: an arthroscopist's perspective of anatomy and pathology, *Clin Orthop* 223:113-125, 1987.
14. Johnson LL: Arthroscopic abrasion arthroplasty historical and pathological perspective: present status, *Arthroscopy* 2(1):55-69, 1986.
15. Johnson LL: *Arthroscopic surgery: principles and practice*, St Louis, 1986, Mosby–Year Book.
16. Johnson LL: Diagnostic and surgical arthroscopy, ed 2, St Louis, 1981, Mosy–Year Book.
17. Johnson LL: Arthroscopy of the shoulder, *Orthop Clin North Am* 11(2):197-204, 1980.
18. Johnson LL: Needlescope. In *American Academy of Orthopaedic Surgeons Symposium on Arthroscopy and Arthrography of the Knee*, St Louis, 1978, Mosby–Year Book.
19. Johnson LL: Comprehensive arthroscopic examination of the knee, St Louis 1977, Mosby–Year Book.
20. Johnson LL: Arthroscopy of the knee using local anesthesia: a review of 400 patients, *J Bone Joint Surg* 58A:736, 1976.
21. Johnson LL: Diagnostic arthroscopy of the knee joint. In *Excerpta Medica*, New York, 1974, American Elsevier.
22. Johnson LL et al: Two percent glutaraldehyde: a disinfectant in arthroscopy and arthroscopic surgery, *J Bone Joint Surg* 64A:237, 1982.
23. Johnson LL et al: Cold sterilization method for arthroscopes using activated dialdehyde, *Orthop Rev* 6:75, 1977.
24. Kaeding CC et al: Bupivicaine use after knee arthroscopy: pharmacokinetics and pain control study, *Arthroscopy* 6(1):330-399, 1990.

25. Klein AH et al: Measurement of brachial plexus strain in arthroscopy of the shoulder, *Arthroscopy* 3(1):45-52, 1987.
26. Lee YF, Cohn L, Tooke SM: Intramuscular deltoid pressure during shoulder arthroscopy, *Arthroscopy* 5(3);209-212, 1989.
27. Matthews LS et al: Anterior portal selection for shoulder arthroscopy, *Arthroscopy* 1:33, 1985.
28. Neer CS II: *Shoulder reconstruction,* Philadelphia, 1990, WB Saunders.
29. Nole R, Munson NML, Fulerson JP: Bupivacaine and saline effects on articular cartilage, *Arthroscopy* 1:123, 1985.
30. Peek R, Haynes DW: Compartment syndrome as a complication of arthroscopy, *Am J Sports Med* 12:464, 1984.
31. Pitman MI et al: The use of somatosensory evoked potentials for the detection of neuropraxia during shoulder arthroscopy, *Arthroscopy* 4(4):250-255, 1988.
32. Reagan BF et al: Irrigating solutions for arthroscopy, *J Bone Joint Surg* 65A:629, 1983.
33. Rockwood CA: Shoulder arthroscopy, *J Bone Joint Surg* 70A:636-640, 1988 (editorial).
34. Rockwood CA Jr, Matsen FA III: The shoulder, Philadelphia, 1990, WB Saunders.
35. Rowe CR: The shoulder, New York, 1988, Churchill Livingstone.
36. Sherpak RC, Schuster H, Funch RS: Airway emergency in a patient during CO2 arthroscopy (letter), *Anesthesiology* 60:171, 1984.
37. Skyhar MJ et al: Shoulder arthroscopy with the patient in the beach-chair position, *Arthroscopy* 4(4):256-259, 1988.
38. Small NC: Complications in arthroscopic surgery performed by experienced arthroscopists, *J Arthroscopy Relat Surg* 4(3):215-221, 1988.
39. Small NC: Complications in arthroscopy: the knee and other joints, *Arthroscopy* 2:253-58, 1986.
40. Smith CF et al: The carbon dioxide laser: a potential tool for orthopedic surgery, *Clin Orthop* 242:43-50, 1989.
41. Smith JA: Personal communication, 1982.
42. Smith JB, Nance T: Laser energy in arthroscopic surgery, In Parisien JS: *Arthroscopic surgery*, New York, 1988, McGraw-Hill.
43. Souryal TO, Baker CL. Anatomy of the supraclavicular fossa portal in shoulder arthroscopy, *Arthroscopy* 6(4):297-300, 1990.
44. Sweeney HJ: Teaching arthroscopic surgery at the residency level, *Orthop Clin North Am* 13:255, 1982.
45. Waldron BD: Technique of shoulder arthroscopy, *Orthop Rev* 17(6):652-655, 1989.
46. Wissinger HA: Personal communication, 1982.

CHAPTER

6 Arthroscopic Surgical Anatomy

Knowledge of surgical anatomy is very important for the arthroscopic surgeon.[1-3,7,14] During arthroscopy the surgeon does not have the benefit of layer by layer exposure and direct visualization of important anatomical structures as during conventional open surgery. Also, the appreciation of arthroscopic surgical anatomy is limited by a two-dimensional image as compared to the three-dimensional view of direct viewing possible during open surgery. The surgeon must substitute instrument palpation skills during arthroscopy for the finger touch possible during open surgery. Therefore arthroscopic surgery requires mental imaging of anatomical structures and their relationships (see Chapter 5). The surgical exposure for arthroscopy is described in terms of topographical anatomy, skin incisions, and portals.

On the other hand, studies of surgical anatomy of the shoulder during arthroscopy have provided a clearer understanding of the shoulder anatomy.[7,17,20,21] Prior conventional surgical exposures and anatomical dissections have limitations. They were performed from the perspective of outside-inward direction. The penetration of the arthroscope by-passes the usual anatomical landmarks and provides an inside view of the anatomical structures in situ.[10,11]

The arthroscopist's "insider's view" was uncharted anatomical territory to the glenohumeral joint, subacromial bursae, and acromioclavicular (AC) joint. Initially, the exploring arthroscopist recognized the intraarticular portion of the biceps tendon, the humeral head and the glenoid fossa (Fig. 6-1). The anterior and posterior joint was seen as a complex array of ligaments, bands, and foramen (Fig. 6-2). The glenohumeral ligaments were not arranged in the same direction, nor did they have the same glenoid insertion that had been previously described.[18,19] Some confusion existed because the superior glenohumeral ligament was rarely seen arthroscopically, the middle glenohumeral ligament was oblique in direction, and the superior portion of the subscapularis tendon was surprisingly a prominent intraarticular structure. Arthroscopic experience, coupled with anatomical dissections, unraveled the anatomical puzzle.[7]

Initial exploration of the subacromial space illustrated an anatomical arrangement that was equally confusing because of difficulty in spatial orientation. It was not common knowledge that the coracoacromial (CA) ligament extended beyond the anterior acromion to its undersurface (see Fig. 6-60). Also, it had been presumed that the free span of the CA ligament was critical structure in impingement syndrome. Instead the actual cause is that the extension of the ligament under the acromion becomes eroded with pressure (see Chapter 7).

The arthroscope has provided a means of increased appreciation and accurate descriptions of shoulder anatomy, heretofore not available. The understanding of the patient's shoulder problems benefits from both the open and arthroscopic perspective of surgical anatomy.

BONY ANATOMY OF THE SHOULDER GIRDLE

The scapular coracoid process, acromion, spine, and clavicle are palpable and important for establishing the site of arthroscopic surgical portals.

Knowledge of the bony anatomy of the shoulder girdle is essential to understanding arthroscopic anatomy, although only small areas of bone are exposed by arthroscopy (Fig. 6-3). Most areas are covered with soft tissue. The scapular glenoid fossa is visualized medial to the humeral head in the glenohumeral joint.

During arthroscopy of the subacromial space, the scapular acromion is visualized only if pathological erosion or surgical debridement of the acromion is present (see Chapter 10). The underside of the acromion is normally covered with the extension of the CA ligament (see Fig. 6-60). The CA joint is immediately medial to the anterior acromial angle but is not visualized during arthroscopic bursoscopy as it too is covered with soft tissue.

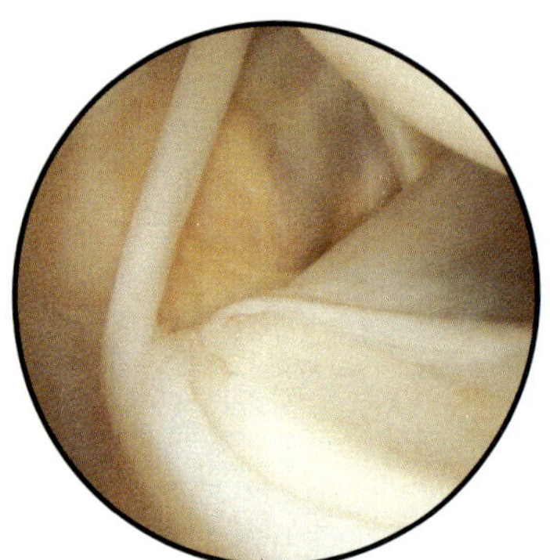

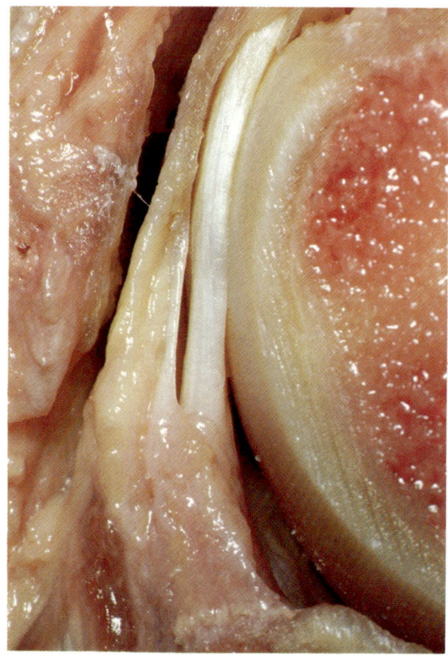

FIG. 6-1 Biceps tendon landmark.

A Arthroscopic view shows an overview of the biceps tendon from posterior as it spans the joint and attaches to the superior glenoid.

B Gross anatomical view of the biceps tendon in relation to the humeral head (cross-sectional view). The rotator cuff is in juxtaposition. The space above the rotator cuff is the subacromial bursa. The acromion forms the roof of the bursa.

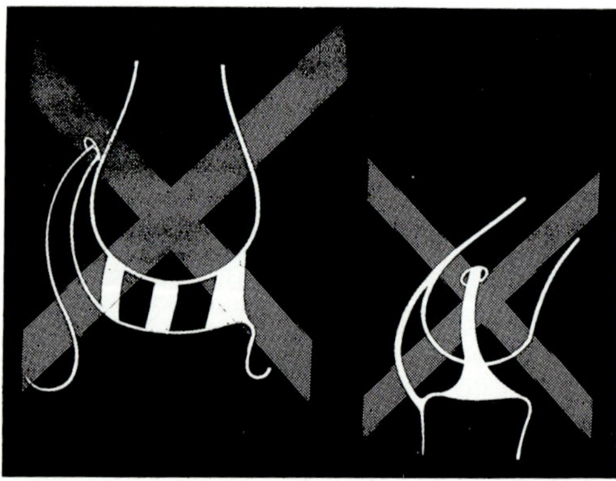

FIG. 6-2 Glenohumeral ligament anatomy revisited. The glenohumeral ligaments are not parallel or in one plane.

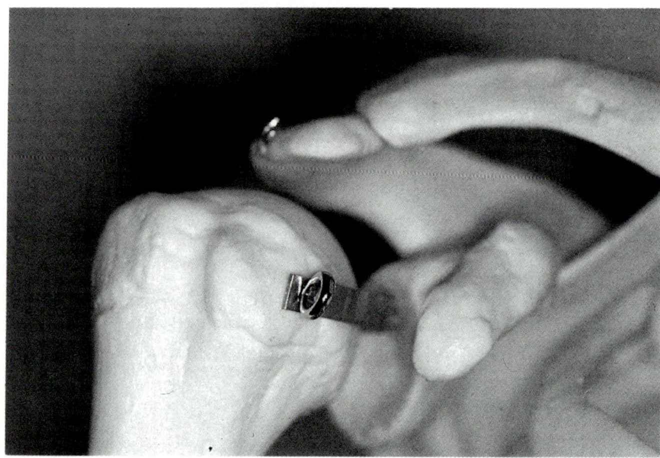

FIG. 6-3 Bony anatomy of the shoulder. Articulated skeleton shows the humeral head to the left, the coracoid process to the right, and the AC joint above.

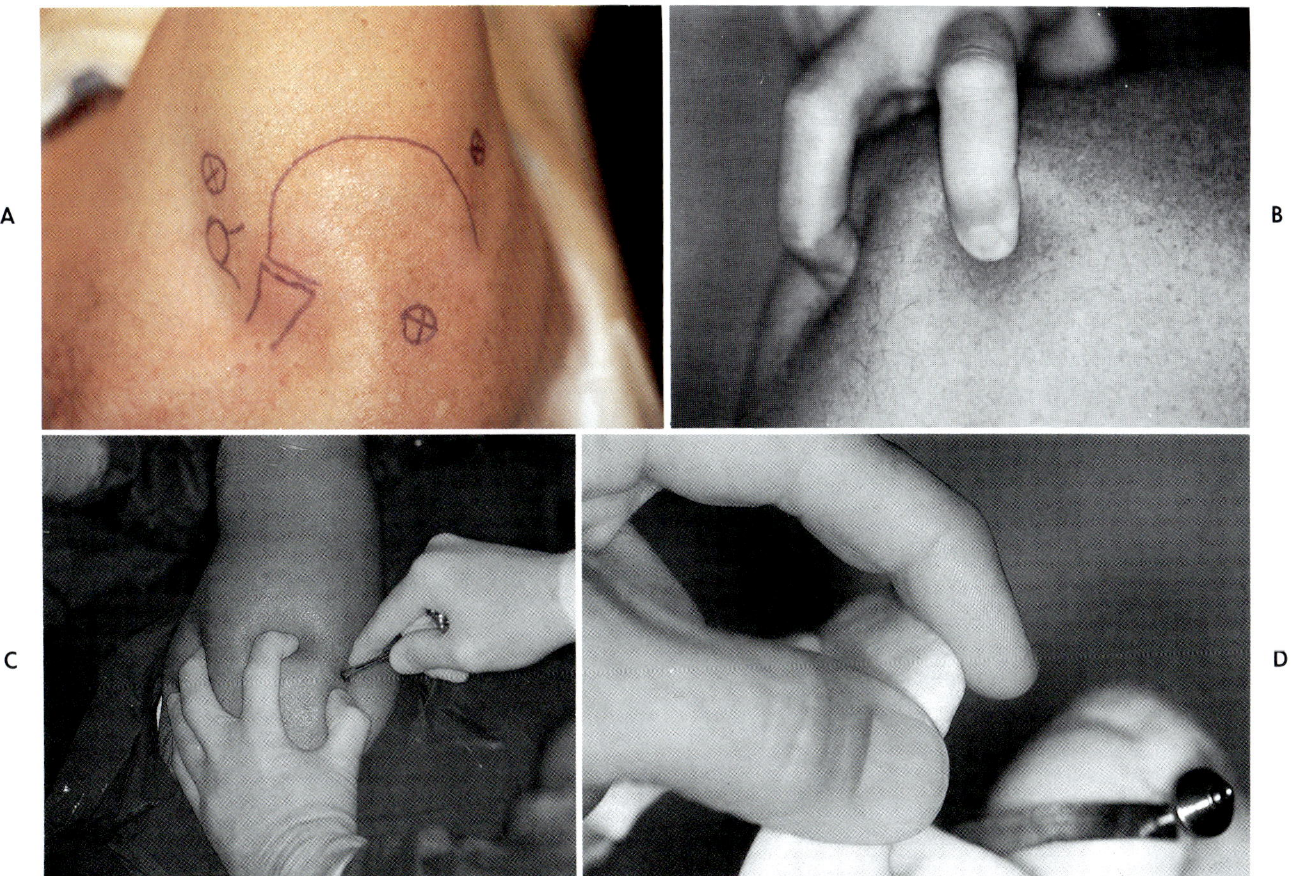

FIG. 6-4 Topographical anatomy.

A Drawing on topographical landmarks on surgical patient show clavicle, outline of acromion, and three standard arthroscopic portals with circled-X.

B Surgeon identifies surgical "soft spot" on his or her body with index finger.

C Capture of the posterior angle of the acromion on the patient. Actual skin incision is displaced posterior to the acromion on the tangential plane of the skin due to interposition of deltoid muscle and subcutaneous fat.

D Capture of the posterior angle of the acromion on the skeleton.

SURGICAL TOPOGRAPHICAL ANATOMY

Topographical anatomical landmarks are the clavicle, acromioclavicular (AC) joint, and the scapular coracoid process and acromion (Fig. 6-4, *A*). The deltoid muscle mass obscures the humerus and glenoid. Subcutaneous fat obscures both the deltoid muscle and the bony landmarks in many patients, but palpation identifies the deltopectoral groove, clavicle, and acromion. Relating the surface anatomy to the deeper anatomical structures is necessary for arthroscopic surgical penetration. Layer by layer surgical exposure is not available to the arthroscopic surgeon, so compensating surgical techniques have been developed (see Chapter 5).

Location of the posterior arthroscopic portal is assisted by the surgeon learning the location of the posterior "soft spot" on himself or herself (Fig. 6-4, *B*). With the right hand on the left shoulder, the index and middle fingers capture the posterior angle of the acromion. Flexion of the index finger 1 cm medial and 1 cm inferior to the posterior corner of the acromion locates the "soft spot."

Capturing the posterior angle of the patient's acromion with the thumb and index finger locates the topographical landmark for penetration of this same "soft spot" on the patient (Fig. 6-4, *C*). The surgeon should then be able to conceptualize the deeper bony structures and their relationships to the glenohumeral joint (Fig. 6-4, *D*).

ARTHROSCOPIC PORTALS (RELATIONAL ANATOMY)

Glenohumeral Joint

Posterior Portal. An optimal posterior entry to the glenohumeral joint passes 1 cm inferior and 1 cm medial to the posterior tip of the acromion (Fig. 6-5, *A*).

The surgeon identifies this area on the patient by capturing the posterior angle of the scapula with his or her thumb and index finger (see Fig. 6-4, *C* and *D*).

The skin incision to approach this point under and parallel to the acromion is displaced posterior by interposing muscle and subcutaneous fat (see Fig. 6-4, *C*). The incision is on the tangential plane of the posterior shoulder contour. This incision may be many centimeters from the acromion, but the plane of passage should be through the "soft spot" 1 cm medial and 1 cm inferior to the posterior angle of the acromion. A position 3 cm inferior to the acromion is too low for proper subsequent arthroscope placement or manipulation (Fig. 6-5, *B*).

The posterior arthroscopic approach requires knowledge of the relational anatomy of the deeper anatomical structures. The arthroscope ideally enters between the teres minor muscle and the infraspinatus tendon (Fig. 6-6). This area is the transition spot of the musculotendinous junction, so neither the muscle nor the tendon is injured at entry. A passage located lower and away from the acromion is dangerously near the supraclavicular nerve; one even lower is too close to the axillary nerve emergence from the quadrilateral space.

Anterior Portal. When the arm is abducted, the neurovascular structures are also moved more lateral. Therefore the anterior portal must be placed superior to the subscapularis tendon. This superior position avoids injury to the neurovascular structures.

Originally, I used a transcutaneous needle from anterior to locate this area. The anterior portal is best established by the method suggested by H. Andrew Wissinger.[23] His suggestion replaces the outside-in method of probing with a No. 18 spinal needle and utilization of the visual landmark of the superior margin of the subscapularis tendon from inside (see Chapter 5). This primary anterior portal is lateral and superior to the coracoid process. It passes through anterior deltoid muscle fiber, superior to the subscapularis, to enter the joint. The portal of entry from the joint perspective is in a triangle formed inferior by the subscapularis tendon, medial by the glenoid fossa, and superior by the thin superior glenohumeral ligament (Fig. 6-7).

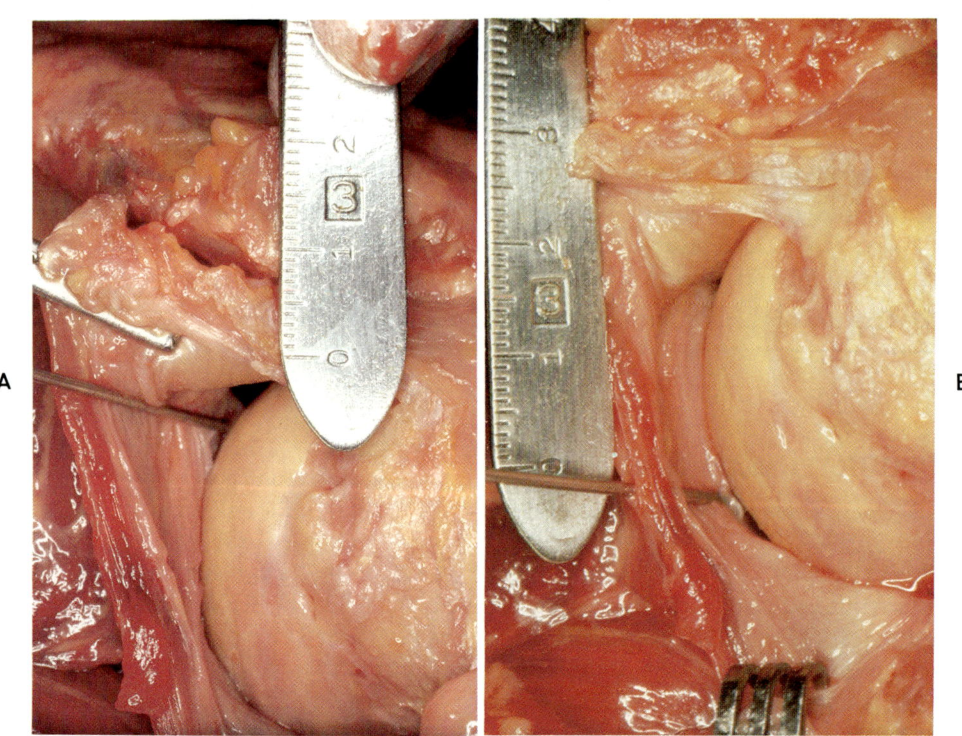

FIG. 6-5 Position of the posterior portal relative to the acromion.

A 1 cm inferior and 1 cm medial.

B 3 centimeters inferior is too low for subsequent optical viewing.

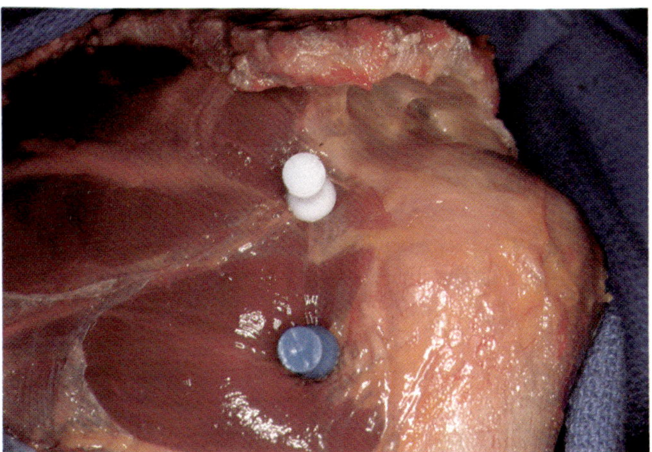

FIG. 6-6 Posterior portal of entry to the glenohumeral joint is between the infraspinatus tendon (white marker) and the teres minor tendon (blue marker).

A

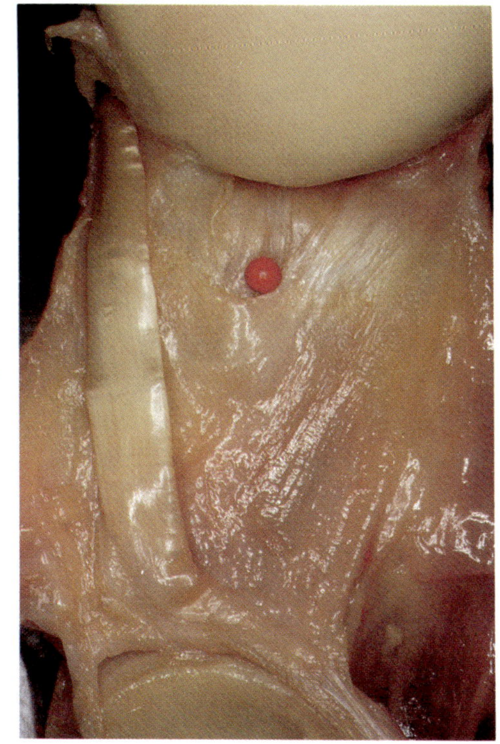

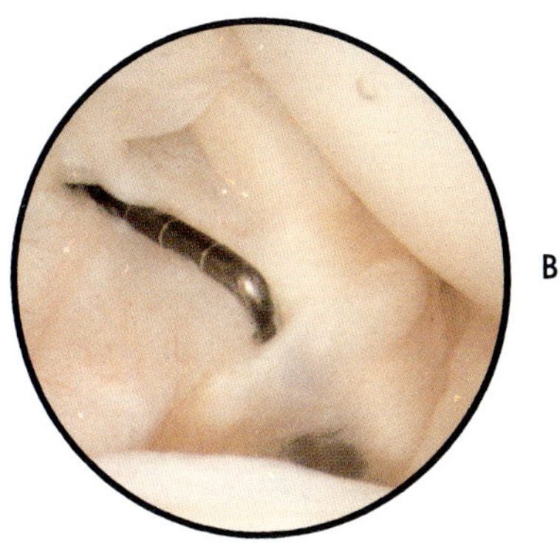

B

FIG. 6-7 Anterior portal is established from inside the glenohumeral joint.

A Gross anatomical specimen shows disarticulated joint with the humeral head superior, the glenoid inferior, and the anterior capsule stretched out. The biceps is to the left. The red marker identifies the internal landmark for placement of the arthroscope and Wissinger rod. It is immediately superior to the subscapularis tendon.

B Arthroscopic view of this same location. The probe is in the portal and spans the area of safe location for anterior portal placement.

Accessory anterior portals. Any area superior to the primary anterior portal may be safely used to approach the glenohumeral joint. Usually the anterior superior portal to the glenohumeral joint is initiated with a No. 18 spinal needle immediately anterior to the midpoint on the anterior acromion. The course varies with the thickness of the soft tissue. The portal track passes through anterior deltoid muscle, through the anterior joint capsule, anterior to the supraspinatus tendon insertion at the greater tuberosity of the humerus. The plane of this portal courses anterior to the glenoid, immediately lateral to the glenohumeral articulation.

Inferior anterior portals. Micheal Gross has reported an upper extremity traction system that uses a sling under the humerus as well as forearm traction.[8] The arm is held in an ADDucted position, but pulled away from the thorax with the sling. With this positioning it is possible to enter the glenohumeral joint from an anterior and inferior approach, but arthroscope placement is from outside to in with the plane of portal close to the humeral head. An inferior approach should not be attempted with the arm in the ABDucted position.

Medial Coracoid Portal. Eugene Wolf has utilized an anterior approach that courses medial to the coracoid process.[24] This places the neurovascular structures at risk, but use of a carefully placed cannula with rotation may displace these anatomical structures to the side during passage. I have inadvertently passed medial to the coracoid with a Wissinger rod for retrograde cannula placement. There were no problems in my patients, but I still avoid this anatomical area. This portal does give a more direct right angle approach to the anterior glenoid neck for ligament fixation, but it is usually not necessary.

Supraspinatus Portal. This approach, popularized by Richard Caspari for arthroscopy, followed the open surgical approach described by Neviaser.[4] This approach is initiated lateral on the top of the shoulder (Fig. 6-8). The bony landmarks are formed by the convergence of the

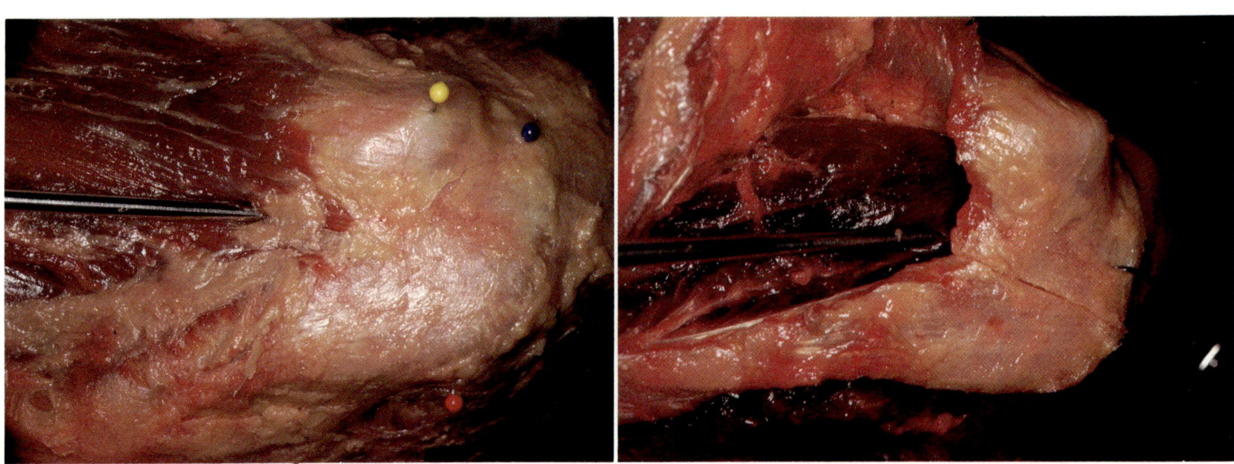

A B

FIG. 6-8 Superior portal is placed through the supraspinatus muscle from the supraspinatus fossa into the posterior aspect of the glenohumeral joint.

A Cannula is placed into supraspinatus muscle of cadaver right shoulder.

B Fascia has been removed from the supraspinatus muscle to show cannula.

C Cannula rests in suprascapular fossa of bony scapula.

D Bony acromion is removed from the gross specimen to show the placement of the cannula through muscle.

E Cross-section of gross specimen shows a No. 18 spinal needle along the course of the superior portal. Notice the position is through the muscle and inferior to the tendon. It rests on the posterior-superior glenoid.

F Position of cannula (demonstrated on a skeleton), coursing into the joint and resting posterior to glenoid.

G Arthroscopic view of inflow cannula resting below posterior glenoid labrum.

clavicle and the scapular spine (Fig. 6-8, *C*).[22] The supraspinatus tendon is not penetrated because the plane is medial to the tendon.

The portal courses through the supraspinatus muscle on an angle into the glenohumeral joint (Fig.6-8, *F*). Typically, the course of this portal is posterior, providing a resting place for a cannula posterior to the glenoid, medial to its posterior lip, in the posterior sulcus (Fig. 6-8, *G*).

This cannula can be redirected toward the anterior aspect of the joint, but the mobility is reduced by bony configuration and visualization is obstructed by the intraarticular course of the biceps brachia tendon.

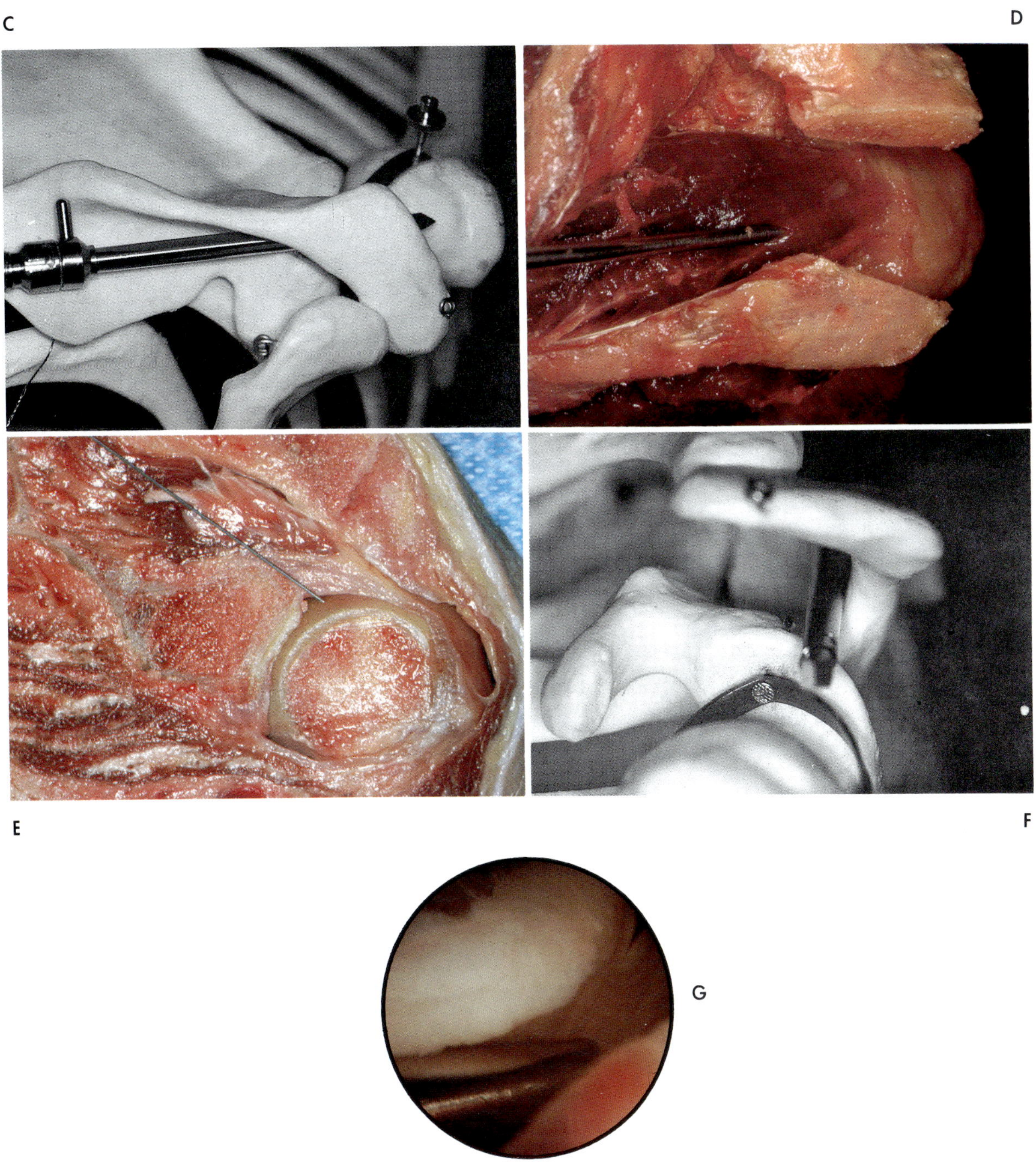

FIG 6-8 ***cont'd*** **For legend, see opposite page.**

Subacromial Space

Posterior Portal. The posterior arthroscopic skin incision utilized for the subacromial space is the same one previously used for the glenohumeral joint. This site is properly positioned for approaching the subacromial space if the arthroscope is withdrawn and cannula redirected toward the underside of the anterior acromion (Fig. 6-9, *A*).

Anterior Portal. This portal courses immediately lateral to the free span of the coracoacromial ligament. It is best established by a Wissinger rod retrograde method from inside to outside under direct vision of the CA ligament (Fig. 6-9, *B*).

Lateral Portal. This portal is initiated with a No. 18 spinal needle that will course inferior to the acromion. The skin incision is on the anterior lateral aspect of the shoulder. The portal enters the subacromial space at an oblique angle from anterior to posterior between the top of the humerus and the underside of the acromion (Fig. 6-9, *C*).

Superior Portal. The skin incision of the Neviaser portal to the glenohumeral joint may be used to direct a cannula into the subacromial space. The cannula and obturator is redirected superior to the supraspinatus muscle to enter the subacromial bursa.

A
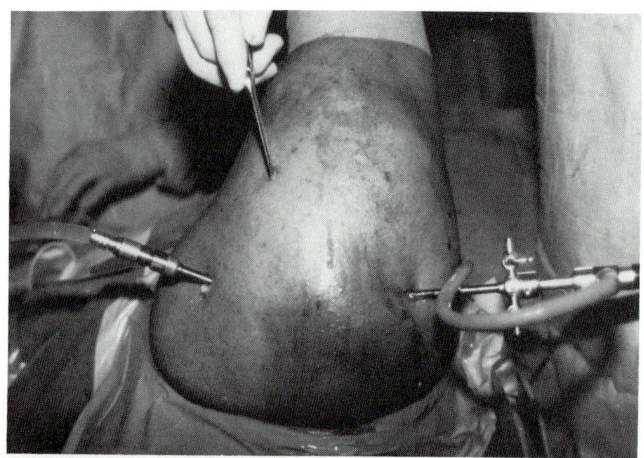

B
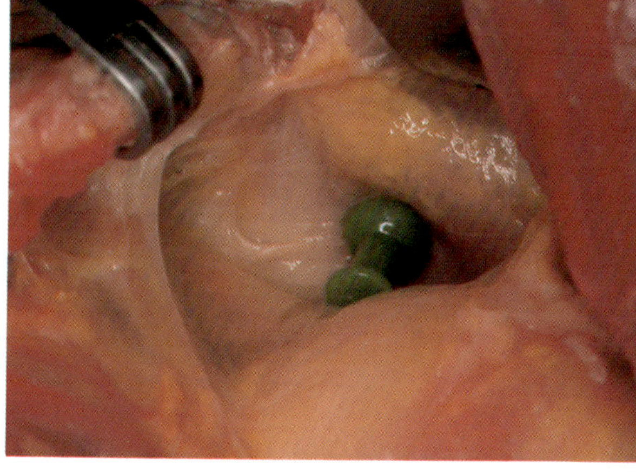

C
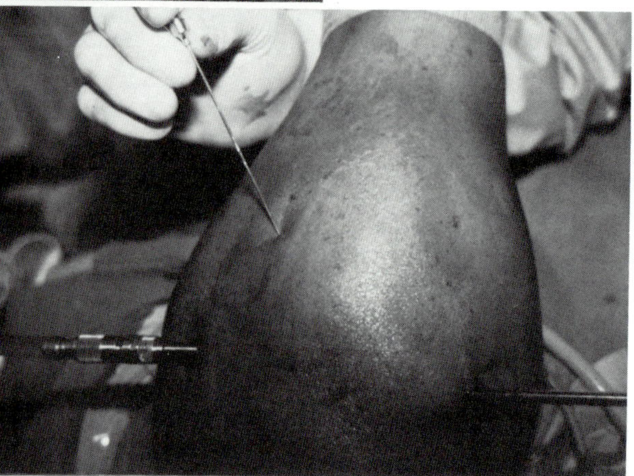

FIG. 6-9 Subacromial space.

A The posterior skin incision used for the glenohumeral joint is used for the subacromial portal placement. The direction of arthroscope cannula from posterior portal to the subacromial space is seen on skeleton.

B Anterior portal landmark for Wissinger rod is immediately adjacent to the free span of the CA ligament. This gross dissection of the subacromial bursa from posterior shows a green marker at the landmark adjacent to the ligament. The retractor is on the posterior acromion. The humeral head is below, covered with rotator cuff.

C Lateral portal is usually anterior topographically, in that the subacromial bursa is an anterior structure. Inflow is anterior. Surgeon is probing from lateral portal.

Acromioclavicular (AC) Joint

This is a small joint and requires topographical palpation, surgical imagination for spacial relationship, and preliminary needle placement to outline its confines. In the pathological joint, a limited debridement is often necessary to gain visual exposure (see Chapter 10).

Transcutaneous Approach. This joint is palpable, especially if accompanying osteophytes are present. The transcutaneous landmarks for the posterior arthroscope portal entry are established by preliminary needle palpation of this small joint (Fig. 6-10). The skin incision position is determined by this method. The anterior transcutaneous portal is established by a Wissinger rod method from interior. The interior landmarks are the bony walls of the joint and the opposite joint wall.

Subacromial Approach. The subacromial approach to the AC joint utilizes the subacromial space topographical landmarks and arthroscopic portals. The location of the AC joint from beneath is facilitated by transcutaneous placement of a No. 18 spinal needle from superior through the joint into the subacromial space (Fig. 6-11). Often the needle will be covered with synovium or soft tissue medial to the subacromial bursae. The needle can be located by palpation with an instrument already in the subacromial bursa. Subsequent debridement of soft tissue in this area will expose the needle tip and the underside of the AC joint. Osteophytes may be palpable on the underside of the AC joint, although they may not be visualized until the soft tissue is removed.

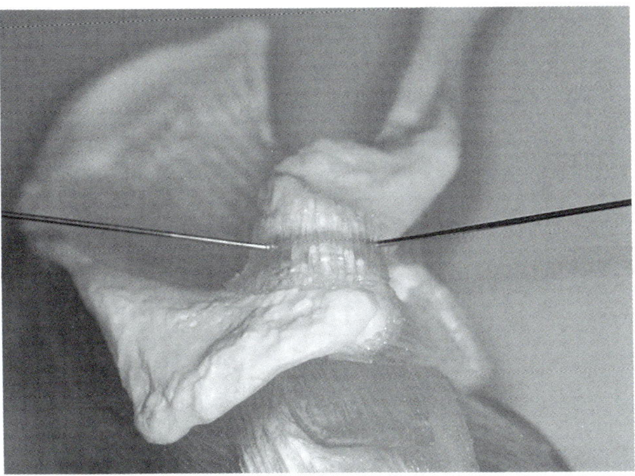

FIG. 6-10 Transcutaneous approach to AC joint. Preliminary needle placement from superior localizes the joint and provides for preliminary distention and cannula placement location. Notice this placement on the skeletal model.

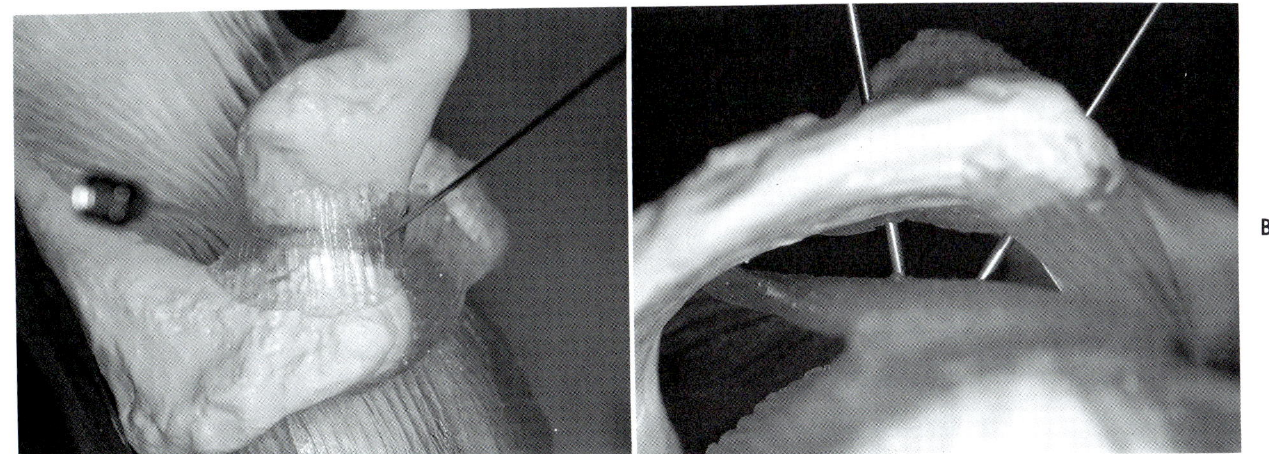

FIG. 6-11 Subacromial approach to the AC joint. Transcutaneous needle placement locates the AC joint from subacromial bursa perspective as demonstrated on a skeletal model.

A Needles seen from above course anterior and posterior through the AC joint.

B Same needles seen within the subacromial space.

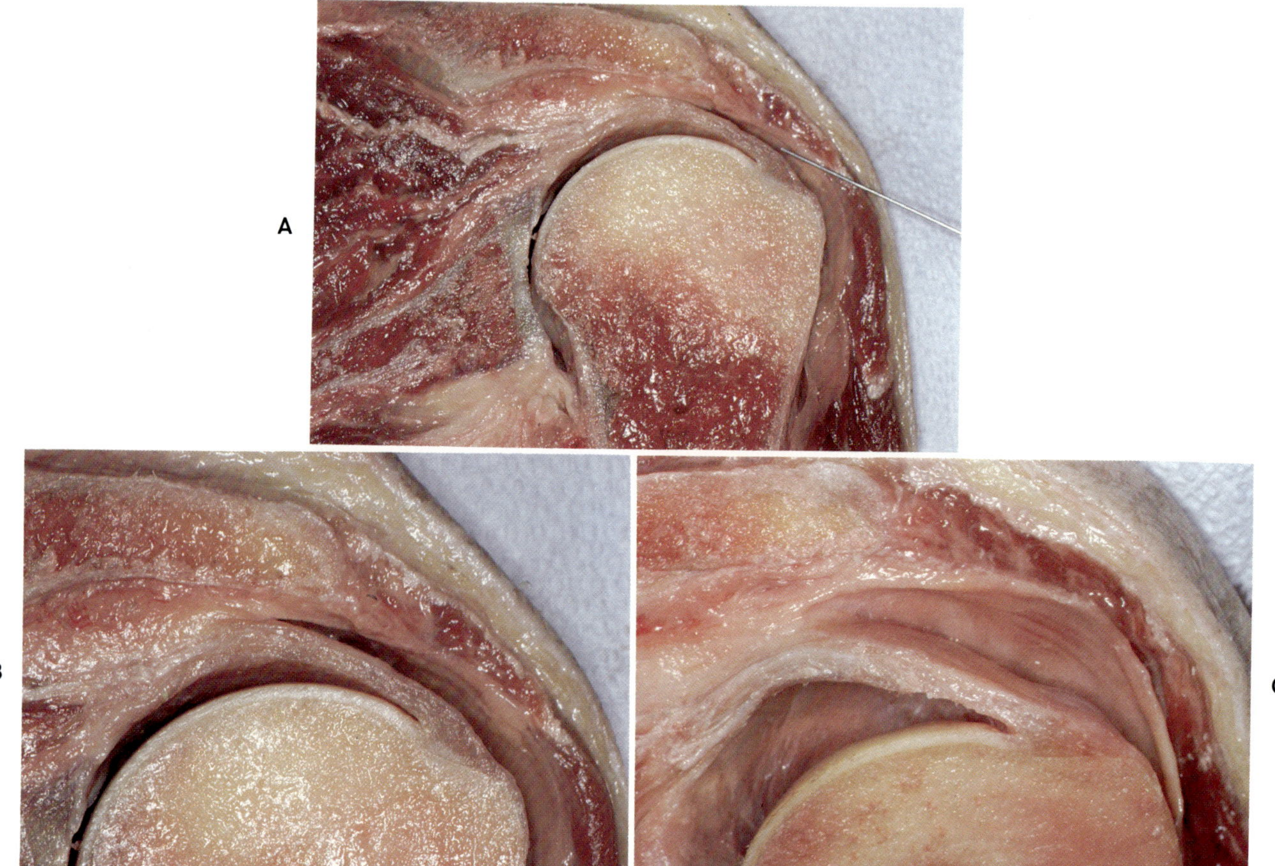

FIG. 6-12 Subacromial bursa in cross sectional anatomy.

A Cross-sectional gross specimen viewed from posterior with needle in the subacromial space.

B A close-up of same specimen without the needle shows the bursa extending from under the acromion to lateral over the humerus when the arm is adducted.

C A closer view of same anatomical relationships.

Bursae

Subacromial Bursa. The subacromial bursa is a normal occurring space anterior and below the acromion (Fig. 6-12). The portals for entry are from posterior as described for the subacromial space. The normal occurring bursa is difficult to identify because of its small size. The subacromial bursa is located immediately posterior to the free span of the coracoacromial ligament. Entry requires the surgeon to palpate the end of the arthroscope immediately beneath the coracoacromial ligament to ensure proper scope location.

Subscapular Bursa. Bursae may exist beneath the scapula, between the subscapularis muscle and the chest wall. Dr. Jerome Ciullo of Detroit, Michigan, has explored these structures arthroscopically. I have no experience with this surgery because I have not seen a patient with a clinical complaint related to this bursa.

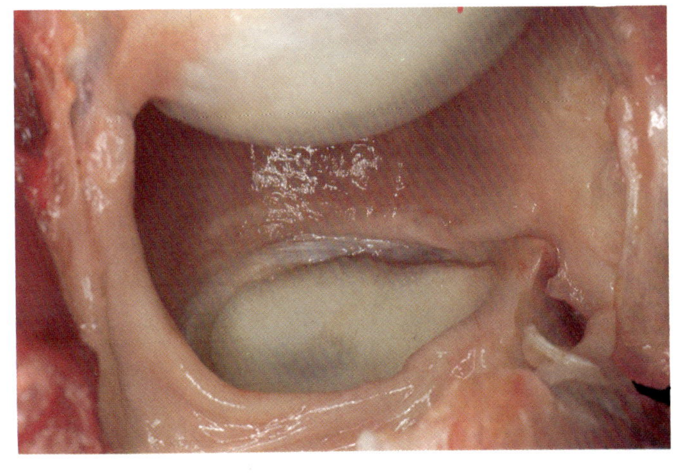
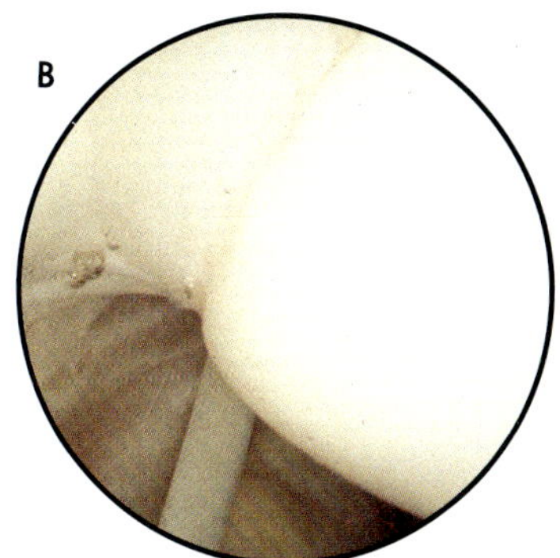
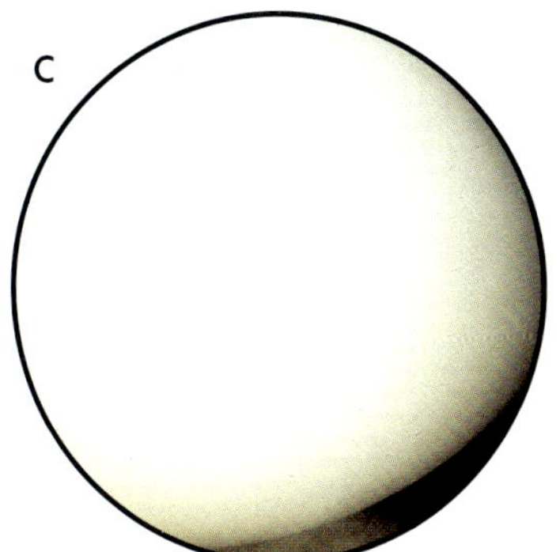
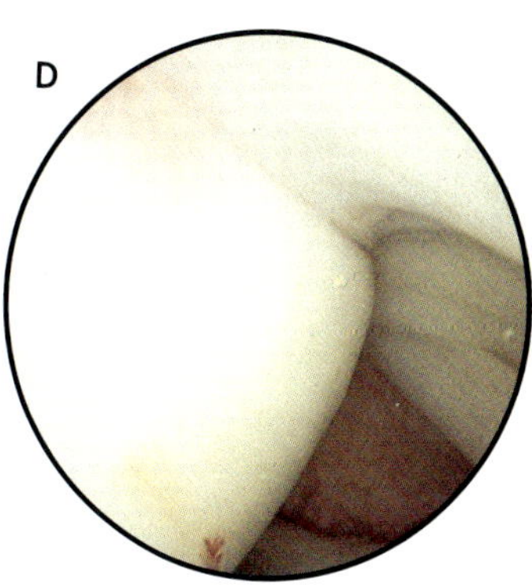

FIG. 6-13 Humeral head.

A Gross anatomical dissection of glenohumeral joint viewed from posterior.

B Arthroscopic view of the biceps tendon is to the left and the ellipse of the superior-articular surface of the humeral head.

C Arthroscopic view of movement of the scope to scan the horizon of the humeral head to the mid portion.

D Arthroscopic view of posterior-inferior aspect of the humeral head.

ARTHROSCOPIC ANATOMY OF INTRAARTICULAR STRUCTURES

Glenohumeral Joint

Articular Surfaces. Viewing from posterior, starting at the biceps tendon, one can move the scope inferiorly to see along the entire glenohumeral joint, with the humerus lateral and the glenoid medial (Fig. 6-13).

Humerus. The humeral head is covered with white articular cartilage. The posterior view shows a transition area from articular cartilage to the synovial reflection (Fig. 6-13, *B*). In children this is a smooth juxtaposition transition. In the adult one sees a "bare" area that is distinguished with small pitting into the humeral neck (Fig. 6-14, *A*). Small vessels are seen entering the small holes on the posterior aspect of the humerus (Fig. 6-14, *B*). This pitted area must not be mistaken for a pathologic Hill-Sachs lesion.

Glenoid. The glenoid articular surface is covered with hyaline cartilage (Fig. 6-15). It is common to see a central thin area (Fig. 6-16). The surface of the thin area is smooth, unlike the surface in degenerative arthritis, from which the central thin area must be differentiated.

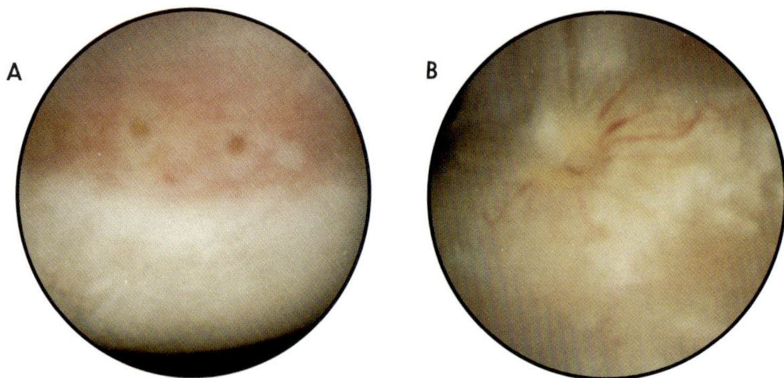

FIG. 6-14 Normal posterior bare area seen between articular cartilage and synovial reflection in adult.

A Arthroscopic view shows articular cartilage below and the punctate areas in bone of bare area.

B Arthroscopic close-up view of punctate area shows surface vessels penetrating into bone through these holes.

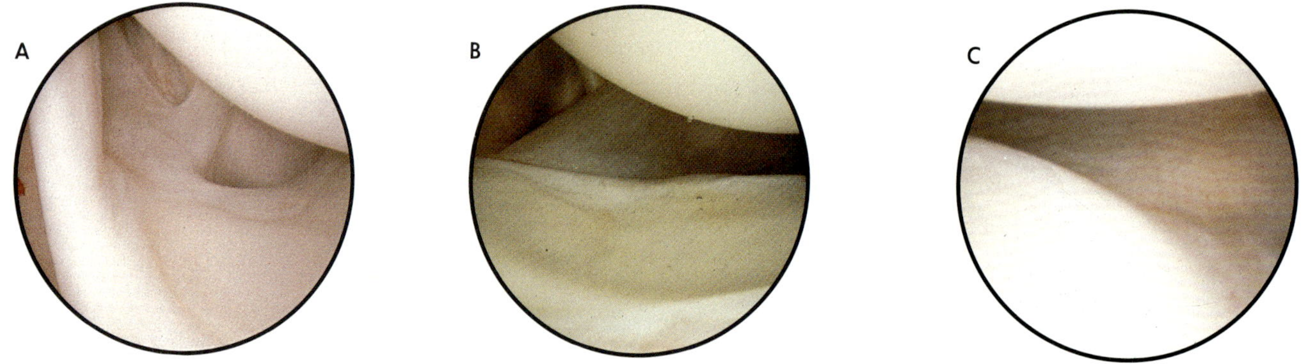

FIG. 6-15 Glenoid fossa.

A Arthroscopic view of superior glenoid fossa with biceps tendon to the left and humerus above.

B Arthroscopic overview of glenoid fossa.

C Arthroscopic view of inferior aspect of glenoid fossa viewed from posterior on the right shoulder.

A

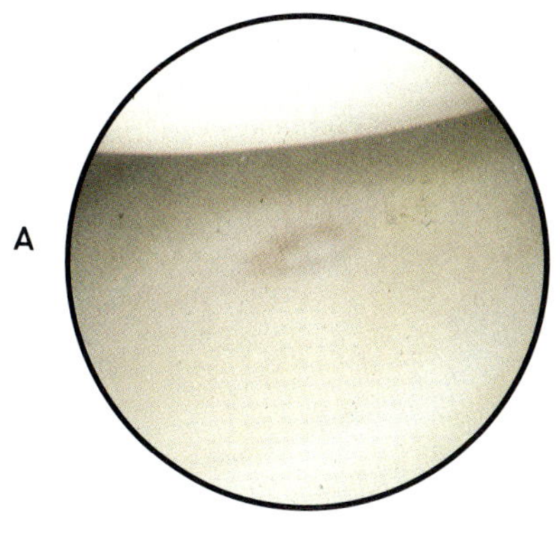

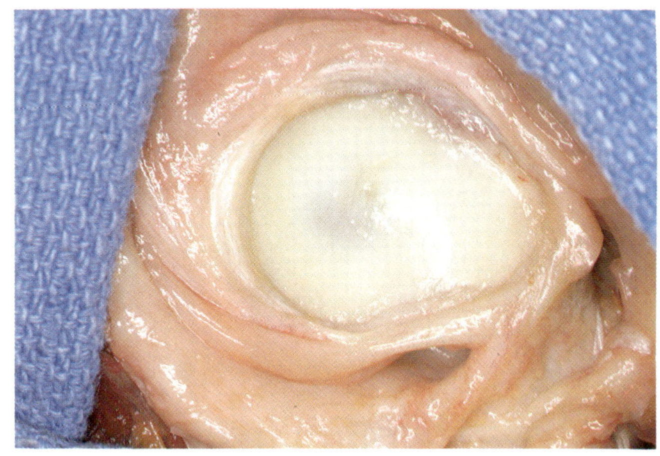

B

FIG. 6-16 Glenoid fossa: normal central thinning of articular cartilage.

A Arthroscopic view of central thin area.

B Gross anatomical specimen of glenoid fossa and thin central area.

A

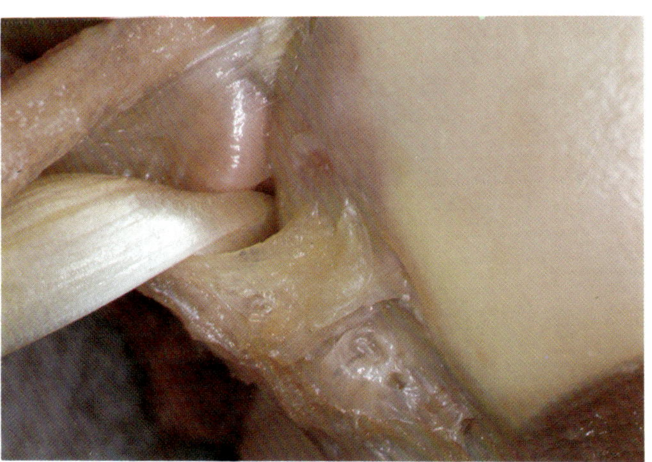

B

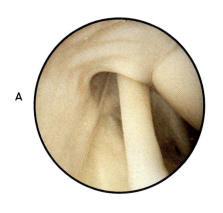

FIG. 6-17 Exit of the biceps tendon into the bicipital groove.

A Arthroscopic view of biceps leaving joint into the bicipital groove.

B Gross anatomical dissection shows this same area.

Superior Region

Biceps brachia. When the joint is entered from a posterior portal, the first and most identifiable anatomical structure seen superiorly is the biceps tendon (Fig. 6-17, *A*). With further superior rotation and movement, visualization can follow along the biceps tendon. With elbow flexion and some external rotation, the scope can go all the way to the exit of the biceps tendon in the shoulder joint (bicipital groove) (Fig. 6-17, *B*).

Vincula of biceps tendon. Returning to the biceps tendon, the scope is rotated to view the superior structures (Fig. 6-18, *A*). The surgeon can see the undersurface of the rotator cuff.

Often fibrous bands are present coursing from the undersurface of the rotator cuff to the bicipital groove (Fig. 6-18, *A* and *B*). I found no description of this glenohumeral joint structure in a medical literature search. I first recorded this observation in a surgical report on June 6, 1986, as an anomalous band.

A subsequent search was made of my data base between January 1, 1986, to October 21, 1991, for cases in which the lesion was mentioned. This query was edited to

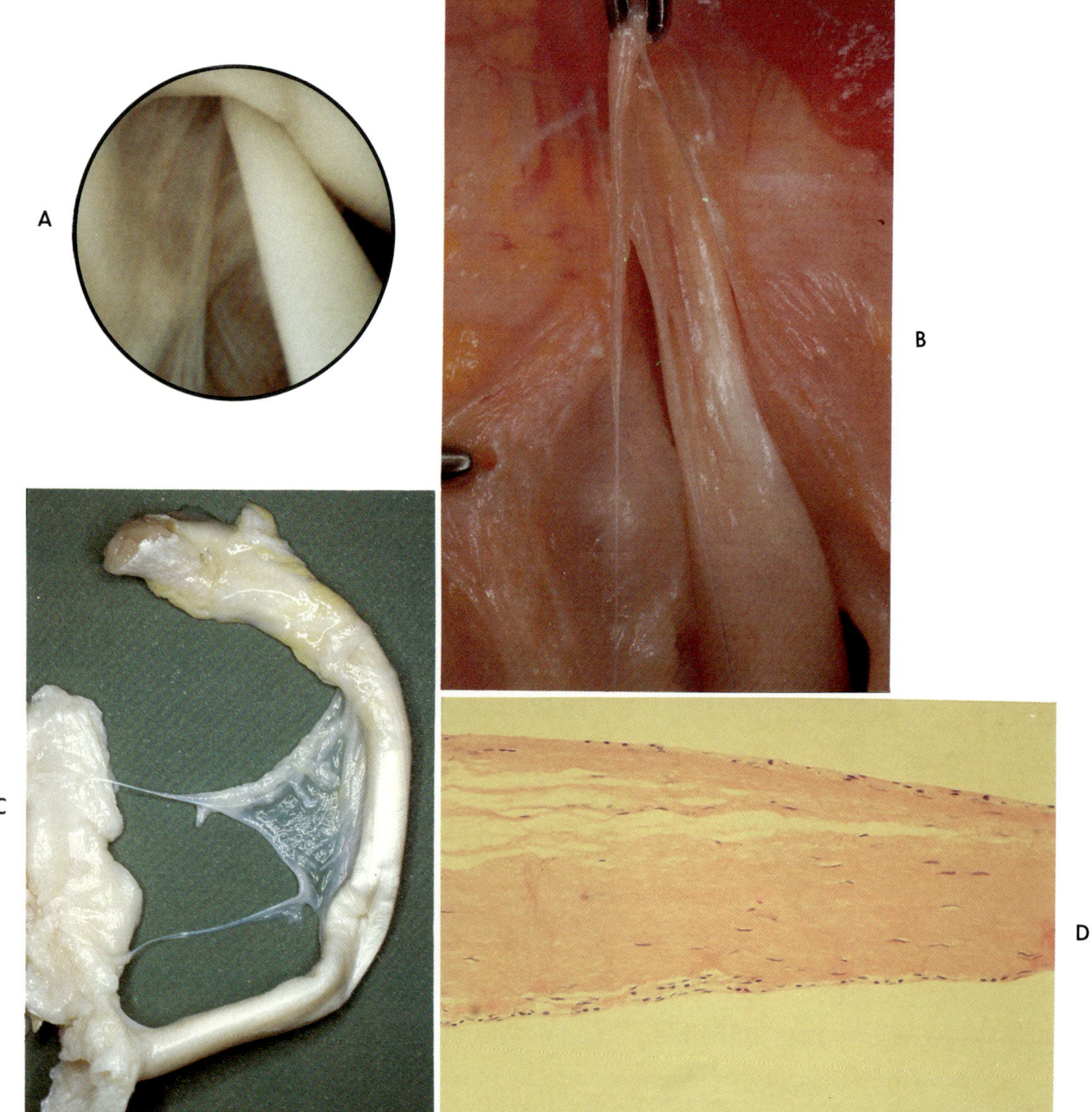

FIG. 6-18 Vincula of the biceps brachia tendon.

A Arthroscopic view of biceps tendon with the fibrovascular vincula coursing from the rotator cuff area and out the bicipital groove.

B Gross dissection of bicipital vincula shows its course along the tendon with attachment to the tendon proper in the bicipital groove.

C Further gross dissection shows the vincula spanning from the rotator cuff to the broad expanse of the biceps tendon.

D Photomicrograph of vincula shows synovial covering over fibrous band with small vessel. (Hematoxylin and Eosin, original magnification ×100.)

remove those cases (not patients) that represented a second look into the same shoulder by subsequent surgery. This created a file that contained 466 cases and 444 patients who had diagnostic arthroscopy. The data base was further shaped by removing those patients who had previous surgery. Those without surgery would offer the best review of unaltered anatomical and pathological anatomy. This group studied contained 411 cases and 390 patients.

The vincula were observed in 24.3% of all shoulders undergoing shoulder arthroscopy in this series (101 cases in 99 patients). Two patients had bilateral shoulder arthroscopy. In 310 cases and 295 patients a vinculum was not seen. Fifteen patients had bilateral arthroscopy. Four patients had arthroscopy of both shoulders, showing one shoulder with and one shoulder without a vinculum. This accounts for the 295 patients plus 99 to equal 394 with four patients in both queries.

There was a single vinculum in 56 shoulders; 2 in 32; and 3 in 12. The vincula were seen to have four bands in one patient. No case had more than four bands.

Those patients with evidence of a vinculum were on the average younger (33 years) than those without one (41 years).

The percentage of men or women in either group, with or without vincula, did not differ. The number of patients with noncaucasian genetic origin was too small to make various comparisons.

The right side had vincula present in 69 shoulders, and the left in 32. The vincula were present in 27% of the right shoulders and 21% of the left shoulders.

The vincula were seen in 27% of the dominant extremity's shoulder; the percentage of frequency in the nondominant extremity's shoulder was the same.

Presence of vincula related to diagnosis. The vincula were identified in 30% of patients with *no* rotator cuff tear. It was seen in only 12% of those with a rotator cuff tear.

The vincula were seen in 23% of those with *no* anterior instability. This is compared to the 27% incidence of those patients with an anterior dislocation/subluxation of the shoulder.

The vincula were seen in 33% of patients with diagnosis other than rotator cuff tear and/or anterior instability. The highest incidence by diagnosis was labrum tear (52%). It was seen in 41% of those patients with impingement syndrome without complete rotator cuff tear.

In the miscellaneous group, the vincula were not seen in the one patient with isolated biceps tendon rupture. They were present in the one normal joint at arthroscopy in which no postoperative diagnosis was made.

Gross anatomy. An anatomical dissection shows the relationship of the vincula to the biceps tendon in the bicipital canal. They course from the undersurface of the rotator cuff obliquely across the joint to parallel the biceps tendon as it exits the glenohumeral joint (Fig. 6-18, *A* and *B*). It was not an extension of either the underlying joint capsule or rotator cuff tendon. The bands were well defined as they spanned the joint. The bands expanded to sheets of tissue surrounding the tendon (Fig. 6-18, *B*). Gross dissection shows the broad expanse of attachment to the biceps tendon (Fig. 6-18, *C*). The attachment at the biceps tendon area was to the peritendon and not to the tendon.

Microscopic anatomy. The microscopic anatomy showed these bands to be fibrous tissue covered with a thin layer of synovium (Fig. 6-18, *D*). No inflammation or neoplasm was evident. Vascularity was minimal.

These structures are analogous to the vincula of the finger flexor tendons. Therefore I have named them the vincula of the biceps tendon. A scientific paper on this topic was published in the *Journal of Shoulder and Elbow Surgery*.[11a]

Superior wall

Underside of rotator cuff. When the glenohumeral joint is distended the undersurface of the rotator cuff separates from the biceps tendon (Fig. 6-19, *A*). A common variation is a transverse band of the capsule that is arcuate in shape (Fig. 6-19, *A* and *B*). This prominence traverses from anterior to posterior approximately 1 cm from the supraspinatus attachment to the humerus. It varies in size and may appear as large as the biceps tendon (Fig. 6-19, *C*).

The tendons of the supraspinatus and infraspinatus muscles are not visualized from beneath the rotator cuff unless a rotator cuff tear is present.[5] The only intraarticular structure of the rotator cuff seen by arthroscopy is the superior aspect of the subscapularis tendon (see Fig. 6-49).

Components of rotator cuff. The underside of the rotator cuff is lined with synovium. The normal synovium is smooth with minimal vascularity.[12] The next layer is capsular tissue (Fig. 6-20). The capsule usually has a smooth contour. Gross anatomical dissections demonstrate the various layers in the area of the supraspinatus insertion to the humerus (Fig. 6-20, *A*). The synovium attaches closest to the articular surface, the capsule more lateral, and the tendon on the greater tuberosity. These structures can be separated by anatomical dissection.

The clinical significance is that the "rotator cuff" is not solely tendon tissue, but three layers: synovium, capsule, and tendon (Fig. 6-20). In rotator cuff tear, for instance, one must recognize both the capsule and tendon detachment. The capsular layer provides the static stability and the tendon provides the dynamic stability to the glenohumeral joint. In the pathological condition, they are often separated from each other (see Chapter 7). What have been identified by imaging techniques or at surgical exploration as intrasubstance tears of the tendon are probably a pathological cleft between the capsular and tendinous layers.

A

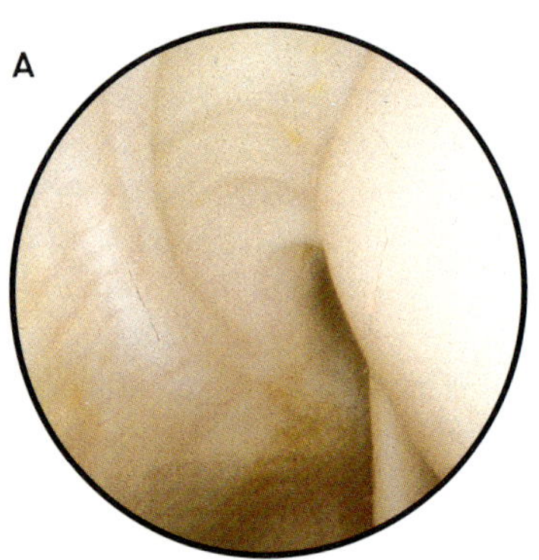

B

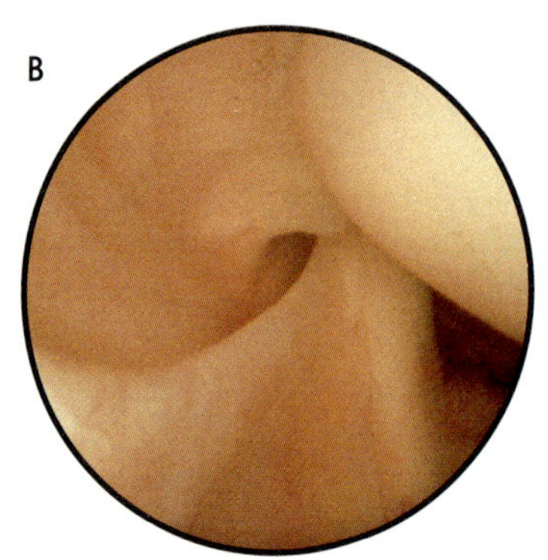

C

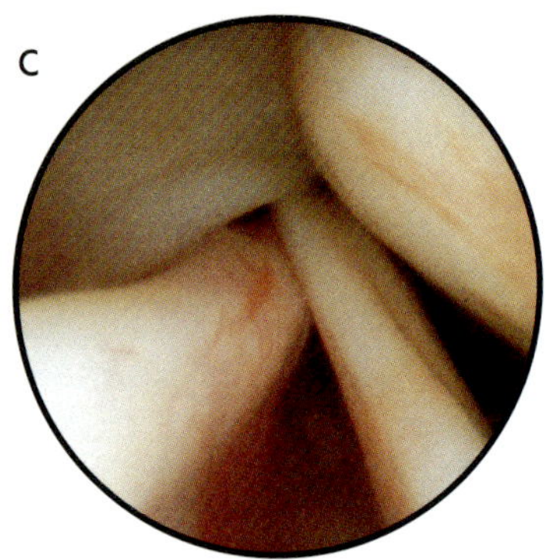

FIG. 6-19 Transverse arcuate capsular band of rotator cuff.

A Arthroscopic view shows the rotator cuff to the left, the humeral head to the right and the biceps tendon deep in the photo at 5 o'clock. Notice the small transverse band of capsular tissue.

B Arthroscopic view of more prominent transverse capsular tissue.

C Massive capsular transverse arcuate band is larger than the biceps tendon that is to the right.

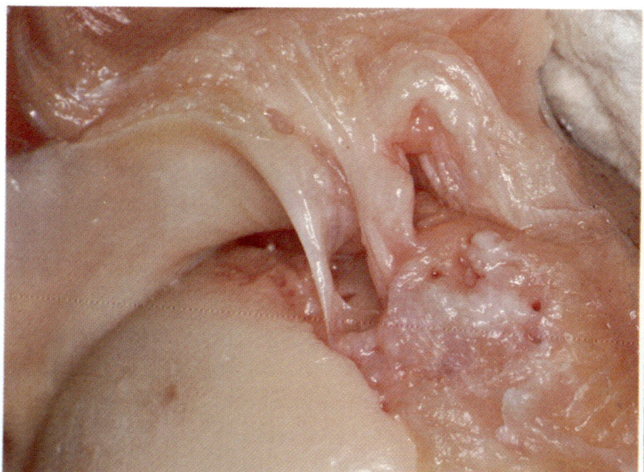

A

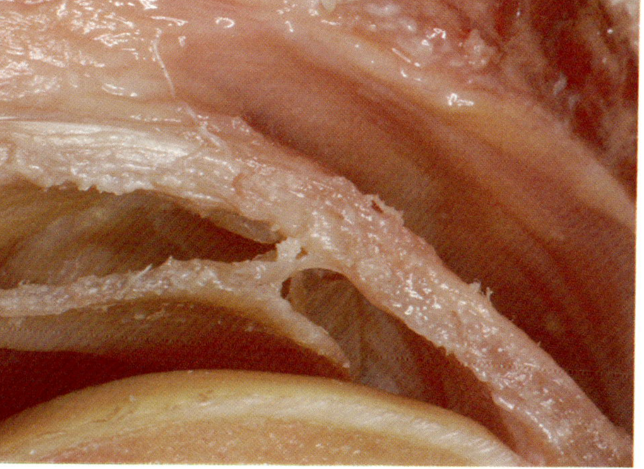

B

FIG. 6-20 Composite rotator cuff: synovium, capsule, tendon. The rotator cuff is composed of three distinct layers in the area of the supraspinatus insertion. These can be separated by anatomical dissection; separation occurs in some pathological cicumstances.

A Gross anatomical dissection shows the humeral head with three distinct areas of tissue insertion. The synovium is next to the articular cartilage. The capsule is next. The tendon attaches on the greater tuberosity.

B This cross-section anatomical close-up of the humeral head below shows the synovial and capsular layer as one, and the thicker tendon layer above. The smooth synovial lined subacromial bursa is above the tendon.

This observation of various layers has clinical significance (see Chapter 9). The partial tear of the rotator cuff identified by incomplete extrusion of dye on arthrogram is in fact an extrusion through only the synovial and/or capsular layers. These layers also have surgical implications. An undersurface debridement by arthroscopy has a good prognosis because most of the capsule is intact and the tendon is unaffected. Intraoperative recognition of the various layers is necessary to reattach both the capsular and tendon portions to the humerus during rotator cuff repair.

Biceps tendon attachment. The biceps tendon is followed to its attachment on the glenoid (Fig. 6-21). The biceps tendon courses posterior across the joint to the glenoid. It attaches into the labrum at the junction of the superior and posterior labrum. The attachment is not directly to bone. The loose attachment is demonstrated by arthroscopic probing (Fig. 6-22). Histological examination shows the tendon-to-bone transition not to be direct in all cases (Fig. 6-23).

A

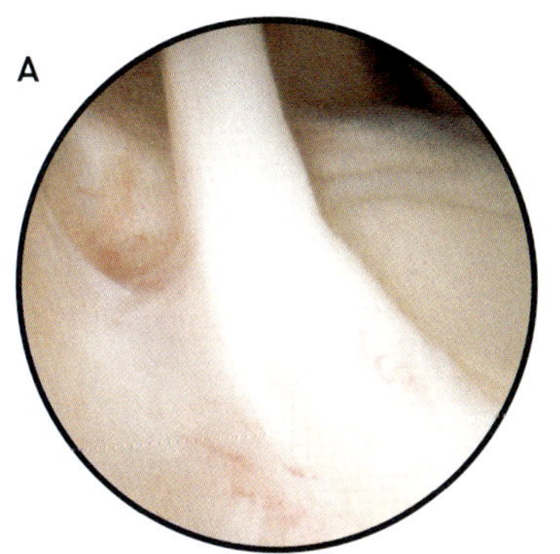

B

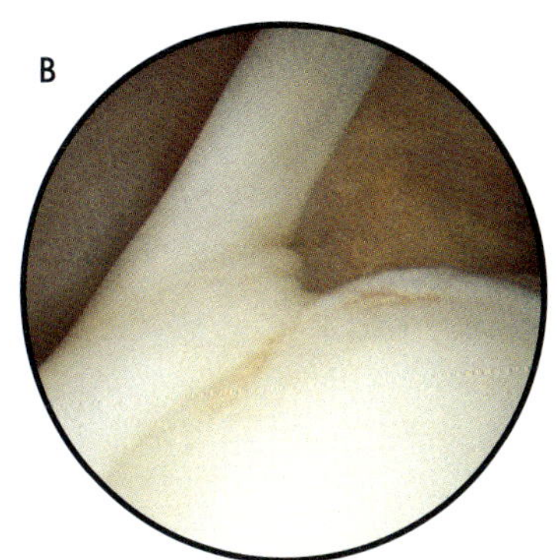

C

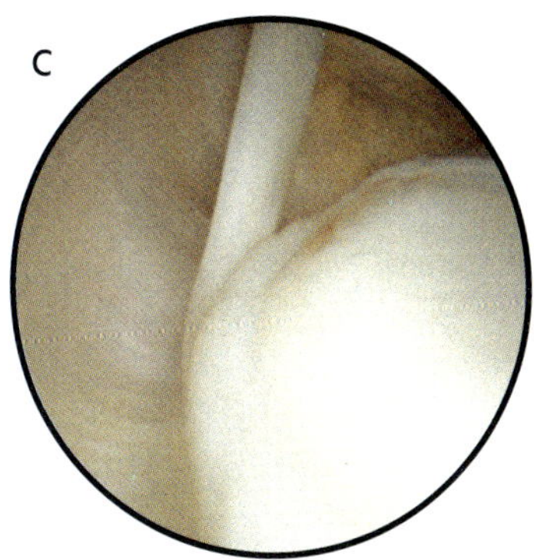

FIG. 6-21 Biceps attachment variations to the superior labrum.

A Arthroscopic view from superior shows oblique attachment to the posterior-superior glenoid blends into the posterior superior labrum.

B Another arthroscopic view from inferior of the biceps tendon demonstrates the oblique course of the tendon.

C Arthroscopic view of biceps tendon attachment superior to the labrum.

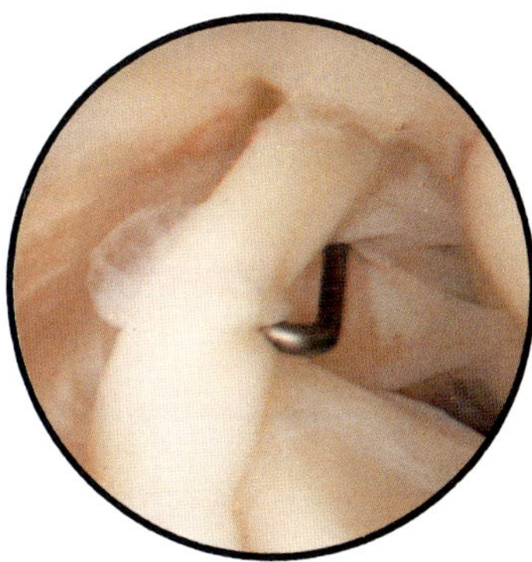

FIG. 6-22 Arthroscopic view of biceps tendon.

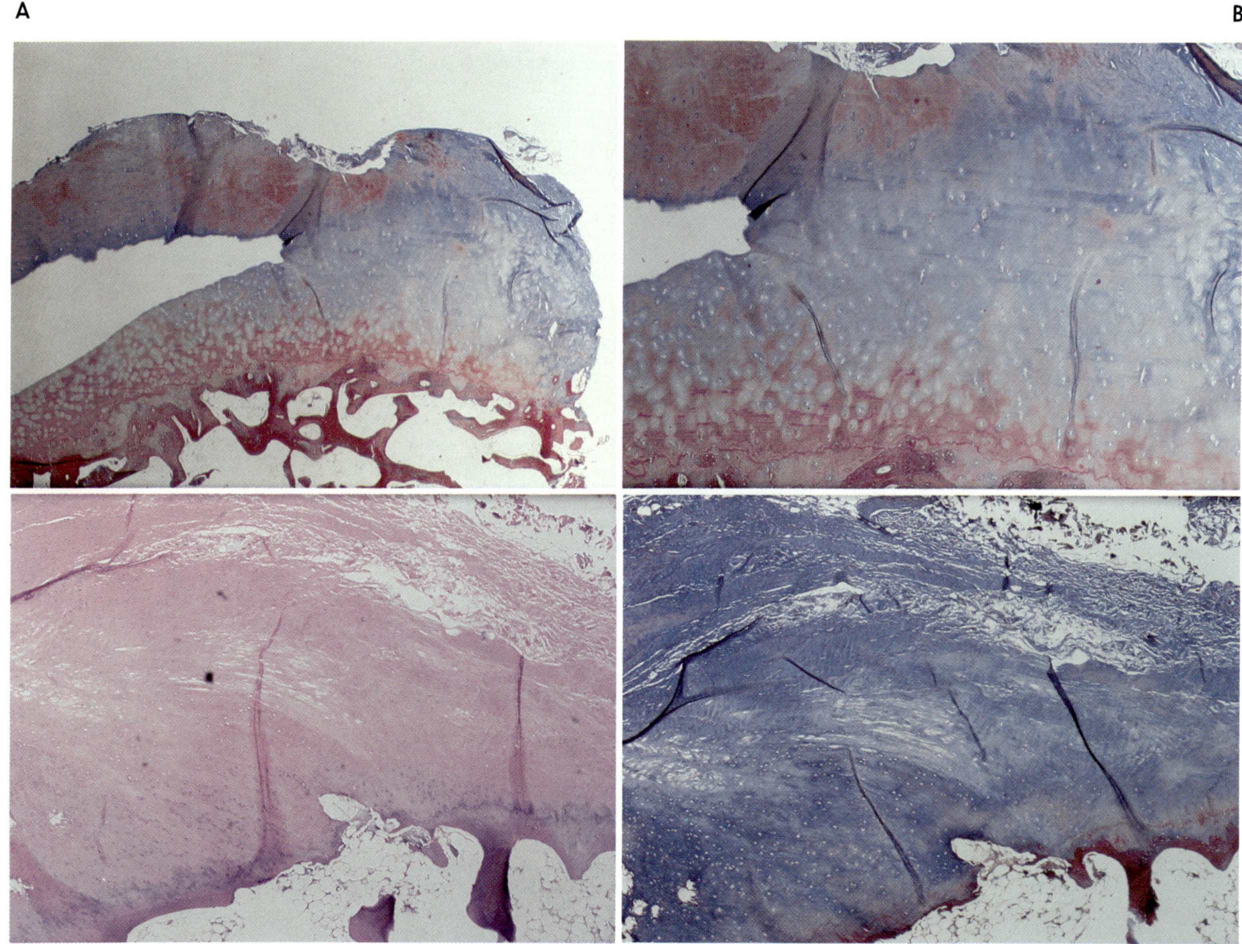

FIG. 6-23 Histological view of biceps tendon attachment to glenoid.

A Photomicrograph of biceps tendon attachment to the glenoid. The tendon is superior and the bone of the glenoid is below. (Trichrome stain, original magnification ×40.)

B Photomicrograph of biceps tendon shows transition into the labral fibrocartilage.

C Photomicrograph of another type of attachment, showing tendon fibers coursing directly into bone. Hematoxylin, original magnification ×100.

D Same section as shown in 6-23, *C,* but with Trichrome staining to show direct attachment of tendon to bone of glenoid. (Trichrome, original magnification ×100.)

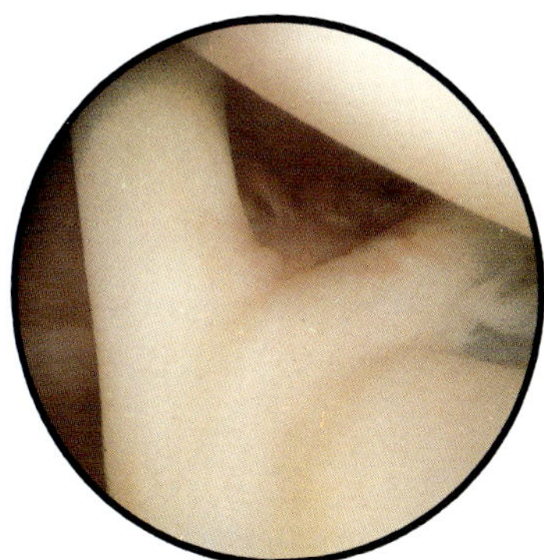

FIG. 6-24 Solid biceps-glenoid junction.

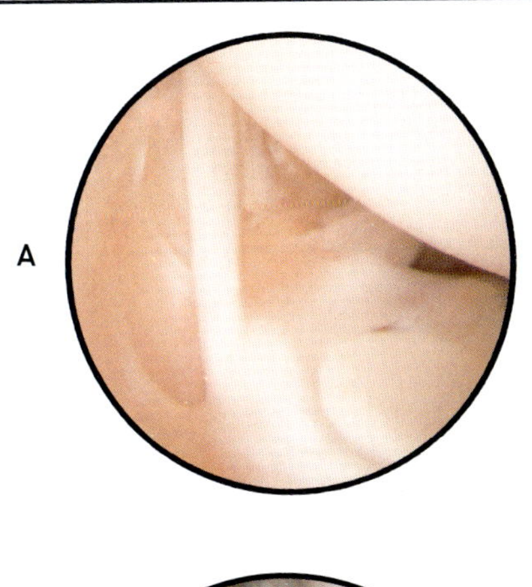

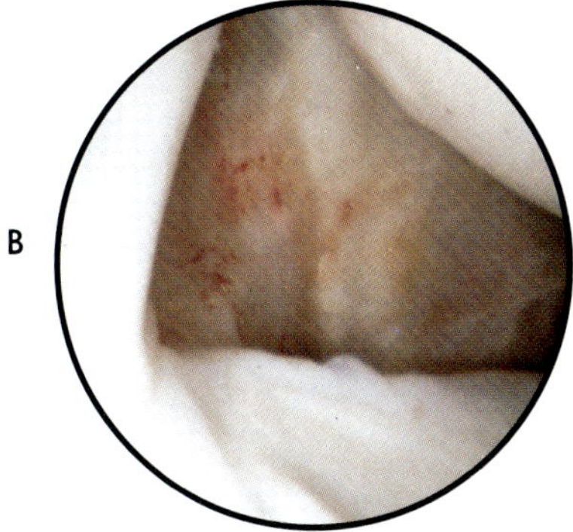

FIG. 6-25 Triangle formed by biceps tendon, humeral head, and glenoid is identified and traversed to view anterior structures.

A Arthroscopic overview of the triangle.

B Arthroscopic view as triangle is traversed.

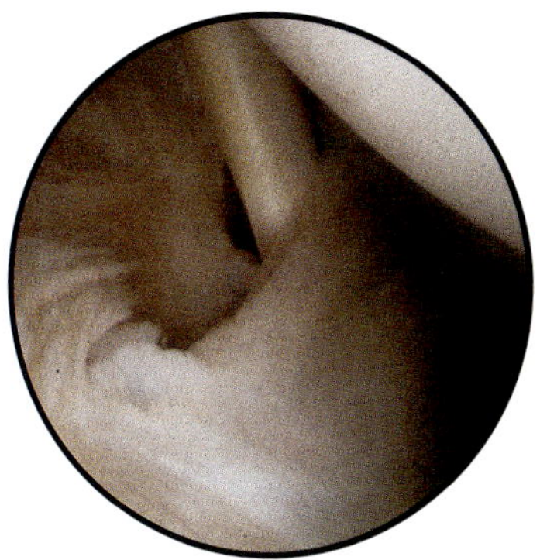

FIG. 6-26 Anterior structures are approached by arthroscope from posterior portal. The most distinct anatomical structure is the superior tendon slip of the subscapularis tendon.

Superior labrum. The superior labrum is a continuation of the connection to the biceps tendon (Fig. 6-24). The labrum is usually well defined. The inner margin of the labrum can be elevated to visualize under the labrum to the superior aspect of the glenoid reflection under the biceps insertion. The superior labrum is wider than other areas of the labrum.

Anterior Region. Starting at the biceps tendon, the scope is positioned to view the triangle that is created by the biceps tendon, the superior humeral head, and the glenoid (Fig. 6-25). The arthroscopic view appears as the scope traverses this triangle (Fig. 6-25, *B*).

From this position the scope penetrates anterior to inspect the anterior region of the glenohumeral joint (Fig. 6-26). The anterior structures are not in the same plane, nor do they have a parallel course (see Fig. 6-2). The anterior region anatomical structures will be described, proceeding from posterior to anterior passing from the glenoid fossa to the anterior glenoid.

Glenoid sulcus. A sulcus is normally present in the central area of the anterior bony glenoid (Fig. 6-27, *A*). The prominent sulcus should not be interpreted as a sign of subluxation or dislocation.

Labrum. The labrum originally was described by Bankart as a fibrous and fibrocartilaginous rim that tore during subluxations or dislocations of the shoulder. Townley[22a] and Moseley and Overgaard[15] have subsequently shown that the labrum is basically a thickening of the fibrous capsular tissues that includes very little fibrocartilage. It is covered with synovium and is continuous with the capsule (Fig. 6-28). Only a small area at the transitional zone with the glenoid surface is composed of fibrocartilage. When the labrum is a well-defined, separate, and movable structure that encircles and covers the glenoid, then the tissue is histologically identifiable as fibrocartilage (Fig. 6-29).

The labrum can appear as a piling-up of synovium and

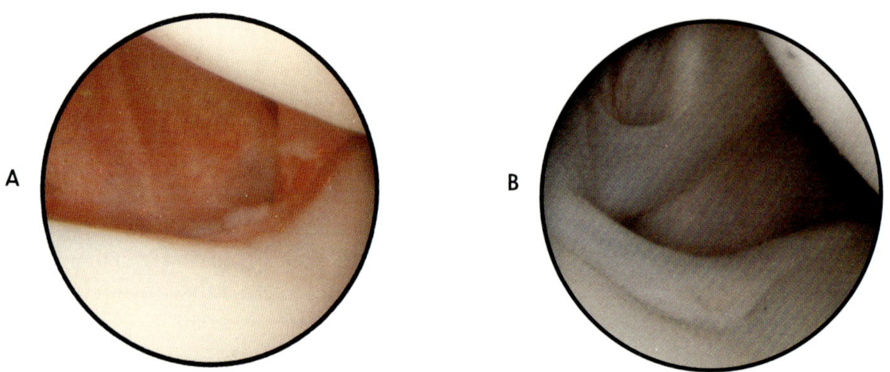

FIG. 6-27 Anterior glenoid sulcus.

A Normal sulcus.

B Prominent sulcus is normal and not to be considered sign of subluxation or dislocation.

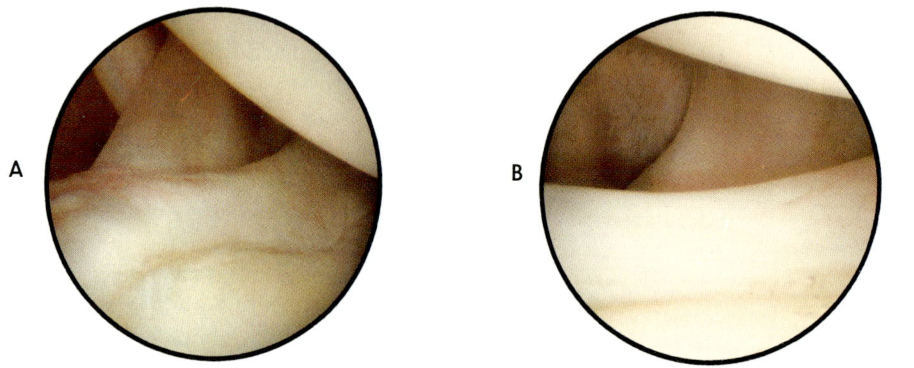

FIG. 6-28 Anterior glenoid labrum.

A Arthroscopic view of small anterior labrum.

B Arthroscopic view of large anterior labrum.

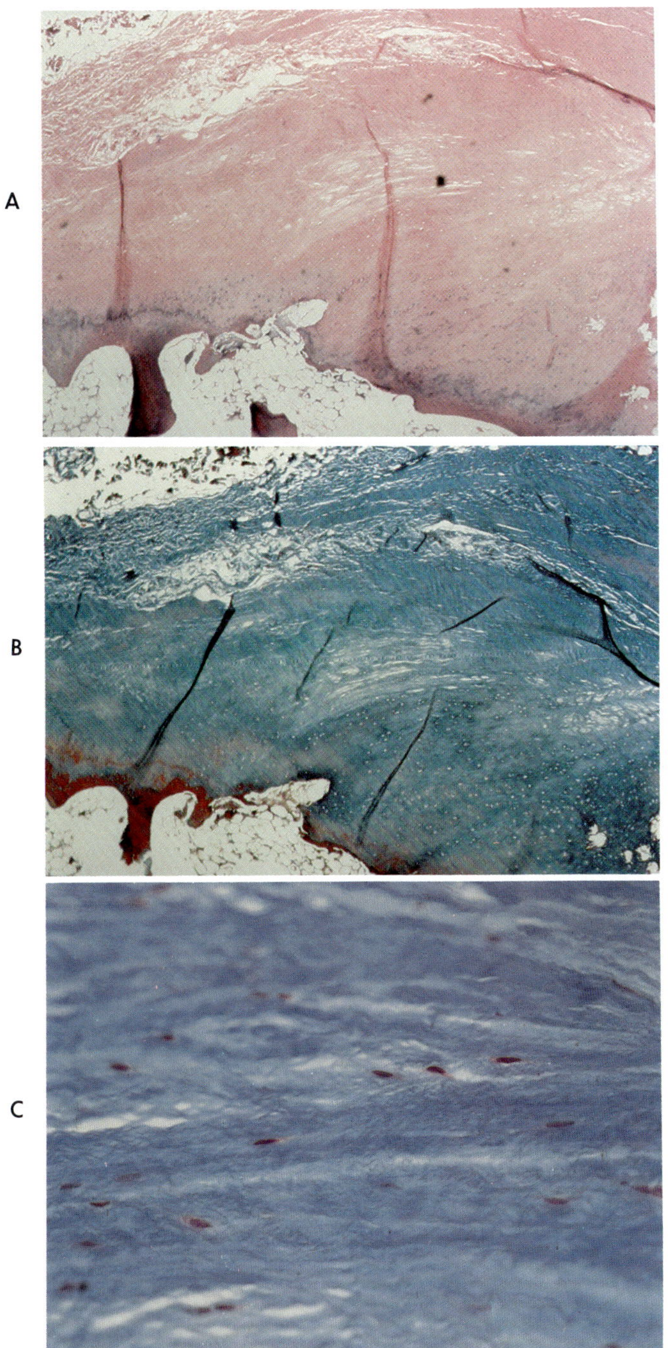

FIG. 6-29 **Histological nature of the labrum.**

A Photomicrograph of labrum attachment to glenoid. Notice the predominantly tendinous nature of the labrum. (Hematoxylin and Eosin, original magnification ×100.)

B Photomicrograph of labrum with stain showing tendon tissue in blue. (Trichrome, original magnification ×100.)

C Photomicrograph of fibrous tissue. (Trichrome, original magnification ×400.)

capsule, especially as seen anteriorly with the shoulder in internal rotation and posteriorly with external rotation. When the shoulder is taken into marked external rotation, the anterior lip tissue flattens out. This type of labrum is composed of fibrous tissue.

Glenohumeral ligament-labrum junction. The labrum varies in its presence and its size (Fig. 6-30). It may be nonexistent, with the ligament attaching directly to the glenoid rim. The labrum may be small, yet defined. Other patients have a large, well-defined labrum with glenohumeral ligaments flowing into the glenoid bone beneath. In such a case, the circumferential tissue is composed of fibrocartilage (Fig. 6-31).

If the glenoid labrum is less distinct, then the transition from articular cartilage via labrum to the anterior glenohumeral ligaments is without definition (Fig. 6-32).

If the labrum is well developed, it may be a continuation of the same configuration that is commonly seen in the superior labrum, with the "lip" elevated off the articular cartilage.[9]

A

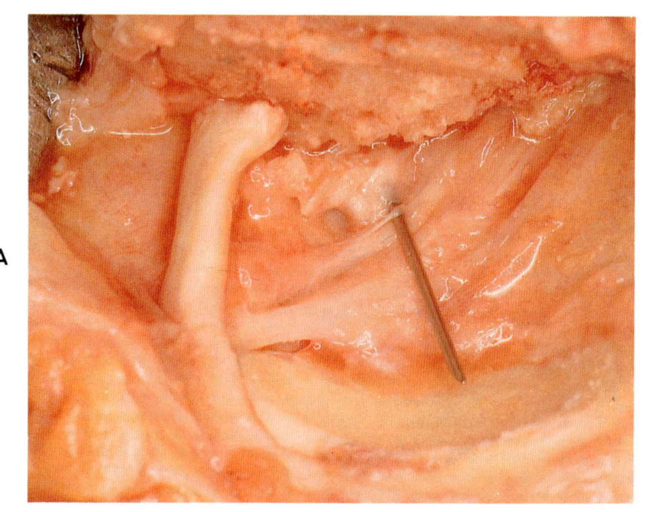

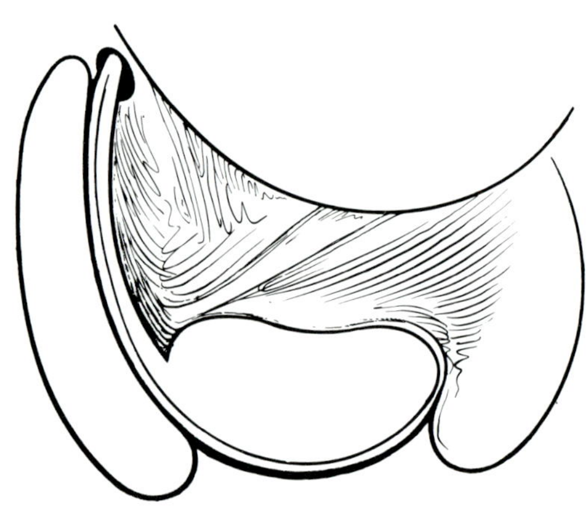

B

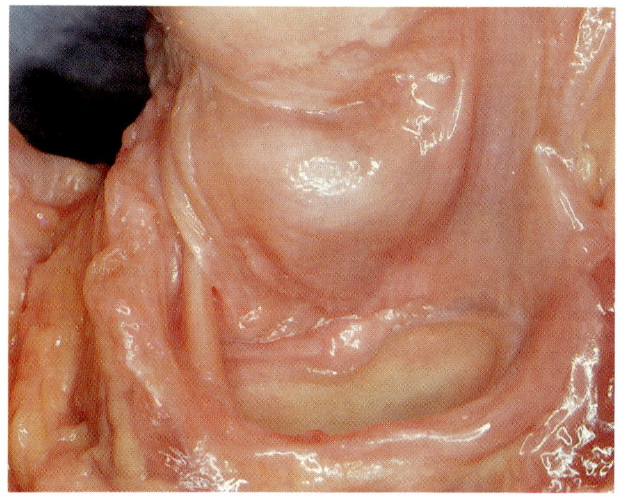

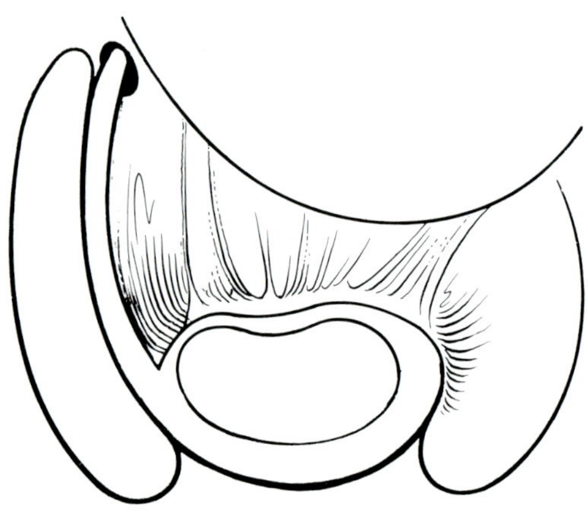

FIG. 6-30 Gross anatomical variations of ligament-labrum attachments.

A No labral definition. Needle points to direct ligament attachment.

B Small labrum.

Continued.

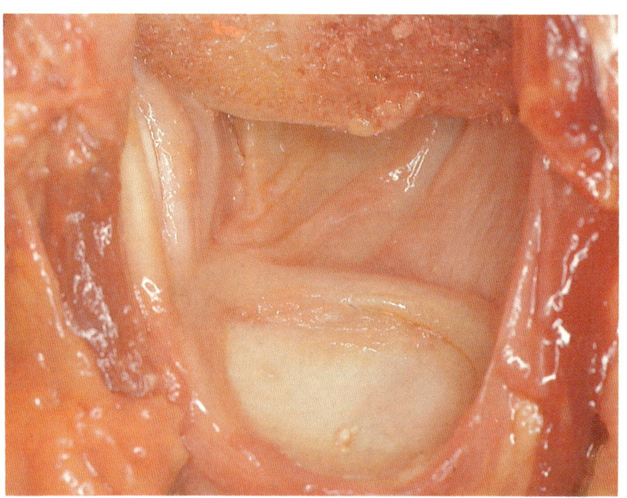

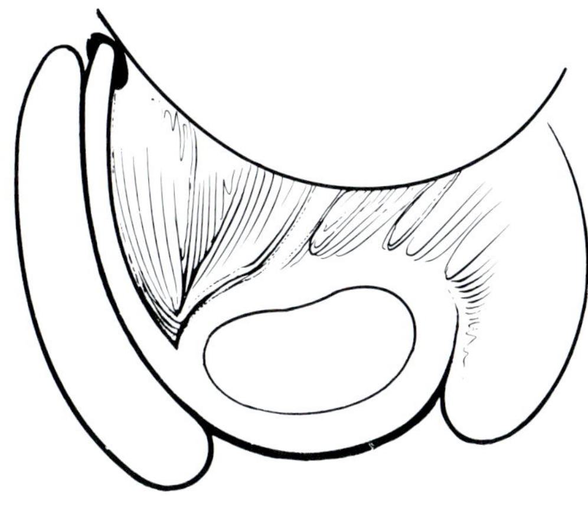

FIG 6-30 *cont'd* Gross anatomical variations of ligament-labrum attachments.

C Well-developed glenoid labrum.

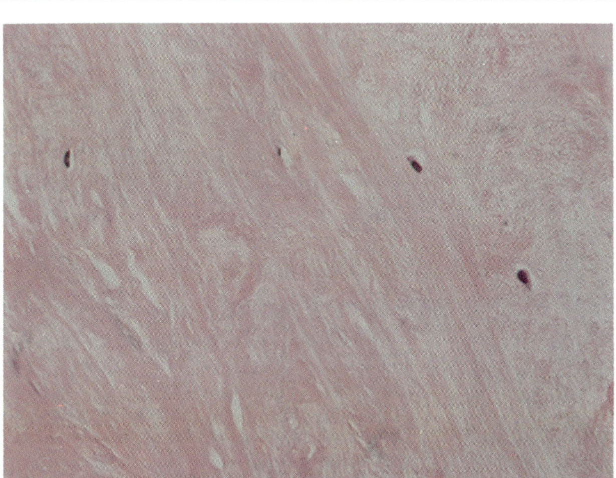

FIG. 6-31 Histological nature of labrum: Fibrocartilage in well-developed type of labrum. (Original magnification ×400.)

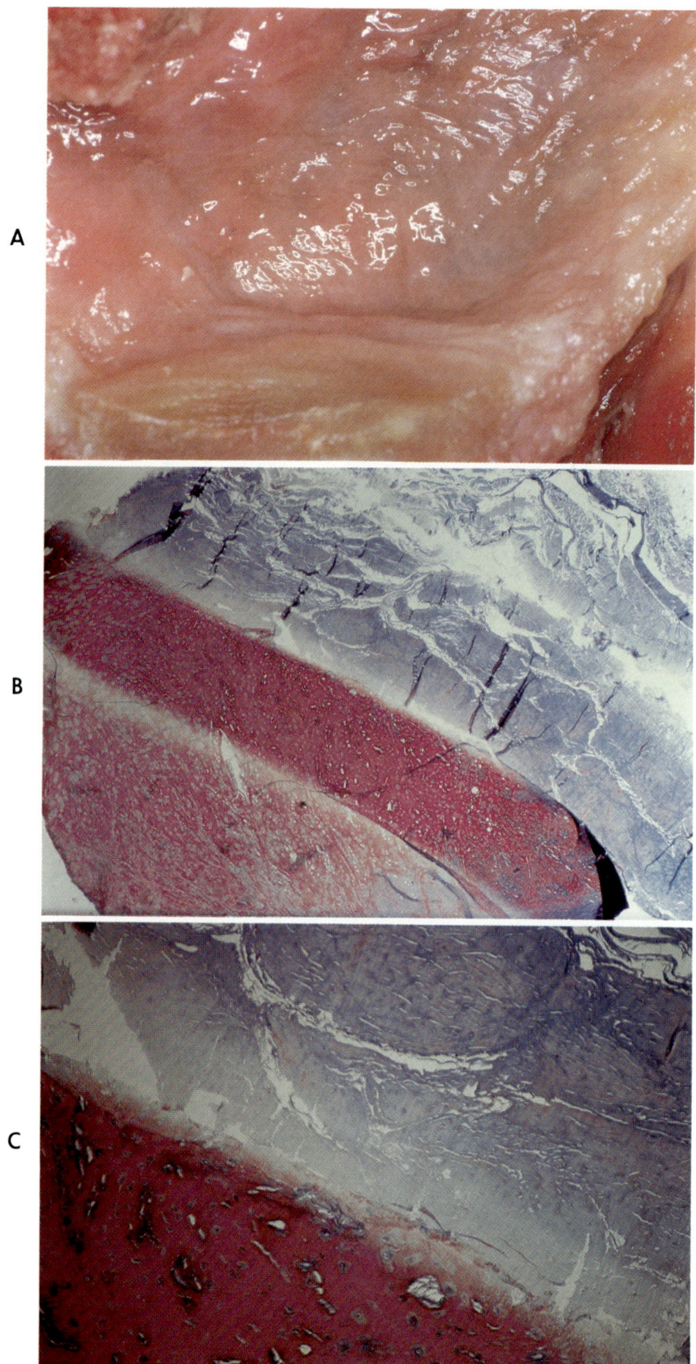

FIG. 6-32 **Junction of ligaments with glenoid.**

A Gross cross-sectional specimen shows the confluence of the glenohumeral ligaments with the anterior glenoid in the right lower portion of the photograph.

B Photomicrograph of the same area shows bone in red and ligament in blue. (Trichrome stain, original magnification ×40.)

C Photomicrograph at higher power shows bone in red and fibrous tissue above. Focal areas of red staining fibrocartilage in the labrum are visible. (Trichrome stain, original magnification ×100.)

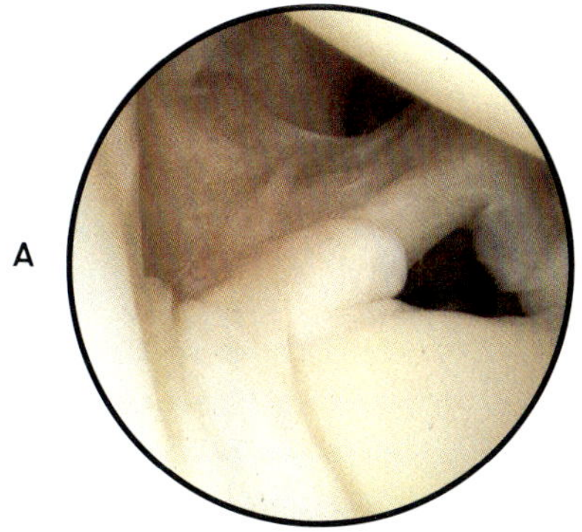

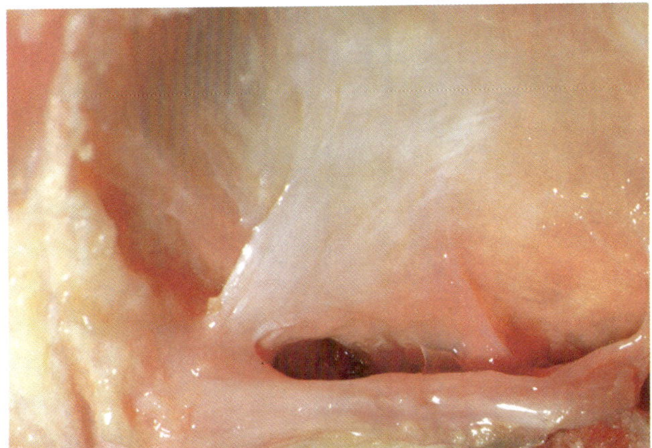

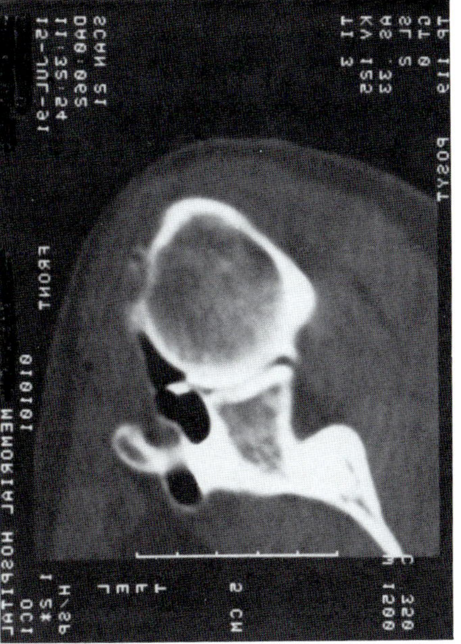

FIG. 6-33 Anatomical variations in anterior wall.

A Arthroscopic view of anterior-superior foramen beneath the obliquely traversing middle glenohumeral ligament and the labrum. This opening connects to the subscapularis bursa.

B Gross anatomical specimen demonstrates a similar foramen.

C MRI shows anterior projection of this anterior band from middle glenohumeral ligament to glenoid.

Variations of recesses and foramen. The areas of greatest anatomical variability are the synovial recesses and foramen at the area of transition of the anterior glenohumeral ligaments to the labrum. These variations are found either superior or inferior to the middle glenohumeral ligament. These openings to the subscapularis bursa (Fig. 6-33) fill with dye on an arthrogram (Fig. 6-34).

Glenohumeral ligaments. The glenohumeral ligaments are not arranged as is suggested in some textbooks on open surgery.[18,19] They are not separate distinct ligaments that run perpendicular to the glenohumeral joint (see Fig. 6-2).

Variations are the rule. The glenohumeral ligaments have considerable variations. Anatomical dissections by Mosely and Overgaard and by others have shown considerable variation in the attachments of these ligaments.[15] The glenohumeral ligaments are not distinct ligaments as seen in the knee joint but are thickenings within the joint capsule (Fig. 6-35). This observation has been demonstrated by O'Brien et al.[16]

Ligaments named from humeral attachment. Ligaments are named for the location of their attachment to the humerus: superior, middle, and inferior. The humeral at-

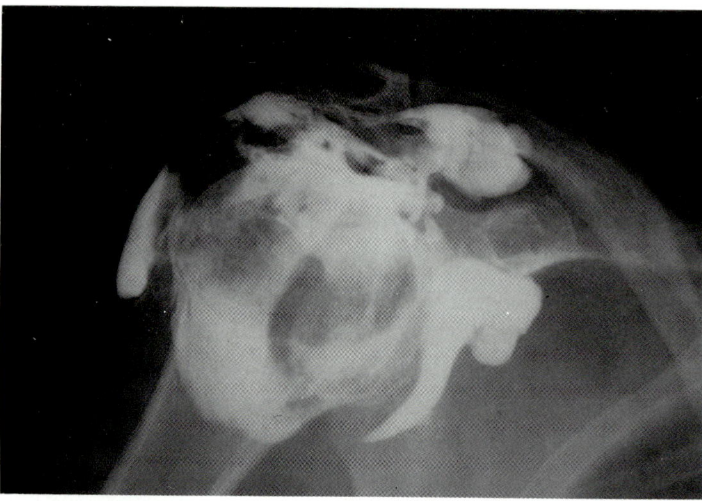

FIG. 6-34 Arthrogram of rotator cuff tear. Dye extravasation into subacromial bursa demonstrates tear. Note dye in bicipital groove and subscapularis bursa.

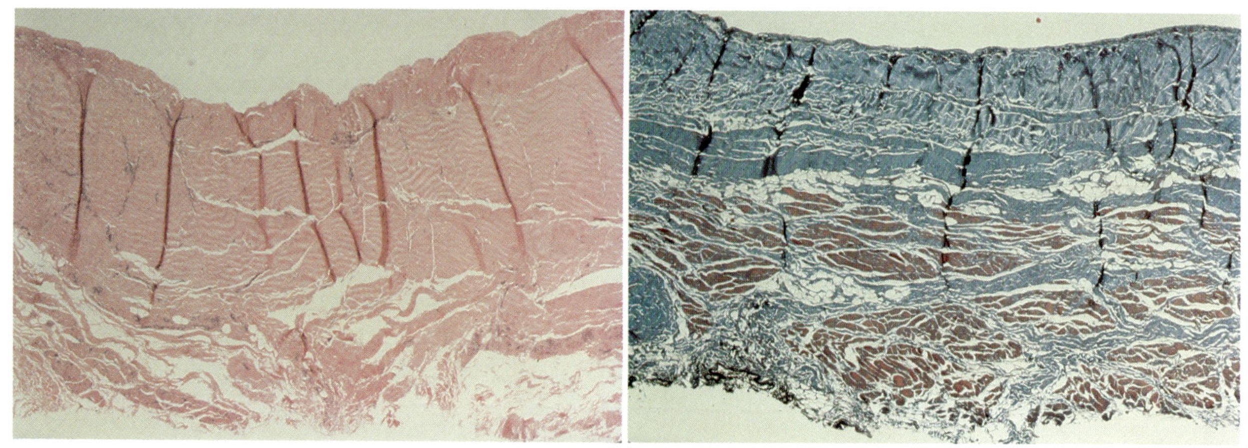

FIG. 6-35 Glenohumeral ligaments are thickenings in capsule.

A Photomicrograph of anterior glenohumeral ligaments shows synovium on top, fibrous thickening in middle and loose connective tissue beneath. (Hemotoxin and Eosin, original magnification ×100.)

B Photomicrograph of another specimen showing synovium on top, dense blue fibrous tissue capsular ligament with subscapularis muscle below. (Trichrome stain, original magnification ×100.)

tachment of the superior ligament is near the fovea capitis or the tip of the lesser tuberosity. The middle attaches on the lesser tuberosity and actually fuses with the posterior aspect of the subscapularis tendon near its attachment. The inferior portion of the ligament attaches on the surgical neck or the medial border in an area of the lesser tuberosity. The inferior glenohumeral ligament comes off the inferior portion of the humerus (Fig. 6-36).

SUPERIOR. The glenoid attachment of the superior glenohumeral ligament is in the superior glenoid tubercle and at an area near the base of the coracoid process. The attachment is not identified arthroscopically because it is

A

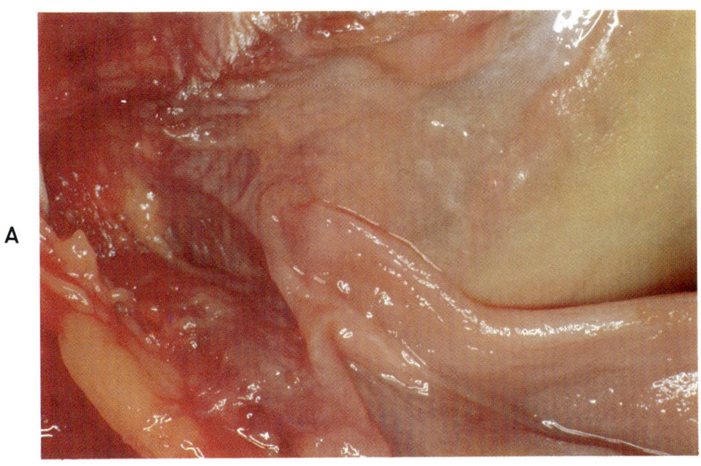

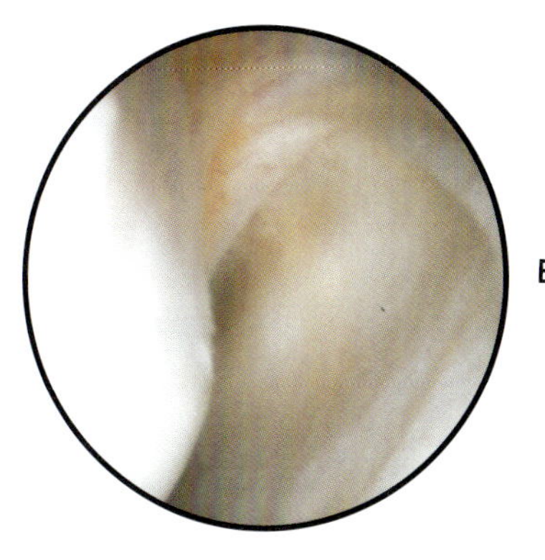

B

FIG. 6-36 Glenohumeral ligament attachment to humerus.

A Gross specimen shows inferior glenohumeral ligament attachment to humerus from anterior perspective.

B Arthroscopic view of normal attachment of inferior glenohumeral ligament in right shoulder view from posterior portal perspective. The humeral head is to the left and the inferior glenohumeral ligament is an arcuate confluence that connects to the anterior humerus.

A

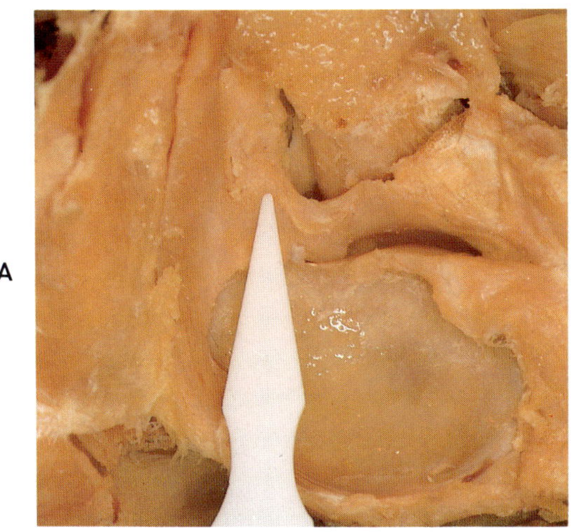

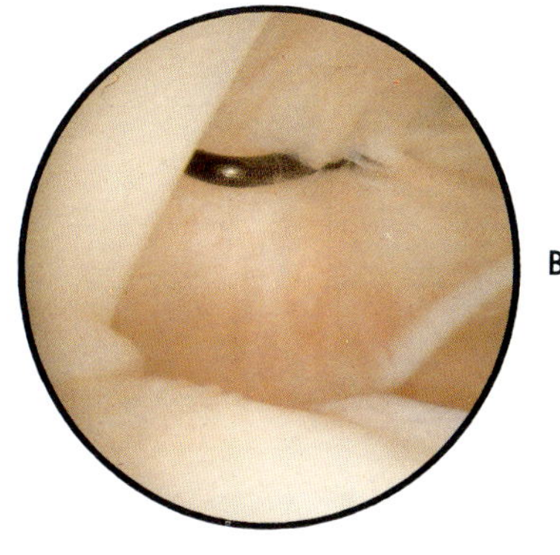

B

FIG. 6-37 Superior glenohumeral ligament.

A Gross dissection to superior glenohumeral ligament.

B Probe on superior glenohumeral ligament.

deep under the synovium. This site is immediately anterior to the biceps tendon (Fig. 6-37).

MIDDLE. The middle glenohumeral ligament attaches to the labrum obliquely and at the middle and superior glenoid (Fig. 6-38). It is a large, fibrous structure that goes down anteriorly on the scapular neck.

INFERIOR. The inferior glenohumeral ligament comes across and attaches on virtually the entire anterior labrum, with a bony insertion on the anterior glenoid neck (Fig. 6-39).[16] The inferior glenohumeral ligaments have been identified by Turkel et al and confirmed arthroscopically by McGlynn and Caspari[14a] as the important structures preventing anterior-inferior dislocations of the shoulder.

Inferior arcuate portion of the capsule. Between the

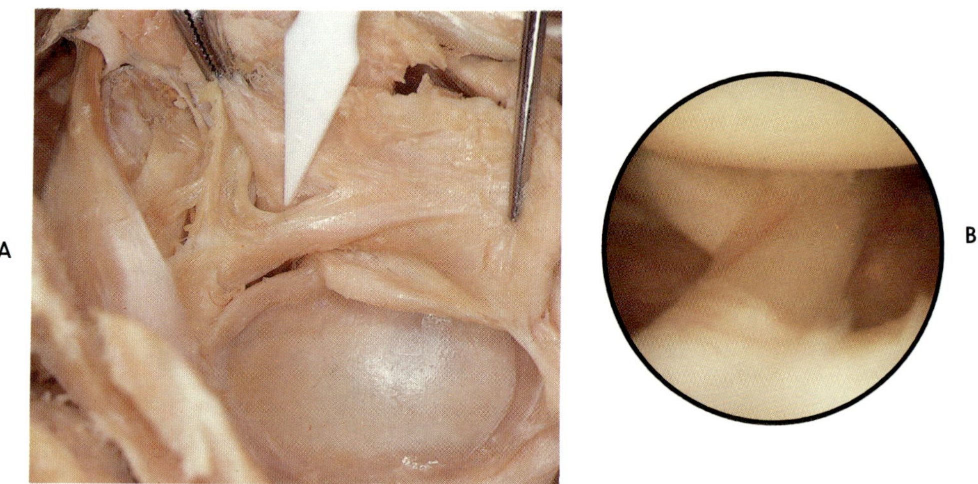

FIG. 6-38 Middle glenohumeral ligament.

A Gross dissection to oblique course of middle glenohumeral ligament.

B Arthroscopic view of middle ligament crossing over superior margin of subscapularis tendon.

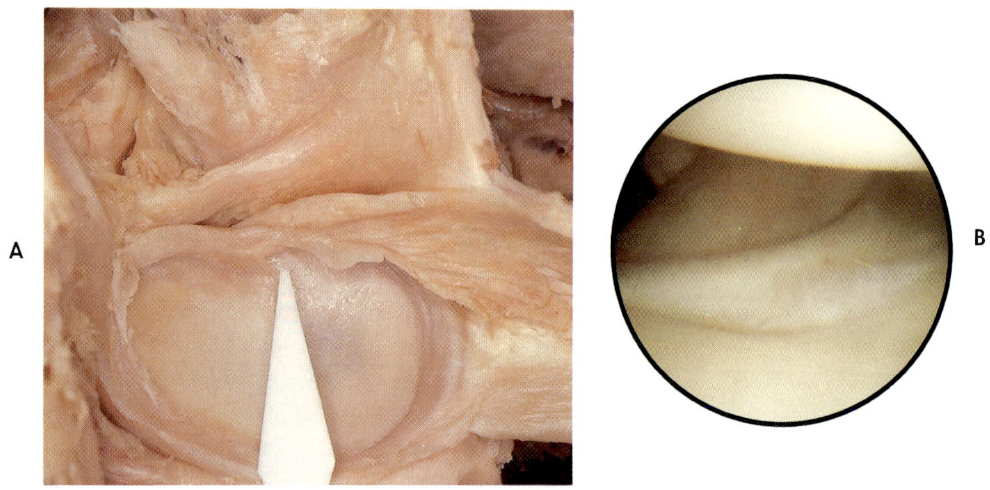

FIG. 6-39 Inferior glenohumeral ligament.

A Pointer is at central sulcus glenoid, showing broad anterior triangular attachment of inferior glenohumeral ligament to entire anterior glenoid.

B Inferior glenohumeral ligament at anterior glenoid sulcus showing broad triangular attachment.

better defined anterior inferior glenohumeral ligament and the occasionally defined posterior inferior ligament is the inferior pouch of the glenohumeral joint. This area is also capsular and ligamentous (Fig. 6-40).

Variations in glenohumeral ligaments

OBLIQUE COURSE. The glenohumeral ligaments have an oblique course across the glenohumeral joint. They take their origin in three locations (superior, middle, and inferior) on the humerus and pass obliquely to a superior attachment on the glenoid. The superior glenohumeral ligament is small, takes its origin from the superior humerus, and attaches to the superior aspect of the glenoid, near the

A 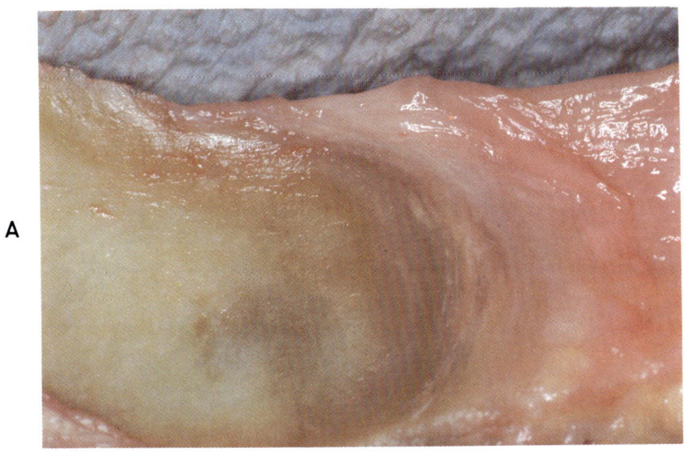

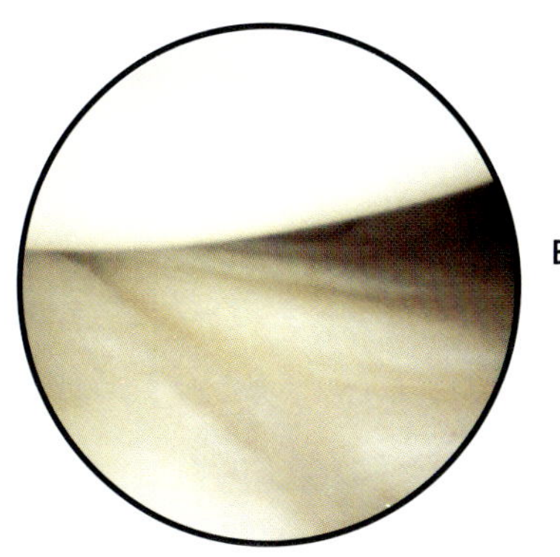 B

FIG. 6-40 Inferior arcuate portion of the capsular ligaments.

A Gross specimen was dissected to demonstrate the glenoid fossa and the inferior ligamentous attachments.

B Arthroscopic view of same area as demonstrated by gross specimen in Fig. 6-44, *A*.

A 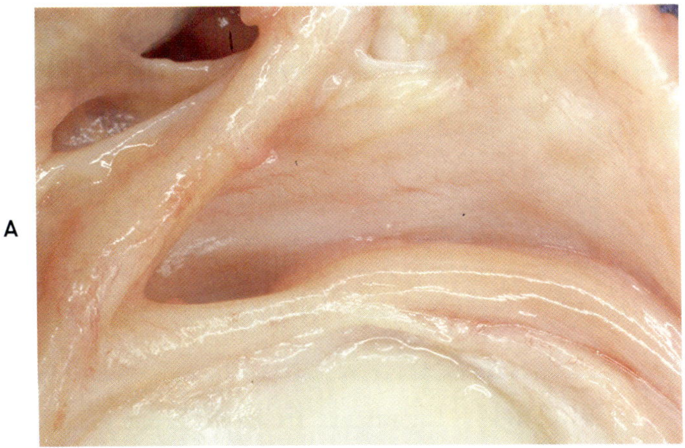

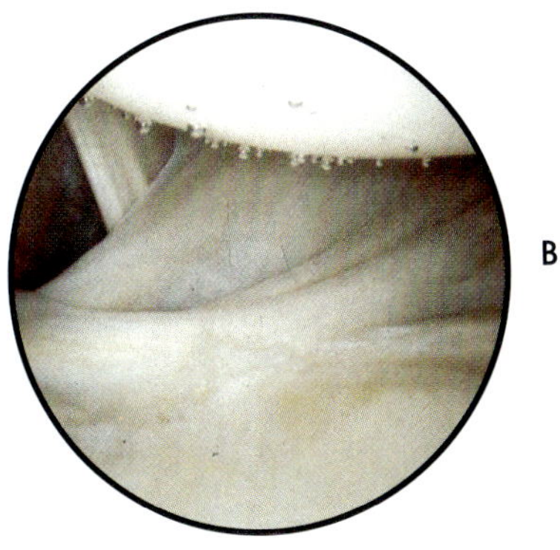 B

FIG. 6-41 Oblique course of glenohumeral ligaments.

A Gross anatomical dissection of the middle and inferior glenohumeral ligaments. The middle ligament crosses the photograph obliquely in left upper corner. It is separated from the inferior ligament by a broad recess. The inferior glenohumeral ligament is anterior and parallel to the anterior glenoid.

B An arthroscopic view of similar configuration of the middle and glenohumeral ligaments as shown in *A*.

biceps tendon (see Fig. 6-37).

The middle glenohumeral ligament attaches to the midportion of the humerus and to the superior aspect of the scapular glenoid along an oblique course (Fig. 6-41).

The inferior glenohumeral ligament traverses from the inferior aspect of the humerus, blending with the labrum into the superior aspect of the glenoid rim (Fig. 6-42). In some specimens it has a triangular shape and attaches obliquely across the entire anterior portion of the glenoid margins. Its bony attachment is on the inferior half of the anterior glenoid neck and is seen clinically only after an avulsion of bone with traumatic anterior dislocation (see Chapter 8).

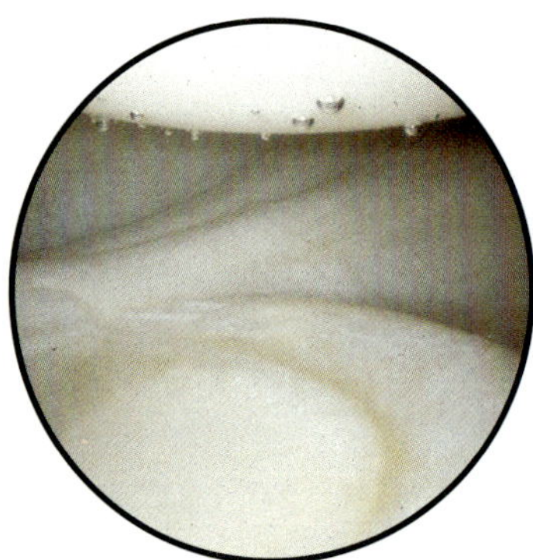

FIG. 6-42 Inferior glenohumeral ligament is prominent, oblique, and triangular.

A

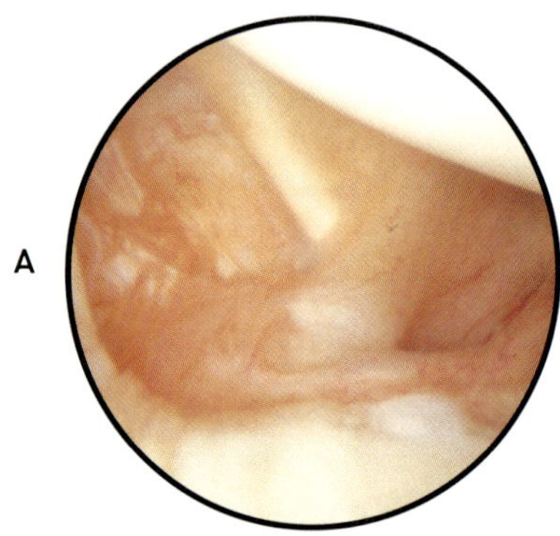

B

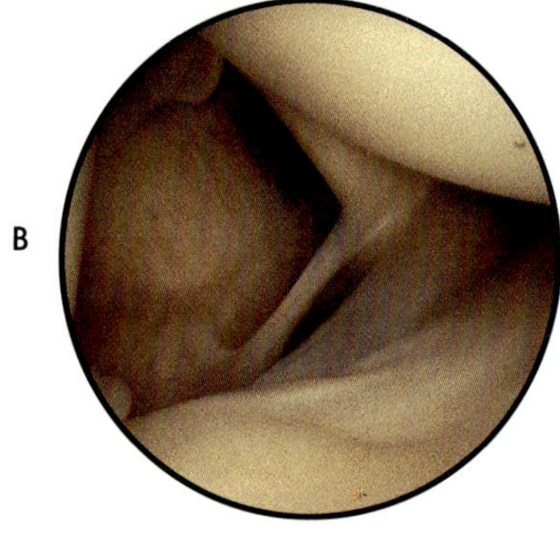

FIG. 6-43 Arthroscopic view of anterior glenohumeral joint from posterior. The humeral head is distracted by intraarticular pressure. The middle glenohumeral ligament is a single thin band crossing obliquely posterior to the superior subscapularis tendon slip.

A Single, thicker band of middle glenohumeral ligament (orange color slide) and small subscapularis bursa.

B Double strand of middle glenohumeral ligament and large subscapularis bursa.

A

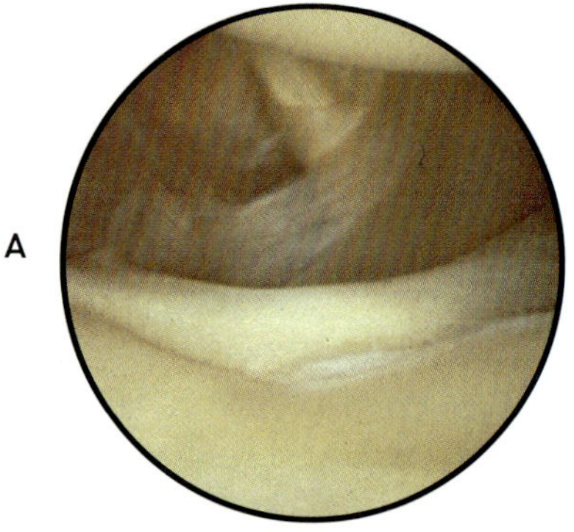

B

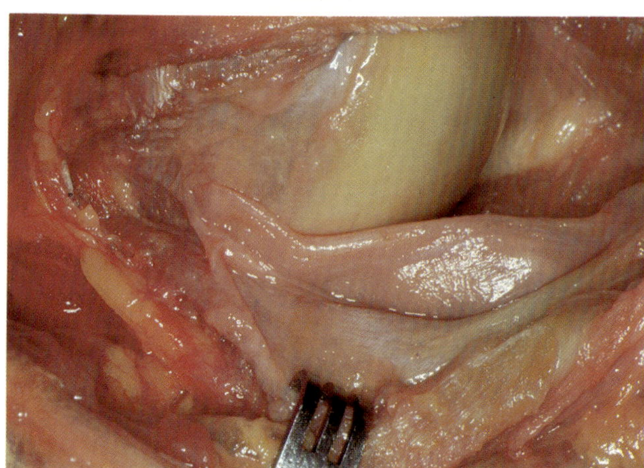

FIG. 6-44 Ligaments are in different planes.

A Arthroscopic view of anterior glenohumeral joint shows the middle glenohumeral ligament in a plane anterior to the inferior ligament.

B Gross anatomical dissection from anterior shows the distinct planes of the middle glenohumeral ligament (retractor) and the deeper (posterior) band of the inferior ligament.

VARIED SIZES. As a result of the varied thickenings, the ligaments vary in size. The superior ligament is rarely developed enough to be visually distinct by arthroscopy. The middle glenohumeral ligament may be represented by a single thin band (Fig. 6-43).

VARIED SHAPES. The superior and the middle glenohumeral ligaments are rectangular or band shaped, and the inferior portion is triangular in shape and attachment (see Figs. 6-41 and 6-42).

VARIED PLANES. The glenohumeral ligaments are not in the same plane. The anterior glenohumeral ligaments are in different planes anterior to posterior and run an oblique course from the humerus to the glenoid. The inferior glenohumeral ligament is posterior and inferior to the middle glenohumeral ligament (Fig. 6-44).

VARIED CONNECTIONS. In some patients, the ligaments may blend with one another to appear as one continuous ligament (Fig. 6-45).

SULCUS OR RECESS VARIATIONS. The ligaments may be confluent but separated by a sulcus or recess. This is not a complete opening into the subscapularis recess (Fig. 6-46). A sack or recess in the inferior portion has been described by Turkel et al.[22b]

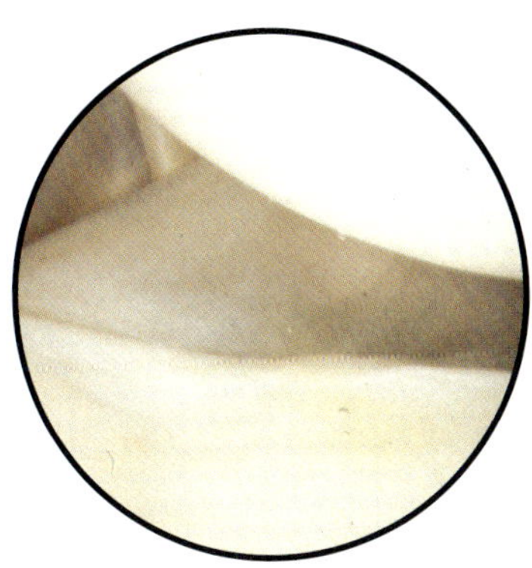

FIG. 6-45 Arthroscopic view shows confluence of middle and inferior glenohumeral ligaments.

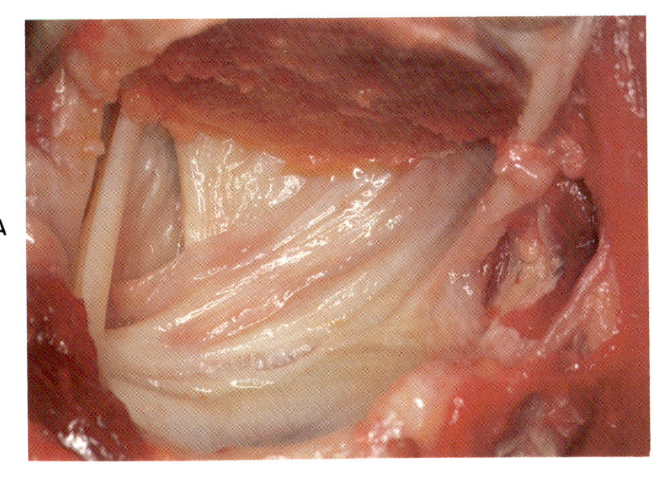

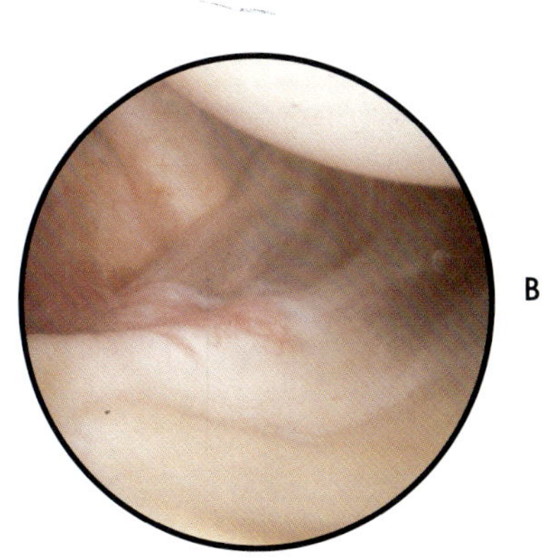

FIG. 6-46 Sulcus or recesses.

A Gross anatomical specimen shows continuous band from inferior to middle glenohumeral ligaments, but definition is provided by sulcus.

B Arthroscopic view of similar configuration with recesses between glenohumeral ligaments.

VARIED OPENINGS. In some patients the ligaments are separated by openings (foramen) into the subscapularis bursa (Fig. 6-47). The most common foramen is found between the superior and middle glenohumeral ligaments (Fig. 6-48). Occasionally one is visible below the middle glenohumeral ligament or in both positions.

IMPORTANCE OF RECOGNIZING GLENOHUMERAL LIGAMENT VARIATIONS. The arthroscopist must bear in mind the possible variations of the anterior glenohumeral ligaments. Normal glenohumeral anatomy is best seen arthroscopically when inspecting the glenohumeral joint in a patient with isolated impingement syndrome. This experi-

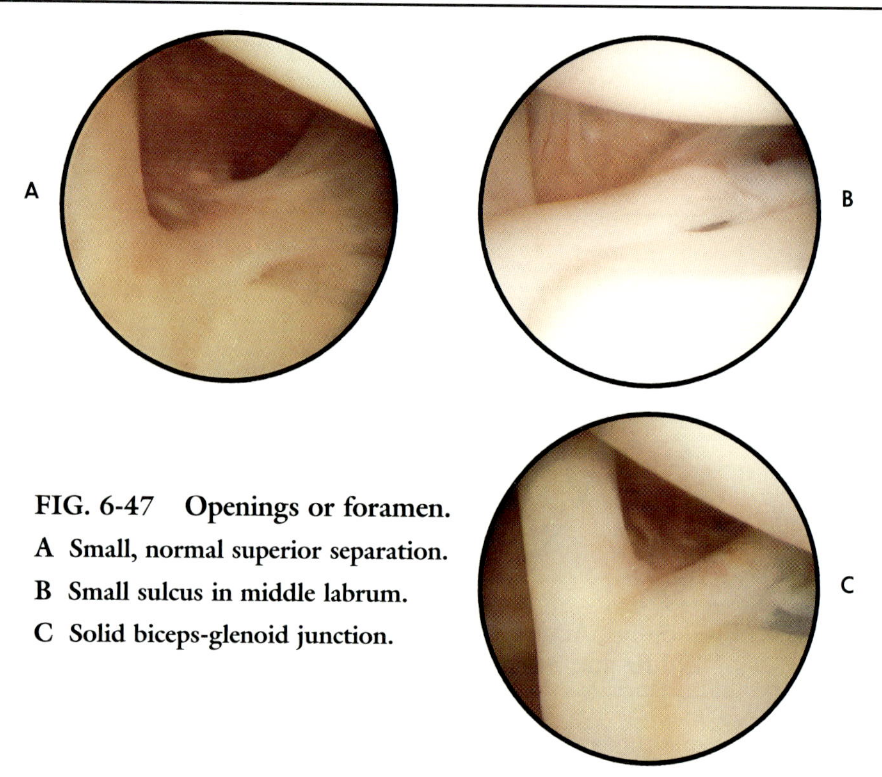

FIG. 6-47 Openings or foramen.
A Small, normal superior separation.
B Small sulcus in middle labrum.
C Solid biceps-glenoid junction.

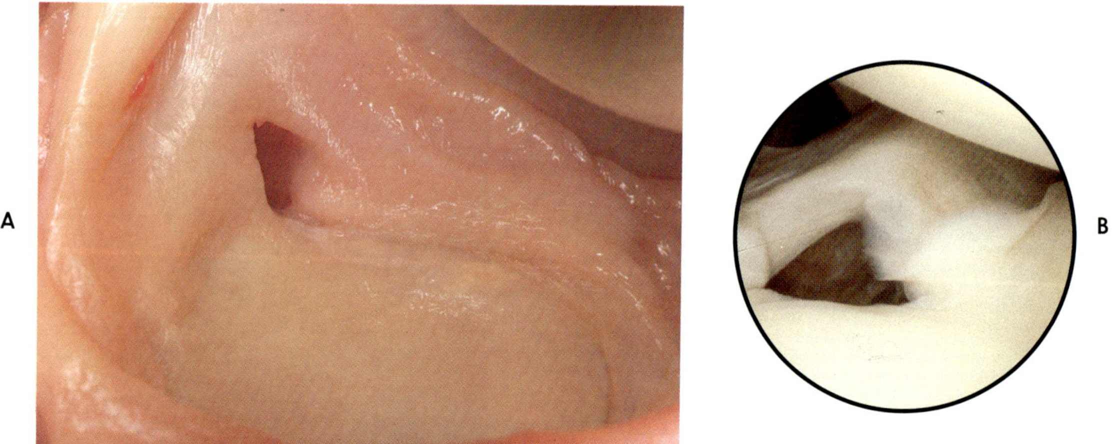

FIG. 6-48 Most common opening or foramen.
A Gross specimen shows superior opening.
B Arthroscopic view shows similar opening as seen in gross specimen.

ence will build the surgeon's knowledge of the normal variations in size, presence, separations from the other ligaments and points of attachment on the anterior bony glenoid. Since no single normal pattern of the glenohumeral ligaments exists, this regular experience will assist the surgeon in determining abnormal ligament structures. This knowledge is especially important in determining subsequent labrum injury and in assessing glenohumeral ligament integrity.

Subscapularis bursa. The subscapularis bursa opening is anterior and superior on the anterior glenohumeral wall (Fig. 6-49). The opening is defined inferiorly by the superior margin of the middle glenohumeral ligament. The anterior margin of the opening is the superior tendon slip of the subscapularis tendon. The opening can be entered from a posterior portal with arthroscope penetration and downward rotation of the inclined lens (Fig. 6-50).

The anterior approach provides a better angle to pene-

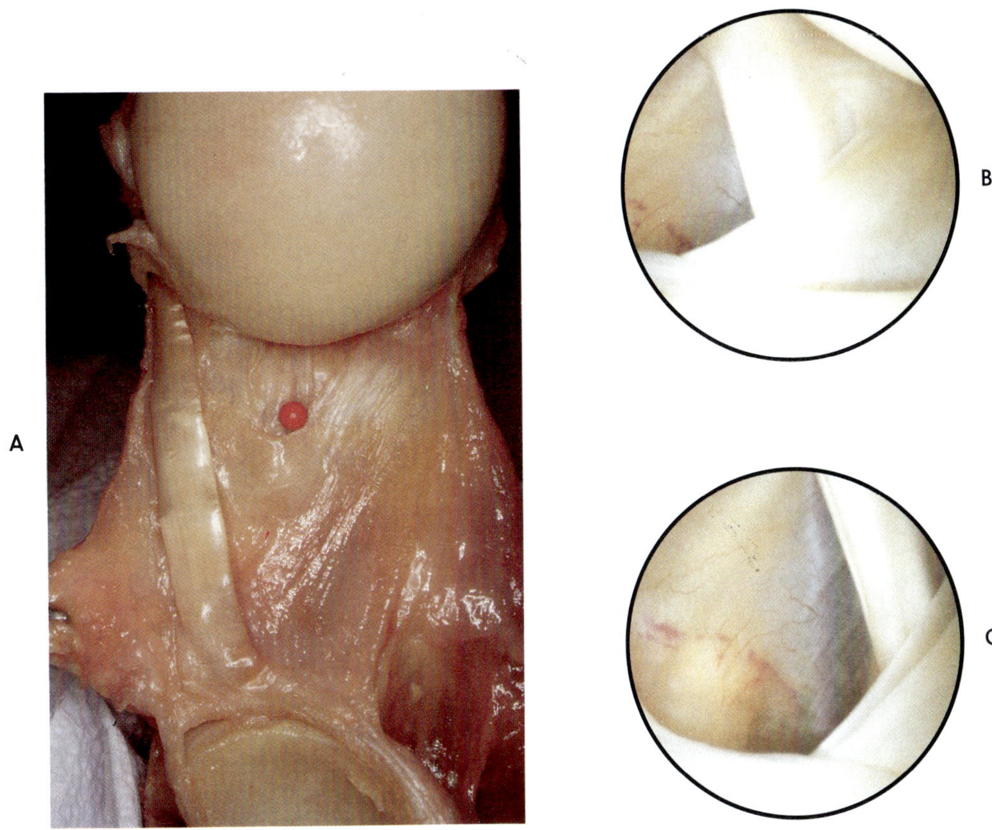

FIG. 6-49 Subscapularis bursa.

A Gross anatomical specimen shows humeral head superior, biceps tendon to the left and a red dot marker in the opening of the subscapularis bursa.

B Arthroscopic view of the opening of the subscapularis bursa with middle glenohumeral ligament inferior, the subscapularis tendon to the right.

C Advancement of the arthroscope shows depths of the subscapularis bursa.

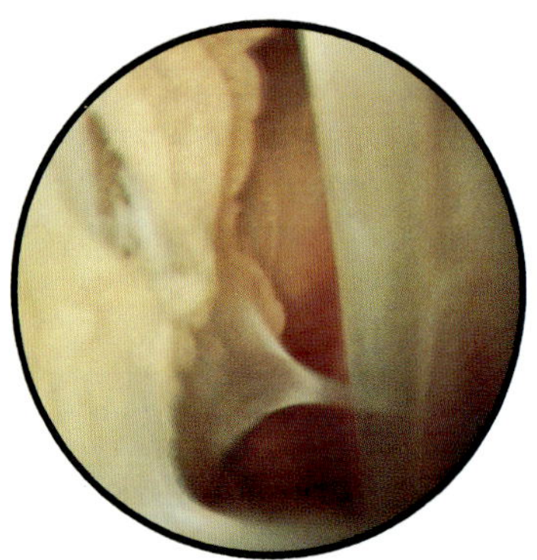

FIG. 6-50 View after penetration of scope into subscapularis bursa.

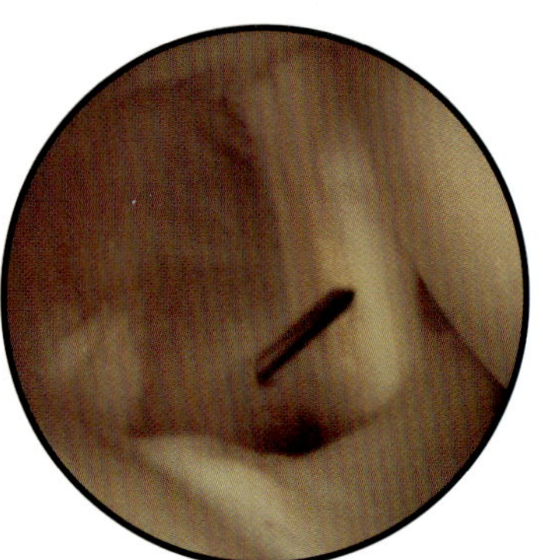

FIG. 6-51 Subscapularis tendon. Arthroscopic view of the needle pointing to the intraarticular portion of the subscapularis tendon.

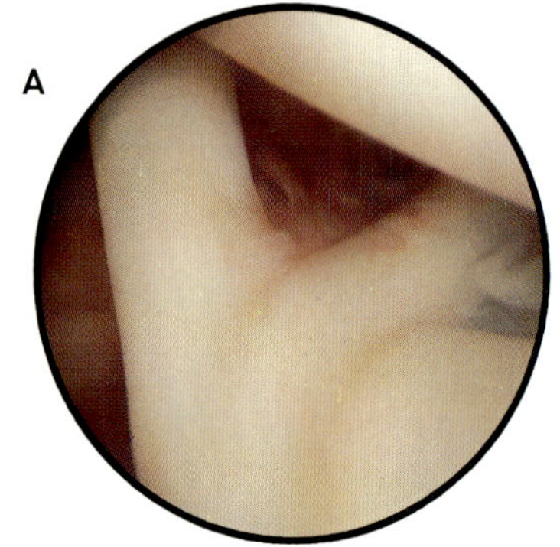

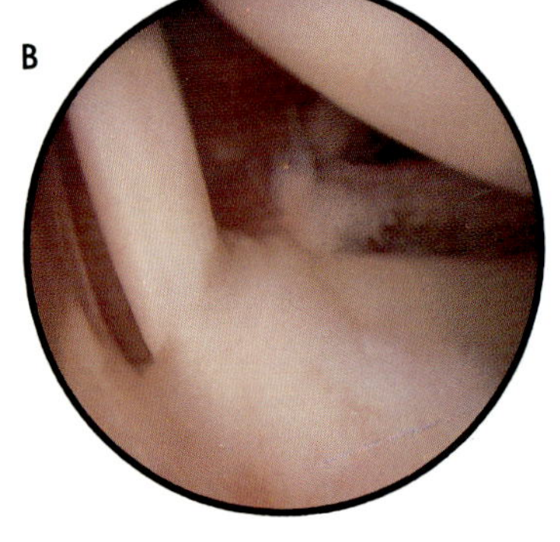

FIG. 6-52 Normal anatomical variations.

A Solid biceps-glenoid junction.

B Labrum wrapped around biceps attachment.

trate the depth of the subscapularis bursa. The subscapularis muscle forms the anterior wall of the subscapularis bursa. This bursa varies in diameter and is as much as 6 cm deep.

Supscapularis tendon. The most distinct anterior wall structure is the intraarticular portion of the superior tendon slip of the subscapularis muscle (Fig. 6-51). This is only a small portion of the broad insertion of the subscapularis muscle on the humerus (Fig. 6-52). The subscapularis musculotendinous junction has thickened tendon slips on its posterior side extending into the subscapularis muscle (Fig. 6-52, *B*). The intraarticular tendinous portion is usually not appreciated in open surgery or by anatomical dissection from the anterior approach.

The subscapularis muscle is found on the anterior wall, deep in the subscapularis bursa (Fig. 6-53). It is seen during arthroscopy only if all of the glenohumeral ligaments are pathologically absent (see Fig. 6-52, *A*).

Gross dissection shows multiple tendon slips in the broad subscapularis (see Fig. 6-52, *B*). These tendon slips look like the bony slips in a turkey drumstick that blend into the muscle. The tendon slips do not attach to the anterior glenoid but are confluent with the subscapularis muscle belly.

Posterior Region. The posterior joint is inspected from both posterior and anterior.

From posterior portal. From posterior, the biceps tendon is followed to its attachment posterior and superior on the glenoid. With slight retraction and moderate distention of the joint, the scope can be moved along the posterior labrum (Fig. 6-54). Slight decompression of joint distention is necessary to see into the posterior sulcus, behind

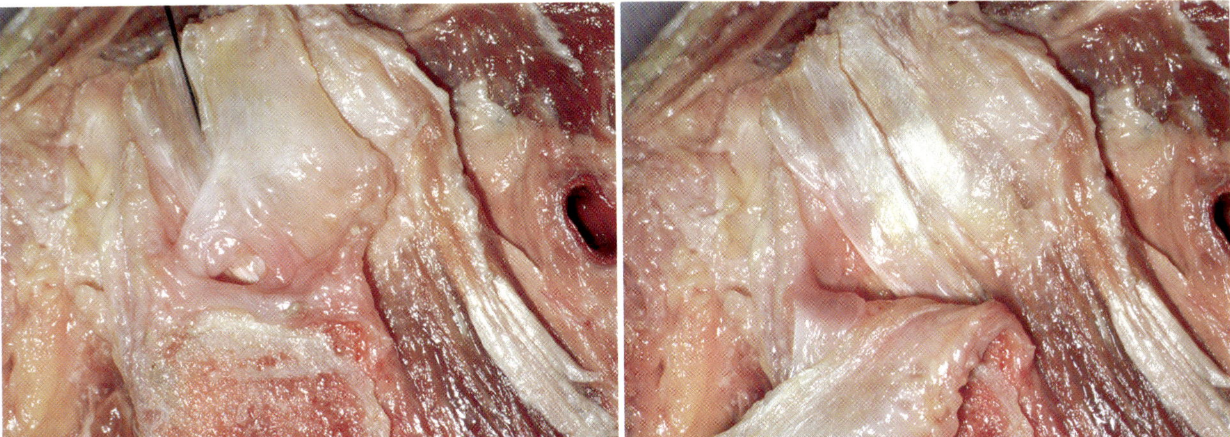

FIG. 6-53 Subscapularis muscle.

A Gross anatomical dissection with cross-section of glenoid shows the anterior glenohumeral ligaments covering the subscapularis muscle.

B Same gross specimen with closer view shows retraction of the glenohumeral ligaments to expose the musculotendinous junction of the subscapularis muscle.

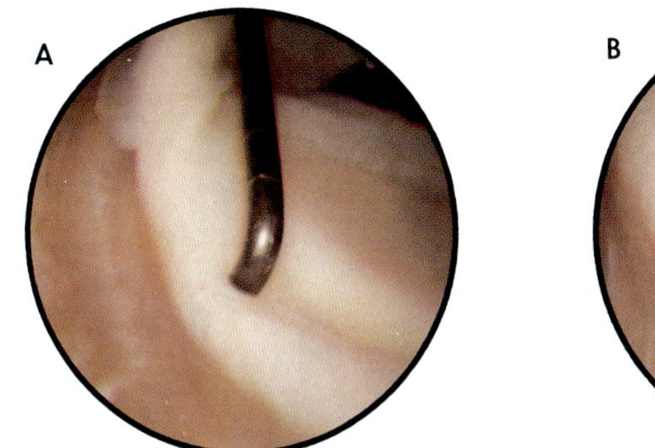

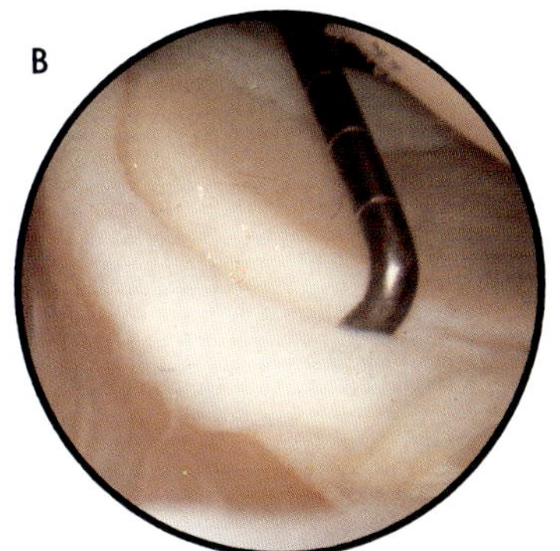

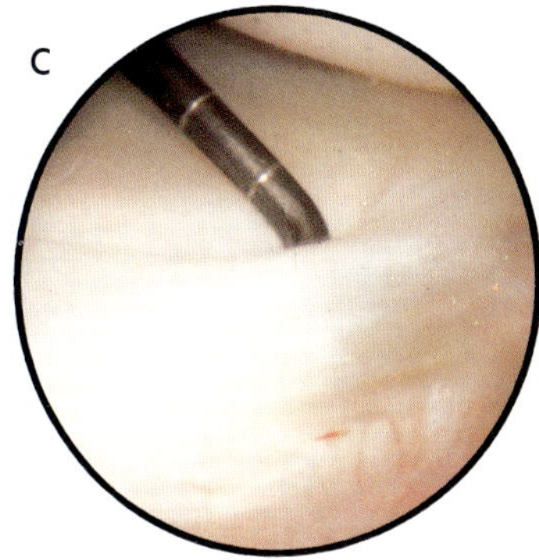

FIG. 6-54 Normal posterior glenoid labrum.

A Probe on continuation of biceps tendon to posterior-superior labrum.

B Probe in normal sulcus at midportion of posterior labrum.

C Probe in sulcus, not tear, of posterior-inferior labrum.

the glenoid rim. This area has normal synovial "veils" extending from the synovium on the posterior reflection of the glenoid (Fig. 6-55). The synovium is normally vascular on the posterior sulcus. The posterior-inferior glenohumeral ligament is prominent in some patients and can be visualized even from the posterior portal (Fig. 6-56).

From anterior portal. The posterior wall and ligamentous structures are best viewed from an anterior arthroscopic portal (Fig. 6-57). The biceps is the best structure for orientation. The biceps courses posterior and inferior to blend into the posterior labrum (Fig. 6-57, *B*). The glenoid surface blends into the posterior labrum. The posterior labrum is less prominent than the anterior labrum (Fig. 6-57, *A*). No central sulcus is present. Over the posterior labrum and behind is the long glenoid fossa. Beyond the fossa is the vertical posterior joint wall. Only the posterior inferior area has definition or thickening in the capsule suggesting a ligament. This is best seen with rotation of the humerus. No posterior extraarticular muscle or tendons are seen from inside. The posterior wall is covered with synovium. Its vascularity is minimal.

Inferior Region. The inferior region is inspected from both posterior and anterior. It is best seen from posterior with scope rotation. The posterior glenoid labrum is followed to the inferior labrum, which has the same contour.

The inferior recess of the glenohumeral joint is covered with smooth synovium. The capsular ligaments form the arcuate portion of the inferior glenohumeral ligaments, both anterior and posterior (see Fig. 6-40).[16]

The Arthroscopic-Correlated Open Anterior Surgical Approach to the Glenohumeral Joint. Detrisac and Johnson[7] correlated the arthroscopic understanding of the glenohumeral ligaments with the classical descriptions of the anterior surgical approach to the glenohumeral joint. They pointed out that the "anterior capsule" of open surgery was the middle glenohumeral ligament.

His anatomical dissections from anterior clear up some of the previous misunderstandings. The interval between the supraspinatus and the superior subscapularis is opened (Fig. 6-58, *A*) to show the extension of the middle glenohumeral ligament. Further dissection reflects the subscapularis muscle from the humerus starting superior (Fig. 6-58, *B*). The "anterior capsule" is exposed. The subscapularis is completely reflected from the humerus (Fig. 6-58, *C*) to show the confluence of the middle glenohumeral ligament with the inferior from anterior perspective.

The next step is to detach the middle and inferior glenohumeral ligaments from the humeral head. When the specimen is rotated, one can see the "anterior capsule" is middle glenohumeral ligament (Fig. 6-58, *D*).

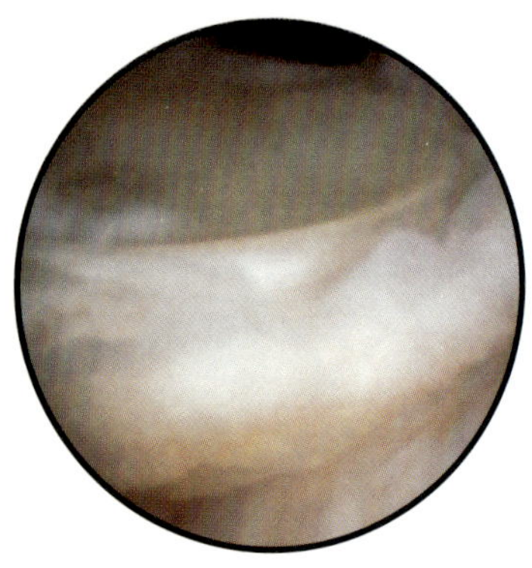

FIG. 6-55 Synovial veils. Arthroscopic view of right shoulder from posterior shows small normal synovial projections from posterior labrum.

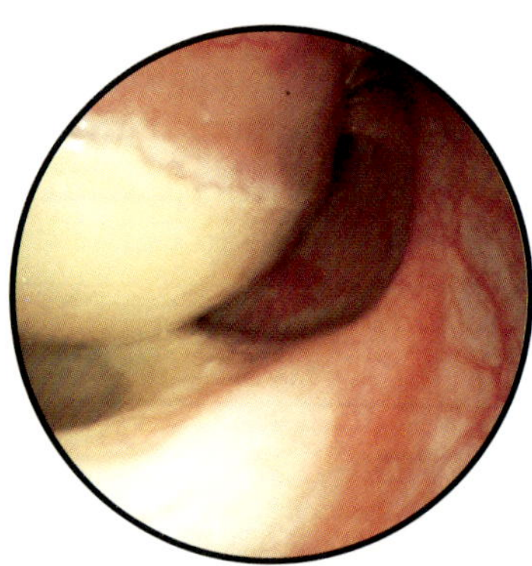

FIG. 6-56 Arthroscopic view of posterior-inferior glenohumeral ligament from posterior portal in right shoulder. Photograph was taken in air medium. The humerus is between 9 and 12 o'clock. The prominent ligament defines the posterior aspect of the arcuate portion of the capsule on its way upward to the humerus.

A

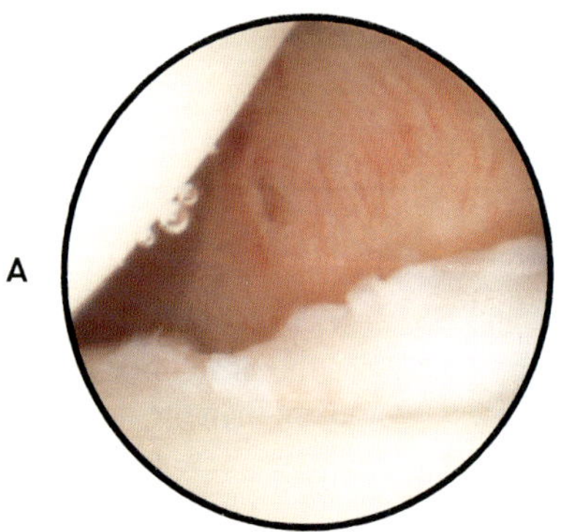

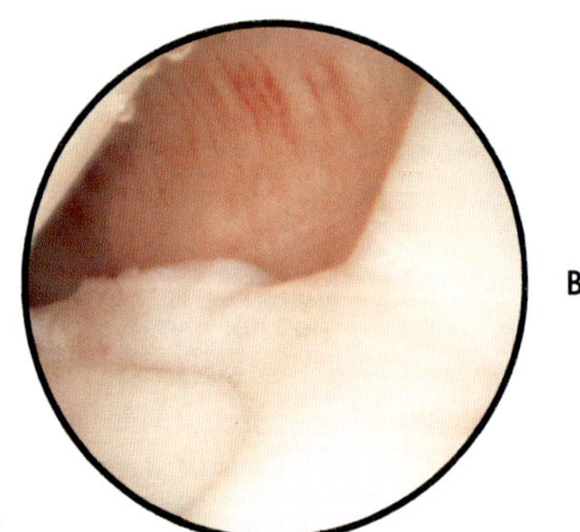

B

FIG. 6-57 Anterior view of the posterior joint wall.

A Arthroscopic view of posterior labrum and joint from anterior portal.

B Biceps labrum attachment from anterior arthroscopic portal.

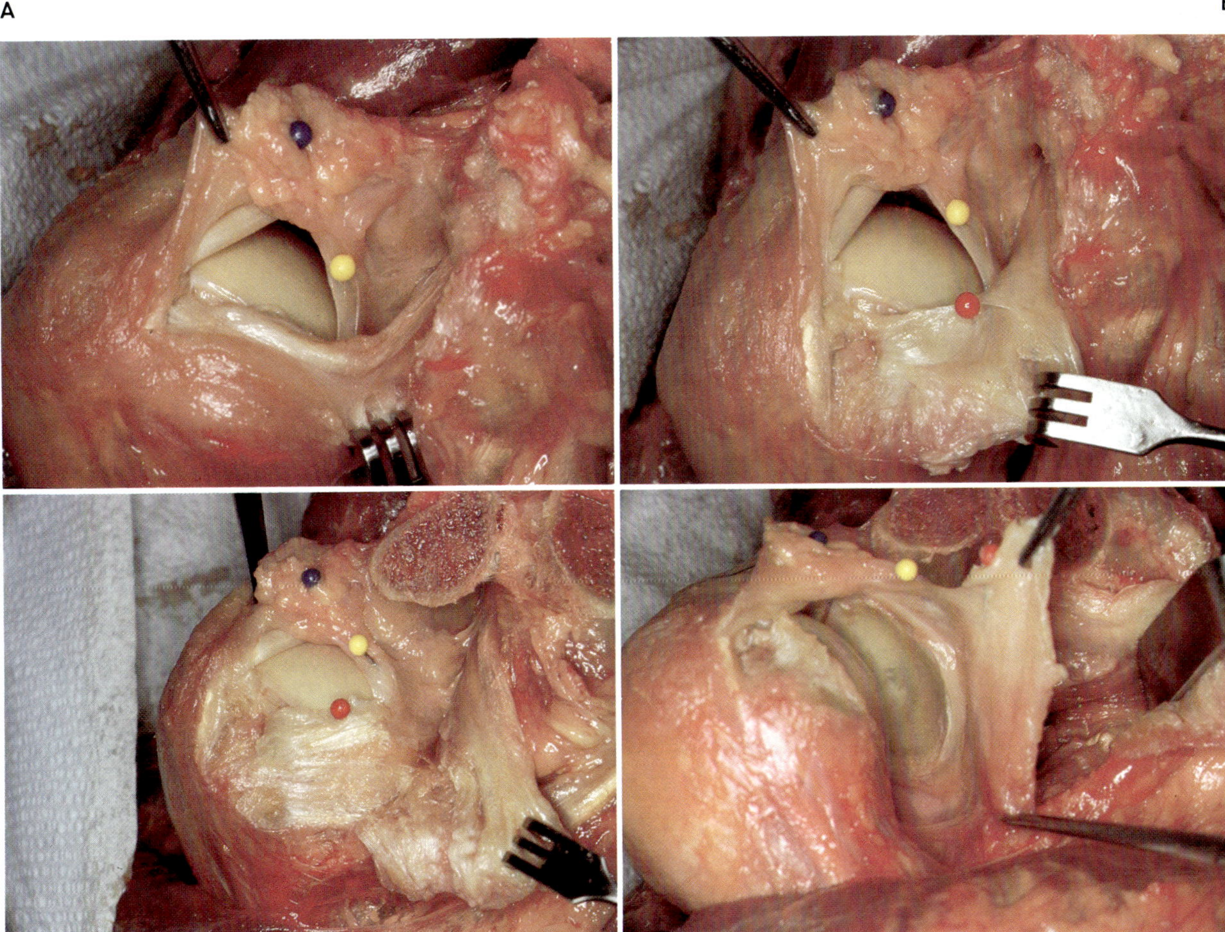

FIG. 6-58 Open anterior surgical approach to the shoulder.

A Gross anatomical specimen of right shoulder viewed from anterior shows blue dot on supraspinatus tendon and yellow dot on superior extension of the middle glenohumeral ligament. The rake retractor is pulling down the subscapularis muscle to widen the interval between the supraspinatus and subscapularis muscles.

B Gross anatomical specimen shows reflection of superior aspect of subscapularis tendon insertion from the humerus. Markers are same color and place as in *A*. Notice the "anterior capsule" with red marker.

C Complete removal and retraction of the subscapularis from the humerus shows the entire intact "anterior capsule." The red marker in on the middle glenohumeral ligament.

D The specimen is rotated and the glenohumeral ligaments are removed from the humerus. The markers are unchanged. Notice that the "anterior capsule" is in reality the middle glenohumeral ligament. In this specimen the middle and inferior glenohumeral ligaments are confluent.

Subacromial Bursa

The normal subacromial bursa is small (Fig. 6-59, *A*).[6,13] It is anterior and immediately posterior to the free span of the coracoacromial (CA) ligament (Fig. 6-59, *B*). The normal bursa is difficult to find and enter. It has a potential volume of less than 5 ml. In the normal state this bursa is similar to bursa in other areas such as prepatellar or olecranon. All are difficult to palpate in the normal uninflamed condition.

The anterior and superior wall is composed of the CA ligament (Fig. 6-60). The free span of the ligament attaches to the underside of the acromion. The normal ligament under the acromion is white, soft, and compressible. David Detrisac and I measured 50 cadaver shoulders, finding that the ligament is typically 1 cm wide, 0.5 cm deep, and 4 cm long on the underside of the acromion.

The subacromial portion of the CA ligament is covered with a smooth, thin layer of synovium with an occasional vessel. The arthroscopic view of the anterior wall shows the ligament traversing the space, with a transverse translucent plica at its base (Fig. 6-61). Normal blood vessels may be present on the ligament, but no vascular reaction is evident (Fig. 6-61, *B*). The yellow subbursal fat is seen beneath the thin bursal lining (Fig. 6-61, *C*).

The normal space has a smooth synovial lining (see Fig. 6-59). Often plica or folds cross the space (Fig. 6-62, *A*). In some cases the folds are circular, outlining the superior aspect of the supraspinatus tendon (Fig. 6-62, *B*). The plica are pathologic, only if separated or fragmented to form a band across the space (see Chapter 7).

The superior aspect of the tendon is smooth and covered with synovium. Small, well-organized vessels may be seen on the superior surface of the rotator cuff tendons (Fig. 6-63).

The supraspinatus tendon forms the bottom of the bursa (Fig. 6-64, *A*). The tendon inserts into the humeral head. A cross-section of a gross anatomical dissection shows the relationships (Fig. 6-64, *B*).

On one occasion I identified a well-developed coracohumeral ligament by arthroscopy in the subacromial bursa. It is more easily identified by open dissection (Fig. 6-65).

The normal subacromial space may be enlarged in patients with activity in throwing sports or swimming, yet such an enlargement is not pathological. No synovitis is present.

In normal patients with a small space, one can place a scope cannula under the acromion and manually create an enlarged false subacromial space with side-to-side motion. This maneuver should be avoided. Distention and arthroscopic inspection show this space but reveal no well-de-

A

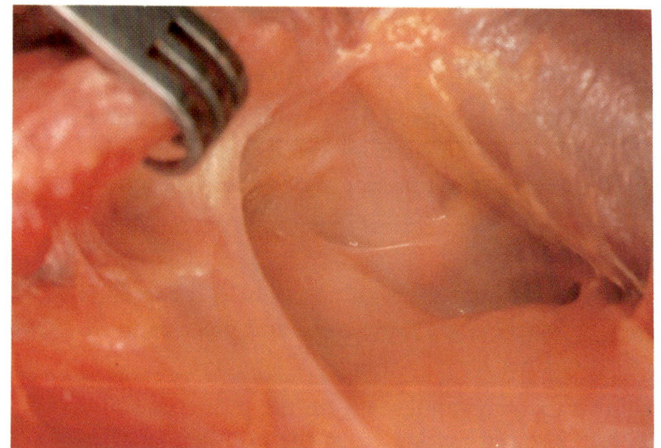

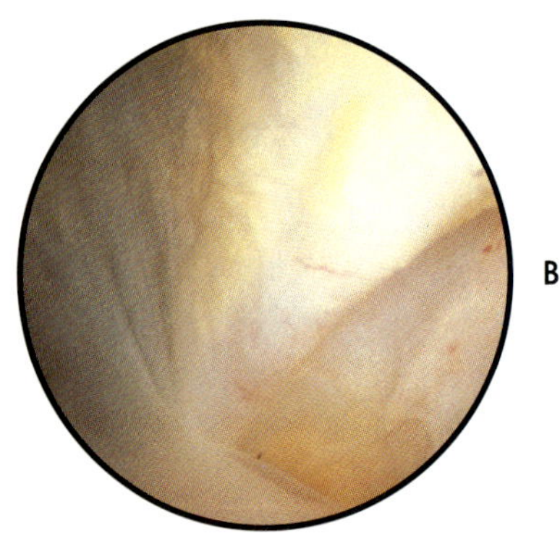

B

FIG. 6-59 Subacromial bursa.

A Close-up of a normal subacromial bursa of a gross anatomical specimen of a right shoulder. The rake retractor is on the acromion. The deltoid muscle is located in the upper right of the photograph. A normal subacromial fold is located below the acromion and forms the posterior and medial aspect of the bursa. The CA ligament is the vertical white structure in the middle.

B Arthroscopic view of CA ligament seen on anterior wall of subacromial bursa.

fined bursa with a synovial lining. The walls of the false space have the appearance of any extraarticular, fluid-descended soft tissues. This maneuver, which tears the bursal lining, causes the surgeon to make an interpretation on poorly defined space and makes obtaining and maintaining adequate surgical exposure technically difficult.

If the subacromial bursa cannot be entered as an identifiable space after multiple tries by an experienced surgeon, it is unlikely that a lesion exists in the area.

Visualization in the subacromial area is facilitated if inflammation of the bursa exists. This occurs with rotator cuff disease, rheumatoid arthritis, or an impingement syndrome (see Chapter 7). When a lesion exists in the area and the bursa is present, entry is technically easy. In fact, a greatly enlarged pathological bursa may be entered inadvertently during an approach to the glenohumeral joint.

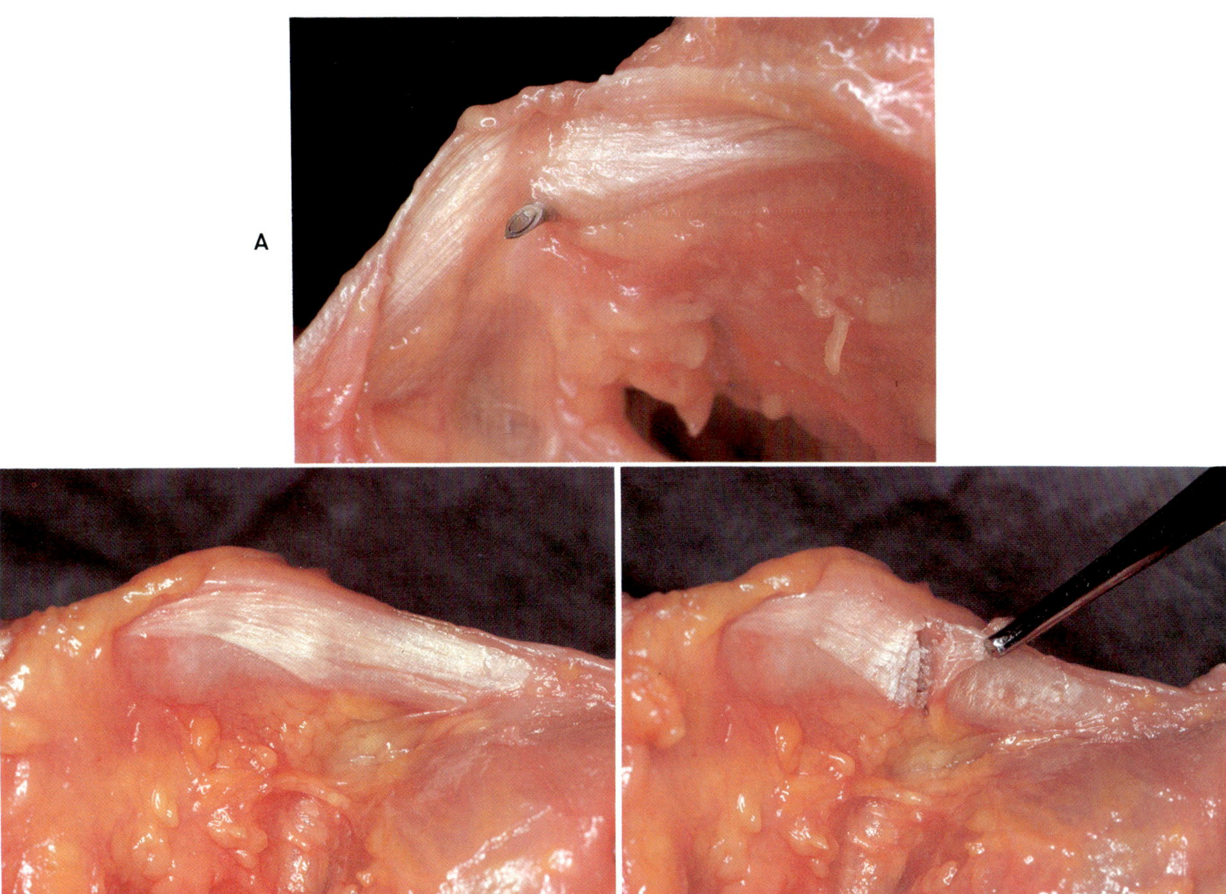

FIG. 6-60 CA ligament.

A Gross anatomical exposure of the CA ligament shows a metal needle through the ligament at the junction of the free span attachment to the underside of the acromion to the left.

B Gross anatomical dissection illustrates entire course of the CA ligament.

C Gross anatomical specimen shows the CA ligament with transection of the ligament at the attachment to the undersurface of the acromion.

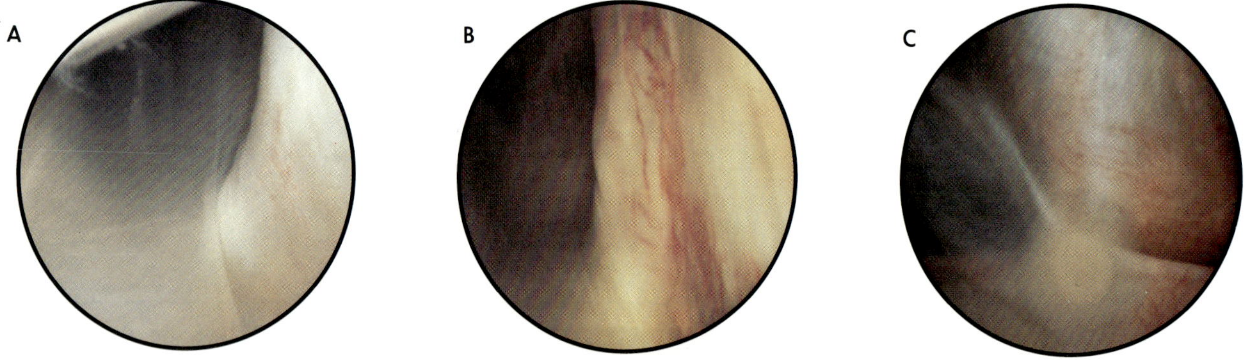

FIG. 6-61 Arthroscopic view of CA ligament.

A The CA ligament is vertical in the arthroscopic view and is covered with a thin synovial plica.

B Arthroscopic view in another patient with a normal bursa shows normal vascular pattern on top on the supraspinatus tendon.

C Arthroscopic view of a patient with smooth synovium, normal vascularity and yellow hue because of normal fat beneath thin bursal lining.

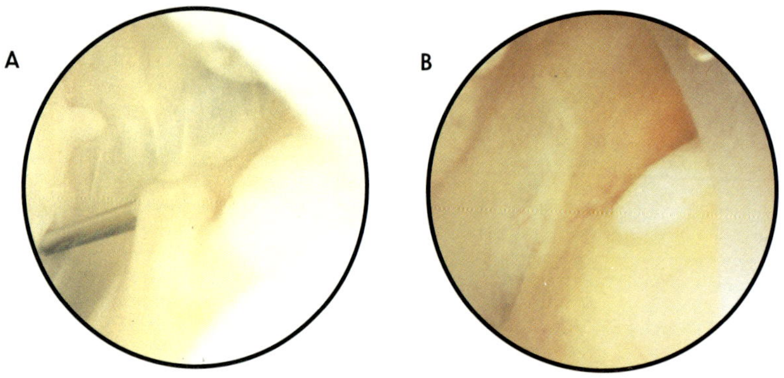

FIG. 6-62 Subacromial bursal folds.

A Arthroscopic view of subacromial bursa shows plica elevated with a spinal needle.

B Arthroscopic view of superior aspect of the rotator cuff circumscribed with a subacromial fold.

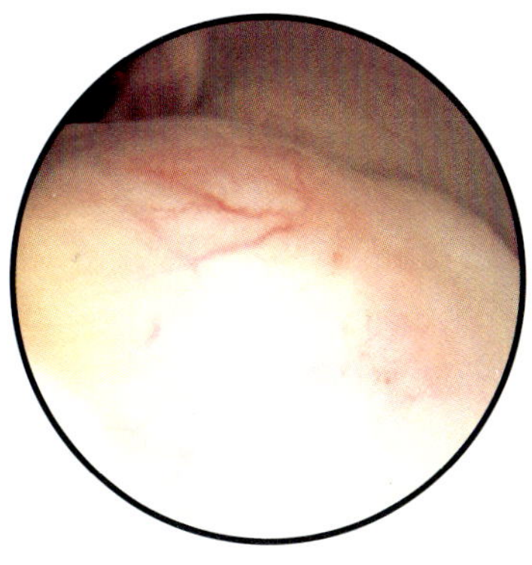

FIG. 6-63 Arthroscopic view of normal vascularity on superior surface of the supraspinatus tendon within the subacromial space.

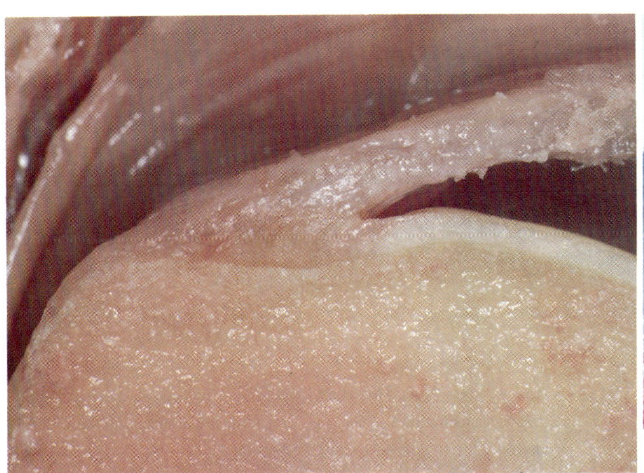

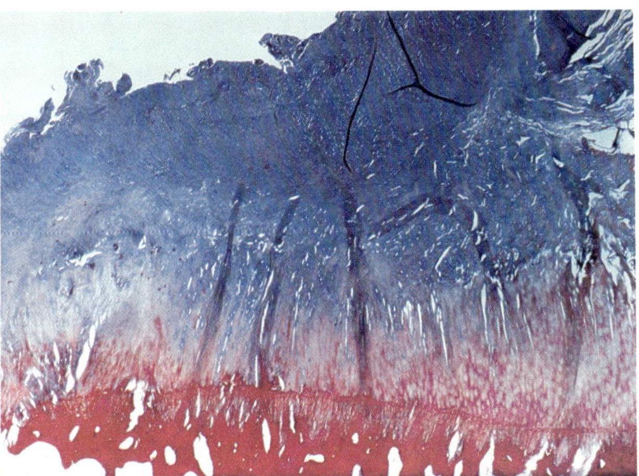

A B

FIG. 6-64 Supraspinatus tendon.

A Gross anatomical cross-section of supraspinatus tendon insertion into the humeral head. The subacromial bursa is superior.

B Photomicrograph of supraspinatus tendon insertion to humerus. Notice the tendon in blue and the bone in red. (Trichrome stain, original magnification ×40.)

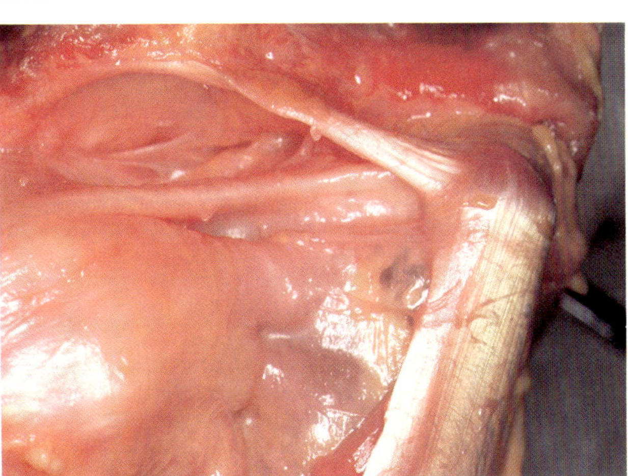

FIG. 6-65 Coracohumeral ligament. Gross anatomical dissection shows the coracoid process with conjoined tendon below and CA ligament above. The CA ligament traverses the floor of the subacromial bursa.

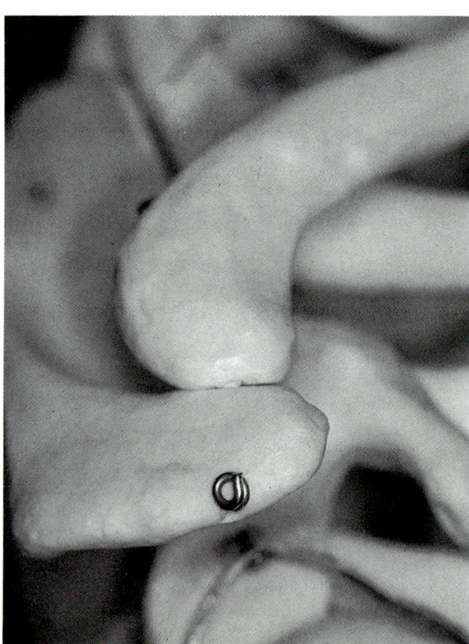

FIG. 6-66 Bony AC joint. Articulated skeleton shows the AC joint from above.

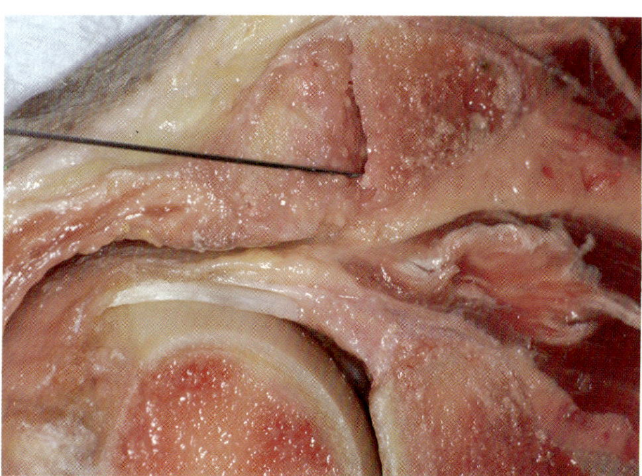

FIG. 6-67 AC joint. Gross anatomical dissection in cross-section shows a needle pointing to the joint. Note the juxtaposition to the subacromial space and the biceps tendon below.

Acromioclavicular Joint

Entering the normal AC joint is difficult. It is small because of its bony confines (Fig. 6-66). The potential space is further decreased by the presence of a normal meniscal disc. I have not seen the normal space arthroscopically, only by anatomical dissection.

The AC joint is immediately superior to the subacromial bursa (Fig. 6-67).

As with the subacromial bursa, the AC joint is more easily and appropriately entered when pathologic (see Chapter 10). In the diseased AC joint, a torn meniscus may not be visible arthroscopically. The view is of articular cartilage on both sides with synovitis.

REFERENCES

1. Andrews JR, Broussard TS, Carson WG: Arthroscopy of the shoulder in the management of partial tears of the rotator cuff: a preliminary report, *Arthroscopy* 1:117, 1985.
2. Andrews JR, Carson WG Jr, Ortega K: Arthroscopy of the shoulder: techniques and normal anatomy, *Am J Sports Med* 12:1-7, 1984.
3. Blachut PA, Day B: Arthroscopy anatomy of the shoulder, *Arthroscopy* 5:1-10, 1989.
4. Caspari RA: Personal communication (with credit to Jules Neviaser), 1984.
5. Clark J, Sidles JA, Matsen FA: The relationship of the glenohumeral joint capsule to the rotator cuff, *Clin Orthop* 254(5):29-34, 1990.
6. Codman EA: Stiff and painful shoulders. The anatomy of the subdeltoid subacromial bursa and its clinical importance: subdeltoid bursitis, *Boston Med Surg J* 154:613-620, 1906.
7. Detrisac DA, Johnson LL: *Arthroscopic shoulder anatomy: pathological and surgical implications,* Thoroughfare, NJ, 1986, Slack.
8. Gross M, Fitzgibbons TC: Shoulder arthroscopy: a modified approach, *Arthroscopy* 1(3):156-159, 1985.
9. Howell SM, Gilanat BJ: The glenoid-labral socket, *Clin Orth Rel Res* 243(6):122-125, 1989.
10. Johnson LL: The shoulder joint: an arthroscopist's perspective of anatomy and pathology, *Clin Orthop* 223:113-125, 1987.
11. Johnson LL: Arthroscopy of the shoulder, *Orthop Clin North Am* 11(2):197-204, 1980.

11a. Johnson LL, Bays BM, van Dyk GE: Vincula of the biceps tendon in the glenohumeral joint: an arthroscopic and anatomic study, *J Shoulder Elbow Surgery* 1(3):162-166, 1992.

12. Lohr JF, Uhthoff HK: The microvascular pattern of the supraspinatus tendon, *Clin Orthop* 254(5):35-38, 1990.
13. Matthews LS, Fadale PD: Subacromial anatomy for the arthroscopist, *Arthroscopy* 5(1):36-40, 1989.
14. Matthews LS, Terry G, Vetter WL: Shoulder anatomy for the arthroscopist, *Arthroscopy* 1(2):83-91, 1985.

14a. McGlynn FJ, Caspari RB: Arthroscopic findings in the subluxating shoulder, *Clin Orthop* 183:173, 1984.

15. Moseley HF, Overgaard B: The anterior capsular mechanism in recurrent anterior dislocation of the shoulder: morphological and clinical studies with special reference to the glenoid labrum and the glenohumeral ligaments, *J Bone Joint Surg* 44B:913, 1962.
16. O'Brien SJ et al: The anatomy and histology of the inferior glenohumeral ligament complex of the shoulder, *Am J Sports Med* 18:449-456, 1990.
17. Richardson AB: Arthroscopic anatomy of the shoulder, *Tech Orthop* 3:1-7, 1988.
18. Rockwood CA Jr, Matsen FA III: *The shoulder,* Philadelphia, 1990, WB Saunders.
19. Rowe CR: *The shoulder,* New York, 1988, Churchill Livingstone.
20. Snyder SJ et al: SLAP lesions of the shoulder, *Arthroscopy* 6(4):274-279, 1990.
21. Snyder SJ, Rames RD, Morgan CD: Anatomical variations of the glenohumeral ligaments, *Arthroscopy* 7(3):328, 1991.
22. Souryal TO, Baker CL: Anatomy of the supraclavicular fossa portal in shoulder arthroscopy, *Arthroscopy* 6(4):297-300, 1990.

22a. Townly CO: The capsule mechanism in recurrent dislocation of the shoulder, *J Bone Joint Surg* 32A:370-380, 1950.

22b. Turkel SJ et al: Stabilizing mechanisms preventing anterior dislocations of the glenohumeral joint, *J Bone Joint Surg* 63A(8):1208-1217, 1981.

23. Wissinger HA: Personal communication, 1982.
24. Wolfe EM: Anterior portals in shoulder arthroscopy, *Arthroscopy* 5(3):201-208, 1989.

CHAPTER

7 Pathologic Anatomy

Recognition of the various intraarticular lesions by arthroscopy directs the surgeon to the nature and magnitude of the problem.[14] This chapter will emphasize the arthroscopic identification of various lesions in the shoulder. Later chapters detail the arthroscopic approach and treatment of these pathologic conditions.

GLENOHUMERAL JOINT

Bone

Hill-Sachs Lesion. The most common disruption of bone seen during arthroscopy is the Hill-Sachs lesion.[4,11] This lesion is a compression fracture of the posterior humeral head following anterior dislocation of the glenohumeral joint (Fig. 7-1). This lesion must be differentiated from the normal posterior bare spot on the back of the humeral head near the synovial reflection (Fig. 7-1).

The presence of a Hill-Sachs lesion confirms the diagnosis of a dislocation; however, the absence of a bony Hill-Sachs lesion does not rule out dislocation. In a very loose-jointed person, a dislocation can occur without injuring the surface or the bone. In some cases the injury is limited to the articular cartilage without evidence of bony injury with the dislocation.

The depth of the Hill-Sachs lesion varies (Fig. 7-2). The original description of this lesion was restricted to bone compression.[11] The magnification provided by arthroscopy may show only articular cartilage disruption following anterior dislocation (Fig. 7-3).

The site of the lesion is posterior, but the exact location varies between superior, inferior, proximal, and distal (Fig. 7-4). The lesion may involve the entire posterior humerus (Fig. 7-5). The compression fracture may be on the juxtaarticular surface of the humeral head (Fig. 7-6).

A

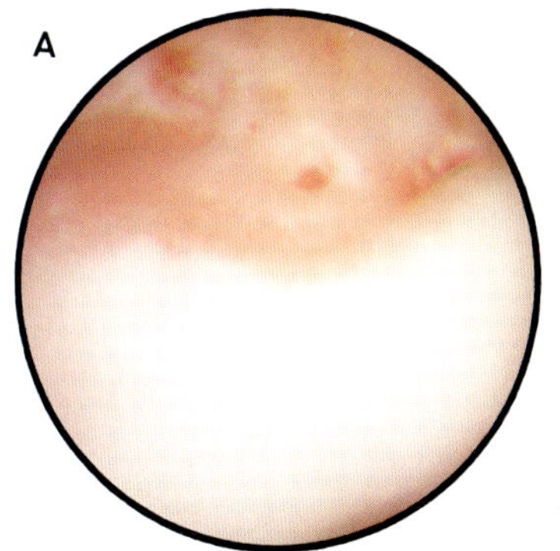

B

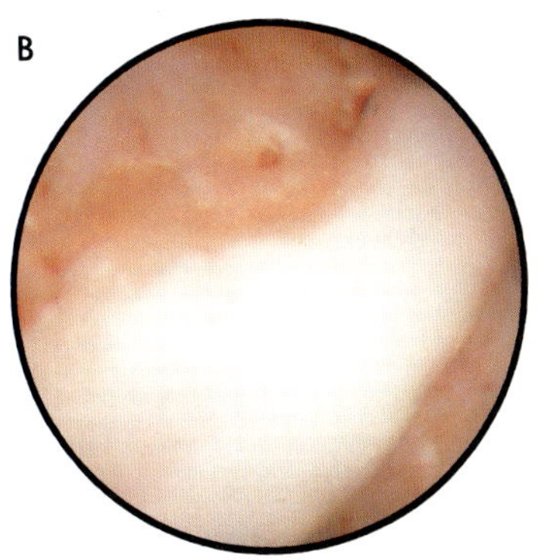

C

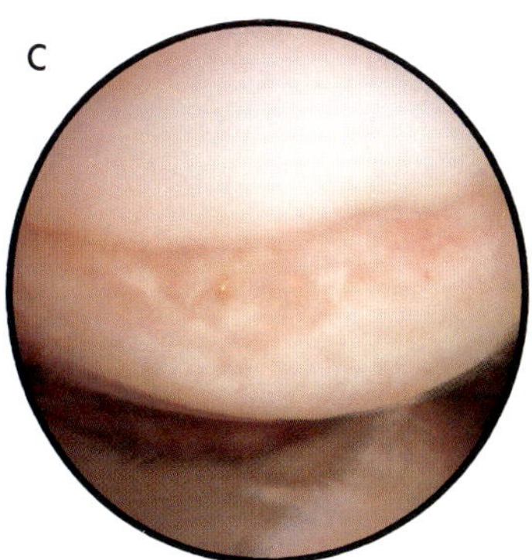

FIG. 7-1 Hill-Sachs lesion with anterior dislocation.

A Normal synovial reflection at margin of articular cartilage in adult.

B Normal synovial reflection and edge of Hill-Sachs lesion.

C Further penetration of scope shows Hill-Sachs lesion.

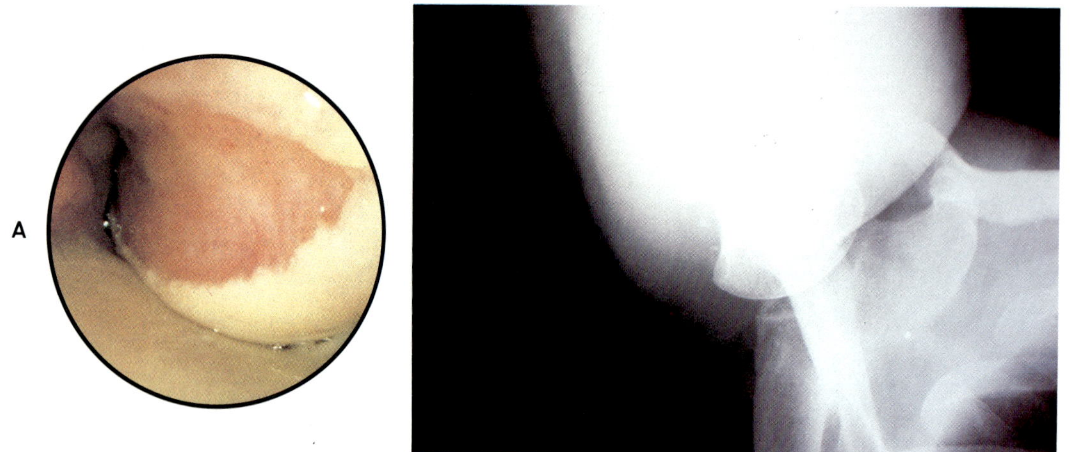

FIG. 7-2 Hill-Sachs lesion. The Hill-Sachs lesion varies in position, size and depth.

A Arthroscopic view from posterior of right shoulder showing large posterior and inferior defect representing compression fracture of the humeral head.

B X-ray view by Stryker technique shows similar large bony defect on posterior humeral head.

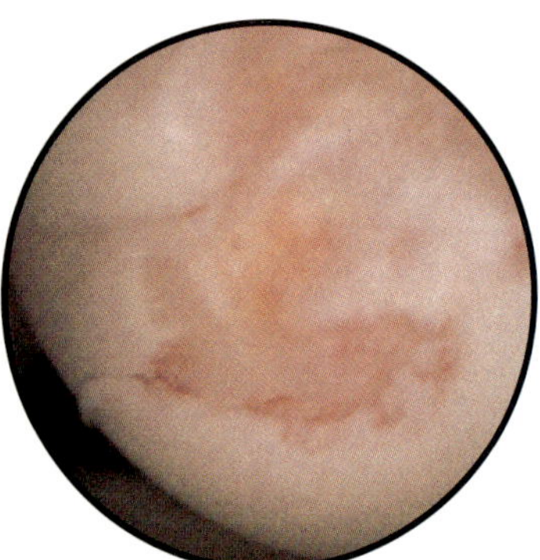

FIG. 7-3 Superficial depth of Hill-Sachs lesion. This arthroscopic view shows Hill-Sachs lesion with loss only of articular cartilage. The x-ray film would be negative for bony defect in this type of case.

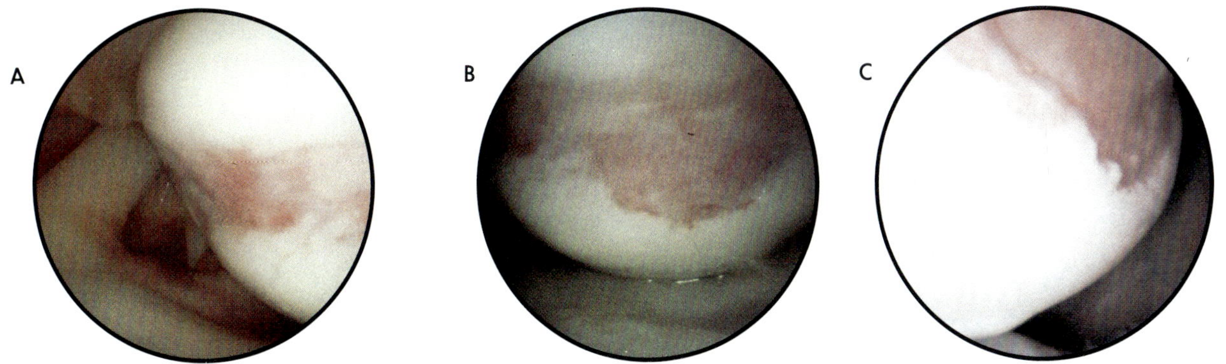

FIG. 7-4 Various locations of Hill-Sachs lesion.

A Arthroscopic view of right shoulder from posterior shows lesion located superior.

B Arthroscopic view of right shoulder from posterior shows lesion central and covering the entire length of the humeral head.

C Arthroscopic view of right shoulder from posterior shows lesion inferior.

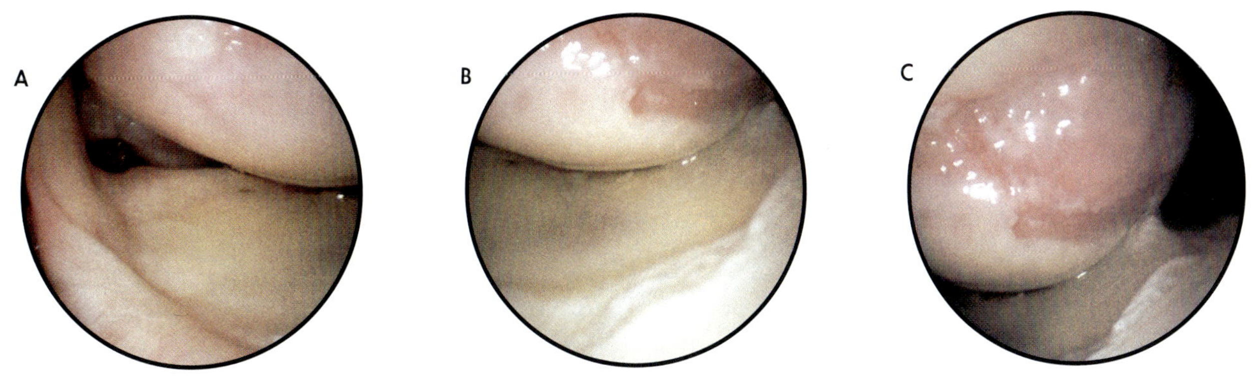

FIG. 7-5 Hill-Sachs lesion over entire length of humeral head.

A Arthroscopic view of right shoulder from posterior shows elipse of superior aspect of lesion.

B Arthroscopic view from posterior of same patient in *A* shows central area envolvement.

C Arthroscopic view from posterior of same patient in *A* shows larger portion of lesion extends to inferior humeral head.

FIG. 7-6 Juxtaarticular position of the Hill-Sachs lesion. This arthroscopic view shows the position of the Hill-Sachs lesion to be opposite the glenoid. Note the articular cartilage remains intact in the area of the compression fracture.

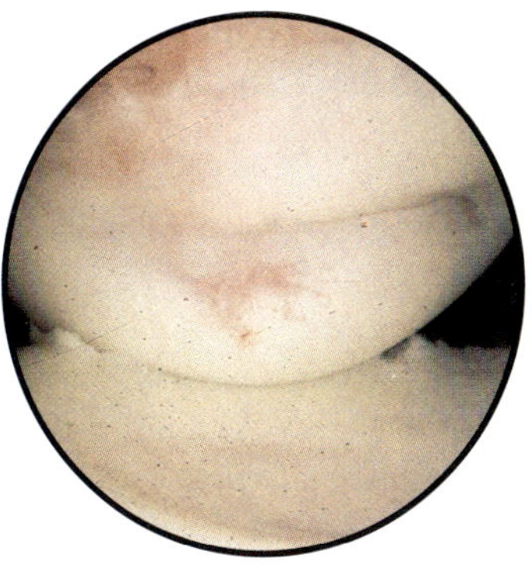

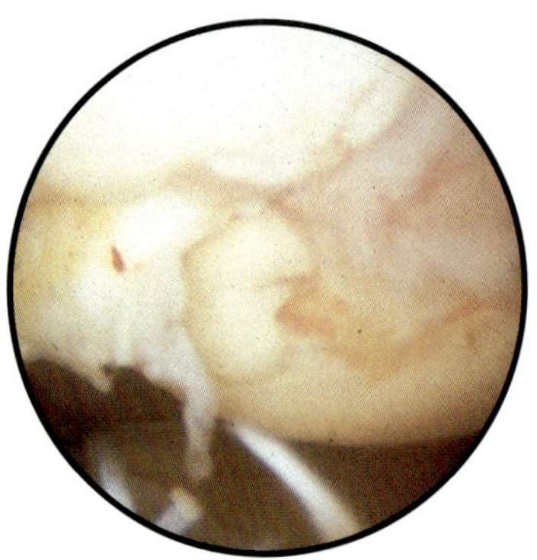

FIG. 7-7 Fragmentation on Hill-Sachs lesion. The Hill-Sachs lesion may have fragmentation, even loosely attached bone or cartilage, as impending loose bodies. Arthroscopic debridement is indicated.

The surface of the Hill-Sachs lesion may be smooth or fragmented (Fig. 7-7). Often large fragments are loosely attached and ready to become loose bodies. This finding is an indication for arthroscopic debridement.

The size of the lesion also varies (see Fig. 7-2); it may be small or large (see Fig. 7-3). The largest lesions may be an indication for a Connolly procedure that transfers the infraspinatus tendon into the large defect (see Fig. 7-2, *A;* also see Chapter 8).

The shape of the lesion varies (see Figs. 7-2, 7-3, 7-4, and 7-6); it may be linear, oval, or round.

In posterior dislocation of the glenohumeral joint the anterior humeral head sustains a compression fracture. This is called a McLaughlin lesion and may be identified by x-ray film.[15a] This condition is uncommon. I have not seen it arthroscopically.

Osteochondritis Dissecans. I have seen a lesion of the glenoid that appears like osteochondritis dissecans as seen in the knee. The shape of the lesion was round. The depth included both articular cartilage and bone of at least 1 cm. The condition in the shoulder may not be the same as the knee, although I am not aware of a previous description in the glenoid. The etiology may not be the same in each case. In the shoulder, the lesion may be traumatic avulsion of bone or secondary to other disease, such as rheumatoid arthritis.

Two of my patients with this condition were throwing athletes. In one, a professional baseball pitcher, the central large fragment was removed. Within 2 months the patient had a subsequent open CA ligament sectioning without acromioplasty by another surgeon. He continued a successful career from age 33 to age 41. An x-ray film taken 8 years after the interventions showed degeneration of the glenohumeral joint as he concluded his career (Fig. 7-8).

The other patient was an amateur baseball player who had an avulsion of the glenoid bone attached to the posterior labrum (Fig. 7-9). The undersurface of the defect appeared like osteochondritis of the knee. A debridement of the fragment and the base plus fixation with staple resulted in healing (Fig. 7-9, *C*).

A third patient with osteochondritis dissecans of the glenoid had severe juvenile rheumatoid arthritis (Fig. 7-10). The glenoid fragment was removed during arthroscopic synovectomy.

I have not seen osteochondritis dissecans of the humerus.

Intraarticular Fracture. The most common intraarticular fracture for the arthroscopic shoulder surgeon accompanies anterior glenohumeral dislocation (Fig. 7-11). This fracture varies in size. The site may be only the avulsion of the anterior glenoid with attached anterior glenohumeral ligaments. In some cases a portion of the articular cartilage may be included (Fig. 7-12).

Arthroscopy may be used in the shoulder as in the knee to evaluate other intraarticular or juxtaarticular fractures to determine the alignment and/or displacement.

Aseptic Necrosis. Aseptic necrosis can occur in the humeral head (Fig. 7-13).[10] This condition is associated with sickle cell disease, lupus erythematosus, alcoholism, and diabetes mellitus. It may be the source of loose bodies. Arthroscopic debridement alone may benefit the early small lesion.

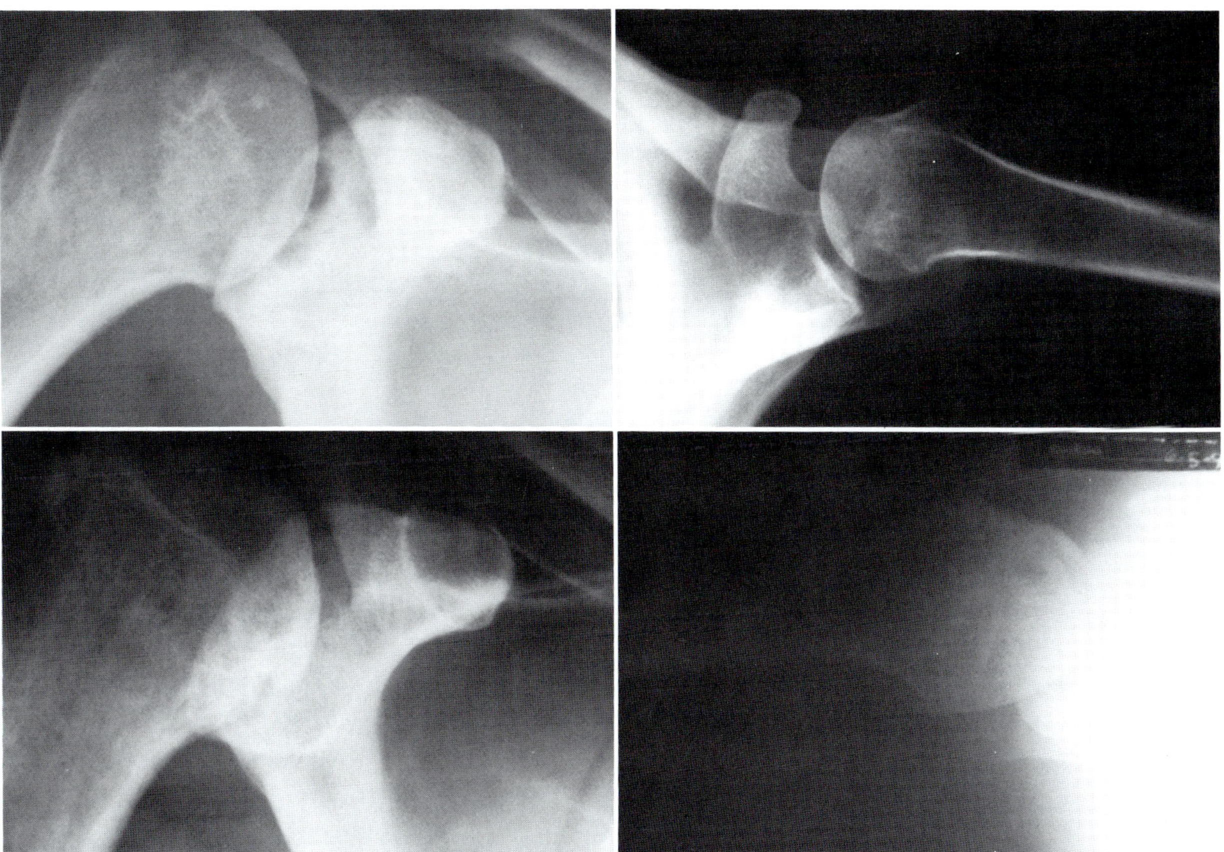

FIG. 7-8 Osteochondritis dissecans of the glenoid: Long-term follow-up. These are shoulder x-ray films of a professional baseball pitcher 8 years after arthroscopic removal of large osteochondral defect in central lower aspect of glenoid. The player performed at an award-winning level in the National League of baseball even at age 33 and for the next 7 years.

A,B Preoperative x-ray films in 1982. Anterior-posterior and axillary views show lytic lesion in glenoid.

C,D Eight years postoperative x-ray film (1990). Anterior-posterior and axillary views show healing of glenoid defect with deformity of humeral head and osteophytes. Patient was still active in professional baseball despite degenerative changes.

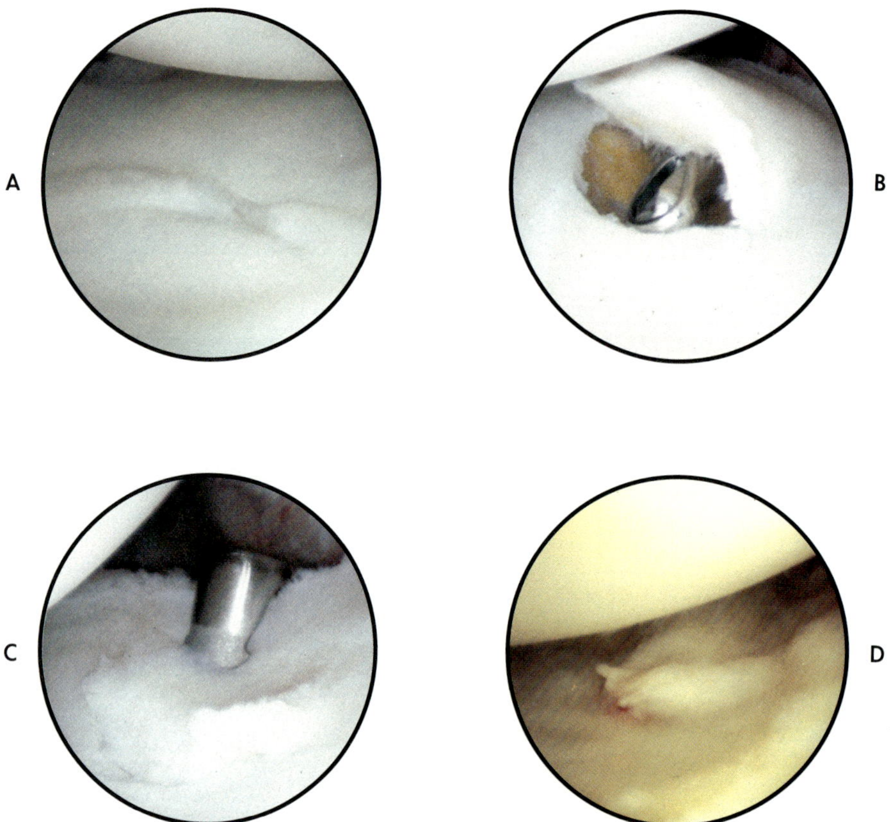

FIG. 7-9 Osteochondritis dissecans of posterior glenoid.

A Arthroscopic view from anterior of avulsion defect of posterior labrum, with bone. Humerus is above. Notice irregular articular surface like osteochondritis dissecans.

B Arthroscopic view from anterior shows defect elevated with full radius resector under the bone. The base was debrided before fixation with metal staple.

C The angle of approach from posterior caused some incongruity of the fixation with the staple.

D Arthroscopic view at 8 weeks at time of planned staple removal. There is some incongruity to the surface. The fragment healed and the patient was rendered asymptomatic after 2 years follow-up.

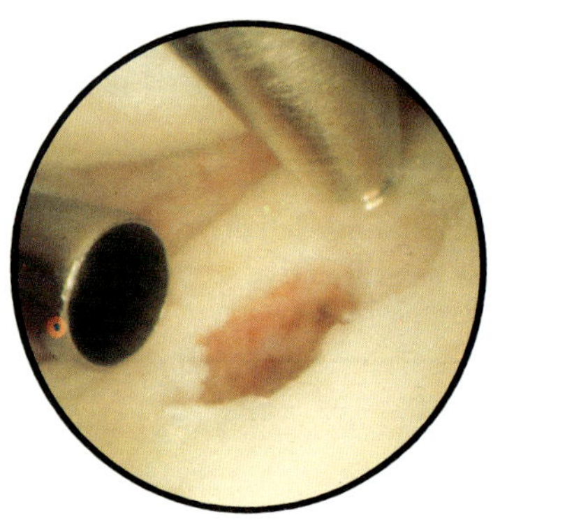

FIG. 7-10 Osteochondritic defect in glenoid.

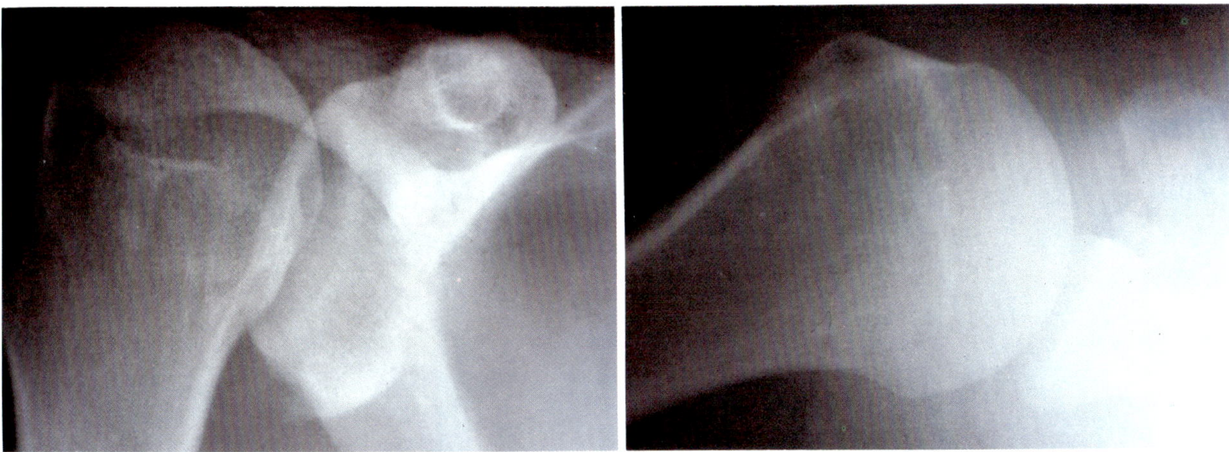

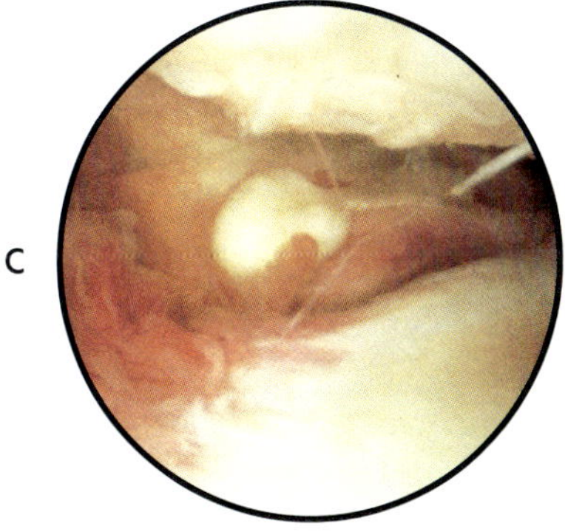

FIG. 7-11 Fracture of glenoid.

A Anterior-posterior x-ray film shows anterior and inferior displaced glenoid fracture.

B Lateral x-ray film shows displaced glenoid fracture.

C Arthroscopic view of displaced anterior glenoid fracture. Note the articular cartilage is still intact on the fracture fragment.

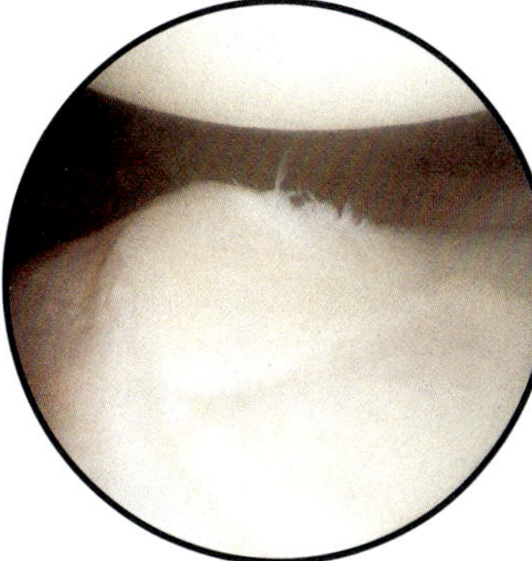

FIG. 7-12 Arthroscopic view shows minimal displacement of intraarticular fracture of the anterior inferior glenoid. The articular cartilage is intact.

A

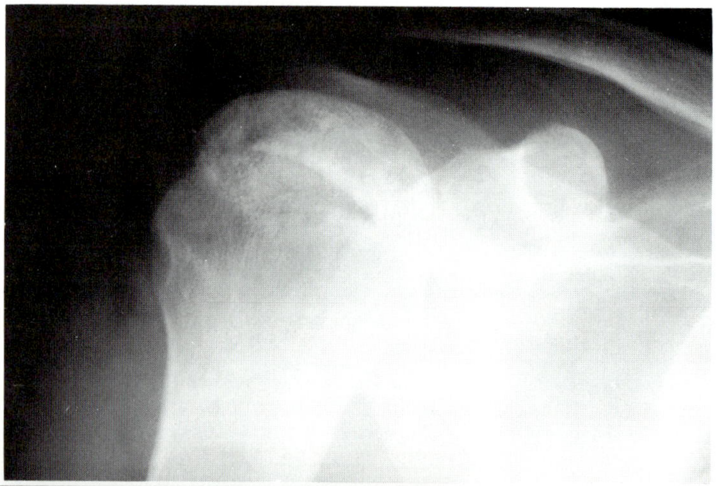

B

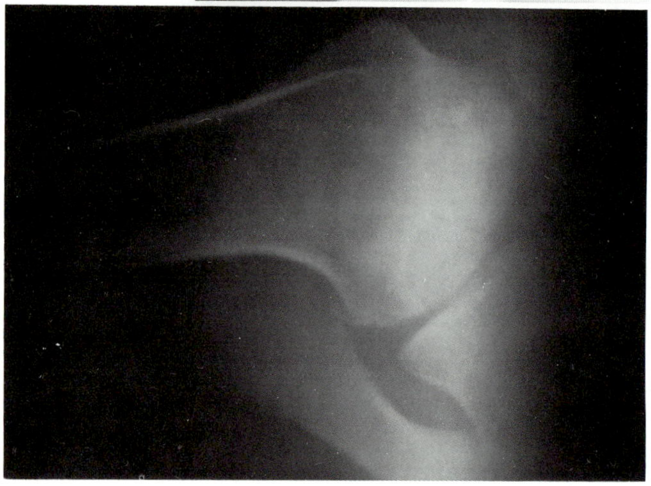

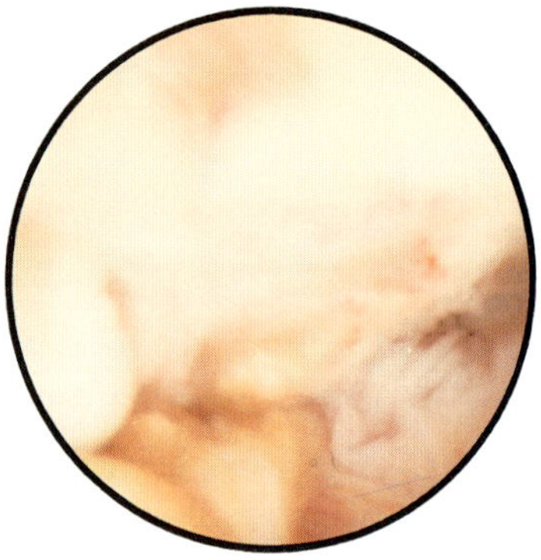

C

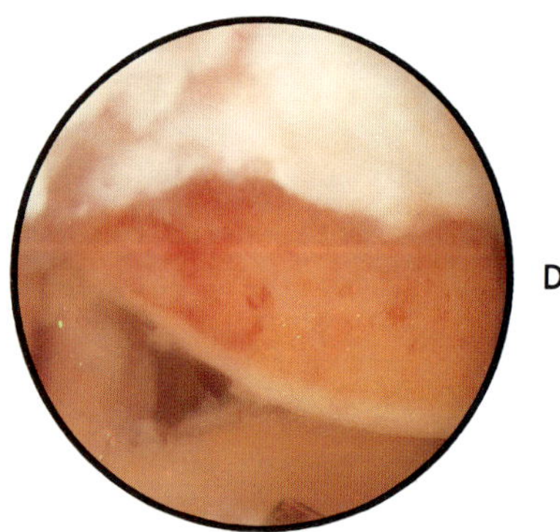

D

FIG. 7-13 **Aseptic necrosis. Although not performed on this patient, arthroscopic bone grafting of small defect is now possible.**

A Anterior-posterior x-ray film of humeral aseptic necrosis.

B Axillary view of large necrotic area. There is no need for arthroscopy in this case.

C Arthroscopic view of another patient with small lesion.

D Postresection area of small lesion. Removed necrotic area to exposed bone.

Articular Cartilage

Recognition of either traumatic or degenerative lesions is important in patient management in that their presence adversely affects the prognosis.

Traumatic. Traumatic lesions of the articular cartilage are commonly visualized by arthroscopy. They are usually partial thickness. Crepitus on physical examination may increase the surgeon's suspicion of the injury. If that bone is not injured, traumatic lesions are not suspected by x-ray examination. The incidence of articular cartilage lesions was high in my diagnostic arthroscopy series of patients with traumatic glenohumeral dislocation. Often the traumatic lesion was on the opposing surfaces of the joint, not just restricted to the expected posterior area of the Hill-Sachs lesion (see Fig. 7-6). This position results in clicking and catching with everyday motion.

Degenerative. Degenerative changes of the articular cartilage secondary to trauma are commonly seen at arthroscopy (Fig. 7-14).[21] The small or superficial lesion may be seen only with arthroscopy, and its presence adversely affects the prognosis (Fig. 7-14, *A* and *B*). The glenoid may be involved in varying degrees and depth (Fig. 7-15).

Fragmentation may occur off the articular surface (Fig. 7-16). Labral fragmentation is also common with degenerative arthritis (Fig. 7-17).

Primary degenerative arthritis is an infrequent reason for arthroscopy (Fig. 7-18).

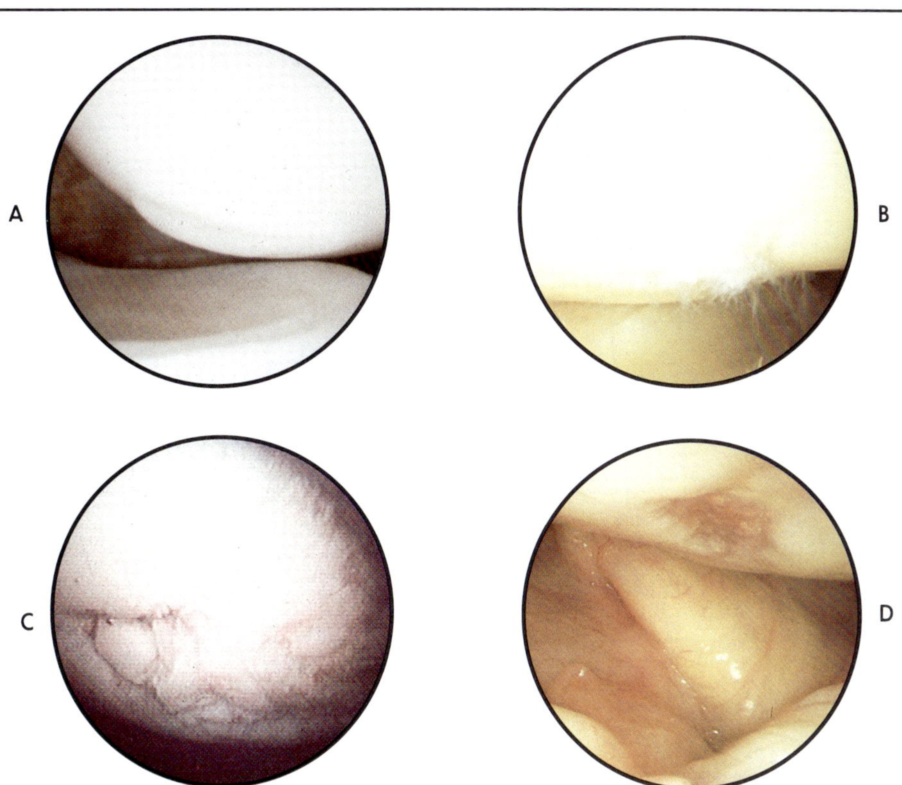

FIG. 7-14 Humeral head degenerative arthritis.

A Arthroscopic view shows degenerative bubble on juxtaarticular aspect of humerus.

B Arthroscopic view shows fibrillation of humeral surface.

C Arthroscopic view shows fragmentation of humeral head.

D Arthroscopic view shows defect with loss of both bone and cartilage on humeral head, following trauma of dislocation. This is not a classic Hill-Sachs lesion because of its anterior position.

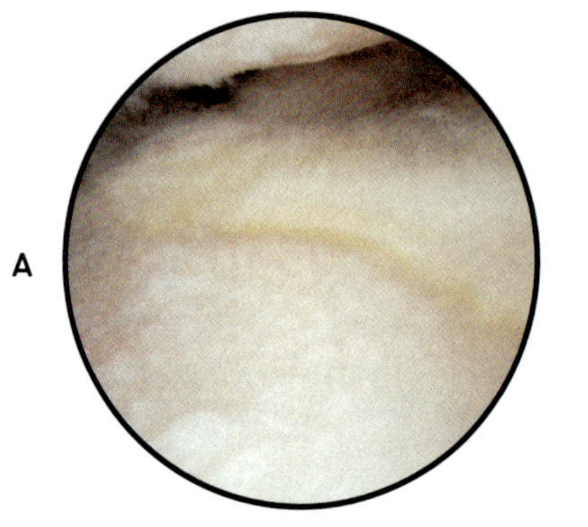

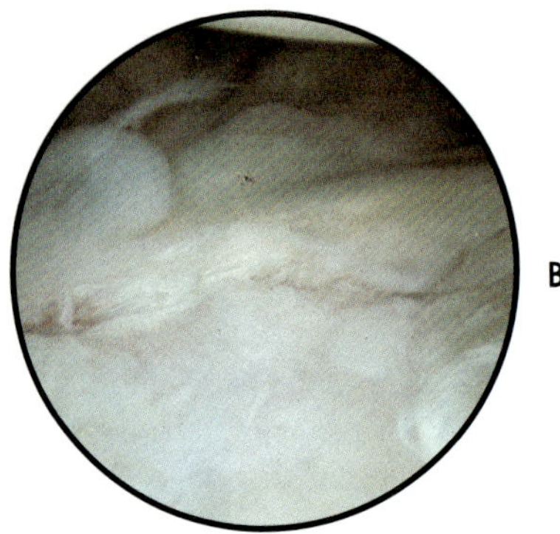

FIG. 7-15 Glenoid degenerative arthritis.

A Arthroscopic view shows thinning of glenoid surface cartilage and patches of repair.

B Arthroscopic view shows greater magnitude of degenerative change with surface disruption and attempts at repair.

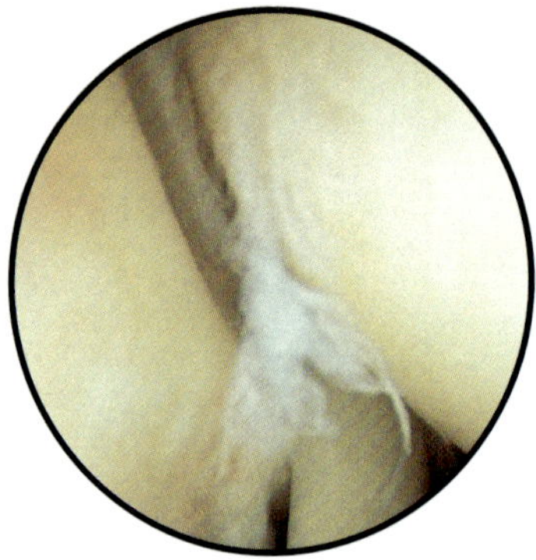

FIG. 7-16 Fragmentation of articular cartilage: Arthroscopic view shows fragment breaking off of posterior-superior humeral head.

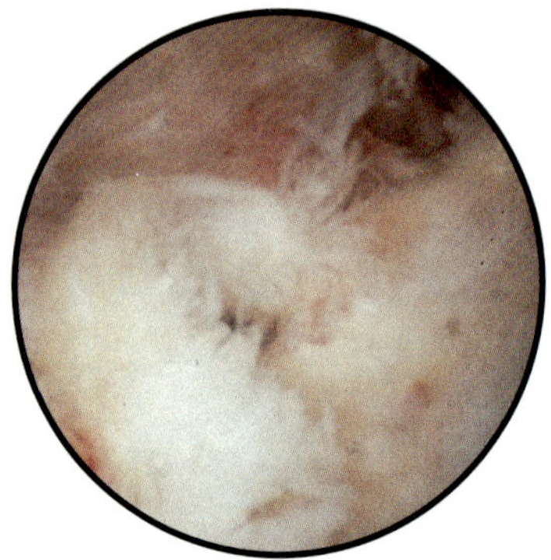

FIG. 7-17 Labral tissue fragmentation: Arthroscopic view of fragmentation of labrum, which can be source of glenohumeral loose bodies.

FIG. 7-18 Degenerative arthritis. (Opposite page.)

A Anterior-posterior x-ray film of degenerative arthritis in shoulder with incongruity of joint surface.

B Axillary view shows fattening of humeral head.

C Arthroscopic view of degenerative synovitis near biceps tendon.

D Degeneration and fragmentation on humeral head.

E Granular degenerative change on humerus.

F Arthroscopic view of exposed bone with natural restored areas of fibrocartilage and recent hemorrhage of surface vessels.

G Arthroscopic close-up of hemorrhage areas on glenoid.

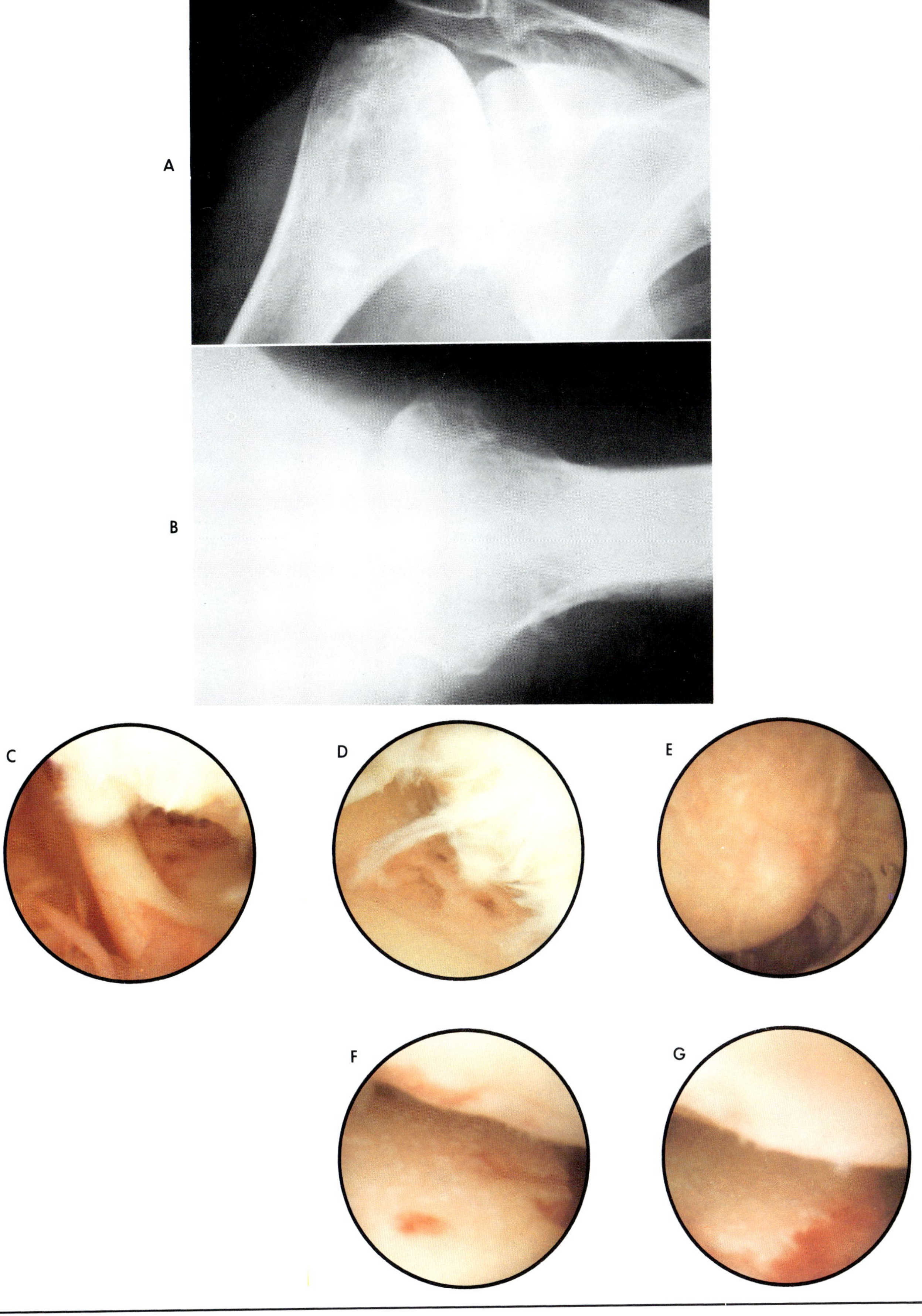
A
B
C
D
E
F
G

Loose Bodies

Loose bodies are common following trauma (Fig. 7-19). They vary greatly in size and shape. The round and smooth surfaces occur with time and exposure, similar to what happens with the tumbling of pebbles on a beach.

These bodies are usually cartilaginous in origin from the articular surface or labrum (Fig. 7-20, *A*). They may originate from a free fragment of rotator cuff, tendon, or ligament (Fig. 7-20, *B*). They may be free-floating small pieces of synovium, as though villi had rubbed off into the joint.

They are usually loose but may be attached to the synovium or even buried in the capsule (Fig. 7-21).

They may reside in any recess, but the subscapularis bursa is the most common site. The surgeon may need to switch to an anterior portal to see to the bottom of the subscapularis bursa (Fig. 7-22).

Vacuuming during diagnostic arthroscopy is necessary to expose hidden loose bodies, because they tend to be multiple (Fig. 7-23).

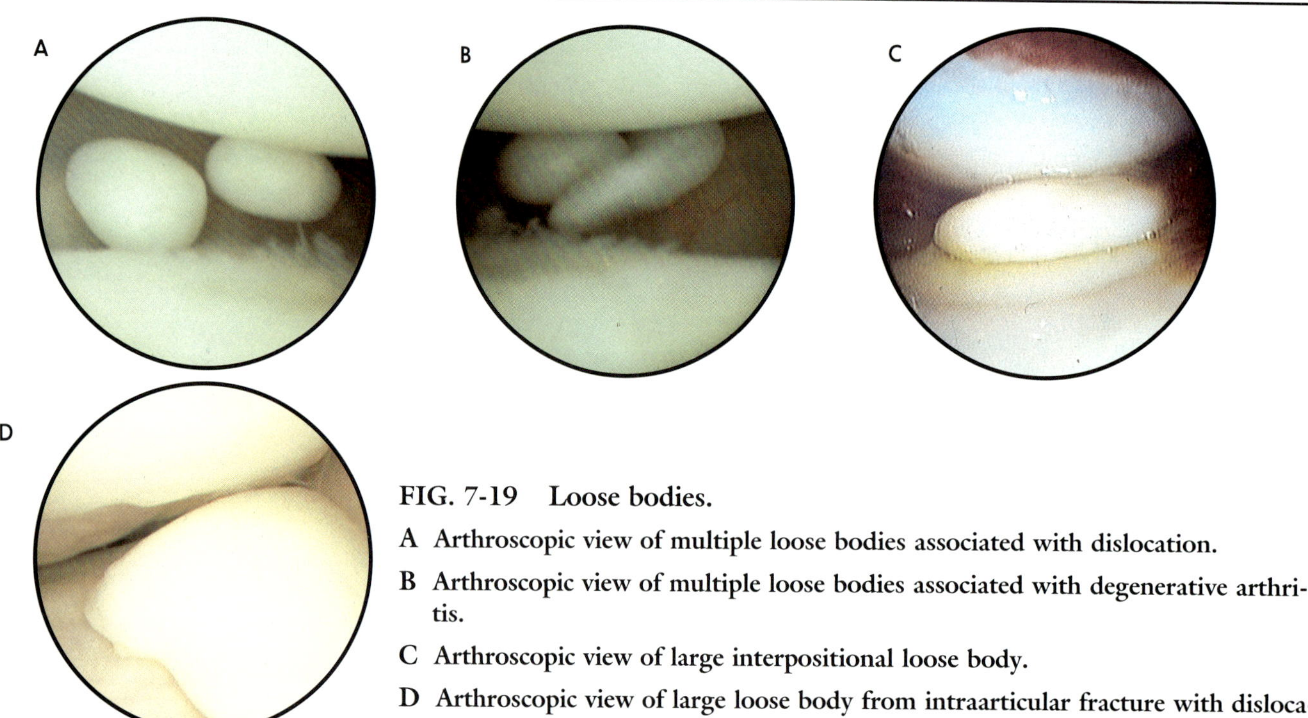

FIG. 7-19 Loose bodies.

A Arthroscopic view of multiple loose bodies associated with dislocation.

B Arthroscopic view of multiple loose bodies associated with degenerative arthritis.

C Arthroscopic view of large interpositional loose body.

D Arthroscopic view of large loose body from intraarticular fracture with dislocation.

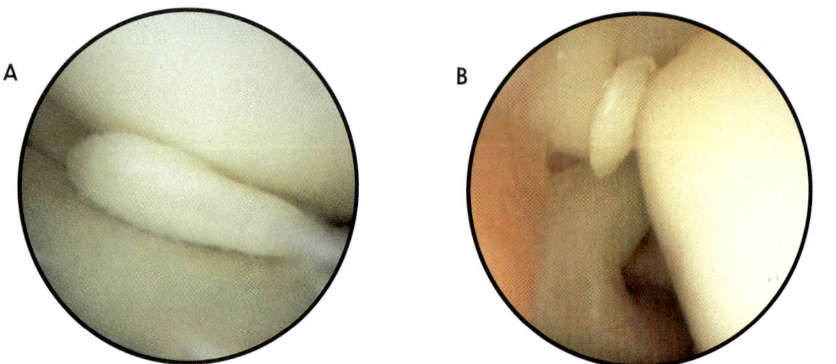

FIG. 7-20 Source of loose body varies.

A Arthroscopic view of attached loose body from labrum.

B Arthroscopic view of loose body of rotator cuff tendinous origin in air medium.

FIG. 7-21 Attached loose bodies. This arthroscopic view shows loose bodies that are attached to the anterior synovium.

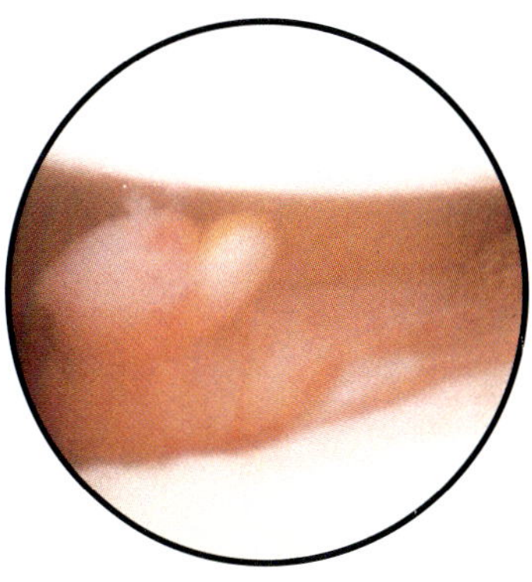

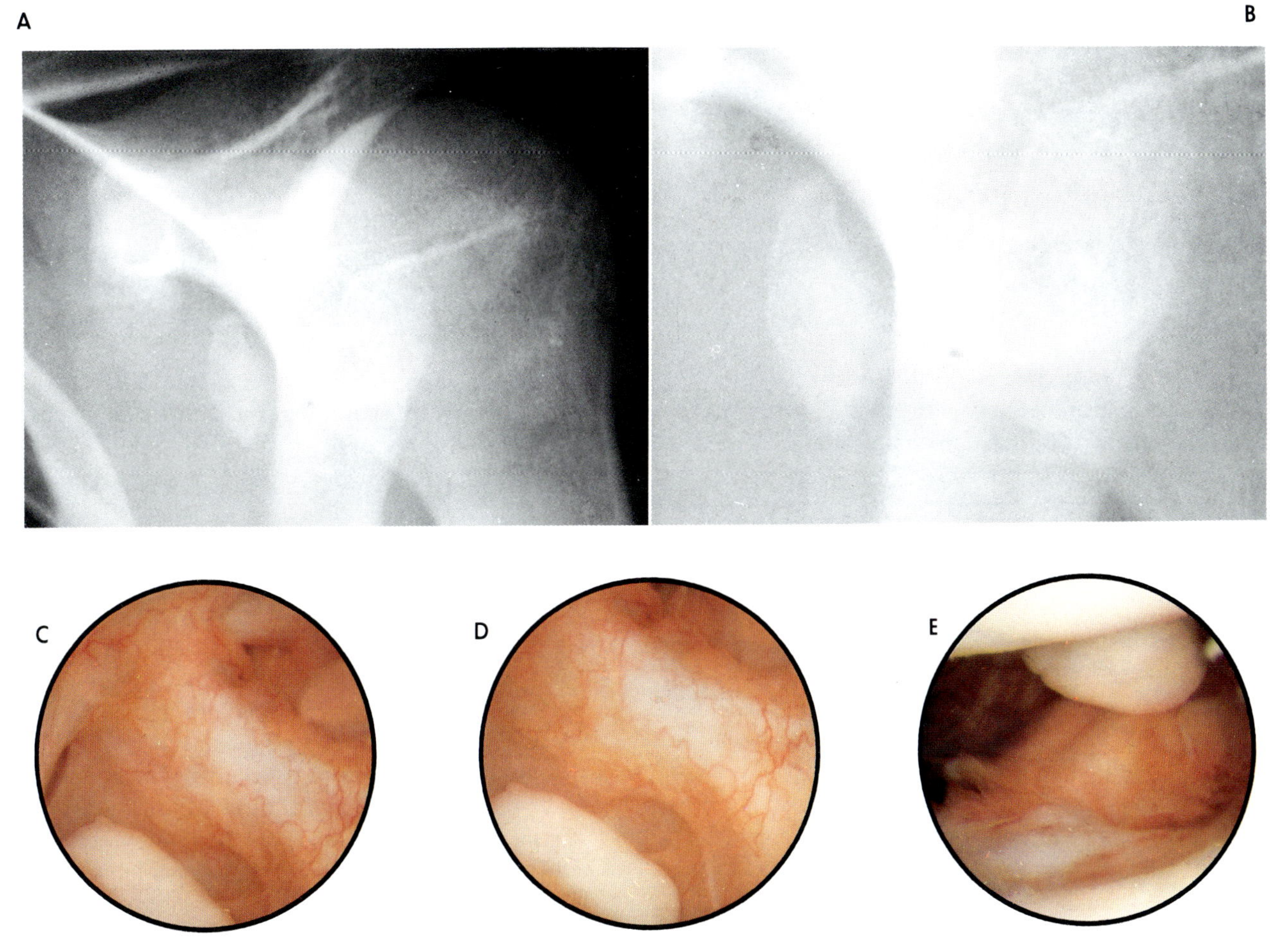

A B

C D E

FIG. 7-22 Loose body in shoulder.

A X-ray film shows large loose body in subscapularis bursa.

B Close-up of x-ray film of large loose body.

C Arthroscopic view of loose body in subscapularis bursa.

D View after penetration of arthroscope into depth of bursa.

E Same loose body mobilized out of bursa with suction attachment to end of arthroscope.

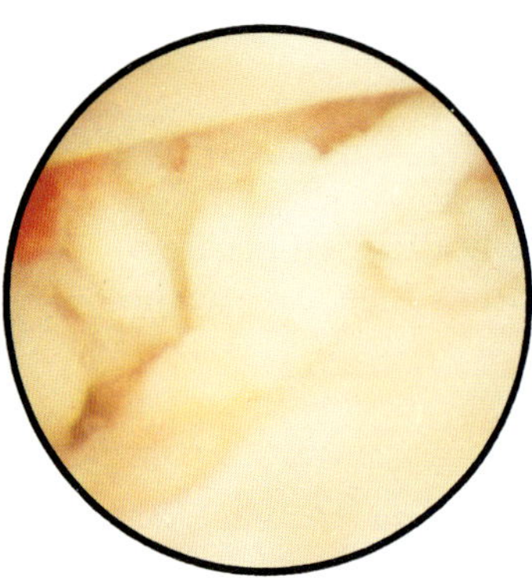

FIG. 7-23 Multiple loose bodies.

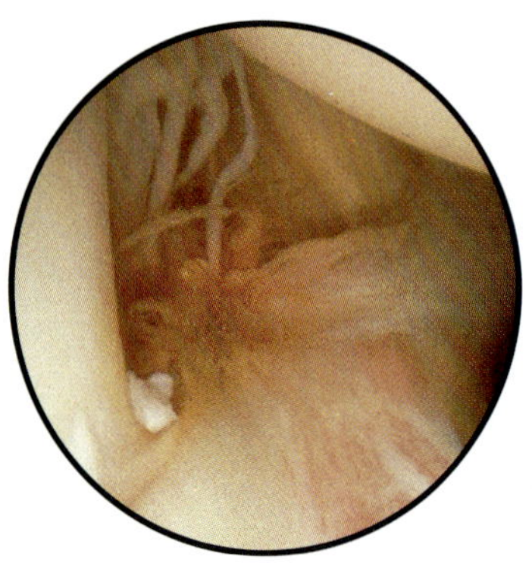

FIG. 7-24 Traumatic synovitis. Arthroscopic view shows traumatic synovitis that is superior to subscapularis tendon and covering area of superior glenohumeral ligament.

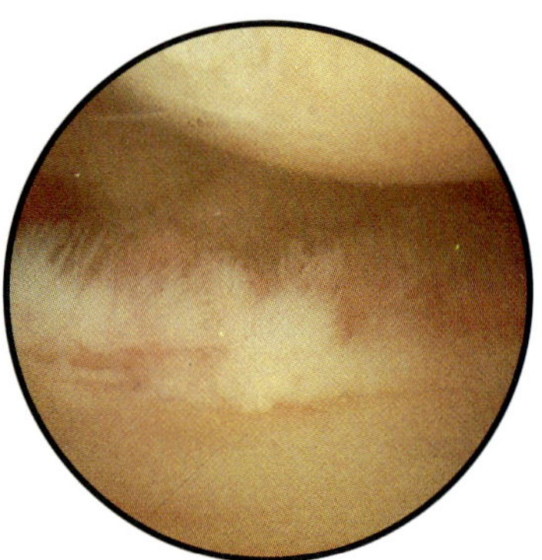

FIG. 7-25 Postoperative synovitis. Arthroscopic view of diffuse postoperative synovitis at 3 weeks following surgery.

Synovium

Types of Synovitis

Traumatic synovitis. Traumatic synovitis is common following anterior glenohumeral dislocations (Fig. 7-24). The area most commonly affected is anterior and superior. The color of the inflamed area is reddish brown. Vascular villi are present.

Postoperative synovitis. Postoperative synovitis may be seen after either open or arthroscopic surgery (Fig. 7-25). The inflamed area in this type of synovitis is red and vascular in origin.

Foreign body synovitis. A foreign body, like a loose or exposed metallic implant, may cause a reactive synovitis (see Chapter 8).

Degenerative synovitis. Synovitis accompanies degenerative arthritis (Fig. 7-26).

Rheumatoid arthritis. Rheumatoid arthritis has a characteristic appearance (Fig. 7-27). The fibrinoid exudate on tips of villi stain positive with methylene blue stain.

Pigmented villonodular synovitis and osteochondromatosis. Pigmented villonodular synovitis and osteochondromatosis are not common in the shoulder (Fig. 7-28). When present, they may be diagnosable only by arthroscopy. They are treatable by arthroscopic means.

Vascular synovitis. The glenohumeral joint has normal abundant and prominent vascularity. The normal state must be recognized so as not to misdiagnose normal (Figs. 7-29 and 7-30). The normal vascular pattern enters the small holes on the bare area of the posterior humerus (Fig. 7-30, *A*). Vessels normally course inside the vincula of the biceps tendon (Fig. 7-30, *B*). A small number of vessels may normally exist on the free span of the CA ligament (Fig. 7-30, *C*). Vessels normally occur on the superior aspect of the rotator cuff tendon (Fig. 7-30 D). The central area over the rotator cuff tendon is usually devoid of vessels. The normal vascularity is without inflammation (Fig. 7-31).

Pathological vascular synovitis usually has accompanying villous formation.

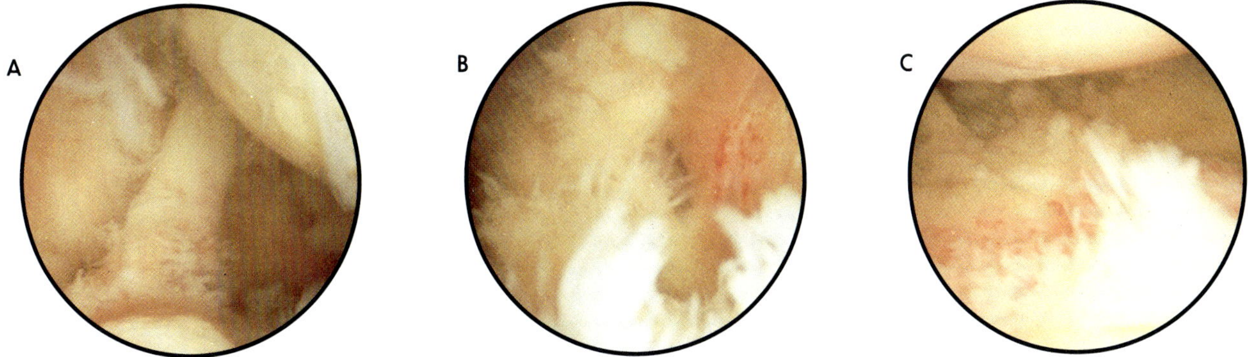

FIG. 7-26 Degenerative synovitis.

A Arthroscopic view of superior glenohumeral joint shows diffuse degenerative synovitis.

B Arthroscopic view of anterior wall shows diffuse synovitis.

C Arthroscopic view shows diffuse synovitis over inferior joint.

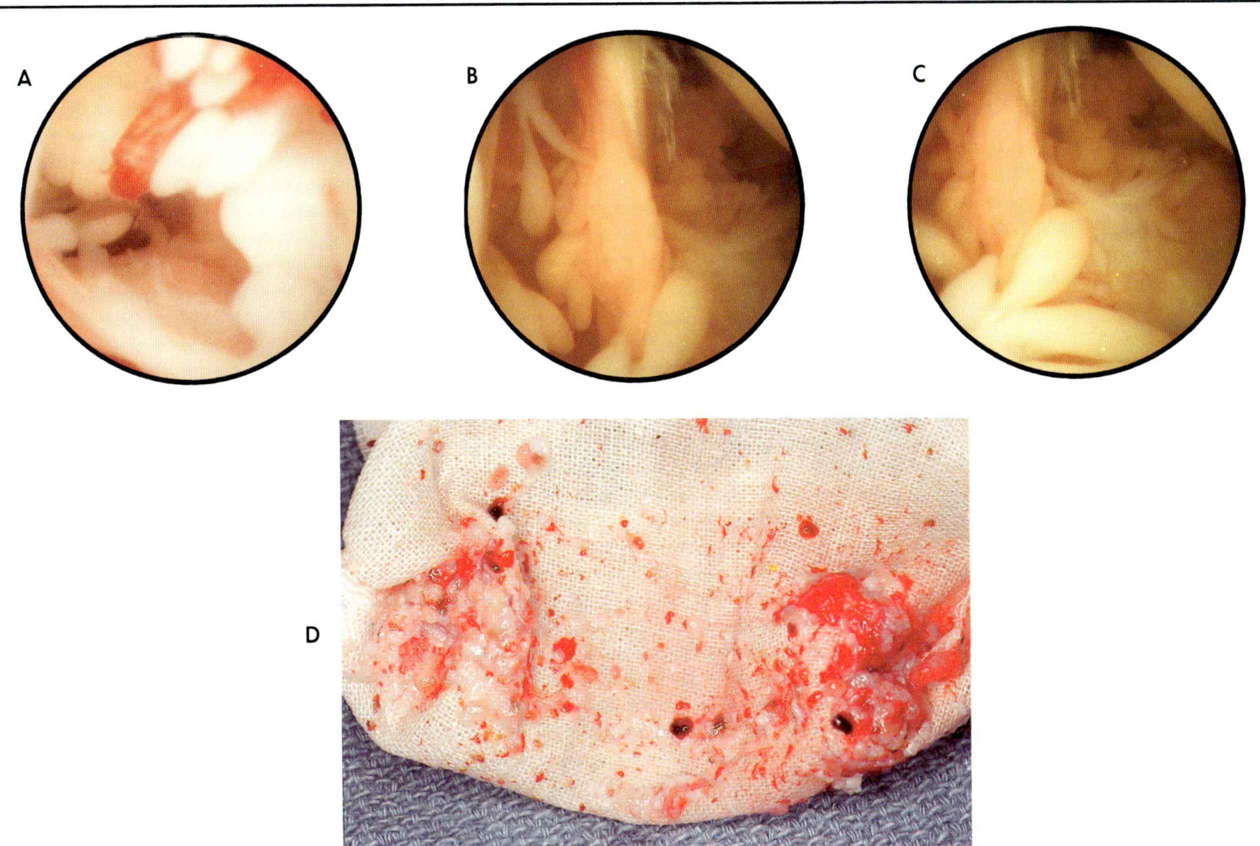

FIG. 7-27 Rheumatoid arthritis.

A Arthroscopic view of synovium with fibrinoid exudate on villi and hemorrhagic changes.

B Marked synovitis on biceps tendon.

C Close-up of dumbbell-shaped fibrinoid exudate on villi.

D Gross pathological anatomical specimen.

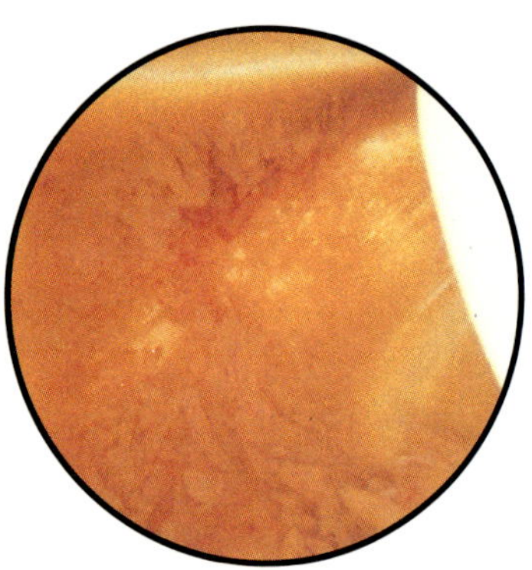

FIG. 7-28 Pigmented villonodular synovitis.

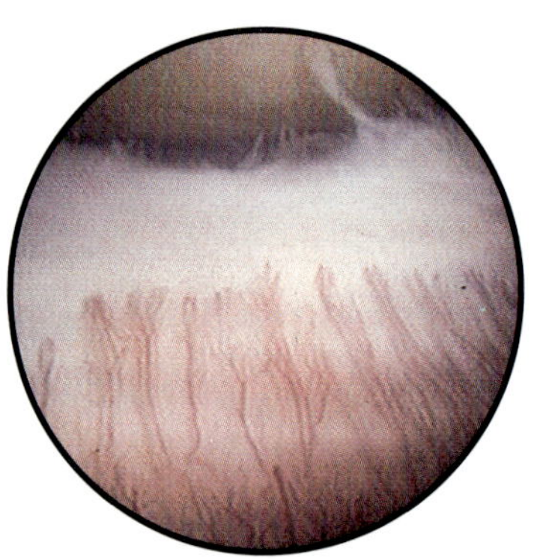

FIG. 7-29 Normal vascular pattern. Arthroscopic view of posterior labrum shows normal vascular pattern on synovium approaching glenoid surface.

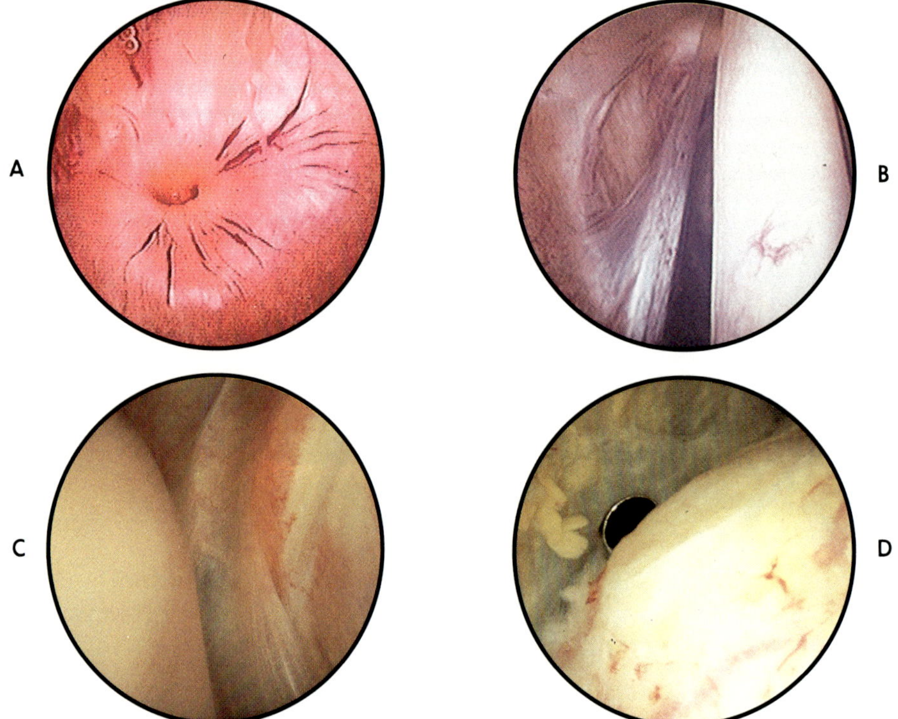

FIG. 7-30 Normal vascular areas seen during shoulder arthroscopy.

A Arthroscopic view of posterior bare area of humerus shows normal small vessels that enter into small holes in bone.

B Arthroscopic view of vessels seen within the bicipital vincula left of biceps tendon.

C Arthroscopic view shows normal vessels on CA ligament within normal subacromial bursa.

D Arthroscopic view of superior aspect of the rotator cuff in subacromial bursa shows vessels on cuff with central area bare of the vessels.

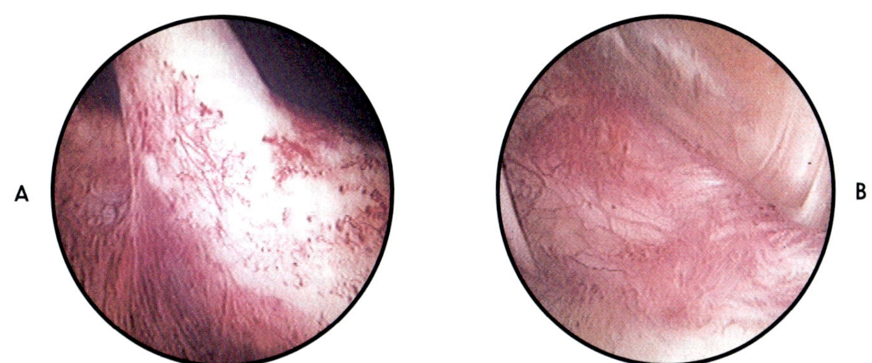

FIG. 7-31 Normal vascularity is without inflammation.

A Prominent but normal vascularity on superior labrum and biceps tendon.

B Normal anterior vascularity but without inflammation.

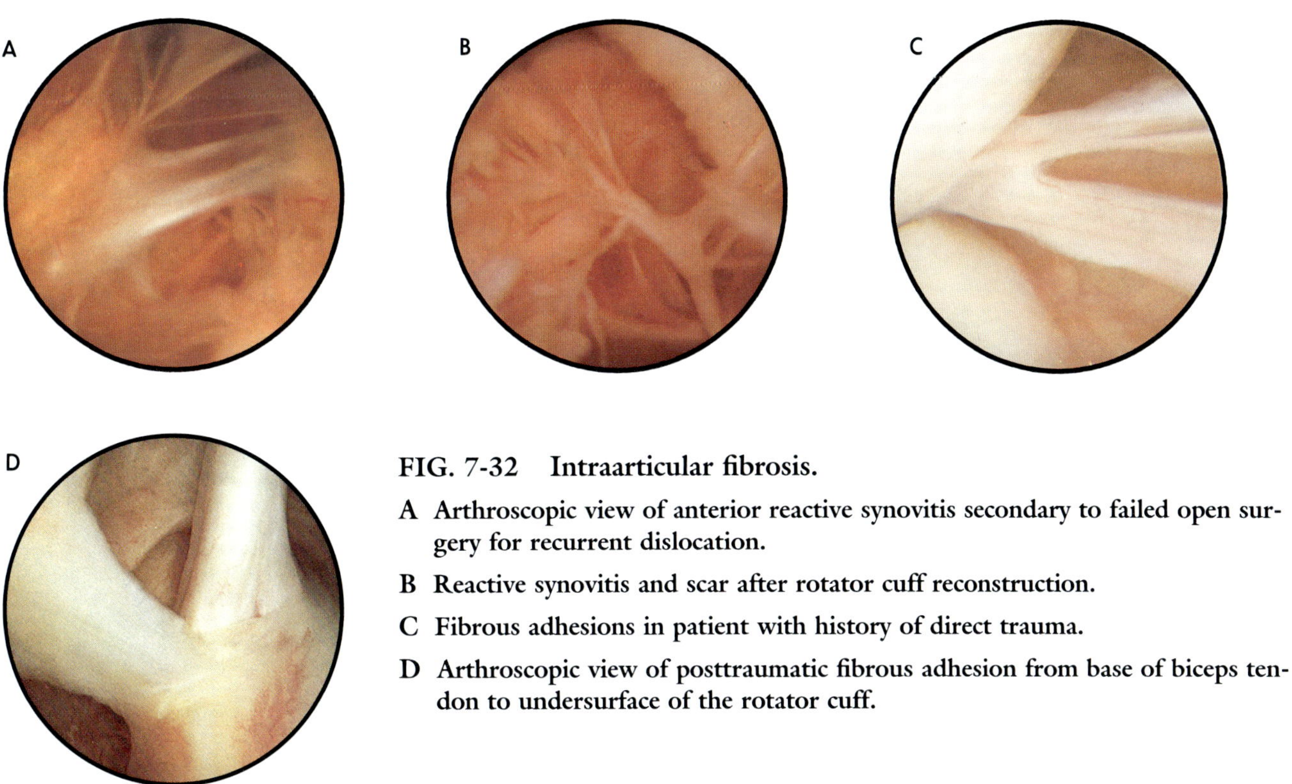

FIG. 7-32 Intraarticular fibrosis.

A Arthroscopic view of anterior reactive synovitis secondary to failed open surgery for recurrent dislocation.

B Reactive synovitis and scar after rotator cuff reconstruction.

C Fibrous adhesions in patient with history of direct trauma.

D Arthroscopic view of posttraumatic fibrous adhesion from base of biceps tendon to undersurface of the rotator cuff.

Fibrosis. A reactive intraarticular fibrosis may result from previous surgery or trauma (Fig. 7-32). The fibrous bands must be differentiated from the normal vincula (see Fig. 7-30, *B*).

Postoperative Findings. Diagnostic arthroscopy after open surgery shows some surprising reasons for continued morbidity. I have seen small fragments of needles broken off in the humeral head. Finding suture material is not unusual after open rotator cuff or instability operations (Fig. 7-33).

I have seen one instance of a patient with previous fascia lata autograft to a large defect in the rotator cuff. The result was a clinical failure. The arthroscopic view showed one prominent band and several small bands of graft (Fig. 7-34). There was no integrity to the graft and little appearance of viability after 2 years in this case.

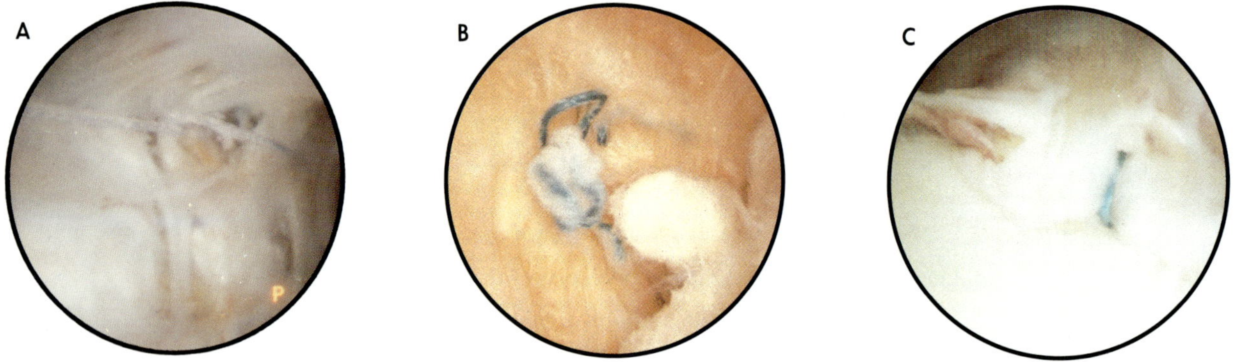

FIG. 7-33 Postoperative findings.

A Suture material evident at intended insertion site.

B Arthroscopic view of loose suture material following failed open rotator cuff repair.

C Arthroscopic view of suture material in anterior glenoid following open Bankart repair. The patient had marked limitation of external rotation requiring arthroscopic release.

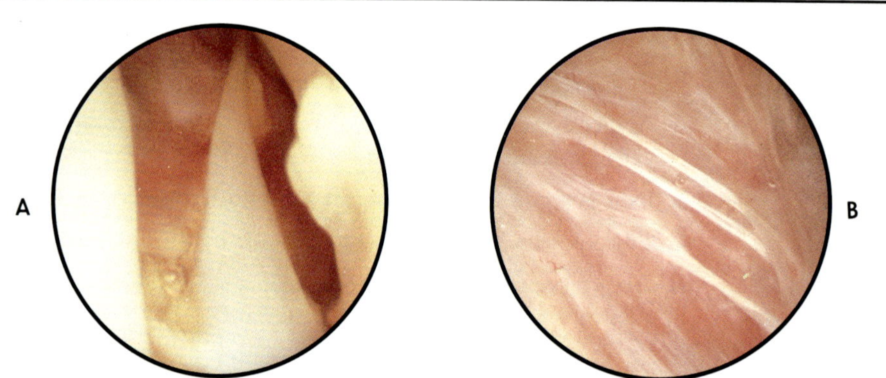

FIG. 7-34 Postoperative findings after fascial graft.

A Arthroscopic view shows thin remnant of previously placed fascia lata graft.

B Arthroscopic view in same patient shows thin thread-like remnants of previous graft.

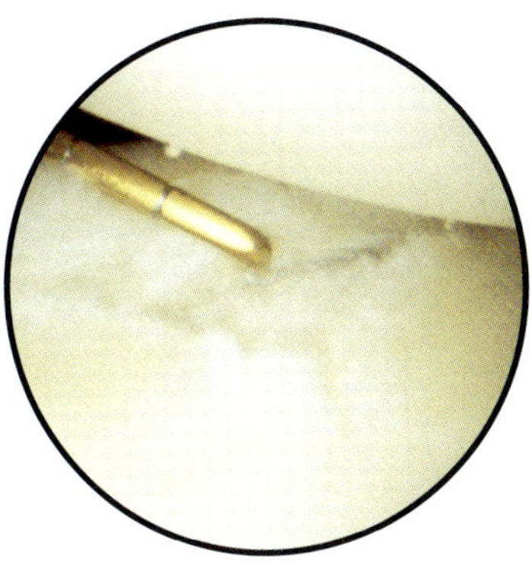

FIG. 7-35 Arthroscopic assessment of labrum. Probing is essential to assessing intraarticular lesions.

Labrum

Anterior labral tears were recognized before arthroscopy through the customary anterior open surgical approach.[20] Nevertheless, arthroscopy has drawn attention to a wide spectrum of labral tears.[12] Other sites for labral tears are more easily recognized by arthroscopy and therefore are more common than previously suspected.

Arthroscopic Assessment. Probing is helpful in determining the extent of the lesion (Fig. 7-35). Other arthroscopic techniques beside probing also help assess the labrum mobility. One is to distend and decompress the joint. This maneuver demonstrates the motion of the glenoid labrum (Fig. 7-36). Another is to first use air medium and then fluid (Fig. 7-37). In addition, small interstitial tears may show up best with injection of dilute methylene blue dye (0.1 ml/60 ml saline) (Fig. 7-38).

A

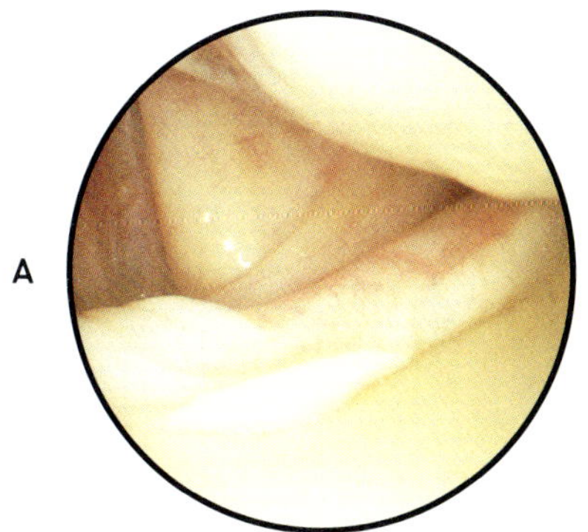

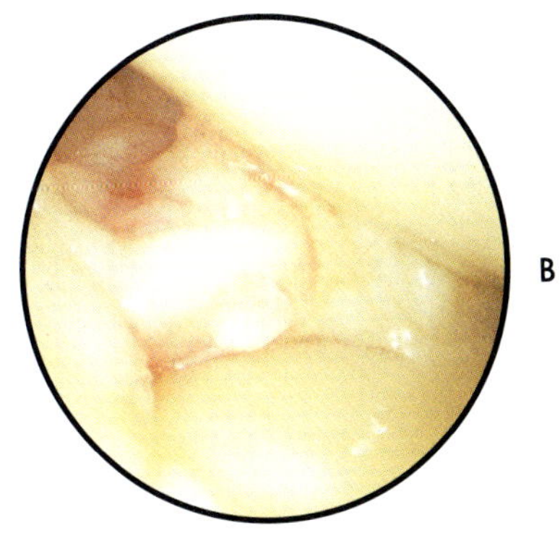

B

FIG. 7-36 Assessment of labrum by distention/decompression.

A Arthroscopic view of anterior capsular ligaments with joint distention.

B Arthroscopic view of anterior capsular ligaments with joint decompression shows the motion of the tissue into the joint.

A

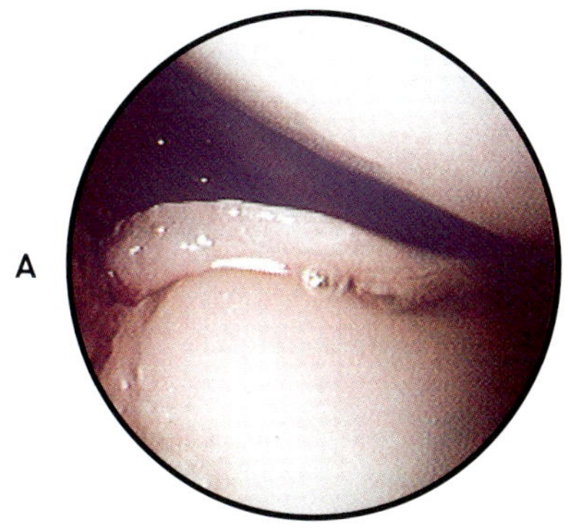

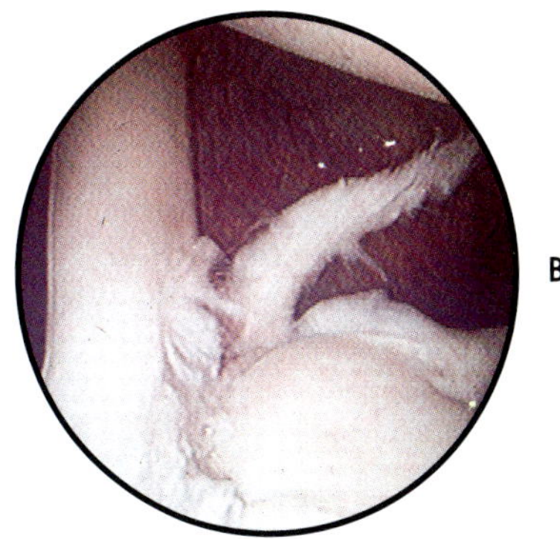

B

FIG. 7-37 Assessment of labrum by air/fluid mediums.

A Arthroscopic view shows labral flap lesion resting on the anterior glenoid in air medium.

B Arthroscopic view shows labral flap moves and floats in fluid medium.

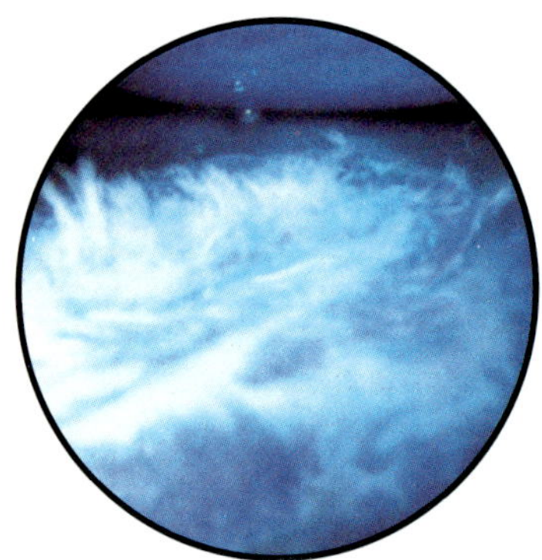

FIG. 7-38 Assessment of labrum by injection of dilute methylene blue dye. Arthroscopic view of posterior labral tear highlights methylene blue dye.

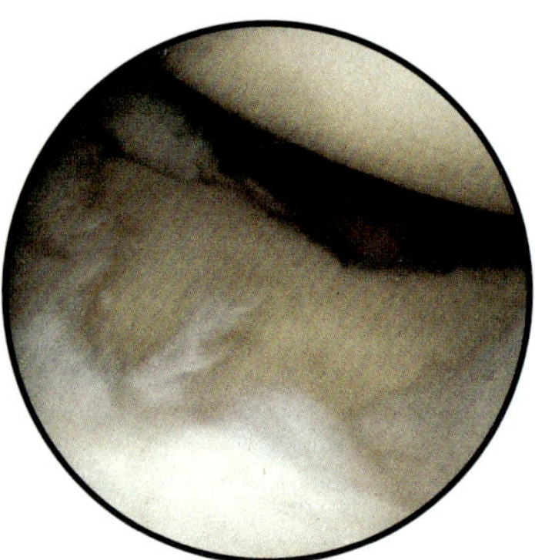

FIG. 7-39 Degenerative labrum. Arthroscopic view shows extensive diffuse fringe degeneration along margins of glenoid labrum.

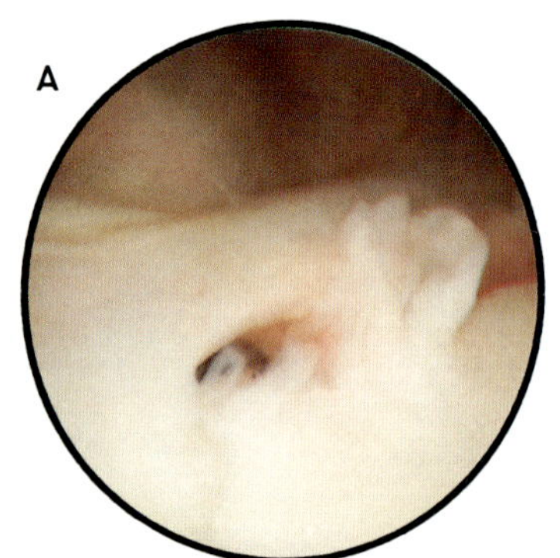

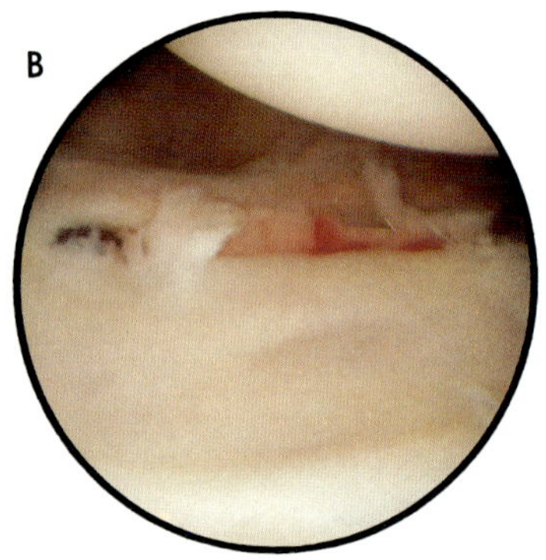

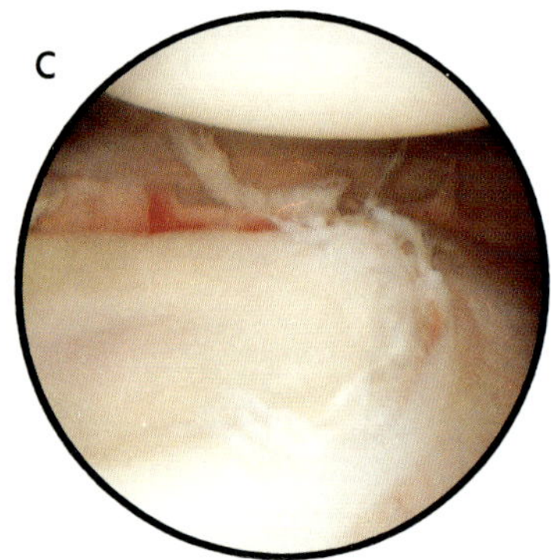

FIG. 7-40 Bankart lesion of glenohumeral ligament dislocation.

A Lesion extends to superior labrum with fragmentation of glenoid articular cartilage.

B Separation of ligament with small labrum and hemorrhage.

C Disruption of inferior labrum is continuous with entire anterior separation.

Determining the nature of the lesion is important in making treatment decisions. Both inspection and arthroscopic probing are necessary. Depending on the nature of the lesion, resection or repair may be indicated (see Chapter 8).

Mechanism of Injury. Aging and tissue attrition are the most common causes of labral tears. These types of tears are degenerative (Fig. 7-39). The other mechanism of labrum injury occurs with trauma, most commonly anterior dislocation. This is the so-called Perthes or Bankart lesion (Fig. 7-40). This and other traumatic lesions are a result of mechanical separation, compression, traction, or a combination of these forces.

The propensity for the anterior labrum to tear can be shown on a cadaver specimen (Fig. 7-41). The labrum is an extension of the glenohumeral ligaments. A contrived illustration shows the redundant extension of the anterior-inferior glenohumeral ligament at the end of the white pointer (Fig. 7-41, *A* and *B*). An incision was made along the glenoid rim, leaving the tissue attached at both ends (Fig. 7-41, *C* and *D*). A correlative arthroscopic view of a labrum tear lends understanding to this process (Fig. 7-41, *E*).

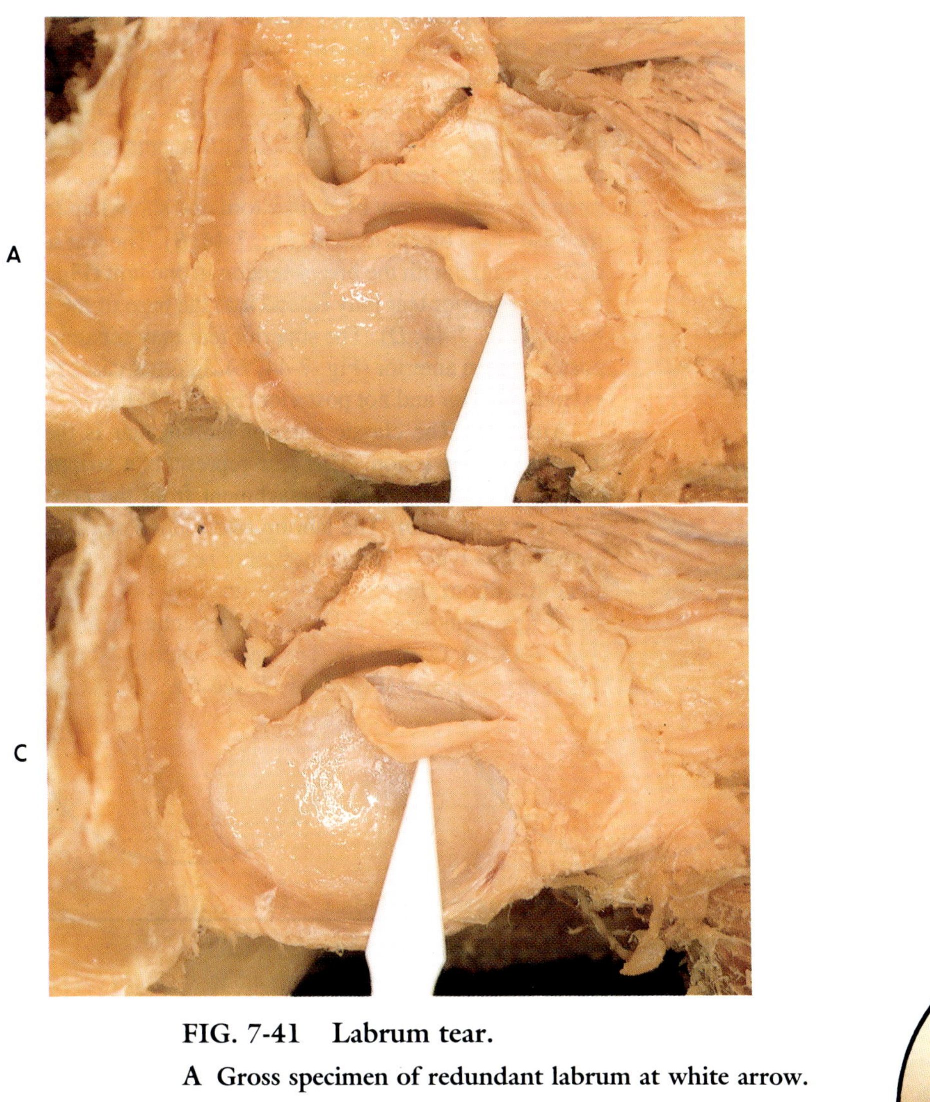

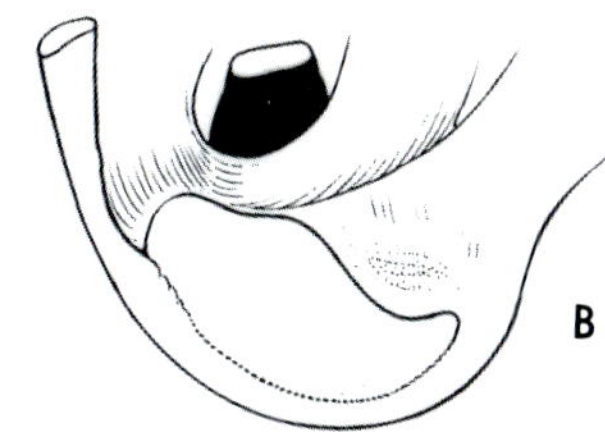

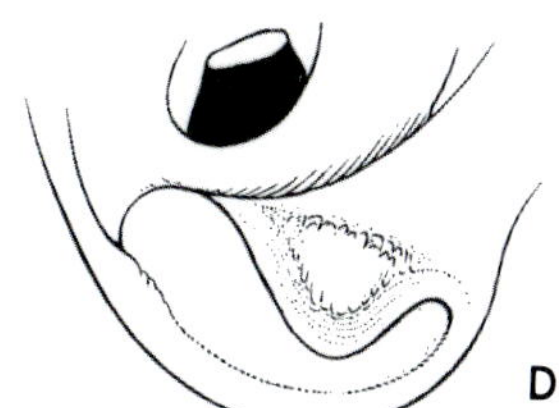

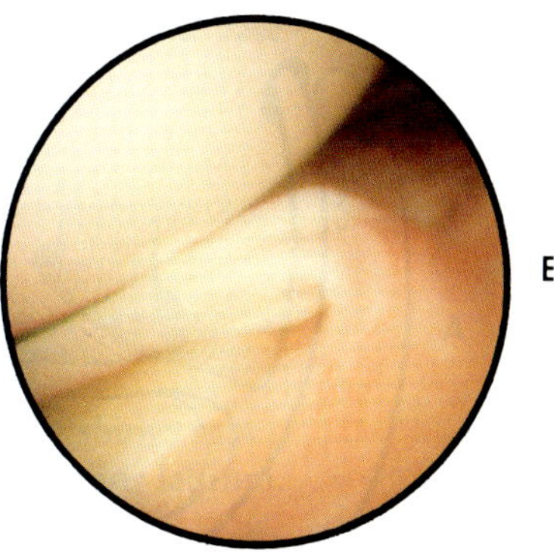

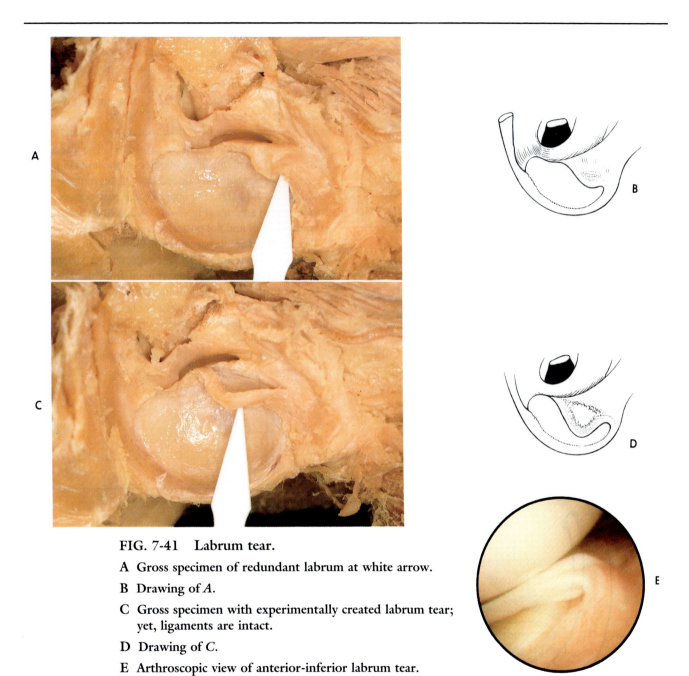

FIG. 7-41 Labrum tear.

A Gross specimen of redundant labrum at white arrow.

B Drawing of *A*.

C Gross specimen with experimentally created labrum tear; yet, ligaments are intact.

D Drawing of *C*.

E Arthroscopic view of anterior-inferior labrum tear.

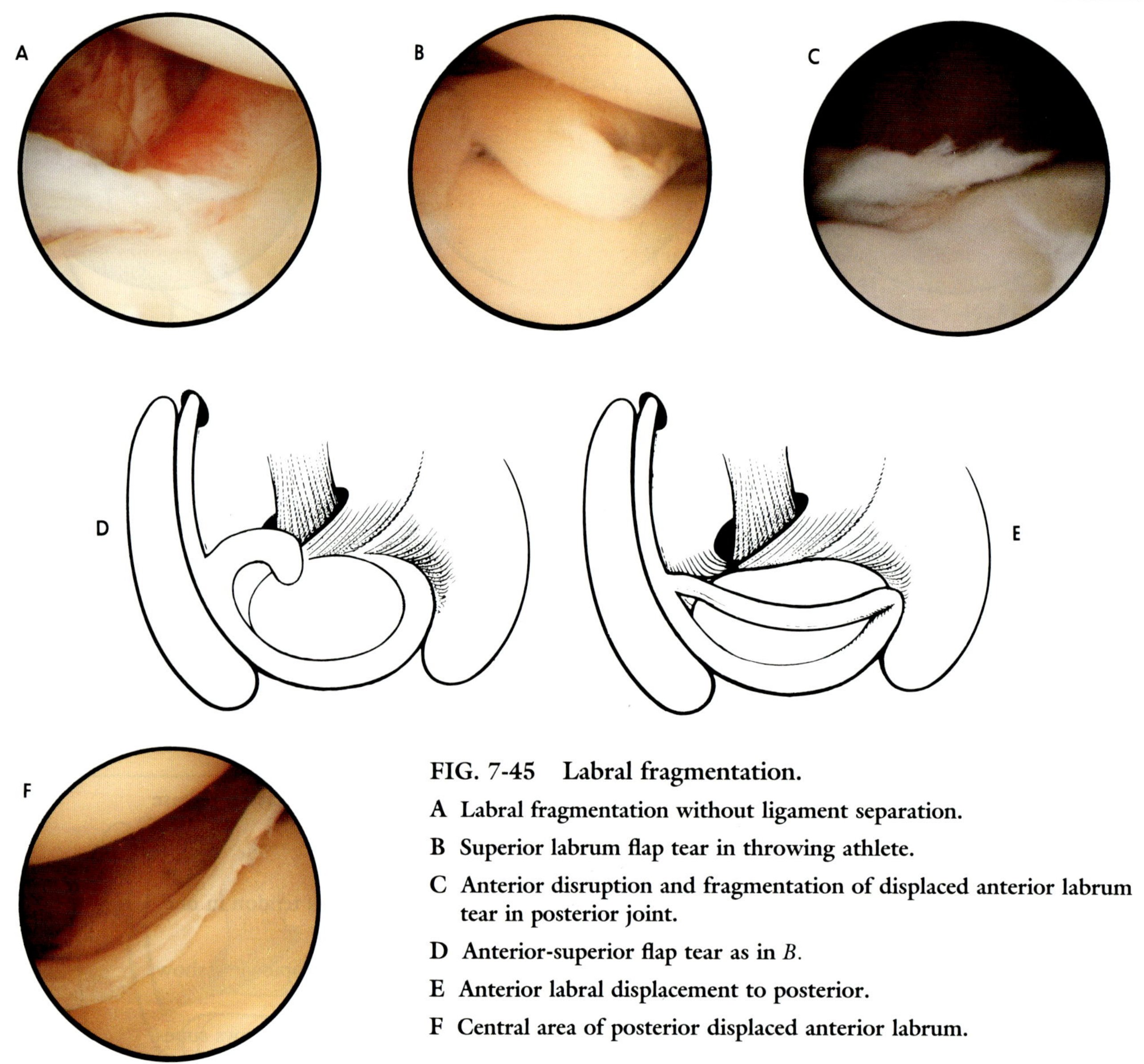

FIG. 7-45 Labral fragmentation.

A Labral fragmentation without ligament separation.

B Superior labrum flap tear in throwing athlete.

C Anterior disruption and fragmentation of displaced anterior labrum tear in posterior joint.

D Anterior-superior flap tear as in *B*.

E Anterior labral displacement to posterior.

F Central area of posterior displaced anterior labrum.

The separation of the labrum occurs in various ways. A classification is proposed in Chapter 8. One way is with the labrum and ligaments intact, in juxtaposition to the glenoid showing the hemorrhage of an acute lesion in the defect (Fig. 7-46, *A*). Another is separation of the labrum with the ligaments, juxtaposition to the labrum, but fragmentation of the labrum (Fig. 7-46, *B*).

The labrum may tear with separation from the glenoid with intact glenohumeral ligaments (Fig. 7-47). Another form of disruption is the separation of the labrum from the glenoid with displacement of labrum, and separation also from the glenohumeral ligaments (Fig. 7-48). The labrum may separate with attached bone (Fig. 7-49). Flap tears occur if the displaced labrum subsequently tears in two (Fig. 7-50).

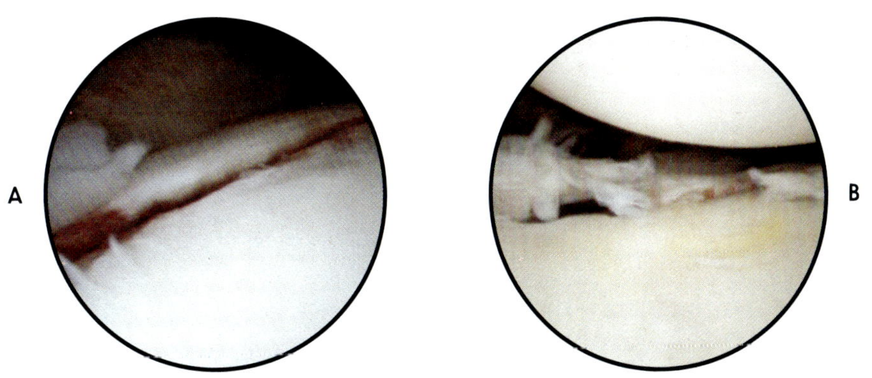

FIG. 7-46 Anterior labral tear without displacement.

A Arthroscopic view shows hemorrhage along line on anterior labral separation. The labrum has not been displaced from the glenoid.

B Arthroscopic view shows fragmentation of labrum with minimal separation from the bony glenoid.

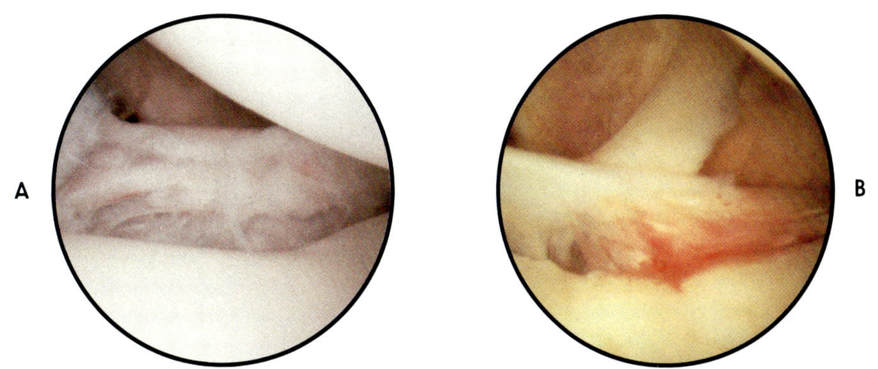

FIG. 7-47 Labrum tear with intact glenohumeral ligaments.

A Arthroscopic view shows tear of labrum away from anterior glenoid with ligaments intact.

B Arthroscopic view shows tear of labrum with intact middle glenohumeral ligament.

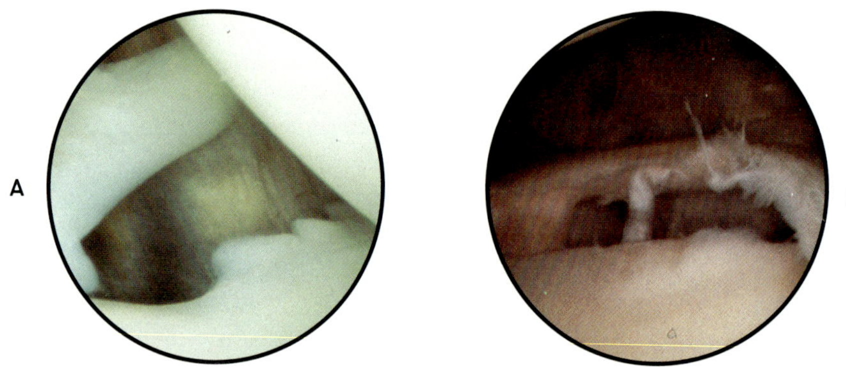

FIG. 7-48 Labrum tear with displacement.

A Arthroscopic view shows labrum tear with anterior displacement with joint distention.

B Arthroscopic view labrum tear with displacement over entire anterior and superior labrum.

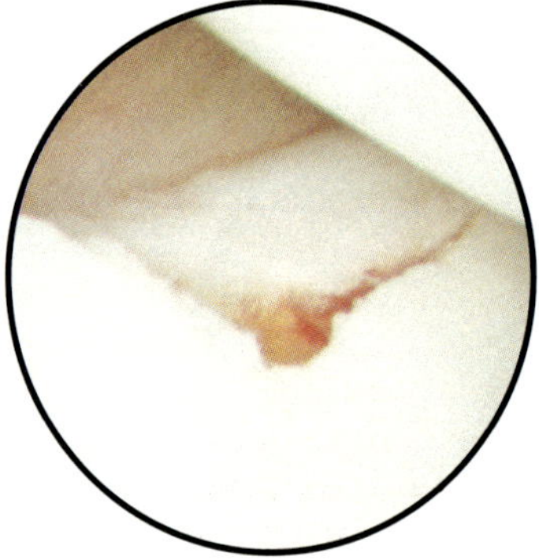

FIG. 7-49 Labrum tear with bone from glenoid. Arthroscopic view shows labrum has torn from glenoid, but with a portion of anterior glenoid bone.

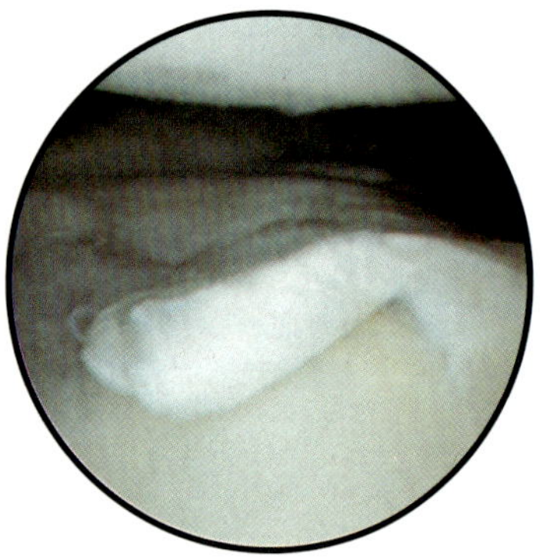

FIG. 7-50 Anterior flap tear of labrum. Arthroscopic view shows flap tear of labrum showing results of progessive fragmentation.

Posterior. The posterior labrum tear manifest with fringe disruption is common in degenerative arthritis (Fig. 7-51).

Traumatic separations occur with traumatic anterior dislocations. These are most common as superficial, interstitial tears (Fig. 7-52). Probing is necessary to determine the depth and mobility of the tear.

Posterior labrum tears occur with subtle anterior instability in throwing athletes. The site includes an inferior component, even though the lesion may extend superior. A flap of labrum may separate with this repetitive trauma (Fig. 7-53). Frank Jobe has observed a "kissing lesion" on the posterior labrum opposite the posterior labrum tear (Fig. 7-54).[13]

The posterior glenohumeral subluxation or dislocation is associated with posterior-superior labral disruption. The posterior-inferior glenohumeral ligament extends superior, blending into the area of this lesion (Fig. 7-55).

A

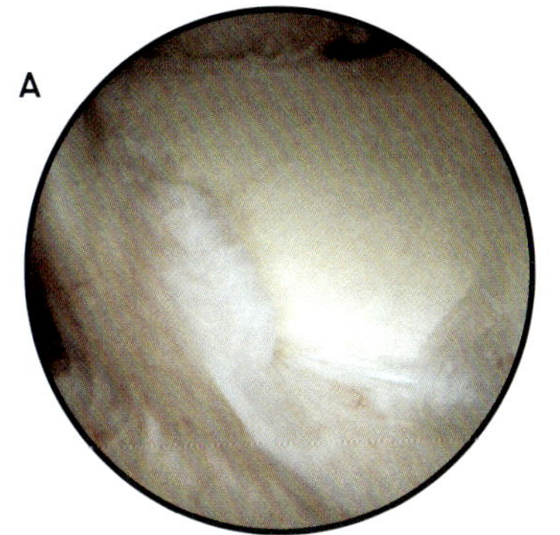

B

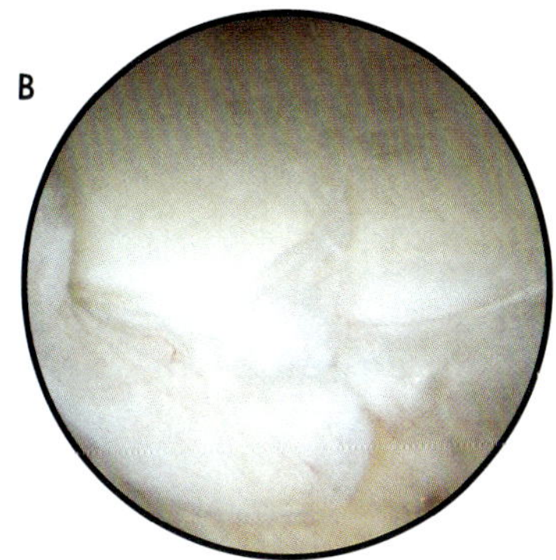

C

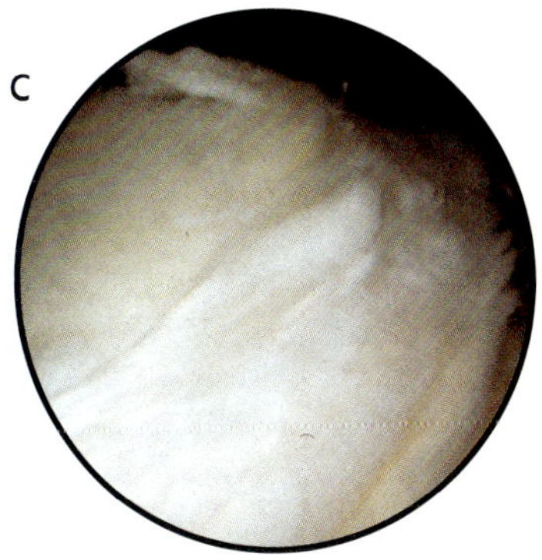

FIG. 7-51 Degenerative posterior labrum tears.

A Arthroscopic view of posterior-superior labrum shows fringe degeneration.

B Arthroscopic view of mid-portion of posterior labrum shows extension of fragmentation.

C Arthroscopic view of posterior and inferior labrum in same patient shows fragmentation of labrum.

A

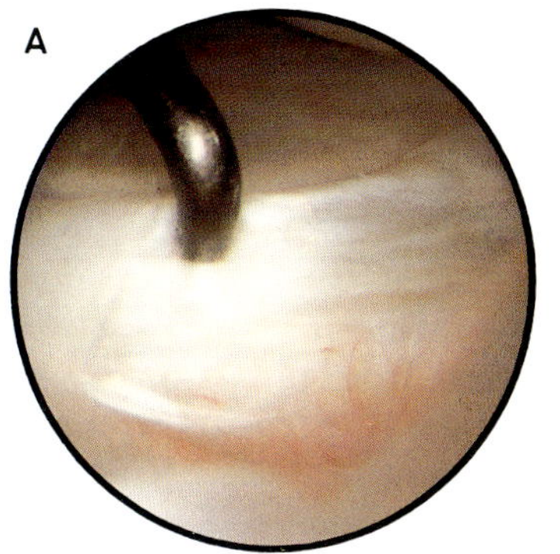

B

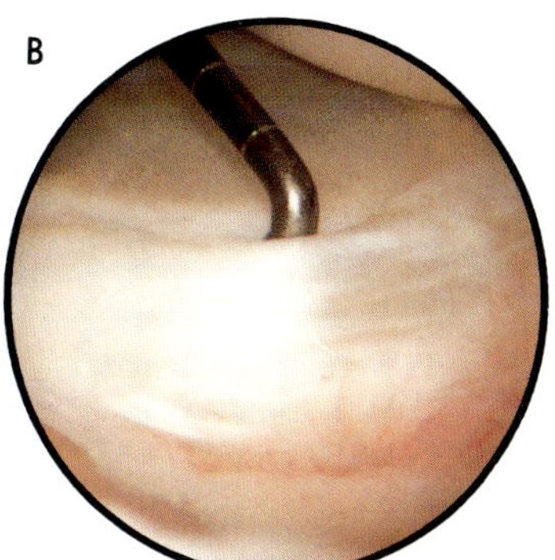

C

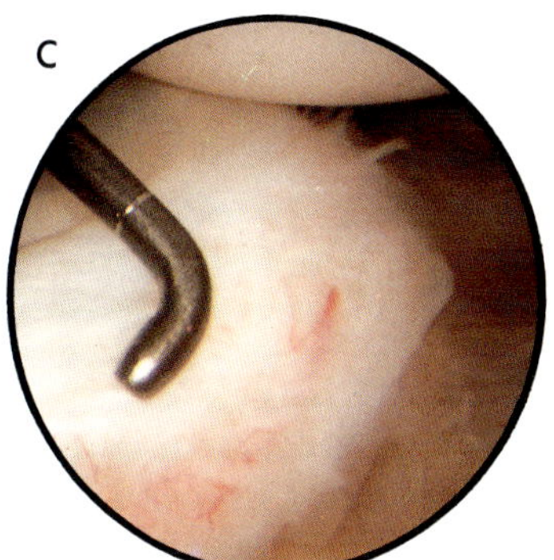

FIG. 7-52 Posterior labrum tears.

A Arthroscopic view of posterior labrum tear with probe at superior separation.

B Probe in normal glenoid labrum interval.

C Palpation of separated fiber of posterior-inferior labrum

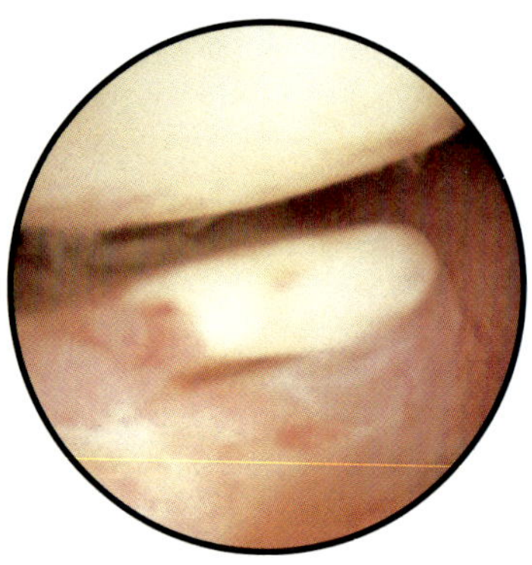

FIG. 7-53 Posterior labral flap tear. Arthroscopic view of posterior inferior flap tear of labrum.

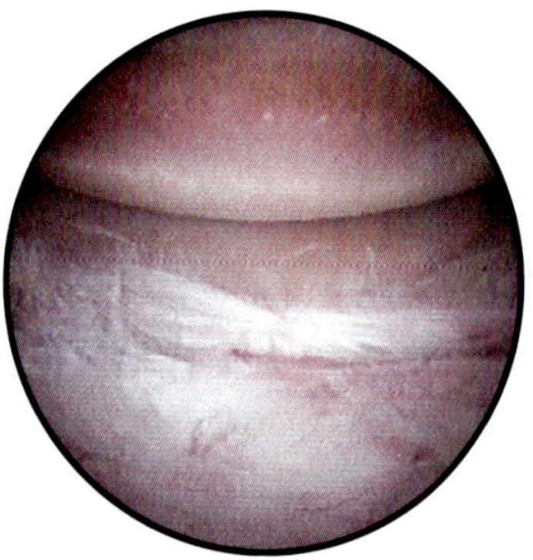

FIG. 7-54 "Kissing" lesion of labral tear and posterior humerus. Arthroscopic view of juxtaposition of posterior humeral and labral lesion.

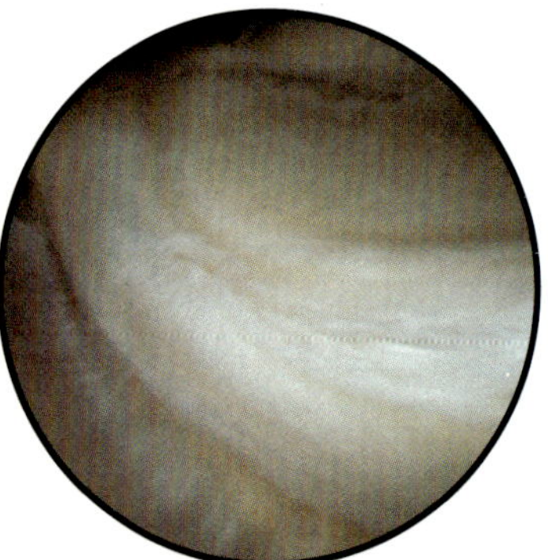

FIG. 7-55 Posterior-inferior ligament/labrum tear. Arthroscopic view from posterior of posterior-inferior ligament extension to area of posterior-superior labrum tear.

Inferior. The inferior labrum tear is associated with anterior and inferior instability (Fig. 7-56, *A*). The tear is traumatic, often showing signs of hemorrhage (Fig. 7-56, *B*). The axillary portion of the glenohumeral ligaments are often stripped from the glenoid (Fig. 7-56, *C*). Fragmentation may be directly inferior without an anterior labrum tear in instability (Fig. 7-56, *D*). Distention shows associated ligamentous laxity when the humerus is elevated away from the glenoid (Fig. 7-56, *D*). In chronic cases the inferior separation is large and covered with regrown synovium (Fig. 7-56, *E*).

Variation in Depth. Labrum tears vary in depth (Fig. 7-56, *D* and *E*). Their length varies. The mobility is determined by probing (see Fig. 7-35). Their clinical significance must be determined in relation to the primary condition and their independent symptom-producing ability, because these factors will direct the treatment.

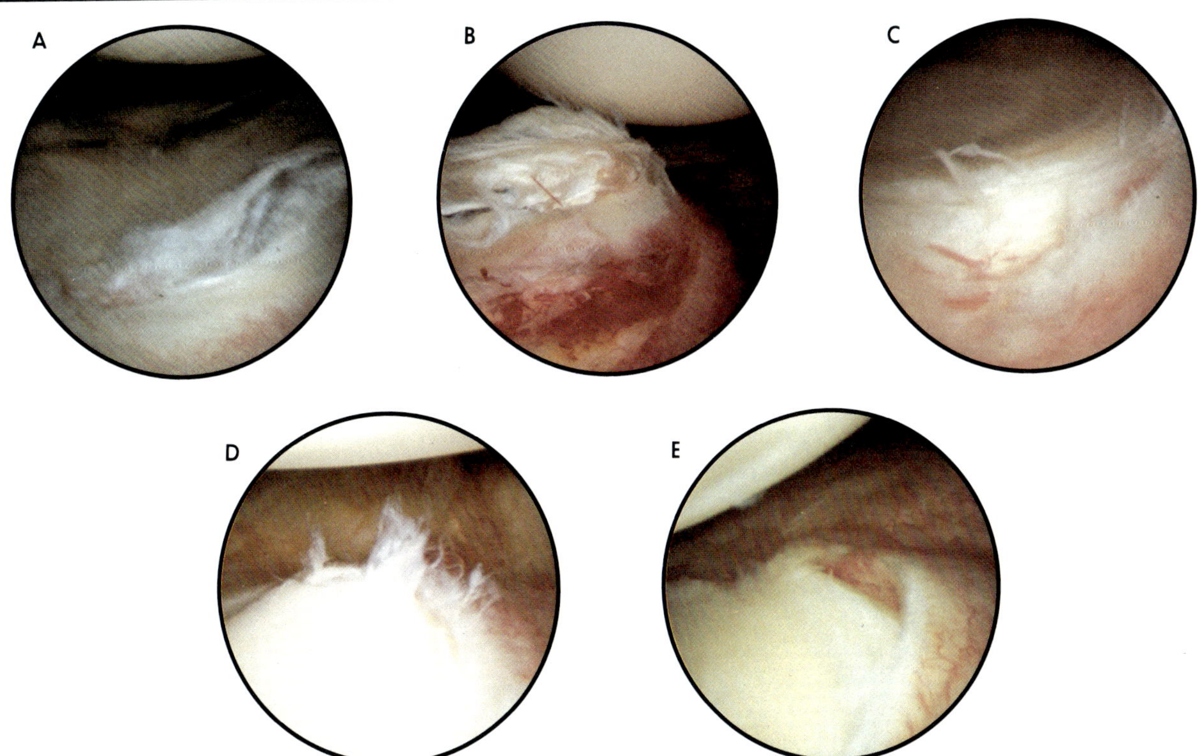

FIG. 7-56 Inferior labrum tears.

A Arthroscopic view of posterior-inferior labral tear.

B Arthroscopic view of acute tear with hemorrhage.

C Arthroscopic view shows stripping of posterior-inferior arcuate portion of glenohumeral ligaments from glenoid.

D Fragmentation of directly inferior labrum tear.

E Chronic direct inferior labrum tear.

Glenohumeral Ligaments

The glenohumeral ligaments may be detached from either the glenoid, humerus, or both areas. The separation from the glenoid varies in type. The separation may appear minimal in the undistended joint (Fig. 7-57, *A*). When the joint is distended, the labrum is moved away from the glenoid, showing the disruption (Fig. 7-57, *B*).

An interstitial glenohumeral ligament tear will show the labrum intact, but with distention the entire anterior ligamentous tissue moves away from the glenoid (Fig. 7-58). This appearance represents an intrasubstance stretching injury of the glenohumeral ligaments. Another difficult diagnostic determination occurs when the glenohumeral ligament attachment to the anterior glenoid has

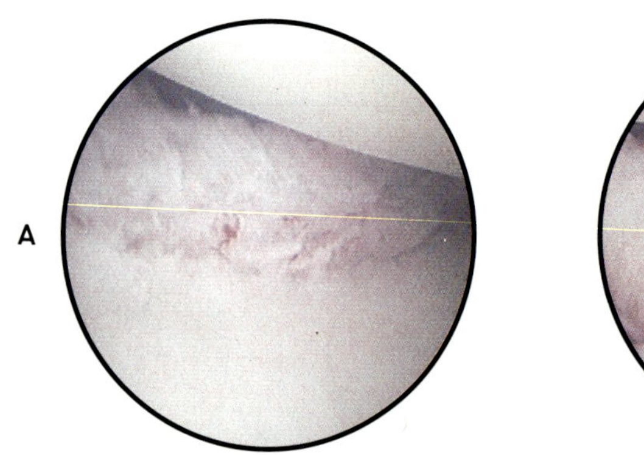

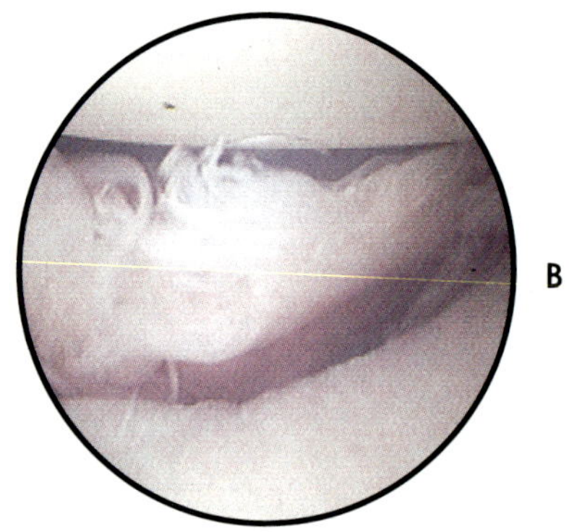

FIG. 7-57 Glenohumeral ligament separation.

A Arthroscopic view in undistended joint does not show the separation of the labrum and the glenohumeral ligaments.

B Arthroscopic view in same patient after fluid distention shows the ligaments to move away from the intended glenoid attachment.

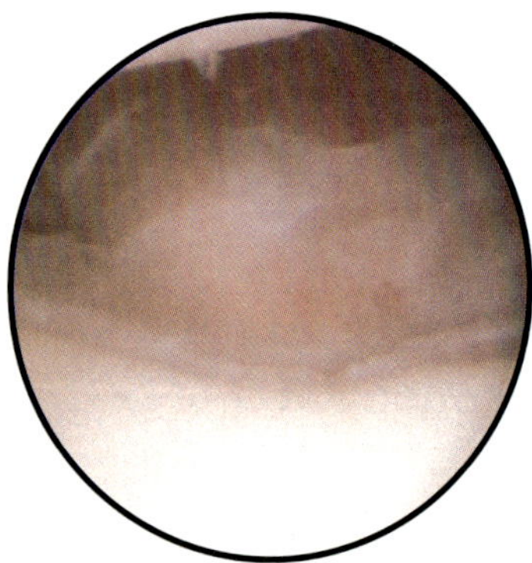

FIG. 7-58 Intrasubstance tear of glenohumeral ligaments. Arthroscopic view shows humerus moved far away from the glenoid with distention, yet no distinct tear or separation is seen in anterior glenohumeral ligaments.

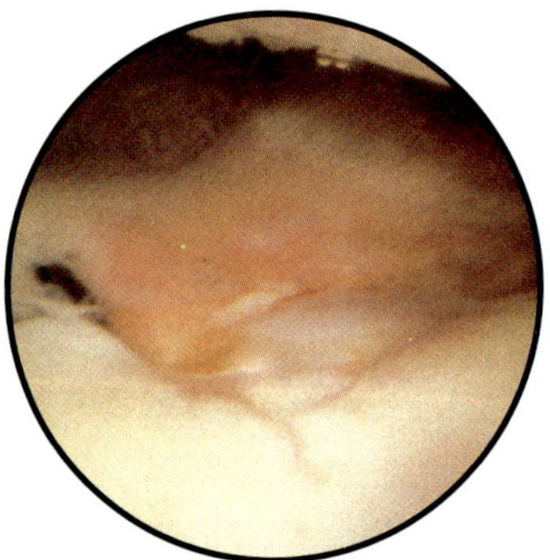

FIG. 7-59 Reattachment of previous glenohumeral ligament tear. Arthroscopic view shows evidence of previous fracture with separation, but healing in situ to the glenoid.

been previously injured, with the labrum uninjured. A fibrous repair has reunited the ligaments to the glenoid (Fig. 7-59) In this case, the labrum appears normal, but there is fibrous tissue filling the gap between the ligaments and the glenoid. In both situations ligamentous laxity is present, which is difficult to distinguish.

In contrast, identifying a separation of the glenohumeral ligaments and labrum is easy when they remain distracted from the glenoid (Fig. 7-60). Recognizing the separation of ligaments and labrum, when they return to rest in juxtaposition to the glenoid, is more difficult (Fig. 7-61).

The site of the tear may be off the glenoid (see Fig. 7-60) The site may be within the substance of the liga-

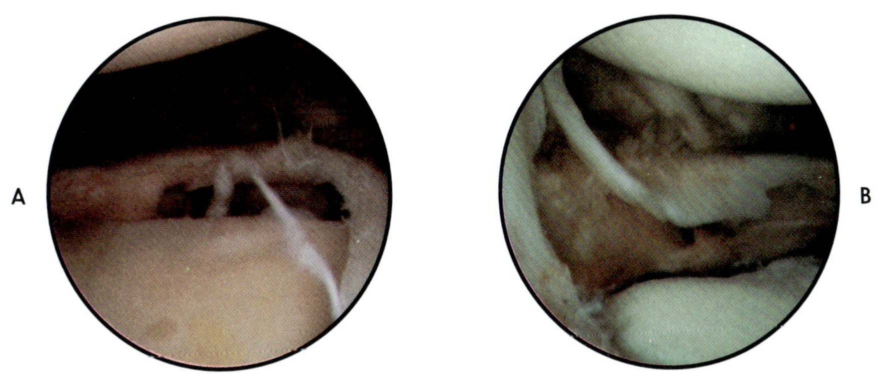

FIG. 7-60 Labrum and ligamentous separation and displacement.

A Arthroscopic view shows circumferential separation and displacement of glenohumeral ligament attachment with labrum.

B Arthroscopic view shows marked anterior separation and displacement of glenohumeral ligaments.

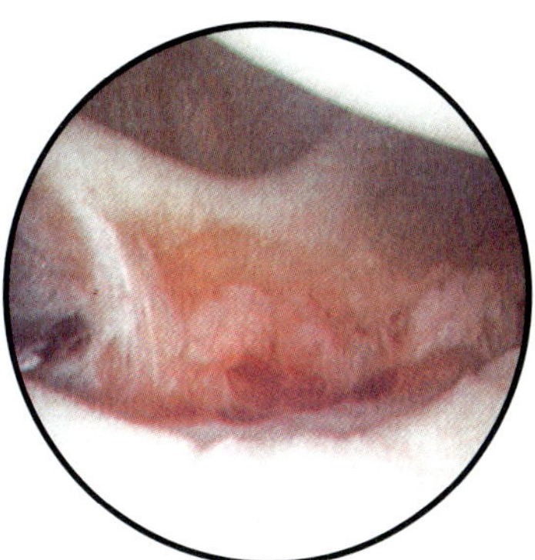

FIG. 7-61 Permanent fixed separation of glenohumeral ligaments. Arthroscopic view shows glenohumeral ligaments displaced a considerable distance from the glenoid and fibrous tissue filling in the defect.

ments (see Figs. 7-58 and 7-59). The detachment may go unrecognized when off the humerus (Fig. 7-62). The injury may be acute (Fig. 7-62, *A*) or chronic (Fig. 7-62, *B*). The chronic tear is more difficult to assess if interval healing has occurred and exact nature of original injury can not easily be determined.

The posterior glenohumeral ligament injury is not as distinct as those that occur anterior. Attenuation or stretching of the posterior ligaments is more common (Fig. 7-63).

A classification of these various tears is described in Chapter 8.

Biceps Tendon

Abnormalities of the intraarticular portion of the biceps tendon are easily identifiable by arthroscopy. Hypervascularity is common on the base of the biceps when a rotator cuff tear exists (Fig. 7-64).

The biceps tendon may be torn or absent (Fig. 7-65, *A* to *F*). The tendon tear varies in configuration. The biceps tear may extend into the superior labrum (Fig. 7-65, *G*). The biceps tendon may have an interstitial bulbus disruption (Fig. 7-65, *H*). The biceps tendon tear is of the erosion type when associated with impingement syndrome and rotator cuff tear (Fig. 7-65, *I*).

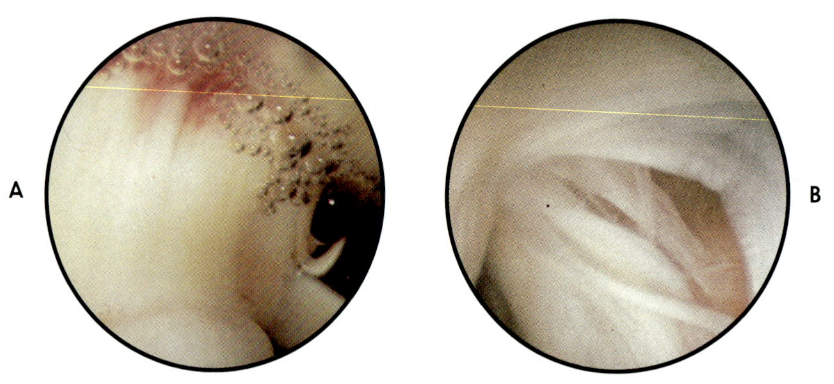

FIG. 7-62 Glenohumeral ligament tear from humerus.

A Arthroscopic view shows acute tear with hemorrhage from humeral attachment of inferior glenohumeral ligament.

B Arthroscopic view of chronic tear with tissue separation of inferior glenohumeral ligament from the humerus. (Courtesy Dr. Eugene Wolf, San Francisco, CA.)

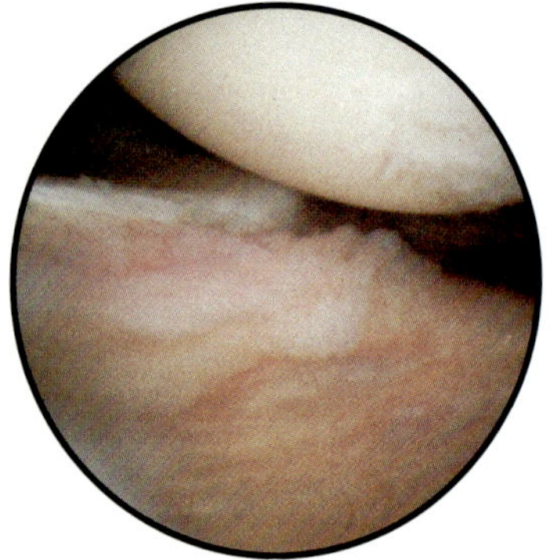

FIG. 7-63 Attenuation of posterior-inferior glenohumeral ligaments. Arthroscopic view shows stripping from the posterior aspect of the glenoid with remaining integrity to the bridge of the ligament.

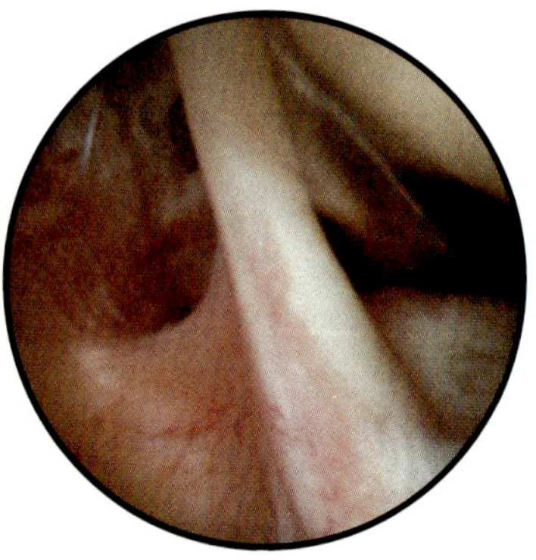

FIG. 7-64 Biceps tendon with hypervascularity. Arthroscopic view of biceps tendon shows hypervascularity at base. This is common site of earliest reaction to joint disease.

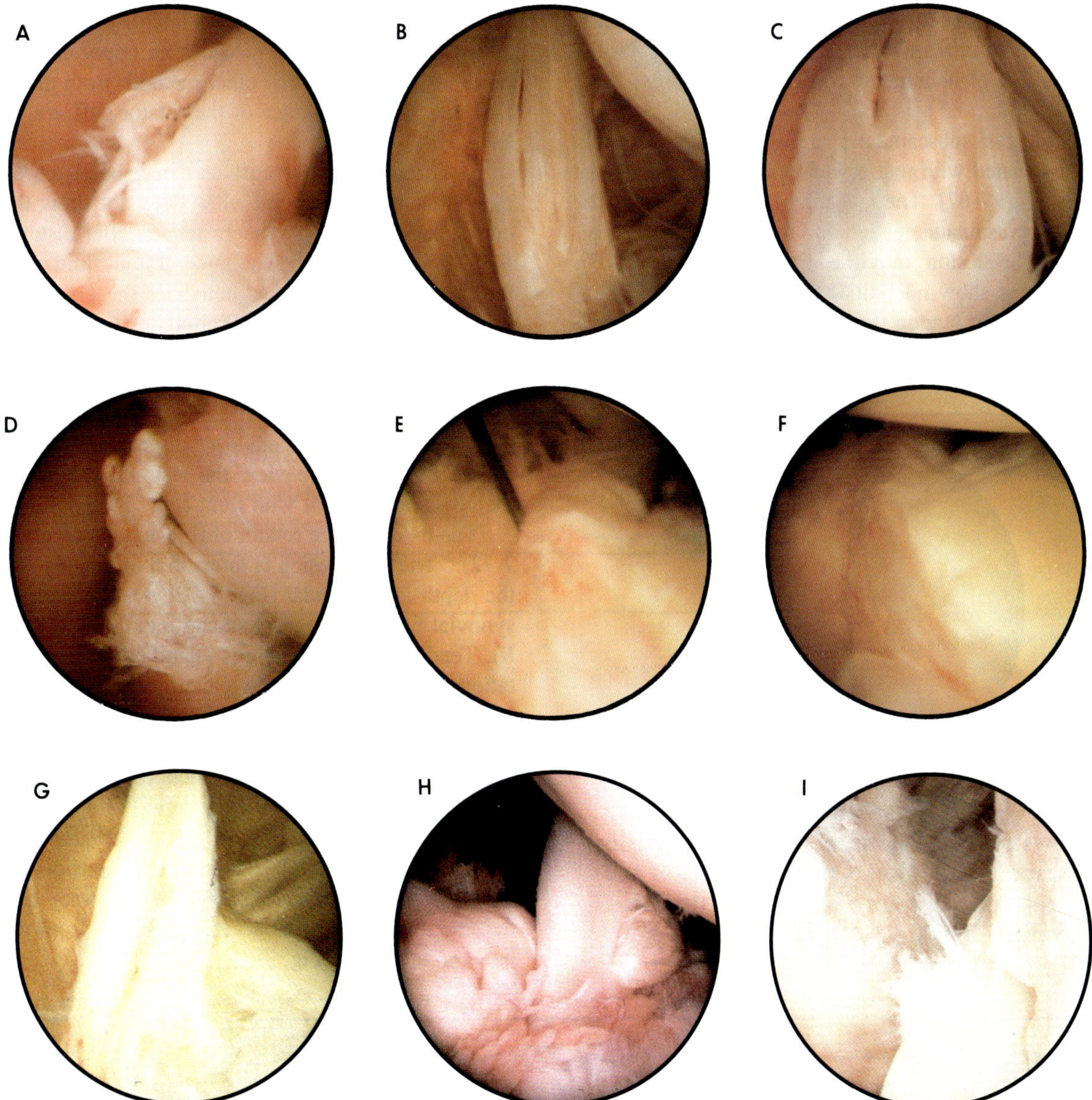

FIG. 7-65 Biceps tendon problems.

A Fragmentation of base of biceps in former throwing athlete.

B Longitudinal separation of fibers in biceps of former throwing athlete.

C Close-up arthroscopic view of longitudinal fiber separations.

D Stump of ruptured biceps tendon. Debridement reduced symptoms.

E Stump of ruptured biceps attached to anterior labrum.

F Absent biceps tendon.

G Biceps tear extension from tear in superior labrum.

H Bulbous biceps tear. Arthroscopic view of biceps tendon with bulbous mass secondary to previous tear.

I Biceps tear adjacent to acromial impingement. Arthroscopic view shows the fragmentation of the superior biceps opposite the acromial imprringement. This is seen with and without complete rotator cuff tear.

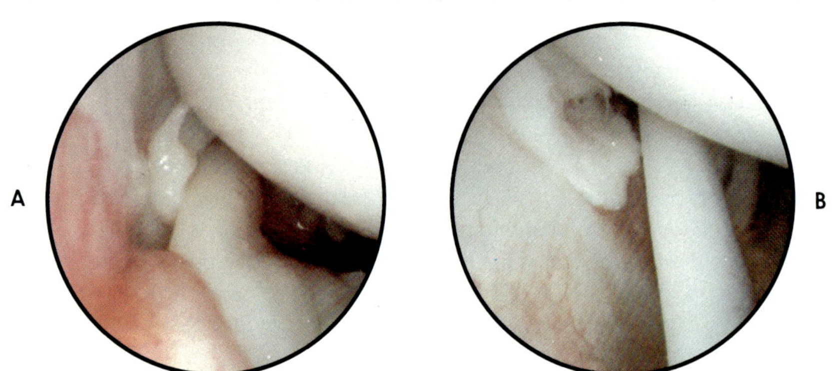

FIG. 7-71 **Assessment of rotator cuff tear with air/fluid medium.**

A Arthroscopic view of rotator cuff tag in air medium shows normal anatomical relationships.

B Same patient after distention with fluid shows the rotator cuff moves away from the biceps and the tear is small and superfical (limited to the synovium and capsule).

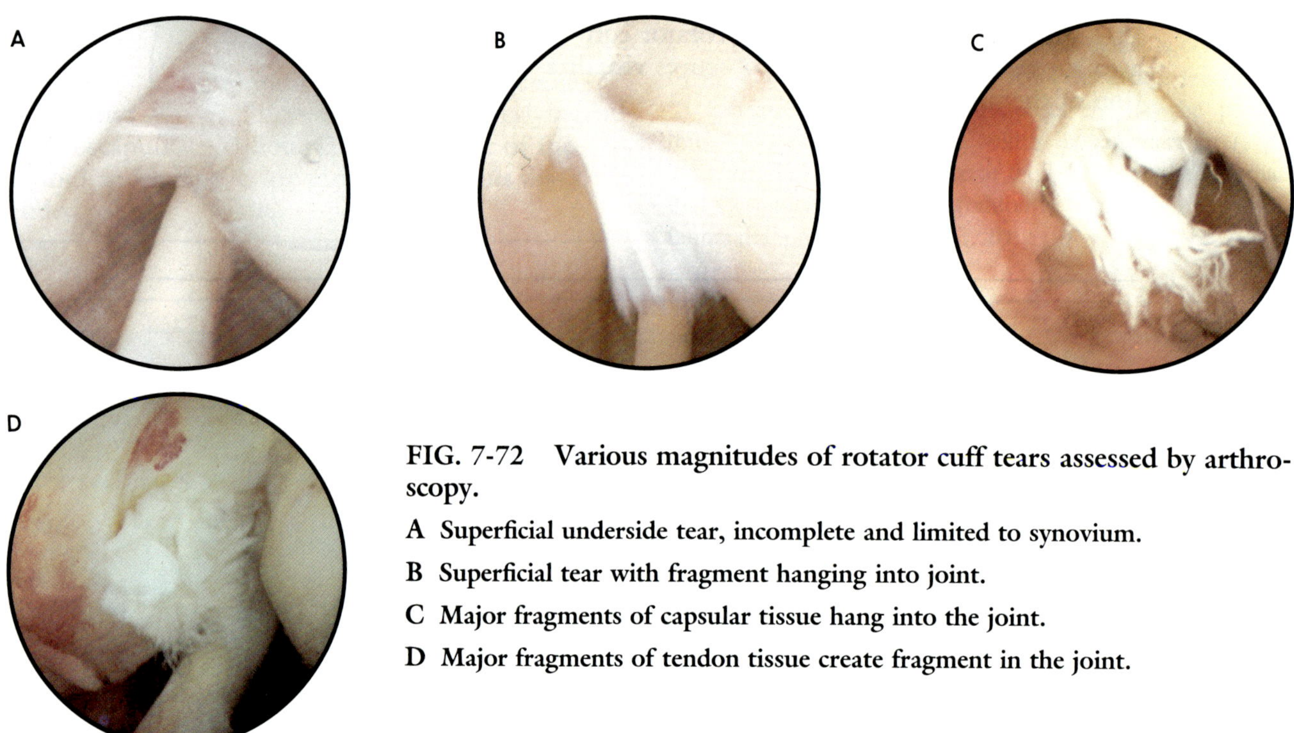

FIG. 7-72 **Various magnitudes of rotator cuff tears assessed by arthroscopy.**

A Superficial underside tear, incomplete and limited to synovium.

B Superficial tear with fragment hanging into joint.

C Major fragments of capsular tissue hang into the joint.

D Major fragments of tendon tissue create fragment in the joint.

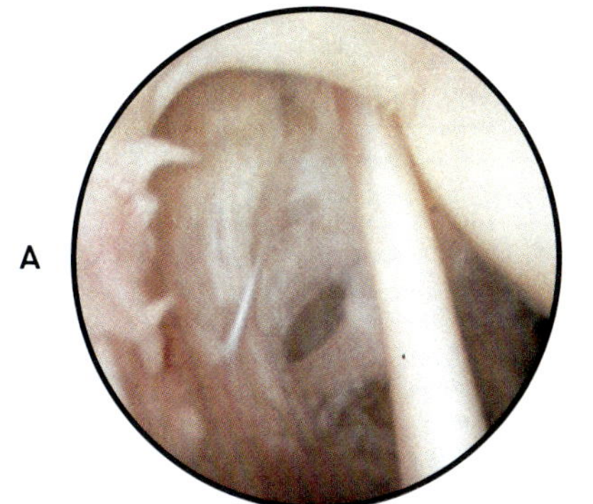

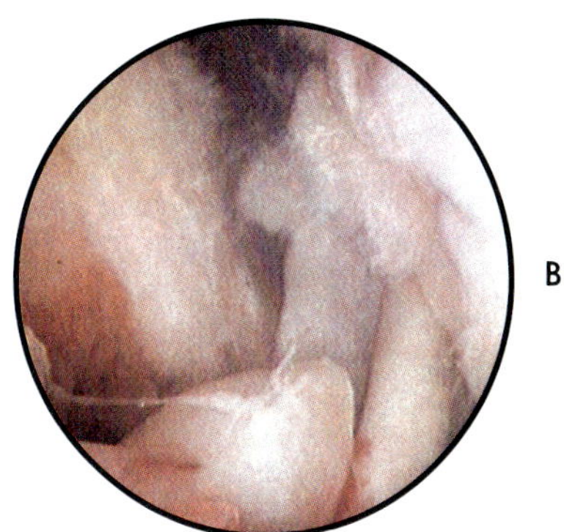

FIG. 7-73 **Large rotator cuff tears.**

A **Arthroscopic view shows a large tear, but incomplete, sparing the tendon above. No communication exists with the subacromial space.**

B **Arthroscopic view of large full-thickness rotator cuff tear seen from the glenohumeral joint side. The biceps tendon is to the right. The cuff is torn, retracted, and thickened. The acromion is visualized through the cuff tear.**

SUBACROMIAL BURSA

In full-thickness lesions the subacromial space may be approached through the rotator cuff tear (Fig. 7-74).

In some cases the inspection of the cuff tear from the glenohumeral side shows no connection with the subacromial space. Subsequent inspection from the superior side shows no complete lesion. In this case a No. 18 spinal needle is placed in the glenohumeral joint before leaving that space. The scope is placed in the subacromial space. Injection of dilute methylene blue dye into the glenohumeral space will find its way by fluid pressure and flow into the subacromial space, thereby demonstrating the connection (Fig. 7-75).

Fibrosis

The earliest sign of pathological change in the subacromial space is fibrosis (Fig. 7-76). The bursal wall thickens. The normal plica tear and become fibrous bands. These bands are separated and fragmented, as opposed to the normal plica that are smooth and attached to the bursal wall (see Chapter 9).

Acromial Erosion

Acromial erosion is the sine qua non of impingement syndrome. Its presence confirms the clinical diagnosis.[2,3] The erosion may exist both with and without a rotator cuff tear. Sometimes the rotator tear is only on the undersurface of the cuff as seen from the glenohumeral view. The rotator cuff tear may be limited only to the superior surface (Fig. 7-77). The cuff lesion may exist without acromial erosion (Fig. 7-77, *A*), or the superior tear may be associated with acromial erosion (Fig. 7-77, *B*).

The expectation of acromial erosion in all cases of rotator cuff tear is erroneous. I have seen superior tears without erosion (Fig. 7-78, *A*). In addition, large and full-thickness tears have been seen without acromial erosion (Fig. 7-78, *A*). Large, multi-layer complete tears usually show associated acromial erosion (Fig. 7-78, *B*).

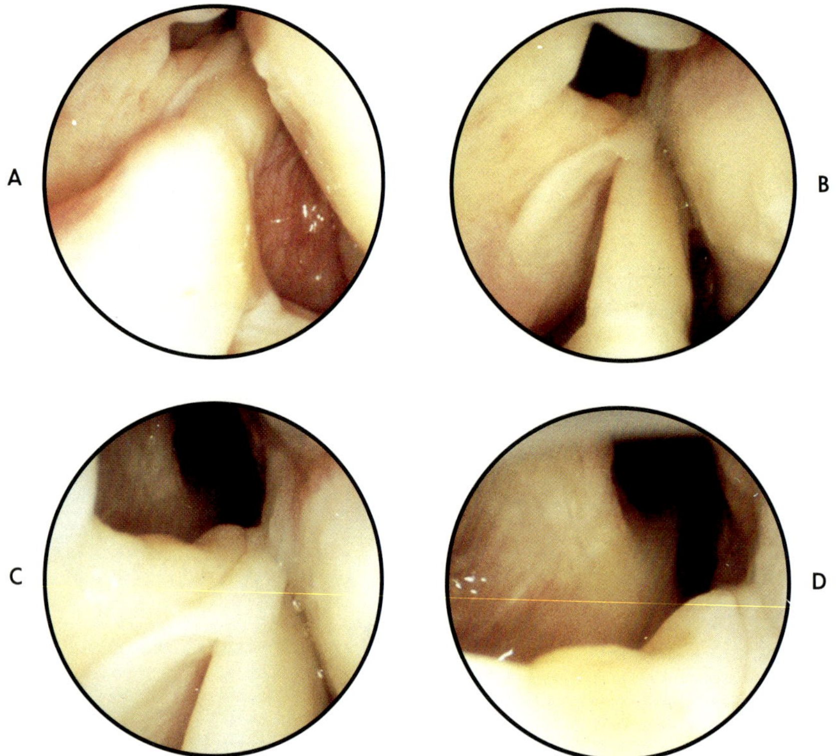

FIG. 7-74 Arthroscopic entry to subacromial space from glenohumeral joint via rotator cuff tear.

A Arthroscopic view shows humerus to right, thickened biceps tendon in middle, and small hole above at about 11 o'clock position.

B The arthroscope is advanced toward the rotator cuff defect.

C The defect appears larger as it is approached with the arthroscope.

D Penetration through the tear with the arthroscope shows the underside of the acromion.

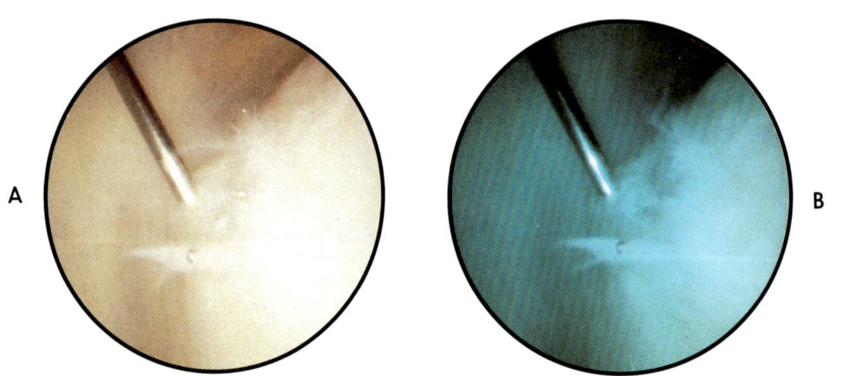

FIG. 7-75 Determination of depth and opening of rotator cuff with methylene blue dye.

A Arthroscopic view of subacromial space shows a needle pointing to roughened area of superior cuff. It cannot be determined if a connection to the glenohumeral joint is present.

B Same patient after methylene blue dye was injected into glenohumeral joint, demonstating the full-thickness lesion and the site of connection.

FIG. 7-76 Subacromial space fibrosis. This arthroscopic view of the subacromial bursa shows inflammation and fibrous bands. These can be differentiated from normal plica by inflammatory signs.

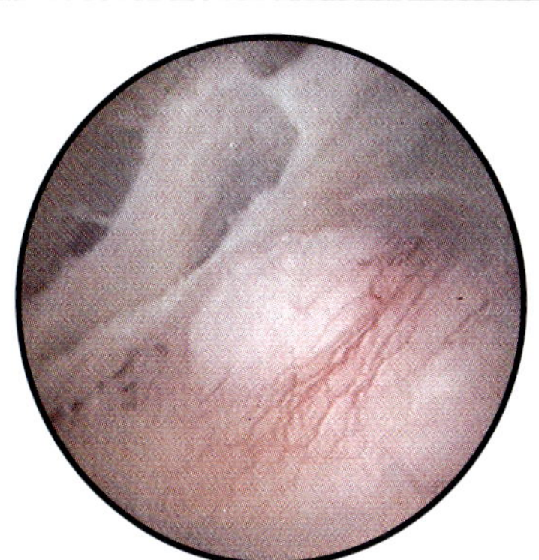

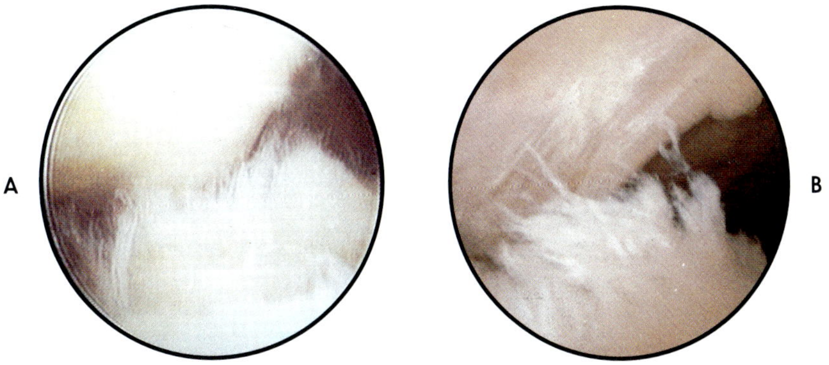

A

B

FIG. 7-77 Superior rotator cuff tear.

A Arthroscopic view shows superior cuff tear below but without erosion under the acromion.

B Arthroscopic view shows both superior cuff tear and erosion under the acromion.

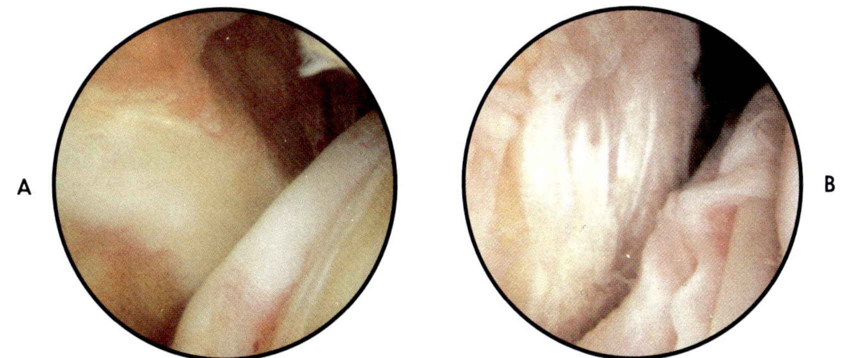

FIG. 7-78 Large rotator cuff tear viewed from subacromial bursa.

A Large rotator cuff tear without acromial erosion.

B Large rotator cuff tear with acromial erosion.

Layered Rotator Cuff Involvement

The extent of the rotator cuff tear may require debridement of the shaggy material to determine the exact nature and location of the tear (Fig. 7-79). After arthroscopic debridement, the tear size and its components are clearly identified (Fig. 7-80, *A*). Further assessment can be made of the mobility of the tear for potential reattachment to the greater tuberosity (Fig. 7-80, *B* and *C*).

This type of intraoperative observation by arthroscopy shows the clear separation of the capsular (static) and tendinous (dynamic) portions of the normal rotator cuff (Fig. 7-80, *B* and *C*). Gross pathological cadaver dissection from older specimens also shows the laminal separation between these two layers (Fig. 7-81). This anatomical area has been thought to represent an intratendinous tear, especially by arthrography, when dye dissects within the cuff and does not enter the subacromial space.[5] The arthroscopic and gross anatomical dissection would show the lesion to be beneath the tendon and above the capsule.[8]

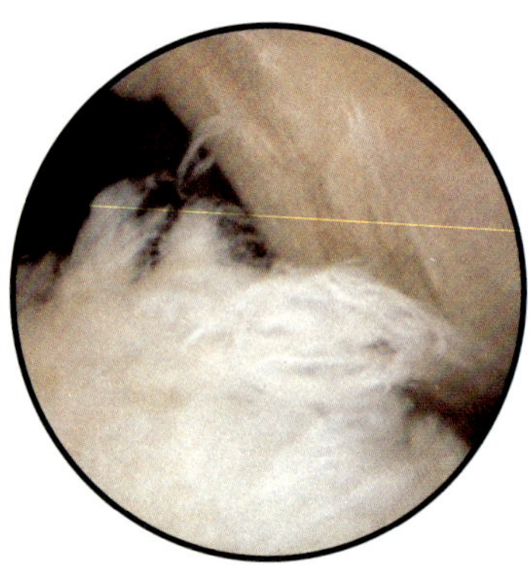

FIG. 7-79 Subacromial view of fragmented rotator cuff tear. Arthroscopic view shows fragmentation of the rotator cuff tear that obscures the very nature of the tear.

Size of Lesion

The size of the lesion varies from small to large. The lesion may be acute or chronic (Fig. 7-82).

Coracoacromial (CA) Ligament

The erosion under the acromion must first disrupt the CA ligament.[22] This is seen with tissue fragmentation by arthroscopy (see Fig. 7-78, *B*). The gross specimen obtained by open acromioplasty shows the disruption of the ligamentous tissue (Fig. 7-83, *A*). The microscopic anatomy demonstrates ligament erosion and the bone beneath (Fig. 7-83, *B*). When the erosion of the ligament is complete, the arthroscopic view shows the exposed undersurface of the acromion (Fig. 7-84, *A*). This view correlates with the gross anatomical cadaver specimen (Fig. 7-84, *B*).

A

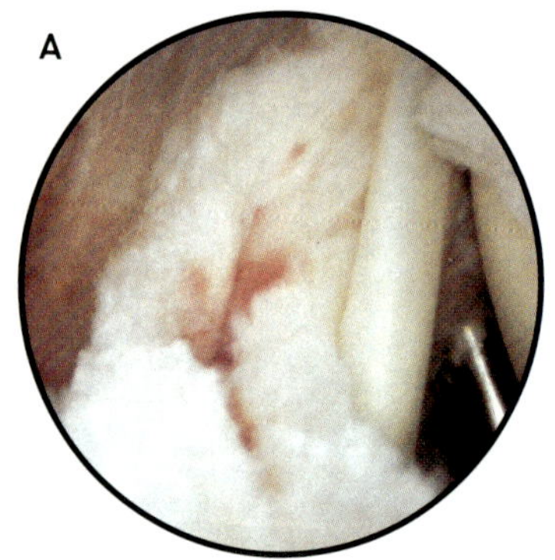

B

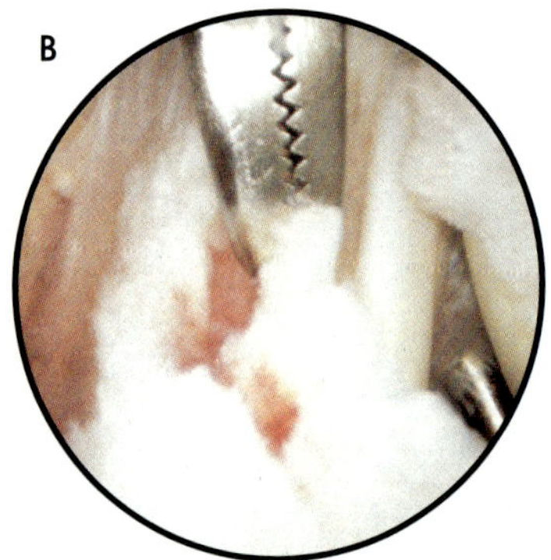

C

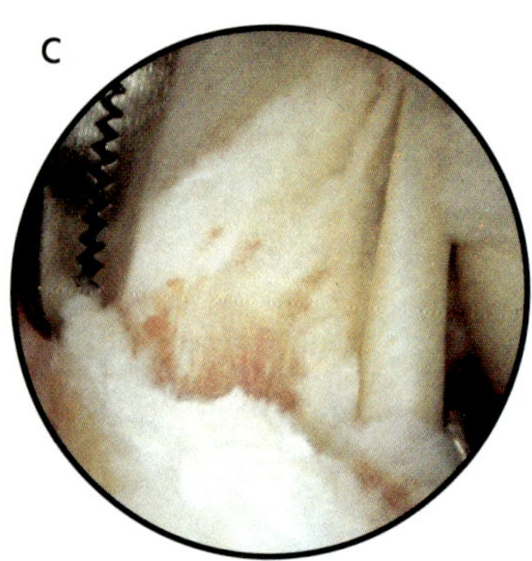

FIG. 7-80 Arthroscopic assessment of components of rotator cuff tear.

A Arthroscopic view of rotator cuff tear after debridement of margins shows biceps tendon to the right, the capsule in middle, and the tendon to the left (superior).

B Arthroscopic view shows grasper on capsular portion.

C Arthroscopic view shows grasper on the tendinous portion of the rotator cuff. Attempts are made to assess possibility of advancement to the greater tuberosity.

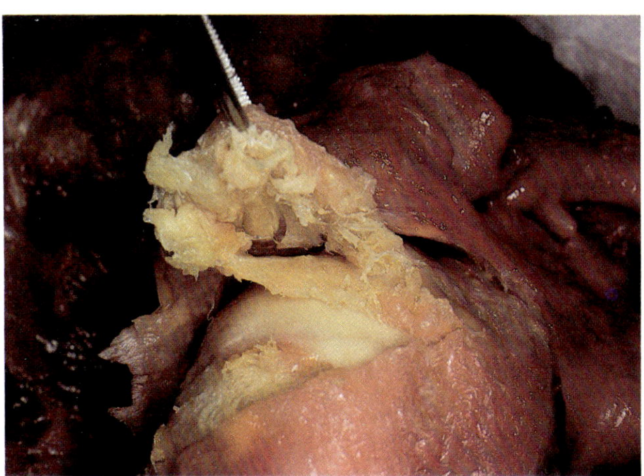

FIG. 7-81 Gross anatomical specimen of intralaminal tear. This gross anatomical dissection of cadaver shoulder shows typical laminar tear of rotator cuff. This opening is not in the tendon, but between the tendon and the capsular portion of the cuff.

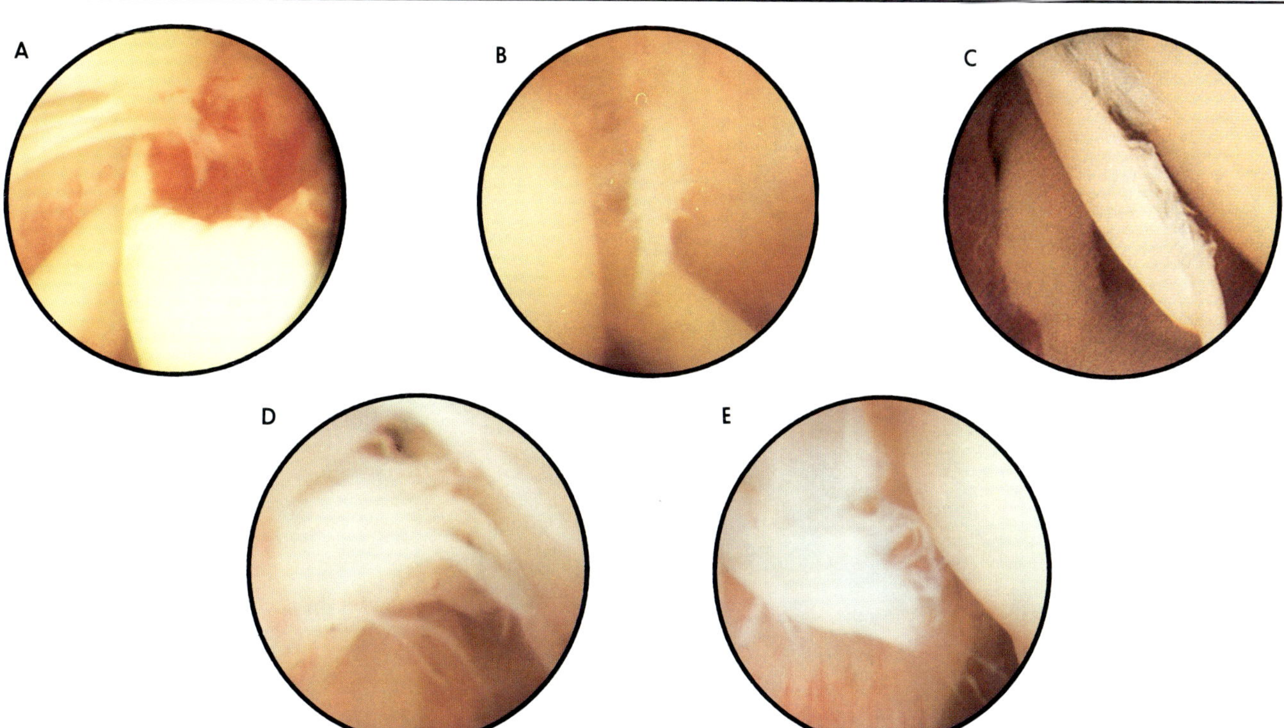

FIG. 7-82 Arthroscopic views of various rotator cuff tears.

A Acute tear isolated to insertion of supraspinatus in professional baseball player.

B Small chronic tear in throwing athlete.

C Large flap tear in laborer.

D Moderate-size tear accompanying anterior dislocation.

E Moderate-size tear in professional woman softball pitcher.

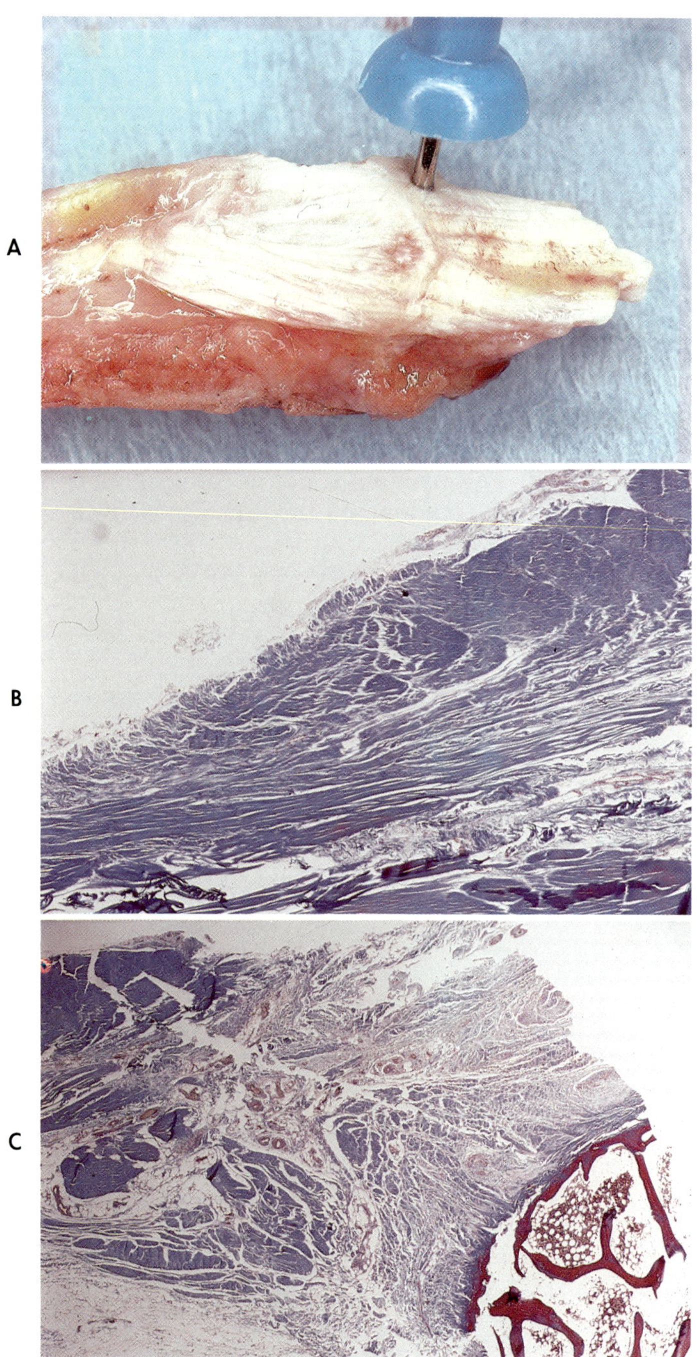

FIG. 7-83 CA ligament.

A Gross specimen shows area of erosion of the CA ligament under the bony acromion.

B Photomicrograph of same specimen shows erosion on CA ligament at bone junction. (Trichrome, original magnification ×20.)

C Photomicrograph of same specimen, but area next to CA ligament attachment to acromion. (Trichrome, ×20.)

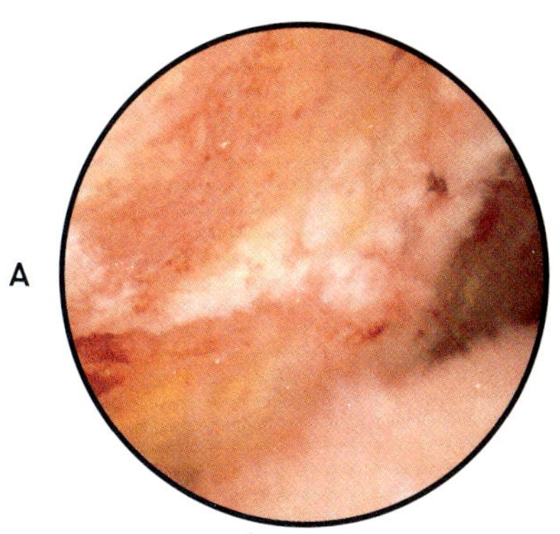

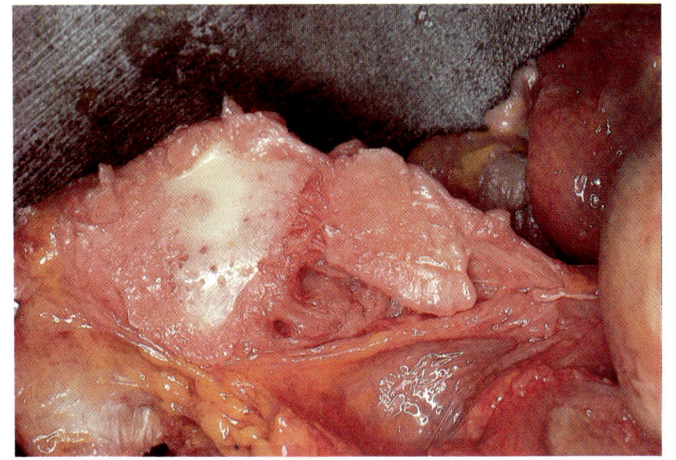

FIG. 7-84 Full-thickness erosion of acromion.

A Arthroscopic view of underside of acromion, when all of the ligament has been eroded.

B Gross anatomical specimen of a similar conditon. Note no soft tissue of the CA ligament is present under the acromion.

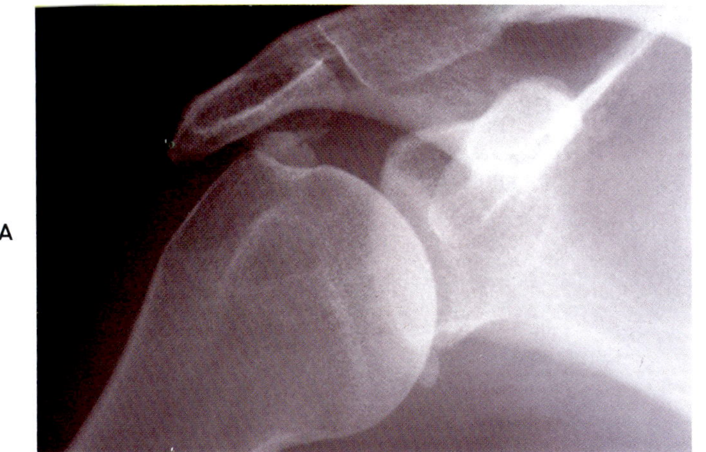

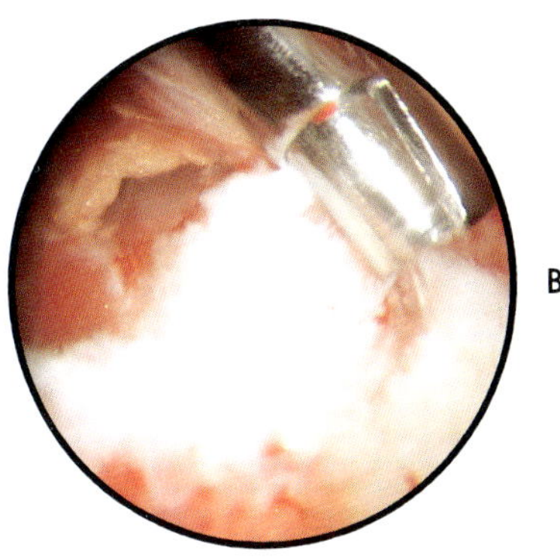

FIG. 7-85 Calcific tendonitis.

A X-ray film confirms the clinical suspicion of acute calcific tendonitis in both superior and inferior lesion.

B Arthroscopic view with cutter in calcium deposit.

Calcific Tendonitis

This condition is clinically suspected by acute pain syndrome and is easily confirmed by x-ray examination (Fig. 7-85, *A*). The condition rarely requires surgery, including arthroscopy. Only those cases that do not respond to conservative measures, including needle aspiration, may come to arthroscopy. In some cases a large calcific mass may limit exposure. The arthroscopic view requires identification with needle puncture and superficial tendon tissue resection to access and remove the calcium (Fig. 7-85, *B*).

Frozen Shoulder

Many etiological explanations have been proposed.[6,7,15-17] The major controversy centers around the existence of intraarticular adhesions as proposed by Neviaser. Contrary to his report, we did not see intraarticular adhesions, but only decreased intraarticular volume (12 ml) and reactive synovitis (Fig. 7-86).[9,19] Subsequent to that report, I have also made it routine to inspect the subacromial bursa. This space was also fibrotic. Small erosions were seen on the undersurface of the acromion, sug-

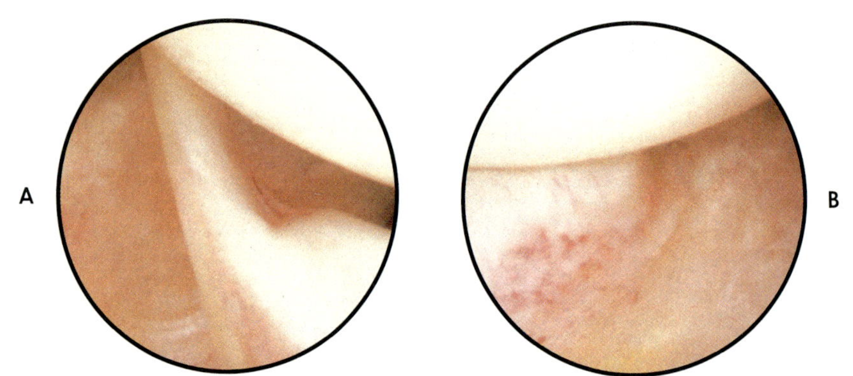

FIG. 7-86 Frozen shoulder.

A Arthroscopic view before manipulation shows diffuse synovial vascularity. No intraarticular adhesions are present.

B Arthroscopic view shows humerus does not move away from the humerus even with maximal distention.

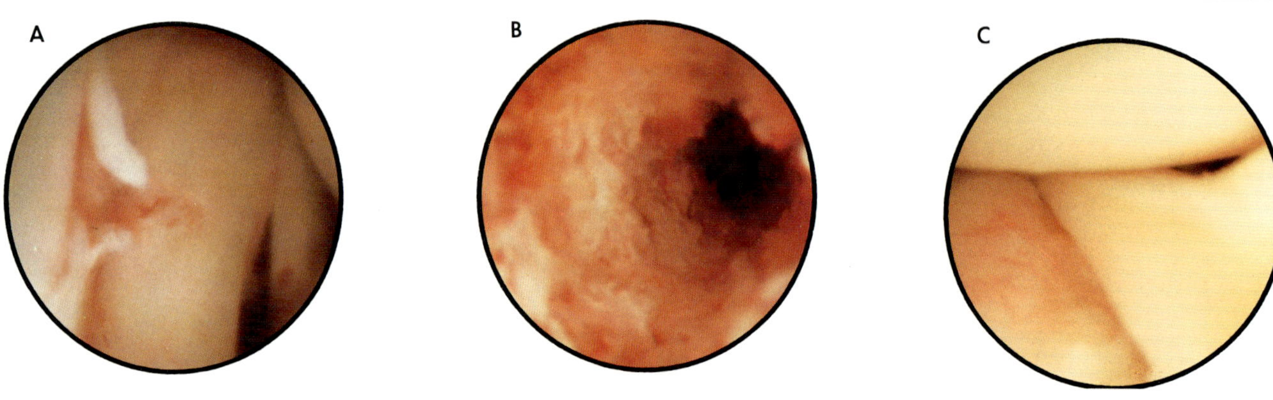

FIG. 7-87 Iatrogenic lesions in glenohumeral joint.

A Injury to rotator cuff with misplaced trocar.

B Hole in humerus caused by incorrect placement and forceful "entry."

C Extravasation of fluid compressing joint from superior.

gesting a component of impingement may accompany frozen shoulder. More case experience would be necessary to demonstrate the association, if any.

Wiley's recently reported arthroscopic findings were similar to those we reported in 1987.[24] The joint capacity was reduced. He demonstated intense synovial vasculitis by photomicrograph.

Following gentle manipulative techniques to regain range of motion, there was hemorrhage seen in the capsular ligaments of the glenohumeral joint (see Chapter 8).

ACROMIOCLAVICULAR JOINT

The acromioclavicular (AC) joint is not easily identified from the subacromial space (see Chapter 10). It is covered by bursal and loose connective tissue. Identification requires probing from beneath to determine if osteophytes are prominent. The use of transcutaneous needles helps identify the joint when combined with subacromial viewing. Visualization of the undersurface osteophytes requires resection of the soft tissue. The bony extension of the acromioplasty shows the osteophytes. The disrupted

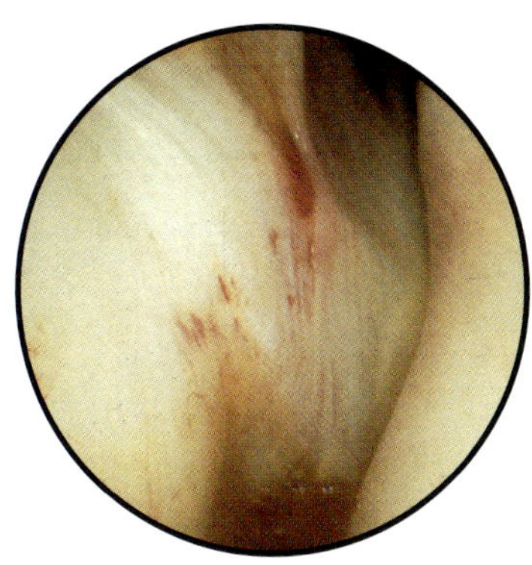

FIG. 7-88 Iatrogenic lesion in subacromial space. Arthroscopic view of hemorrhage on normal CA ligament produced by arthroscope cannula penetration.

meniscus is identified after the acromial bone has been removed. The meniscus will be a flap or even absent (see Chapter 10).

Transcutaneous inspection of the AC joint may show synovitis, especially with degenerative arthritis (see Chapter 10). After the intraarticular debridement of soft tissue, the bone is exposed. Juxtaarticular cysts are exposed with initial bony resection. The osteophytes are not easily seen from this surgical approach because they are covered with thick capsular tissue.

IATROGENIC LESIONS

The transcutaneous passage of the arthroscope cannula and trochar may result in intraarticular trauma (Fig. 7-87). The surgically induced trauma should not be mistaken for a pathological condition like rotator cuff tear (Fig. 7-87, *A*).[18] The postoperative morbidity is greater following bony penetration (Fig. 7-87, *B*).

Technical difficulty can occur with extravasation of fluids. Inadvertent extravasation may be misinterpreted as leakage from a rotator cuff tear. The fluids escaped via arthroscopic portals. The iatrogenic equalization of pressure on each side of the rotator cuff may lead to misinterpretation of a rotator cuff tear (Fig. 7-87, *C*).

Inadvertent injury to the the subacromial space and CA ligament with instrumentation or the arthroscope cannula may occur during entry and must be differentiated from the erosions of the impingement syndrome (Fig. 7-88).

References

1. Andrews JR, Carson WG Jr, Mcleod WD: Glenoid labrum tears related to the long head of the biceps, *Am J Sports Med* 13(5):337-341, 1985.
2. Bigliani LU, Morrison D, April EW: The morphology of the acromion and its relationship to rotator cuff tears, *Orthop Trans* 10:228, 1986.
3. Bigliani LU et al: The relationship between the unfused acromial epiphysis and subacromial impingement lesions, *Orthop Trans* 7:138, 1983.
4. Calandra JJ, Baker CL, Uribe J: The incidence of Hill-Sachs lesions in initial anterior shoulder dislocations, *Arthroscopy* 5(4):254-257, 1989.
5. Cotton RE, Rideout DF: Tears of the humeral rotator cuff: a radiological and pathological survey, *J Bone Joint Surg* 46B 314-328, 1964.
6. DePalma AF: Loss of scapulohumeral motion (frozen shoulder), *Ann Surg* 135(2):193-204, 1952.
7. DuPlay S: De la periarthrite scapulohumerale, *Rev Frat Med* 53:226, 1896.
8. Fukuda H, Hamada K, Yamanaka K: Pathology and pathogenesis of bursal-side rotator cuff tears viewed from En Bloc histological sections, *Clin Orthop* 254(5):75-80, 1990.
9. Ha'eri GB, Maitland A: Arthroscopic findings in frozen shoulder, *J Rheumatol* 8:149-152, 1981.
10. Hayes JM: Arthroscopic treatment of steroid-induced osteonecrosis of the humeral head, *Arthroscopy* 5(3):218-221, 1989.
11. Hill HA, Sachs MD: The grooved defect of the humeral head: a frequently unrecognized complication of dislocations of the shoulder joint, *Radiology* 35:690, 1940.
12. Hopkinson WJ, Ryan JB, Wheeler JH: Glenoid rim fracture and recurrent shoulder instability, *Complications in Orthopedics* March/April:36-40, 1989.
13. Jobe F. Personal communication, 1991.
14. Johnson LL: The shoulder joint: an arthroscopist's perspective of anatomy and pathology, *Clin Orthop* 223:113-125, 1987.
15. Lippman RK: Frozen shoulder, periarthritis, bicipital tenosynovitis, *Arch Surg* 47:283-296, 1943.

15a. McLaughlin HL: Posterior dislocation of the shoulder, *J Bone Joint Surg* 34A:584, 1952.

16. Neviaser JS: Adhesive capsulitis of the shoulder, *J Bone Joint Surg* 27:211-222, 1945.
17. Neviaser TJ: Adhesive capsulitis, *Orthop Clin North Am* 18(30):439-443, 1987.
18. Norwood LA, Terry GC: Shoulder posterior subluxation, *Am J Sports Med* 12:25, 1984.
19. Ogilvie-Harris DJ, Wiley AM: Arthroscopic surgery of the shoulder: a general appraisal, *J Bone Joint Surg* 68B:201-207, 1986.
20. Perthes G: Uber Operationen bei Habitueller Schulterluxation, *Deutsch Ztschr Chri* 85:199-227, 1906.
21. Samelson RL, Prieto V: Dislocation arthropathy of the shoulder, *J Bone Joint Surg* 65A:456, 1983.
22. Sarkar K, Taine W, Uhthoff HK: The ultrastructure of the coracoacromial ligament in patients with chronic impingement syndrome, *Clin Orthop* 254(5):49-54, 1990.
23. Snyder SJ et al: SLAP lesions of the shoulder, *Arthroscopy* 6(4):274-279, 1990.
24. Wiley AM: Arthroscopic appearance of the frozen shoulder, *Arthroscopy* 7(2):138-143, 1991.

CHAPTER

8

The Glenohumeral Joint

This chapter will address the various diagnoses that affect the glenohumeral joint. The diagnoses will be discussed according to the basic surgical procedural categories: incisional, excisional, debridement, repair, reconstructive, and fusion. Each of these has an arthroscopic counterpart.

The American Medical Association's publication of Current Procedural Terminology (CPT codes) for shoulder arthroscopy provide a somewhat different category of surgical procedures (see box). Recognition in this publication indicates that this surgical procedure has a patient benefit and is performed by many surgeons in many and varied geographical places. These codes provide a generalized terminology for surgical billing purposes. The CPT codes for 1992 do not include some of the surgical procedures that have been performed for years by many surgeons. Most notably lacking is the arthroscopic repair of glenohumeral instability. At present, no specific codes are given for arthroscopic acromioclavicular (AC) resection or shoulder fusion. It may take several years after an operation is known for it to receive a CPT code. The operation must meet the critieria of being performed by many doctors in many and varied geographical regions. In addition, new procedures are considered only once a year for CPT code designation.

CURRENT PROCEDURAL TERMINOLOGY (CPT) CODES FOR THE SHOULDER

29815 Arthroscopy, shoulder, diagnostic: with or without synovial biopsy (separate procedure)
29819 Arthroscopy, shoulder, surgical: with removal of loose body or foreign body
29820 Synovectomy, partial
29821 Synovectomy, complete
29822 Debridement, limited
29823 Debridement, extensive
29825 With lysis and resection of adhesions with or without manipulation
29826 Decompression of subacromial space with partial acromioplasty with or without coracoacromial release
29909 Unlisted procedure, arthroscopy

DIAGNOSTIC ARTHROSCOPY

Routine Diagnostic Arthroscopy

A diagnostic arthroscopy should precede or accompany all open shoulder surgery. I recognize this opinion is not shared by everyone, but the arguments against this position are weak and without reasonable medical substantiation. Those who argue against routine arthroscopy say they are able to make a clinical diagnosis that is so accurate that the diagnostic arthroscopy would add nothing to their subsequent decision making and planned open surgical intervention. In my opinion, a diagnostic arthroscopy would at least confirm their clinical judgement. The patient benefit to routine diagnostic arthroscopy is real. Diagnostic arthroscopy may demonstrate an additional or different diagnosis. Arthroscopy has the potential to enhance any surgeon's understanding of the condition under treatment. At the very least the surgeon could use this opportunity to improve his or her arthroscopic skills.

Arthroscopy provides greater access for visualization of the glenohumeral joint than any open operative procedure short of disarticulation. Arthroscopy provides the benefit of magnification. The joint lavage possible in an arthroscopic medium provides for the mobilization and removal of loose bodies. My diagnostic arthroscopy series on glenohumeral dislocations showed many additional lesions that are often not visible by the standard open procedure. The pathological lesions in traumatic anterior dislocation are global in nature. Most of the additional lesions (i.e., loose bodies and labral tears) are amenable to simple arthroscopic debridement. The arthroscopic debridement is more accurate and thorough than what is possible by open surgery, if open surgery indeed revealed the lesion in the first place. Inspection of the subacromial space is another benefit without extending the open surgical incision.

My perception of the real reasons to reject arthroscopy before a planned open procedure is lack of surgeon's expertise with arthroscopic techniques and/or additional consumption of time to perform the arthroscopy, redrape, and/or reposition the patient. This surgical judgment appears to place the doctor's convenience over the potential patient benefit. In experienced hands arthroscopy is performed with dispatch. Redraping is usually not necessary and repositioning takes only a few moments (see below).

These arguments against diagnostic arthroscopy preceding or accompanying open surgery are reminiscent of the 1970s when arthroscopy was first introduced into knee surgery. The argument is no longer valid because diagnostic arthroscopy is an integral part of any surgery on the knee, open or arthroscopic. The sole exception perhaps is total knee replacement, which in reality is an internal amputation of the joint.

Biopsy

Arthroscopically monitored biopsy as a sole procedure is uncommon in shoulder surgery. Biopsy is usually combined with diagnostic arthroscopy, as in synovitis of undetermined etiology. The practice of biopsy in known rheumatoid arthritis seems unnecessary. Biopsy is useful for research purposes. An arthroscopic biopsy should not be considered to require a lesser skill level than arthroscopic surgery. The management of complications of diagnostic arthroscopy and biopsy often requires operative skills.

OPERATIVE ARTHROSCOPY

Trauma

Description. Trauma may result from a direct blow or be secondary to instability. The articular cartilage can be disrupted by a direct blow to the side of the shoulder or with traumatic dislocation. The rotator cuff, biceps tendon, and labrum are subject to tearing by the same mechanism. The bone may be fractured with the same type of mechanisms (i.e., anterior glenoid or Hill-Sachs lesion) (Fig. 8-1).

When the traumatic lesion occurs on the margins of the glenoid, Stephen Snyder[106] has coined the mnemonic G.A.R.D. lesion for Glenoid Articular Rim Divots (Fig. 8-2). He has categorized three grades. Grade 1 involves articular cartilage alone; Grade 2 is cartilage with bone; Grade 3 is all bone.

Treatment. The treatment varies with the potential to reattach lesion. Cartilage lesions are usually debrided. Reattachment is attempted when a significant piece of bone is detached with or without articular cartilage.

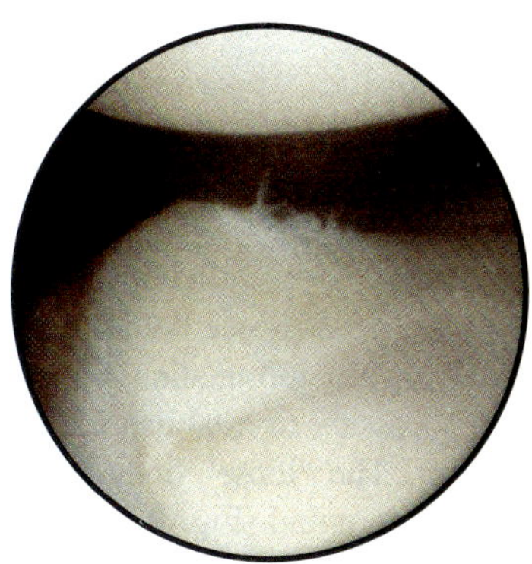

FIG. 8-1 Fracture: Arthroscopic view of fracture of inferior glenoid. The fracture is undisplaced. A line of disruption of the articular cartilage is visible.

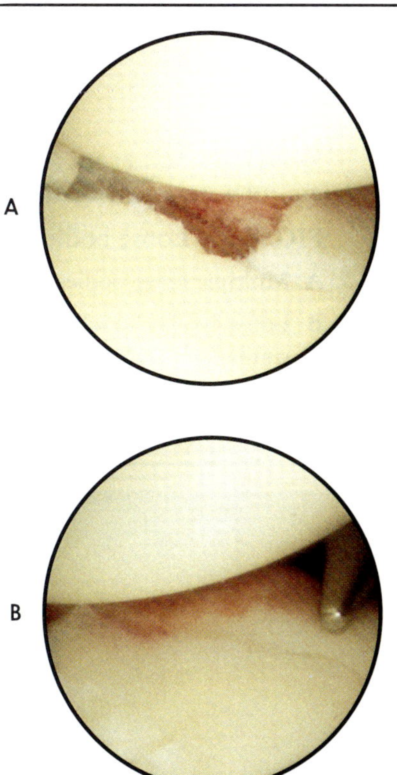

FIG. 8-2 Glenoid articular rim divot (left).

A Arthroscopic view of defect from avulsion fracture of both articular cartilage and bone on anterior-inferior margin of the glenoid following trauma.

B Arthroscopic view of same patient showing intact labrum immediately superior to the rim defect.

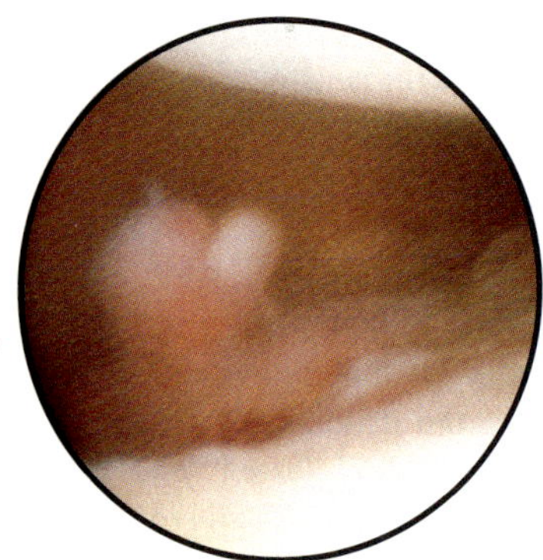

FIG. 8-8 Avulsion fracture: Arthroscopic view shows the displaced bone covered with synovium and prominence of fragmentation on its superior surface.

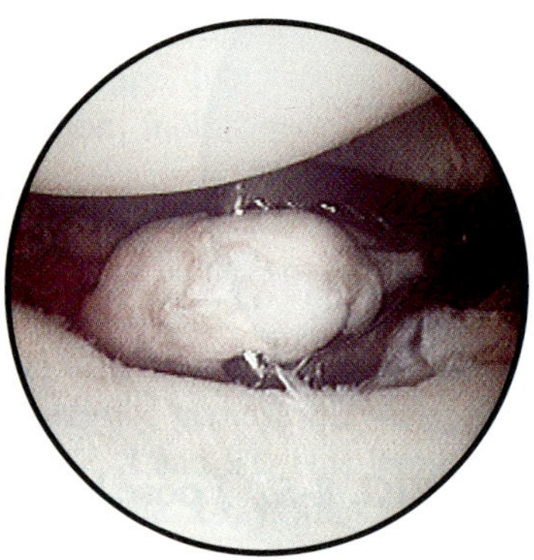

FIG. 8-9 Arthroscopic view of large loose body grasped by Jaws forceps. Large fragments should be removed at conclusion of the procedure to reduce incisional leakage.

view may be required to identify this fracture at the anterior-inferior glenoid location (see Chapter 1). The arthroscopic view may show the avulsion of the anterior glenoid (Fig. 8-8).

Treatment. Small loose bodies are removed by washing out with flow of fluids. A cannula placed within the joint provides the conduit. The arthroscope cannula can be used to remove loose bodies. This is accomplished by maximally distending the joint, followed by quick removal of the arthroscope. The loose bodies will wash out of the joint. Suction can be applied to the end of the cannula. This procedure can be repeated, alternating viewing and cleansing until no other loose bodies are visualized.

When many loose bodies exist additional cannulas are required. The second cannula is for inflow. The third cannula is for removal of loose bodies with motorized instrumentation. A rotation cutting suction instrument can act as a vacuum cleaner as it is moved about the joint. A full-radius cutting head has a smooth contour and is best for soft fragments. Hard fragments may require changing to a more aggressive cutter head.

Larger pieces may have to be broken up to be removed. A large cutter (5.5 mm) will fragment and remove cartilaginous loose bodies. A large bony loose body can be held in place with a transcutaneous No. 18 spinal needle and subject to grinding with an abrader burr. Both of these techniques avoid opening a larger arthroscopic portal wound, whose leakage could compromise distention and subsequent additional surgery. If a large loose body is to be removed with the forceps method, this task should be deferred until the end of any arthroscopic procedure to prevent leakage during the procedure (Fig. 8-9).

Attached "loose" bodies are not mobile. If small, they can be grasped and removed with rotation of the instrument to free them from their soft tissue attachment. When they are large, the attachment is advantageous, in that the loose body can be resected by motorized instrumentation without requiring an additional means of holding the fragment in place. Large bony fragments can be resected by breaking though the outer shell, followed by removal of the inner bone until only a shell remains. Finally, the shell can be fragmented into small pieces for removal.

Surgical judgment must be exercised in treatment of anterior glenoid fracture with dislocation. This bony avulsion may be a small, thin fragment attached to the labrum or glenohumeral ligaments. When small, the piece may be excised and the ligament or labrum reattached to the glenoid. When the bony avulsion is large, the entire capsular/bone unit should be saved. Open surgery is often required to repair this type of injury. A large comminuted fragment may be arthroscopically resected, but followed with an open surgery to repair the defect with a bone graft or transposition of the coracoid process, as in a Bristow procedure.

Labrum Tears

Description. The labrum can be thought of as the O ring of the shoulder; it is circumferential. Therefore tears may occur anywhere on the circle (Fig. 8-10). When the labrum tear is only superior, it is associated with throwing athlete and rotator cuff problems (Fig. 8-11, *A*). When inferior, it is associated with anterior glenohumeral ligament instability problems (Fig. 8-11, *B*).

Labrum tears are commonly associated with trauma to the glenohumeral joint.[66] The most common occurrence is with anterior traumatic dislocation. In this case a variety of types of tears occur (see Chapter 7). The lesion may be a complete disruption of the anterior labrum, looking very

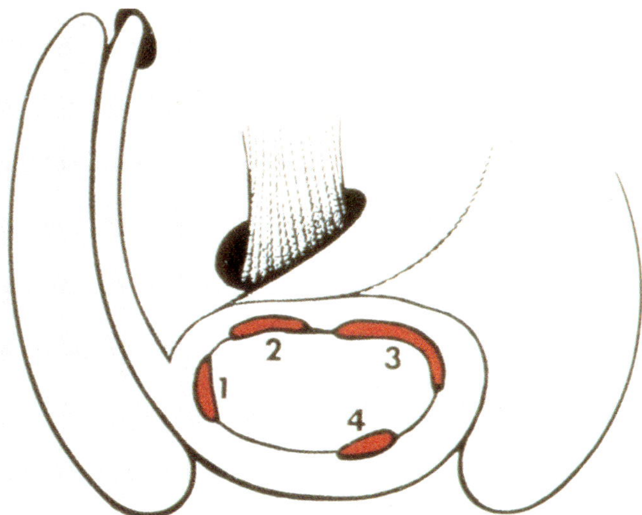

FIG. 8-10 Labral tears: Graphic shows circumferential locations of various tears. *1,* superior; *2,* anterior-superior; *3,* anterior-inferior; *4,* posterior-inferior.

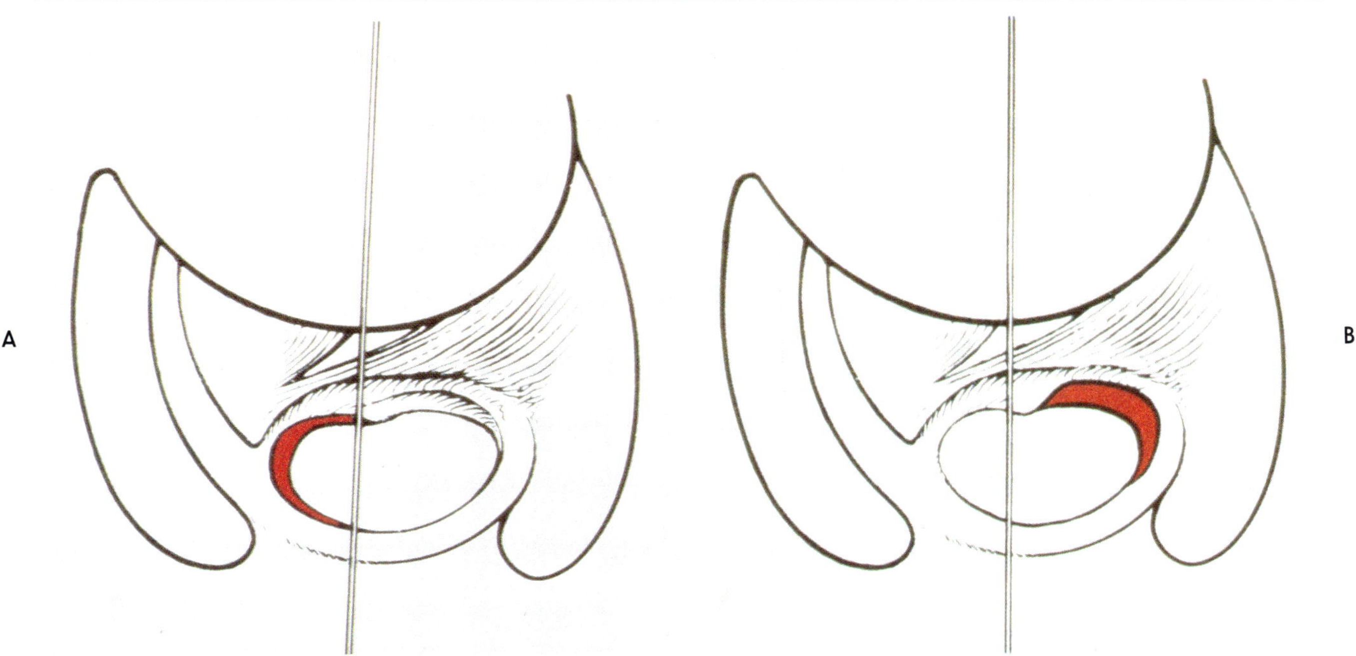

FIG. 8-11 Location of labral tear varies with condition.

A The labral tear located only superior on the labrum is associated with throwing athletes and rotator cuff problems.

B Labral tear on inferior aspect of glenoid is associated with glenohumeral instability problems.

much like a bucket handle tear of the knee joint meniscus (Fig. 8-12, *A*). The tear may be a flap anterior, superior, or inferior (Fig. 8-12, *B* and *C*). Anterior dislocations also have inferior and posterior labrum tears (Fig. 8-13, *A* and *B*).

Labrum tears are common with degenerative arthritis or aging (Fig. 8-14).[56] This may be considered a finding similar to the fringe degeneration observed on the inner margins of knee joint meniscus. This type of tear is small and probably self-limiting in producing symptoms. Kohn studied 106 right shoulder joints from autopsy material within 24 hours of death. There were 67 male and 39 female cadavers ranging in age at death from 1 month to 95 years with the average age 54 years. Fissuring occurred in 76%, and detachment or fragmentation occurred in 50%. In only 16% of the shoulders were no degenerative labrum changes seen at average age 54 years, emphasizing their common occurrence with aging.

Another type of labrum tear is interstitial. This type is probably produced by a traction injury on the capsular ligaments. It is most commonly seen posterior and inferior with anterior-inferior dislocations (see Fig. 8-13). Diagnosis may be determined by computed tomography.[54,98]

Treatment. Surgical treatment of fragmented lesions is limited debridement of the torn tissue, although the clinical significance of isolated lesions is yet to be determined.[56] A careful debridement with motorized instrumentation is indicated for separated degenerated tears (Fig. 8-15).

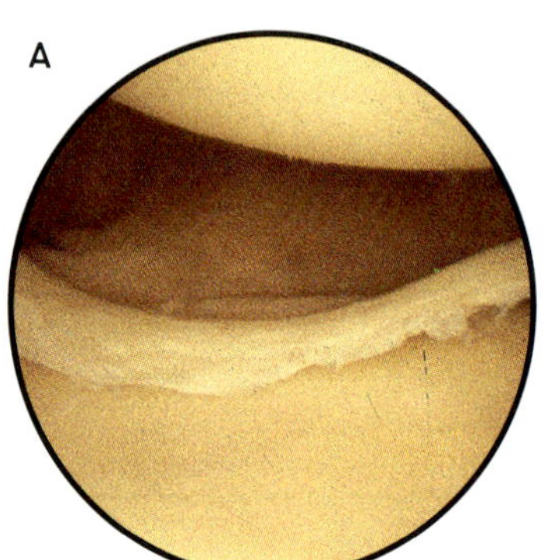

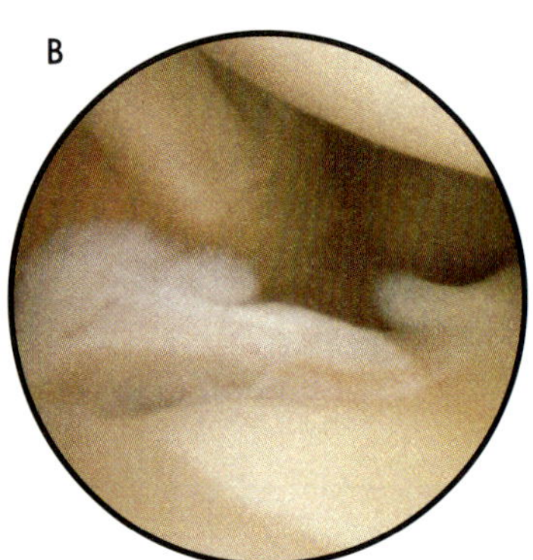

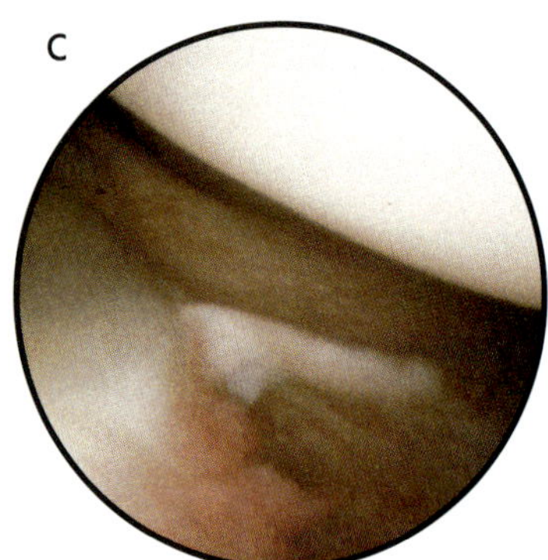

FIG. 8-12 Various labrum tears (right).

A Bucket handle type of tear with ligaments intact.

B Anterior-superior flap tear.

C Anterior-inferior flap tear.

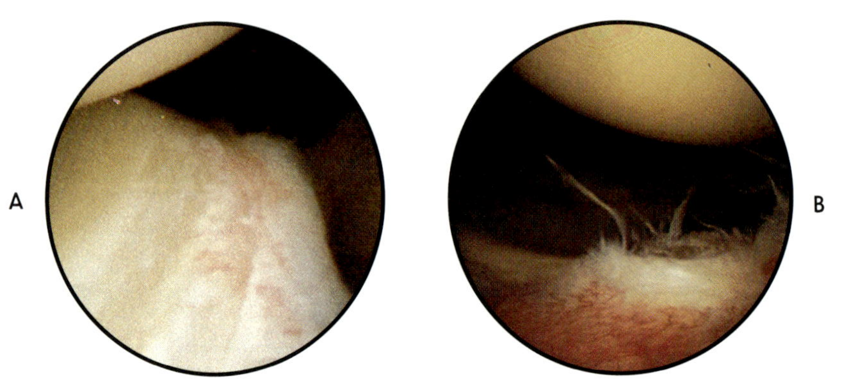

FIG. 8-13 Inferior labrum tear.

A Direct inferior tear associated with sulcus sign.

B Posterior-inferior tear often associated with anterior instability problems.

Care must be taken to minimize the debridement of labrum tears, in that they do represent an extension of the glenohumeral ligament. They also provide a means of static stability to the glenohumeral joint by their physical prominence and effectual widening of the glenoid surface.[43]

If possible, the labrum should be incorporated in capsular ligament repairs or reconstructed. Arthroscopic stapling has been reported by Yoneda et al[124] for superior glenoid labrum tears.

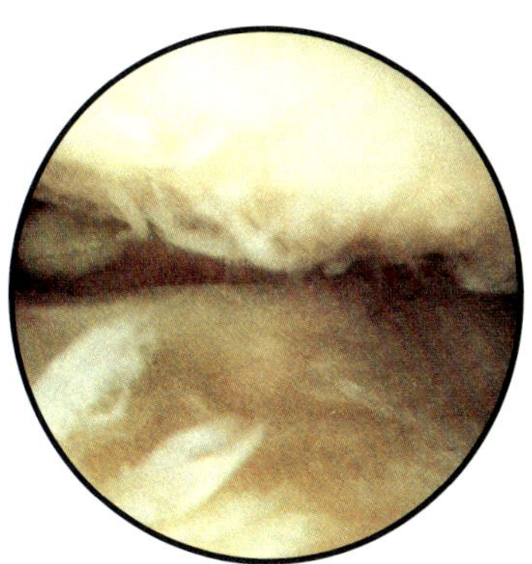

FIG. 8-14 Degenerative labrum tear: This arthroscopic view of patient with diffuse degenerative arthritis shows extensive degenerative labrum fragmentation.

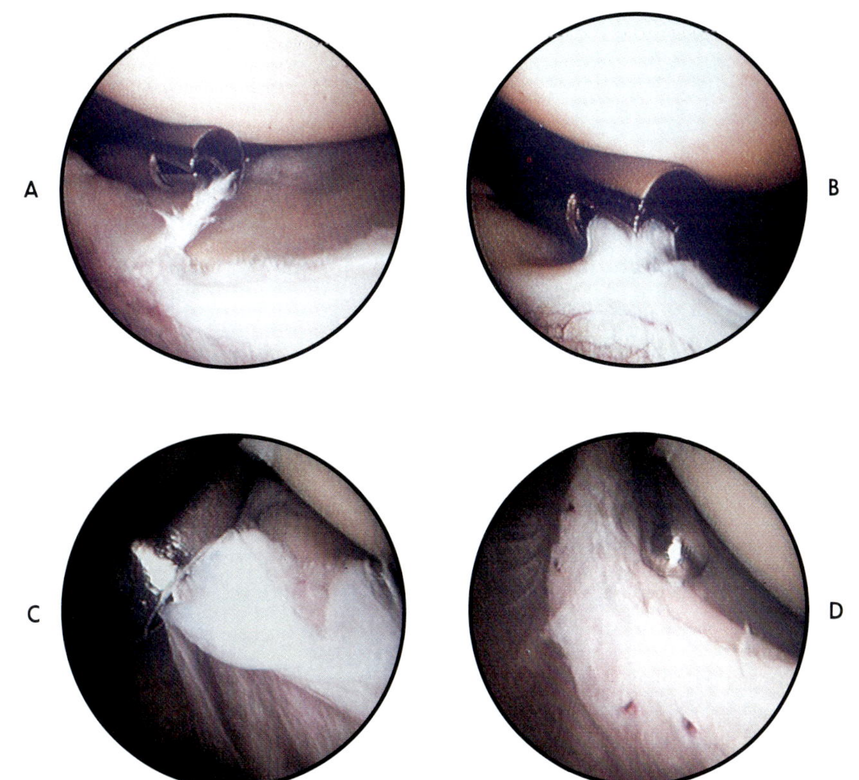

FIG. 8-15 Arthroscopic debridement of labrum tear.

A Labral flap moves toward motorized cutter under force of suction.

B Debridement is initiated.

C Fragment is mobilized with cutter and mobile pieces are removed.

D The final clean up is with full-radius cutter to smooth rim posterior and superior on glenoid.

Biceps Tendon Tears

Description. Tears of the biceps tendon usually accompany rotator cuff tears (see Chapters 7 and 9). This tendon disruption on the superior surface is part of the impingement process of the head against the acromion.

In throwing athletes the biceps tendon tear is traumatic in origin (Fig. 8-16, *A*).[4] It may be associated with a superior labrum tear. The labrum tear may separate the labrum from the biceps tendon at the base or extend longitudinally into the tear.[107] In chronic cases of biceps tearing in throwing athletes, a longitudinal separation of the fibers may have occurred (see Chapter 7).

Intraarticular rupture of the biceps tendon often leaves a stump of biceps attached to the superior aspect of the glenoid (Fig. 8-16, *B*). If long enough, this stump will cause joint irritation.

Treatment. Surgical treatment of biceps tendon tears usually involves partial or complete debridement. In partial traumatic tears, the resection is limited to the torn fibers without disrupting the tendon continuity. In longitudinal tears a motorized instrument with a small orifice can remove the degenerative fibers while preserving the major remaining bands of tendon. The instrument can be placed in between the fibers and manipulated during resection.

In complete tears the stump is resected to the level of the labrum. The stump of biceps is often enlarged, requiring preliminary sectioning with knife blade before debridement with motorized instrumentation. In some cases I have

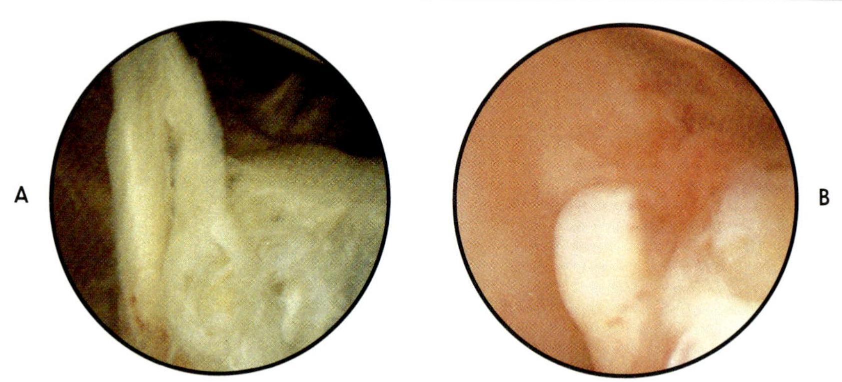

FIG. 8-16 Biceps tendon tears.

A Fragmentation of biceps tendon is extended into the superior labral tear. This is typical of throwing athlete's lesion.

B Stump of biceps tendon remains after rupture or prior open surgical resection. The stump produces joint irritation.

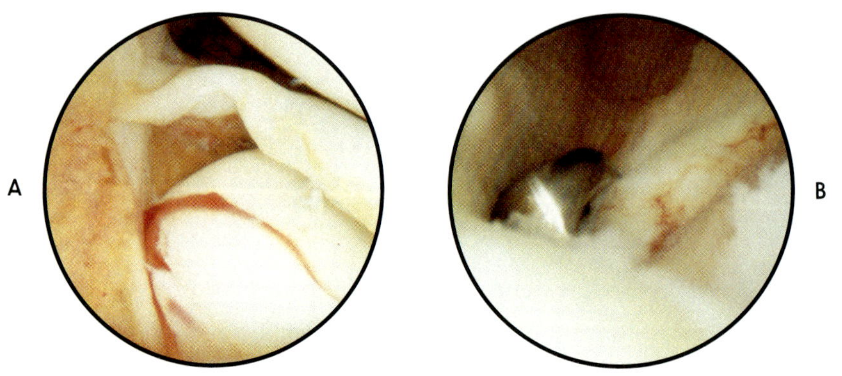

FIG. 8-17 Surgical reconstruction of labrum tear.

A Arthroscopic view shows complete separation of labrum from posterior and superior glenoid, yet attached to base of biceps tendon.

B Immediate postsurgical attachment of the torn labrum to the superior glenoid with metallic staple.

simply resected the stump with a knife blade and removed it with forceps.

A surgical repair may be performed when the biceps can be restored to the glenoid.[124] I have repaired this type of lesion with a metallic staple when detachment extended into the posterior labrum (Fig. 8-17). A second look showed healing to the previously abraded rim of glenoid. I have performed the same procedure for separation directly at the base of the biceps tendon, but without union of the labrum and tendon to the glenoid at staple removal at 8 weeks. Repairs of this type of lesion may be better performed with suture techniques. The use of a biodegradable implant would provide the same fixation without requiring a second look (see Chapter 11).

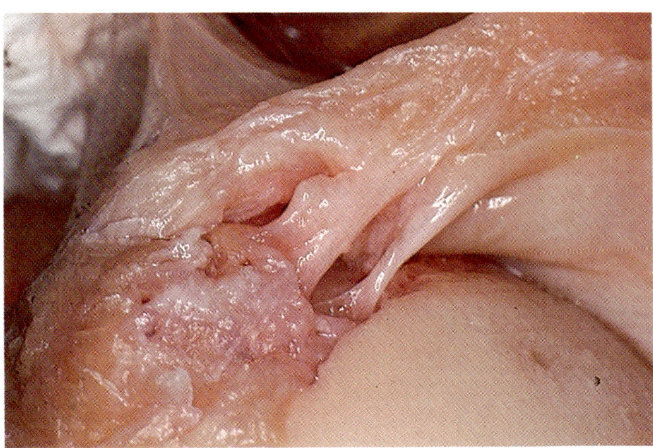

FIG. 8-18 Three-layered "Rotator Cuff": This gross anatomical dissection shows clearly the three layers to the rotator cuff area. The tendon is above, the capsule in the middle, and the synovium is next to the humeral articular cartilage.

Rotator Cuff Tears

Description. The "rotator cuff" has three distinct layers; synovial, capsular, and tendinous. This anatomy is important in understanding the nature and treatment of rotator cuff tears (Fig. 8-18).

The undersurface tear of the rotator cuff is limited to disruption of the synovial and/or capsular layers. When tears extend into the tendinous portion of the cuff, a communication into the subacromial bursa usually results (see Chapter 9).

Partial-thickness tears are usually small (Figs. 8-19 and 8-20, *A*). Care must be taken to examine the extent of the lesion. Often an extension of a "pita bread" type lesion extends posterior from the easily visualized anterior and superior opening in the supraspinatus tendon area (Fig. 8-20).

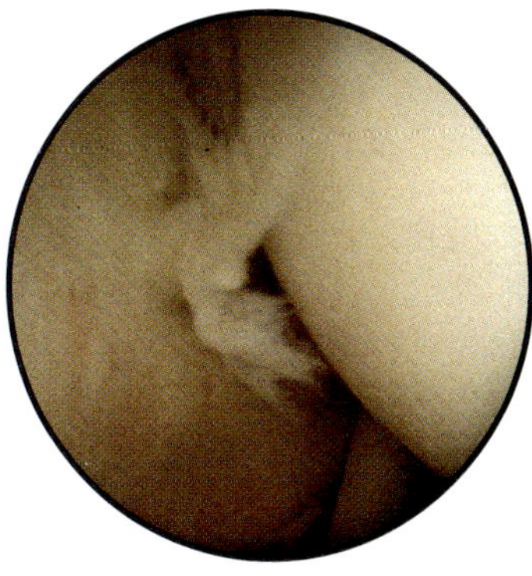

FIG. 8-19 Partial rotator cuff tear: Arthroscopic view of synovial and capsular fragmentation hanging into the joint with partial cuff tear.

A

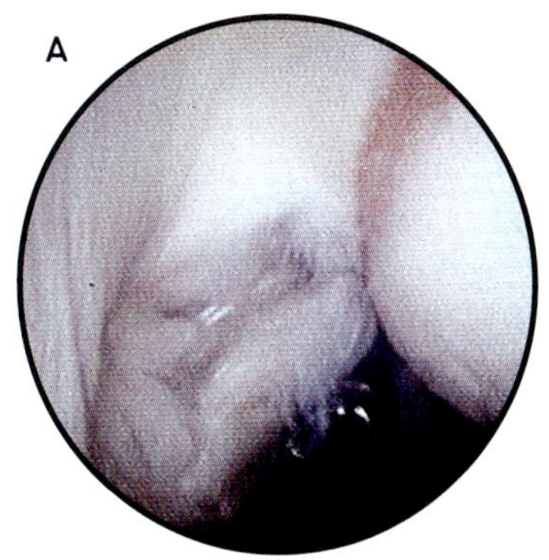

B

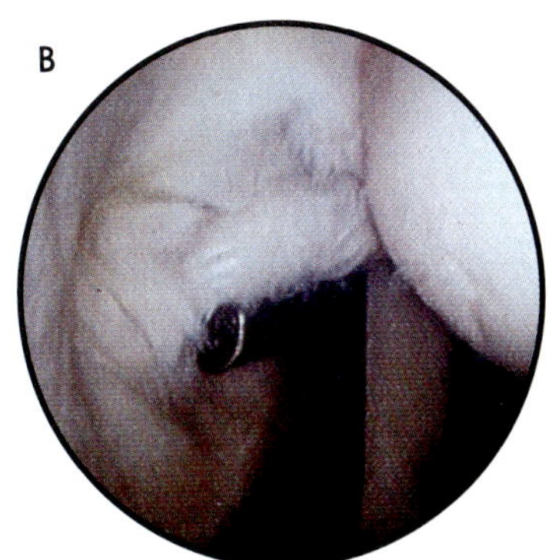

C

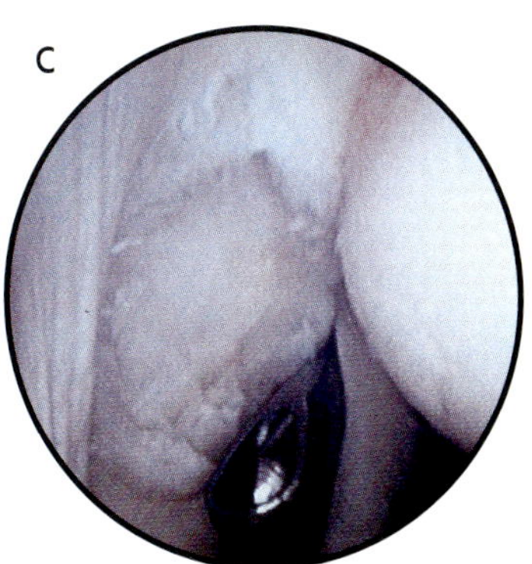

FIG. 8-20 Debridement of partial rotator cuff tear.

A The undersurface rotator cuff tear is located near supraspinatus attachment to the humeral greater tuberosity. This is arthroscopic view.

B Debridement is initiated to determine the depth and extent of the lesion.

C After debridement of the partial tear, the flaps have been removed and the base is smooth. No communication to the subacromial space exists.

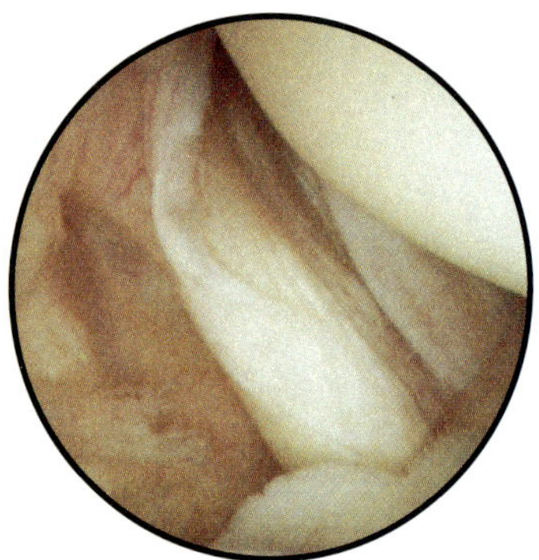

FIG. 8-21 Subscapularis tendon tear: Arthroscopic view of tear and deformity of the superior margin of the subscapularis tendon.

An isolated superficial tear in the area of the infraspinatus tendon attachment is not common in my experience.

The subscapularis tendon is often deformed, torn, or frayed with rotator cuff disease (Fig. 8-21) (see Chapter 9). Diagnostic attention should be given to the interval between the subscapularis and the supraspinatus tendon to ensure this interval has not lost its integrity and widened. Tearing of this interval may also occur with traumatic anterior-inferior dislocation of the shoulder. Recognition of interval widening is an indication for surgical closure.

Further diagnostic testing in determining the extent of rotator cuff tears can be performed with use of methylene blue dye. Dye is injected into the glenohumeral space and simultaneous inspection of the subacromial space will determine the potential connection of a full-thickness defect if dye flows from one space to the other (see Chapter 9).

Treatment. Surgical treatment of the partial-thickness small underside lesion of the rotator cuff is usually effective in relieving symptoms (see Fig. 8-20). Care must be taken to ensure that the lesion has not penetrated into the subacromial bursa and that erosion of the acromion does not exist.

When acromial erosion exists with a partial-thickness, underside rotator cuff tear, the cuff is debrided and an arthroscopic acromioplasty is performed. I do not take these underside rotator cuff lesion alone as a reason for routine acromioplasty, even in patients with positive physical examination signs of impingement. I reserve acromioplasty for patients who have confirming arthroscopic evidence of impingement by subacromial erosion findings (see Chapter 9).

Degenerative Arthritis

Description. Arthroscopic debridement procedures are limited to those patients without bony architectural changes. When the humeral head is incongruous to the glenoid, the range of motion is limited (Fig. 8- 22). I have performed debridement procedures on this type of patient, but without benefit; the patient still complains of pain at the point of mechanical restriction of motion. This type of patient will eventually be a candidate for total shoulder arthroplasty.

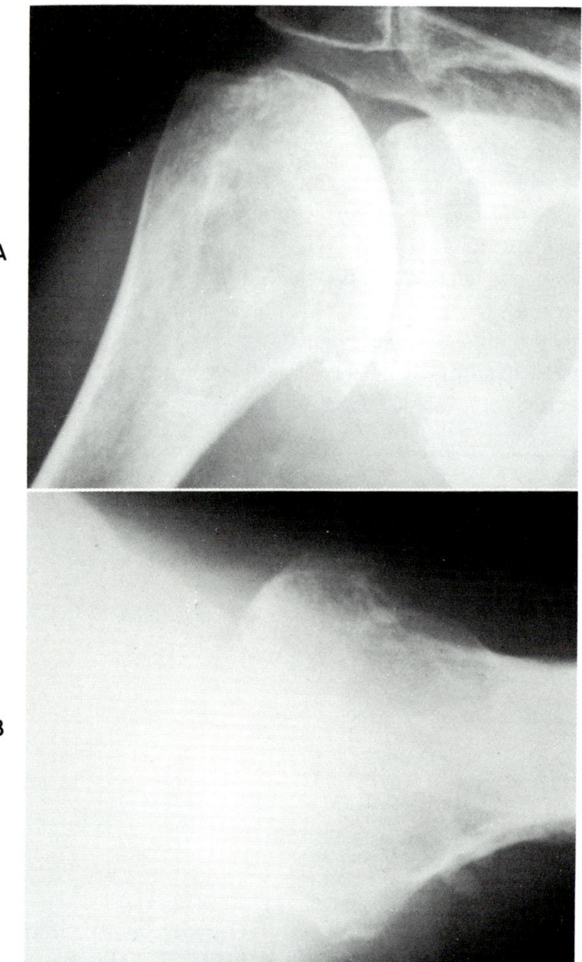

FIG. 8-22 Degenerative arthritis.

A Anterior-posterior x-ray film of degenerative arthritis in shoulder with incongruity of joint surface.

B Axillary view shows fattening of humeral head.

On the other hand, when a patient has degenerative arthritis with preservation of motion, an arthroscopic debridement has given relief of pain. The diagnostic arthroscopic picture is one of fragmentation and associated synovitis (Fig. 8-23).

Treatment. The arthroscopic debridement procedure includes removal of any and all loose bodies, complete synovectomy, and chondroplasty. The debridement should

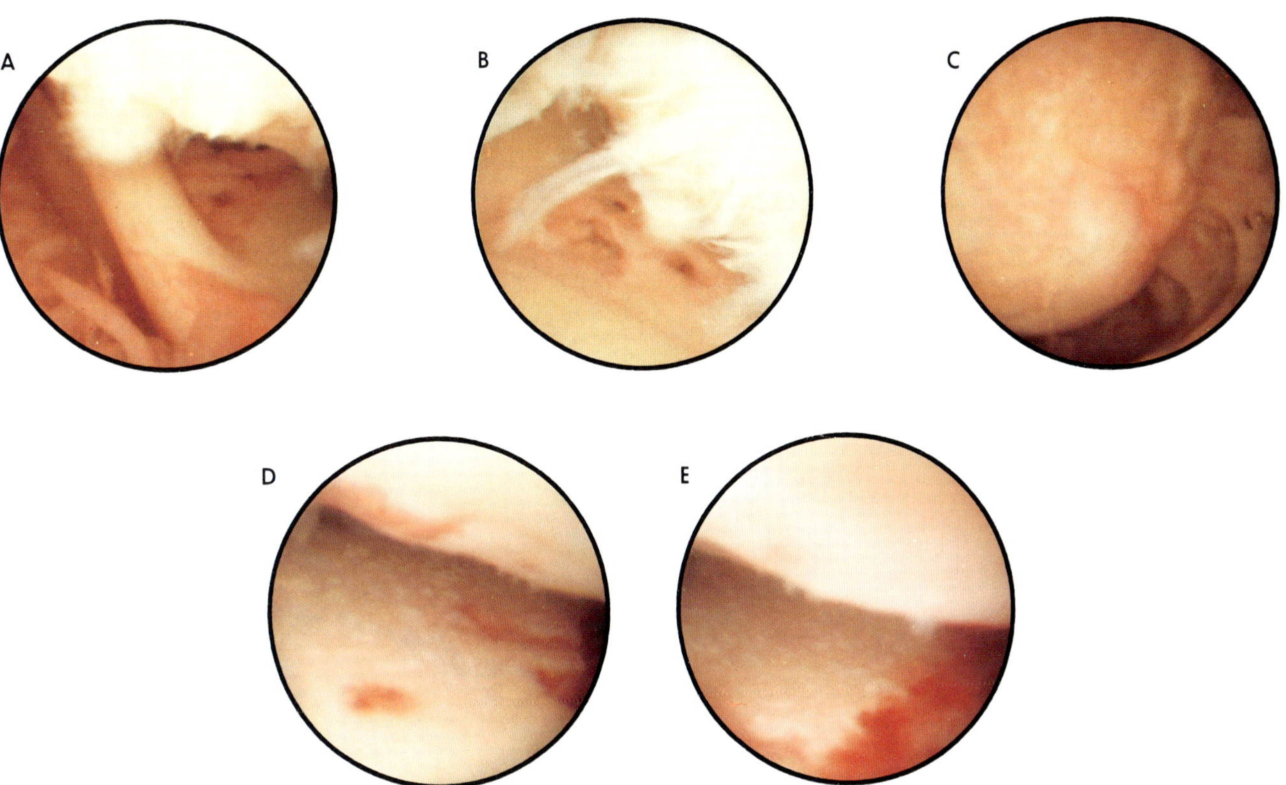

FIG. 8-23 Degenerative arthritis.

A Arthroscopic view of degenerative synovitis near biceps tendon.

B Degeneration and fragmentation on humeral head.

C Granular degenerative change on humerus.

D Arthroscopic view of exposed bone with natural restored areas of fibrocartilage and recent hemorrhage of surface vessels.

E Arthroscopic close-up of hemorrhage areas on glenoid.

be restricted to the level of articular cartilage involvement. A partial-thickness lesion should not be converted to a full-thickness lesion by abrasion.[49] Areas of exposed bone will require abrasion arthroplasty. Drilling into bone is unnecessary as the blood supply is within the bone cortex.

Resection of osteophytes is difficult because they are not accessible. The glenoid rim is covered with labrum and capsule. On the humeral side the larger osteophytes are usually inferior and not safely technically approachable. The removal of osteophytes, even if possible, will not improve motion, in that associated bony incongruity of the articular surfaces plus capsular fibrosis produces the restricted motion.

Osteochondritis Dissecans

Description. This is not a common lesion in the shoulder. The three cases I have seen have been on the glenoid surface. I am not sure that it is the same condition as seen in the knee (see Chapter 7).

Each of my cases has a different location, underlying disease, or attachment. Such variety makes it difficult to say this is osteochondritis dissecans, but similarities do exist.

A lesion similar to that seen in the knee has been recognized on three occasions in my practice.[51] The first case involved rheumatoid arthritis, and a small fragment was removed at arthroscopic synovectomy. The base of the lesion was filled with granulation tissue (Fig. 8-24). The second patient was a professional baseball pitcher with a painful shoulder. A large fragment was removed by arthroscopy (Fig. 8-25). The player continued his successful career. The preoperative and postoperative plain film x-rays (8-year follow-up) are illustrated in Chapter 7 (see Fig. 7-8). The third patient was also a throwing athlete,

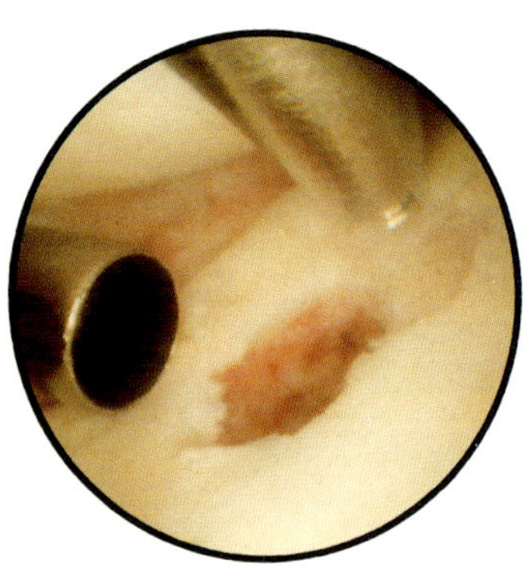

FIG. 8-24 Osteochondritis dissecans in glenoid.

but recreational rather than professional. In this case the bony fragment was elevated with the posterior labrum (Fig. 8-26, *A*). An arthroscopic debridement was performed on the base, and fixation was provided with a metallic staple. A planned second procedure removed the metal staple and demonstrated the healed fragment (Fig. 8-26, *B*).

Treatment. The arthroscopic surgery consisted of removal in two cases and repair in one case. The use of biodegradable implants should provide a more effective method of treatment in the future (see Chapter 11).

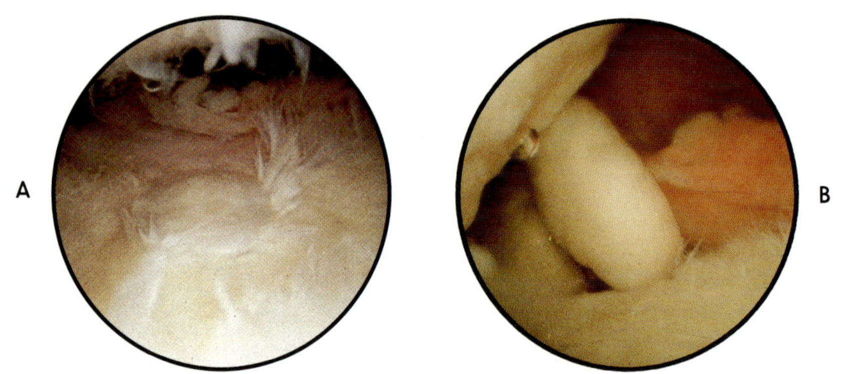

FIG. 8-25 Osteochondritis dissecans.

A Arthroscopic view of defect in central area of glenoid. Associated degenerative arthritis is present.

B Loose body associated with osteochondritic lesion of glenoid.

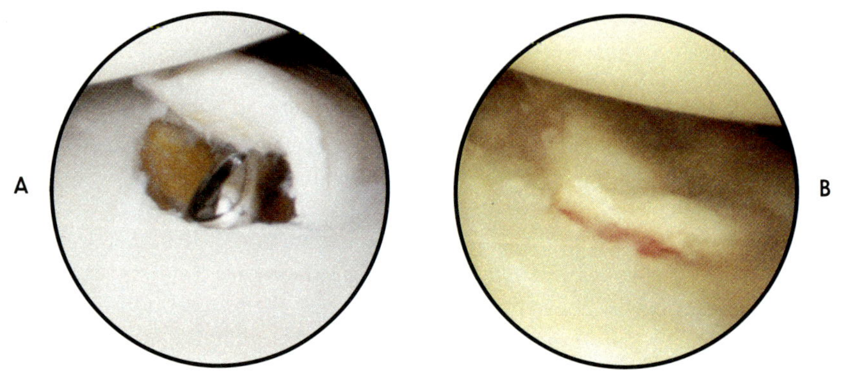

FIG. 8-26 Osteochondritic lesion with attached posterior labrum.

A Arthroscopic view at time of repair. The defect is elevated with motorized instrument during debridement of the base of the lesion. The defect was reduced and held with a metal staple.

B Arthroscopic view of healed defect at time of planned staple removal (8 weeks).

Aseptic Necrosis

Description. Aseptic necrosis can occur in the humeral head (Fig. 8-27). It may accompany sickle cell disease, lupus erythematosus, alcoholism, and diabetes mellitus. It has been reported in the humeral head following steroid treatment.[40] Fragmentation of the these areas may produce loose bodies.

Treatment. Arthroscopic debridement is beneficial in a small early lesion.[40] Transcutaneous bone grafting of the defect may be considered. The larger lesions require prosthetic shoulder arthroplasty.

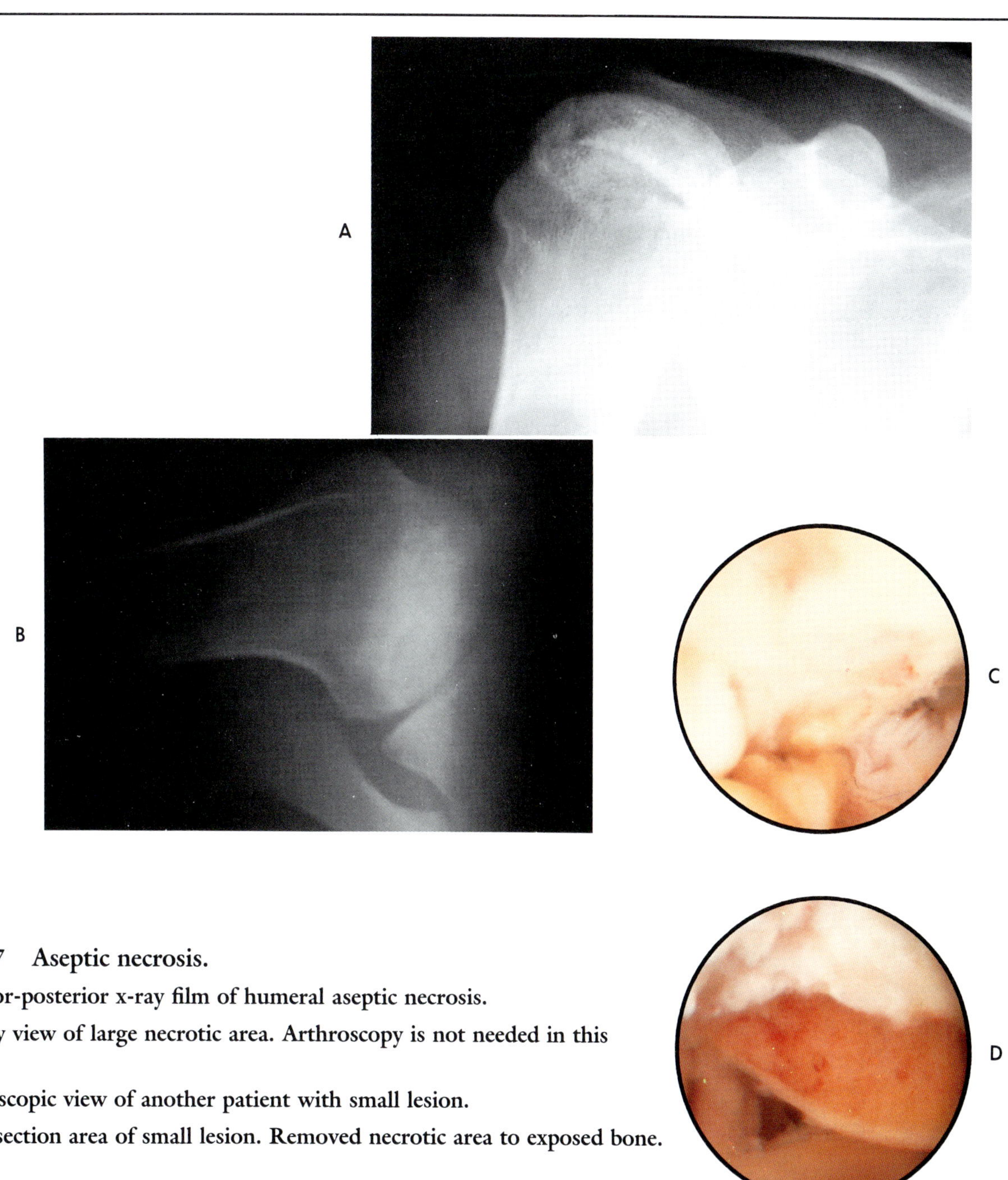

FIG. 8-27 Aseptic necrosis.

A Anterior-posterior x-ray film of humeral aseptic necrosis.

B Axillary view of large necrotic area. Arthroscopy is not needed in this case.

C Arthroscopic view of another patient with small lesion.

D Postresection area of small lesion. Removed necrotic area to exposed bone.

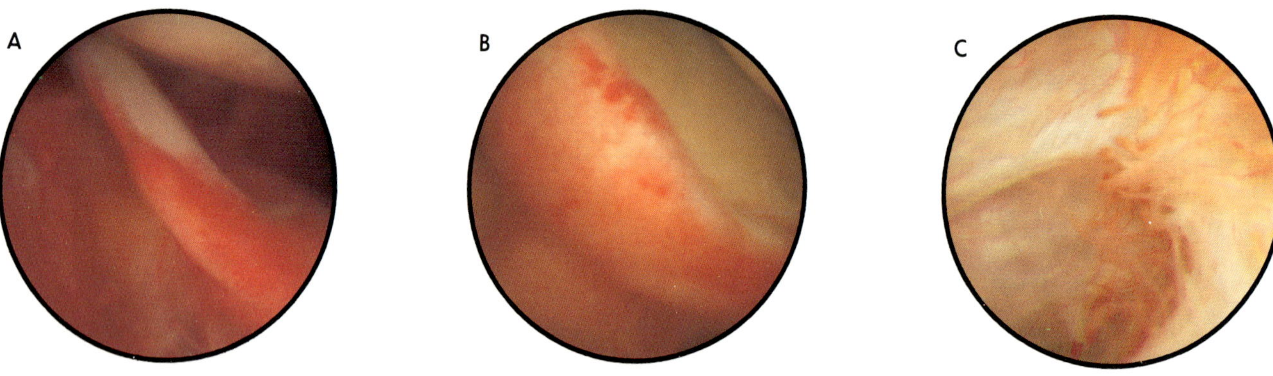

FIG. 8-28 Inflammatory synovitis.

A Arthroscopic view of synovitis on biceps tendon.

B Arthroscopic view of vascular inflammatory synovitis on posterior-superior glenoid labrum.

C Subscapularis bursa synovitis in painful shoulder of competitive swimmer.

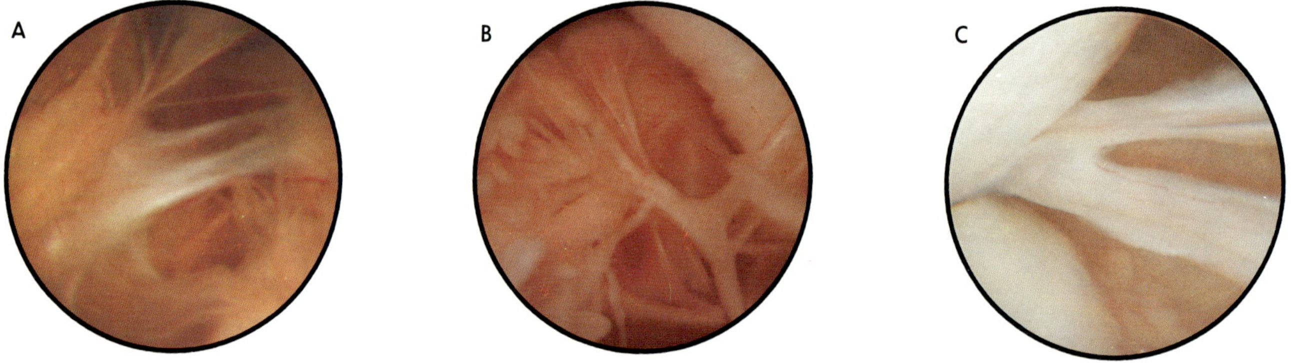

FIG. 8-29 Reactive synovitis and fibrosis.

A Arthroscopic view of anterior reactive synovitis secondary to failed open surgery for recurrent dislocation.

B Reactive synovitis and scar after rotator cuff reconstruction.

C Fibrous adhesions in patient with history of direct trauma.

Inflammatory Synovitis

Description. Inflammatory synovitis is common with frozen shoulder, impingement syndrome, and with overuse syndrome in athletes (Fig. 8-28).

Treatment. Arthroscopic surgical treatment would be performed with partial synovectomy, usually limited to the villa and synovium, but not including the capsule as in rheumatoid arthritis.

Nonspecific Synovitis and Fibrosis

Description. Previous surgery and trauma are the common causes of reactive synovitis and fibrosis (Fig. 8-29). This condition can exist with a chronic loose body, degenerative arthritis, a juxtaarticular metallic implant, and overuse.[32]

Treatment. Arthroscopic surgical treatment is directed to the underlying cause. Local synovectomy and intraarticular adhesiolysis is indicated.

Rheumatoid Arthritis

The shoulder joint is especially suited anatomically for arthroscopic synovectomy (Fig. 8-30). By contrast the open surgical exposure is of considerable magnitude and the resultant access to the synovial lining is restricted. The arthroscopic approach by-passes open intervention and provides maximal access for complete synovectomy. A patient benefit may be achieved even in later stages when degenerative changes also exist. In the severe case the synovectomy is combined with debridement of loose articular debris. The synovectomy is facilitated with interchanging of arthroscope and instrumentation portals (see Chapter 5).

An assessment can also be made of the rotator cuff, which is often involved in rheumatoid disease. The cuff is often so thin that it is not amenable to repair. An arthroscopic acromioplasty may be included in the procedure.

The postoperative morbidity of arthroscopic synovectomy is minimal and the procedure can be performed on an outpatient basis. Immediate postoperative active mobilization of the shoulder is possible.

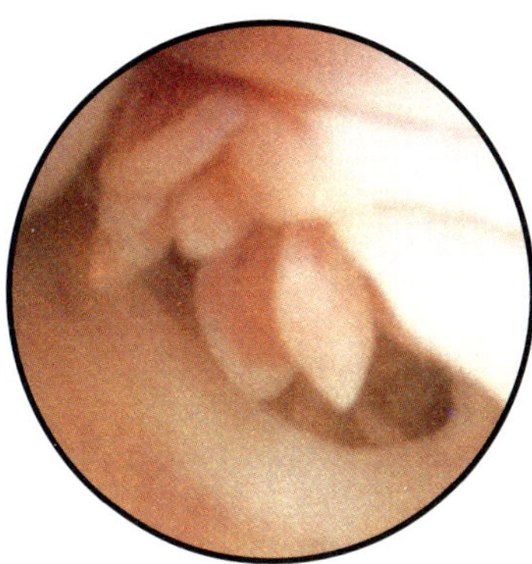

FIG. 8-30 Rheumatoid arthritis: Arthroscopic view of proliferative synovial villa.

Infection

Septic arthritis of the glenohumeral joint is uncommon.[88] The usual postoperative infection following open surgery would be the most common presentation for the surgical practitioner. In this case the infection would be in multiple spaces and best treated by open exploration of the previous wound and drainage, plus antibiotic therapy.[88]

An infection following arthroscopic surgery of the glenohumeral joint would be localized and amenable to arthroscopic treatment as with the knee joint. Arthroscopy provides a means of culture, debridement, and placement of closed irrigation tubing. Because of the rarity of the condition, I have no personal experience with arthroscopic treatment of infection of the shoulder joint.

GLENOHUMERAL JOINT INSTABILITY

The use of the term *instability* is nonspecific. Further definition is required in patient assessment and treatment. The most common instability of the glenohumeral joint is that produced by trauma and in the anterior-inferior direction.

Although not as common, the other instabilites are important to recognize in the differential diagnosis. Their etiology is different and the treatment must be individualized. The posterior instabilities will be discussed later in this chapter.

Step-by-Step Differentail Diagnosis

I look at this sorting process as though it were a conical paper cup filled with all the diagnostic possibilities. When the cup is full of liquid, we have all cases that present with the shoulder "going out." I start the process by eliminating cases that are not indicated for surgery of any type. Subsequently, I work toward those that are amenable to arthroscopic surgical correction.

I remove from consideration those cases identified as functional or emotional causes.[91] The sorting process includes the voluntary dislocator. I like the word *intentional* to describe this type of person, because it is a stronger indication of the mechanism than is the word *voluntary*. I use the word *DISLOCATOR* for one who causes the problem and *DISLOCATION* for the inadvertent condition. One type of patient will reproduce his or her intentional instability by passive force (Fig. 8-31). Another type of voluntary and intentional dislocator will reproduce the instability by active muscle contraction (Fig. 8-32). Plain film x-rays taken in both the reduced and dislocated position are helpful for comparison (Fig. 8-33).

I eliminate those candidates with posterior or multidirectional instabilities whose surgical treatment would be a posterior capsulorraphy or open capsular shift procedure.

I now am left with those patients under reasonable suspicion of having traumatic anterior glenohumeral instability. The medical history, patient interview, imaging techniques, and finally arthroscopy will further eliminate those with only subluxation.

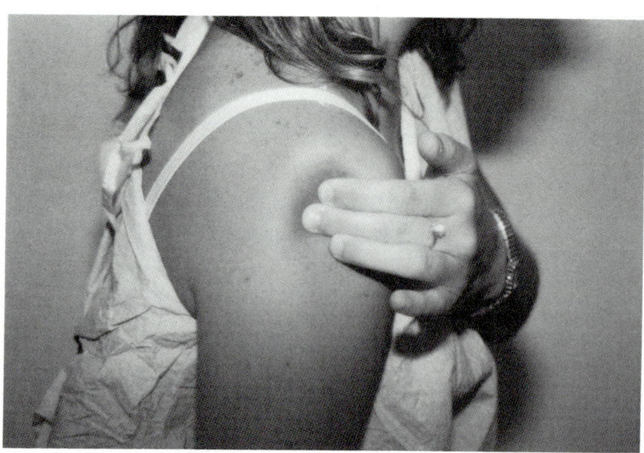

FIG. 8-31 Intentional and voluntary anterior instability: Clinical photograph of patient reproducing direct anterior instability with passive force. She is also able to reproduce this motion with voluntary muscle contraction.

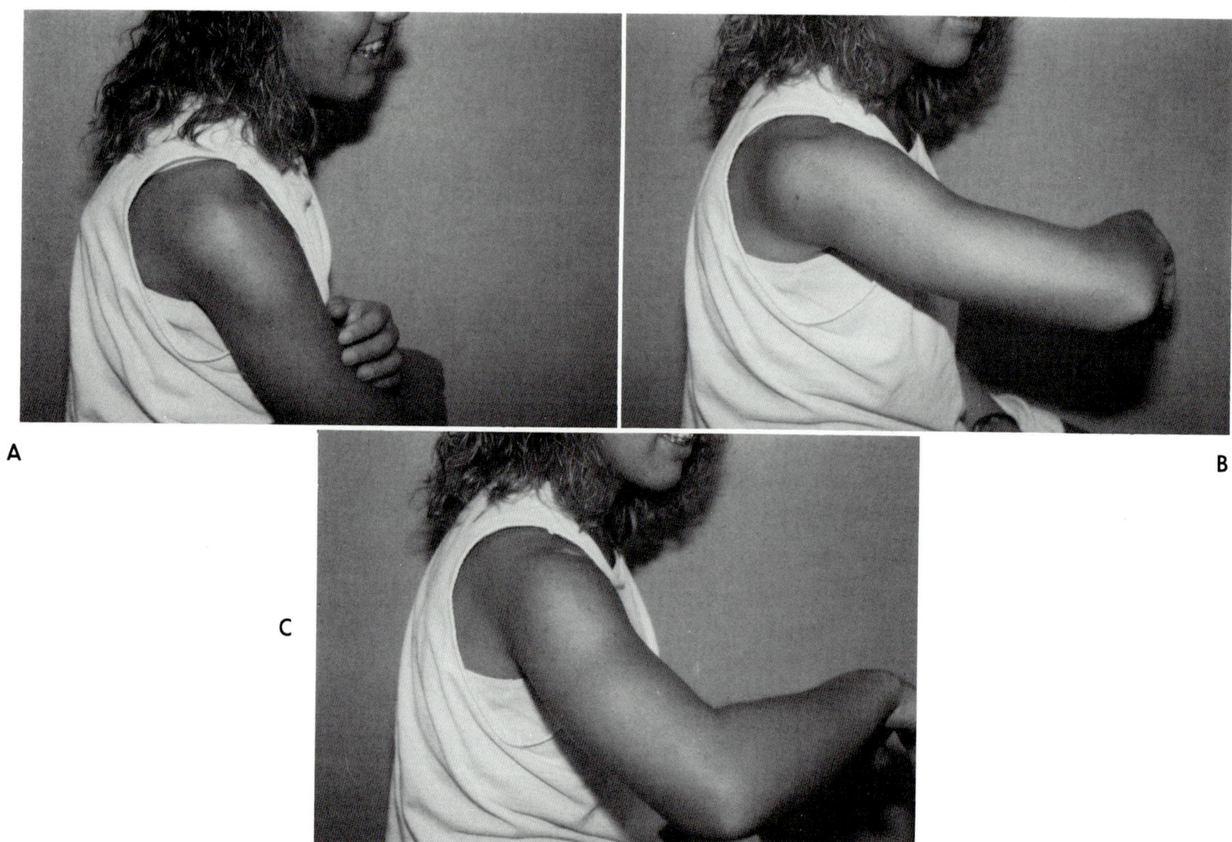

FIG. 8-32 Intentional and voluntary posterior instability: Patient is able to reproduce the motion that produces the instability and causes "pain." This is often demonstrated to the delight of the patient and the consternation of the parents.

A The arm is held in slight flexion and adduction. The muscles selectively and slowly contract. The humeral moves posterior.

B The arm is then elevated and posterior glenohumeral subluxation is complete.

C The arm is moved posterior and the humeral head reduces with a sudden thud.

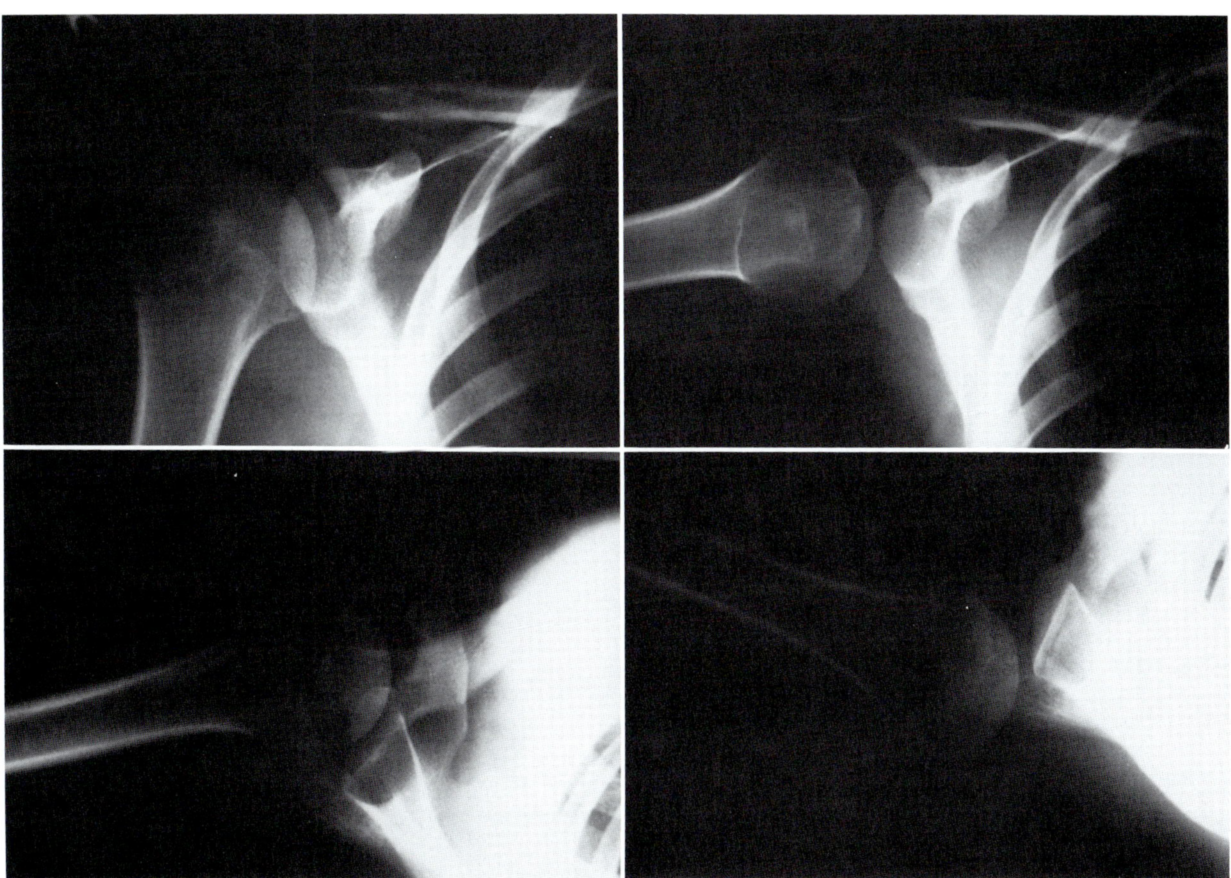

FIG. 8-33 Correlative plain film x-rays: X-ray films confirm the posterior position of the arm in this type of patient.

A Anterior-posterior view with arm at rest and shoulder reduced.

B Anterior-posterior x-ray with arm adducted and shoulder subluxed. This correlates with Fig. 8-32, *B*.

C Axillary view in resting position. Shoulder reduced.

D Axillary view in subluxed position. Shoulder is posterior. This x-ray film correlates with Fig. 8-32, *B*.

Subluxation or Dislocation? The surgeon must differentiate between subluxation and dislocation. Subluxation is a partial disengagement of the joint. Many of the medical, historical, and physical examination findings may be the same for subluxation and dislocation. The classical means of identifying a dislocation by history of "going out" and "someone had to put it in" do not discriminate one from the other. The physical examination findings of "apprehension" and "instability" are present in both conditions. Even the examination under anesthesia is not reliable, even with previous documented dislocation. The arthroscopic findings vary considerably in shoulder instabilities. Therefore a list of criteria must be established for differentiation.

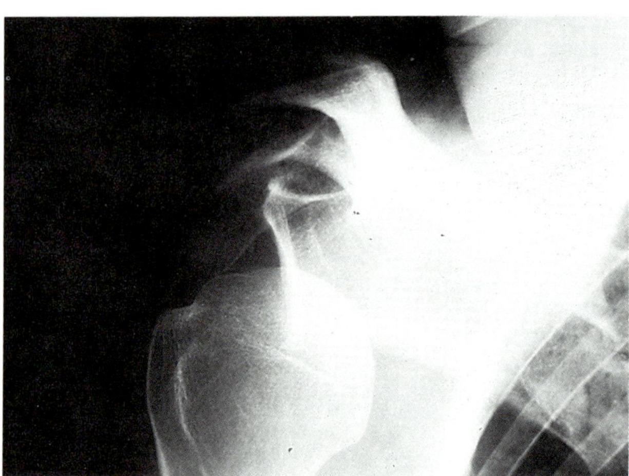

FIG. 8-34 X-ray film gives positive proof of "instability" being a dislocation.

The diagnostic sorting procedure for a patient with suspicion of traumatic anterior dislocation of the shoulder is established per the following protocol:

I. Dislocation (complete disengagement of the humerus on the glenoid) (Fig. 8-34)
   A. Absolute evidence
      1. X-ray evidence with both AP and axillary views
         a. Immediately after injury/before reduction
         b. Physical examination stress test reproduces dislocation
   B. Circumstantial or indirect evidence
      1. Medical history with typical description
         a. Need for manual reduction
         b. Supported by medical observer
      2. Physical examination (clinical)
         a. Decreased external rotation
         b. Manual dislocation
      3. X-ray evidence
         a. Hill-Sachs lesion (Figs. 8-35 and 8-36)
         b. Fracture of anterior-inferior glenoid
      4. Examination under anesthesia
         a. Reproduction of dislocation
      5. Arthroscopic findings
         a. Hill-Sachs lesion
         b. Perthes' (Bankart) lesion
   C. Anterior capsular ligament deficit
      1. Site
         a. Superior
         b. Middle
         c. Inferior

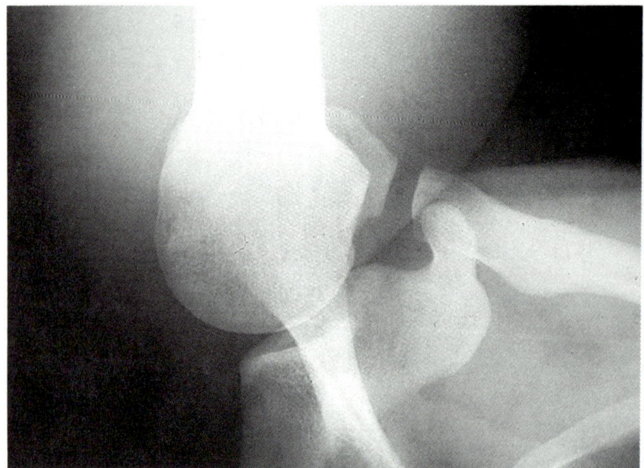

A

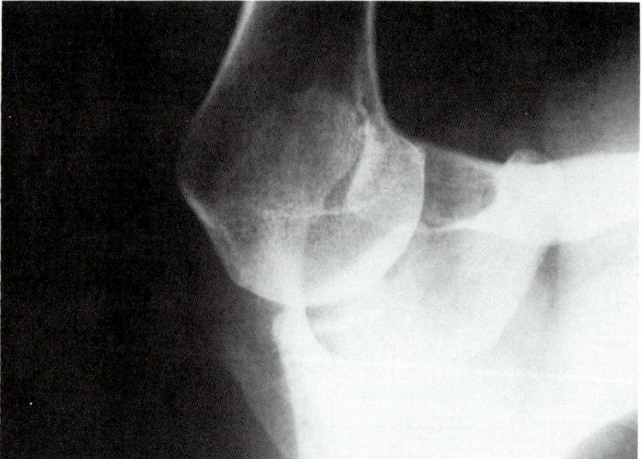

B

FIG. 8-35 Stryker X-ray: This view shows the defect of the Hill-Sachs lesion.

A Normal opposite shoulder.

B Defect seen on posterior aspect of affected shoulder humeral head. Film was reversed to permit exact positional correlation.

2. Type
    a. Tear
    b. Stretch
    c. Laxity
    d. Contracted
    e. Absence

D. Labrum tear
    1. Anterior-inferior
    2. Posterior-inferior

E. Rotator cuff tear
    1. Partial
    2. Complete

F. Subscapularis tendon tear

G. Glenoid fracture

H. Loose body

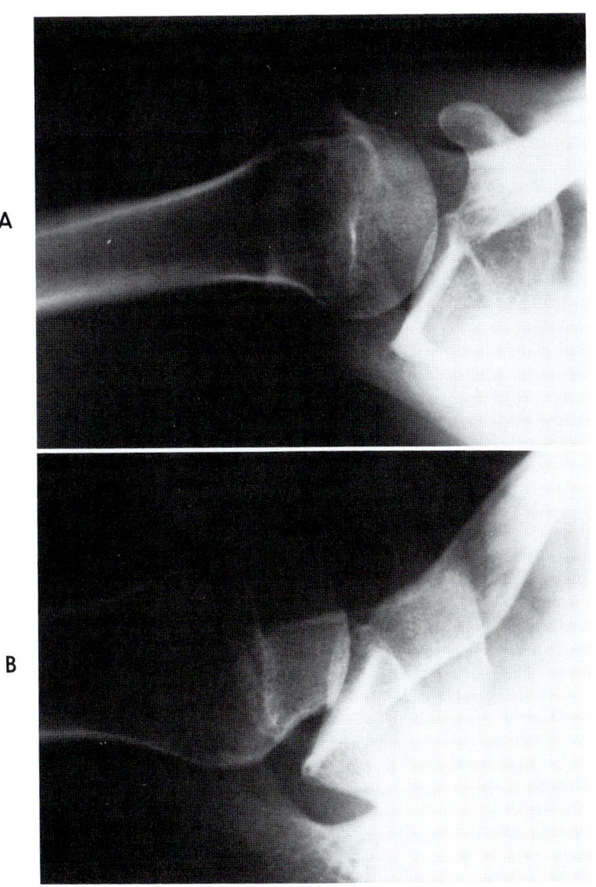

FIG. 8-36 Axillary X-ray: This view shows not only the defect in some cases but the direction of movement.

A Normal opposite shoulder.

B Defect in humeral head contacts the juxtaarticular surface of the glenoid.

II. Subluxation

A. There are no absolutes for this diagnosis; it is a diagnosis of elimination

B. Circumstantial or indirect evidence
    1. Medical history of "going out" or "going out and back in"
    2. Physical examination
        a. Unable to dislocate
        b. Apprehension present or absent (Fig. 8-37)
        c. May be able to reproduce
    3. No x-ray evidence
        a. Dislocation
        b. Hill-Sachs lesion
        c. Glenoid fracture
    4. Examination under anesthesia
        a. No dislocation
    5. Arthroscopic findings
        a. No Hill-Sachs lesion
        b. Anterior labrum/ligament injury present
        c. Excessive joint distraction with distention

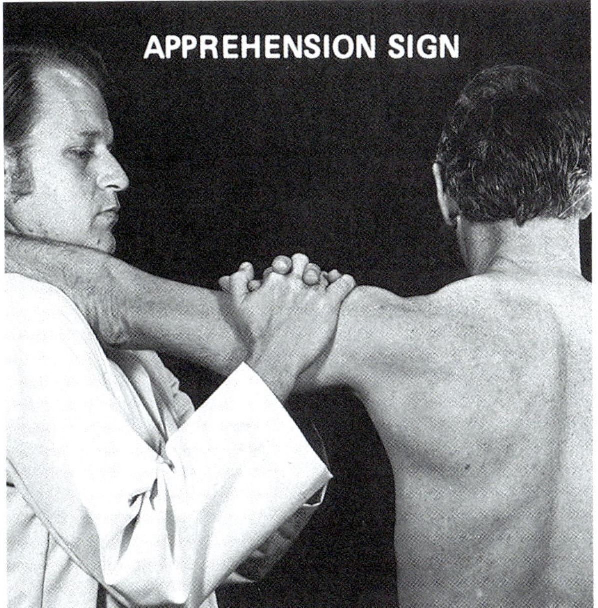

FIG. 8-37 Apprehension test: This clinical test is valuable in assessing anterior and inferior instability. It is performed in a gentle manner, creating the end point of minimal displacement and expression of apprehension by the patient. (Courtesy John Feagin, Durham, North Carolina.)

Medical History Factors

Focusing on trauma concerning shoulder instability is common. The pitfall of this approach is that other types of instabilities may also have a traumatic aspect. The patient with a multidirectional instability may fall, resulting in a traumatic episode with anterior displacement. A patient with a voluntary dislocation of the shoulder may also present after a traumatic episode. A careful medical history of sequences of events plus the patient's demonstration of reproduction of the mechanism and direction is important to the differential diagnosis (see Figs. 8-31 and 8-32).

Another factor to assess is the magnitude of the translation. Was this a partial (subluxation) or complete (dislocation) event? Often the patient feels the shoulder went out, but how far was not known. It may have gone out and spontaneously reduced, suggesting a subluxation, but in reality it dislocated.

Physical Examination Factors. The range of motion is important in evaluating a patient with glenohumeral instability. The important motion is external rotation at the side and in 90 degrees abduction. In patients with tissue laxity, the motion will be greater than normal on both sides and they will have hypermobility of both elbows. The shoulder of a throwing athlete also shows increased range of motion on the throwing arm as compared to the other arm. A patient with subluxation will have increased motion of the affected shoulder, and also the opposite shoulder.

It may be somewhat surprising to find the physical examination of a patient with a well-documented history of anterior traumatic history includes nonconfirming tests of shoulder stability. The only finding may be a restricted range of motion.

Table 8-1 Range of Motion (Average Degrees)

	At the side		90 degrees ABD	
	Dislocated	**Normal**	**Dislocated**	**Normal**
Clinical Examination				
Active external rotation	43°	54°	96°	110°
Anesthetized				
Passive external rotation	57°	69°	95°	116°

Clinical study. Over a period of time I examined 30 consecutive patients with traumatic anterior dislocations for stability and range of motion both in the office and during anesthesia. The average age in this group was 25 years. There were 27 men and 3 women. The average number of dislocations was 7.5.

These patients were evaluated preoperatively for instability and external range of motion with the arms at the side and at 90 degrees abduction position. The same tests were performed with the patient under general anesthesia. The diagnosis of dislocation was confirmed at arthroscopy.

On clinical examination, all patients had apprehension, but no patient was manipulated to the point of dislocation. Under anesthesia, 8 were stable, 6 were subluxed, 13 were

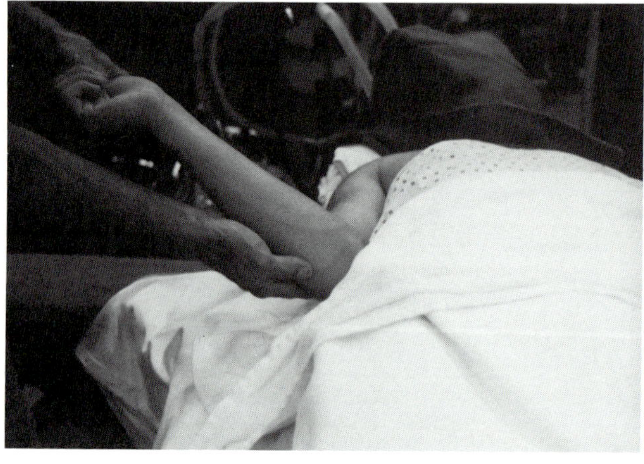

A

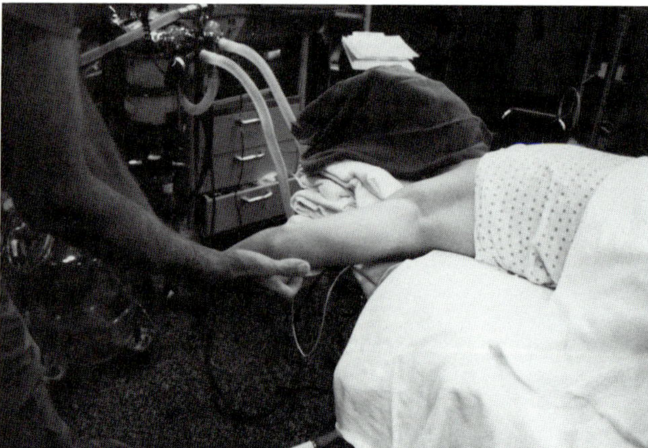

B

FIG. 8-38 Examination of passive range of motion under anesthesia. This is a valuable opportunity for evaluation and learning. Assessing range of external rotation is critical in anterior shoulder instability. Testing is performed from two different starting positions.

A Passive external rotation motion is evaluated with arm adducted to the chest wall and elbow touching the lateral abdomen.

B Passive external rotation motion is evaluated with the arm abducted 90 degrees.

dislocated, and in 3 the result was not recorded. In my hands, the assessment of instability in the office or under anesthesia was not a reliable test for glenohumeral dislocation. On average, the involved shoulder showed less external rotation than the normal opposite side at both positions and under both conditions (Table 8-1). The external rotation motion with both arms was greater under anesthesia, but still showed the relative restriction of the affected shoulder. It seemed, therefore, that the limited external rotation of the involved side on physical examination is not solely due to pain or apprehension, since external rotation was also limited under anesthesia. The restriction of external rotation under anesthesia at 90 degrees abduction was a common finding in chronic traumatic anterior dislocation. It is probably due to the repeated trauma to the anterior capsule and resultant fibrosis and contracture of the glenohumeral ligaments.

Value of examination with anesthesia. The examination under anesthesia provides another opportunity for evaluating the patient and a learning experience for the surgeon.[4,20]

I first evaluate the passive range of external rotation in two positions (Fig. 8-38). This approach provides an opportunity to compare these results to the clinical evaluation.

I perform two physical tests for instability (Figs. 8-39 and 8-40). I compare one shoulder to the other in that contralateral side involvement often occurs.[78] The asympto-

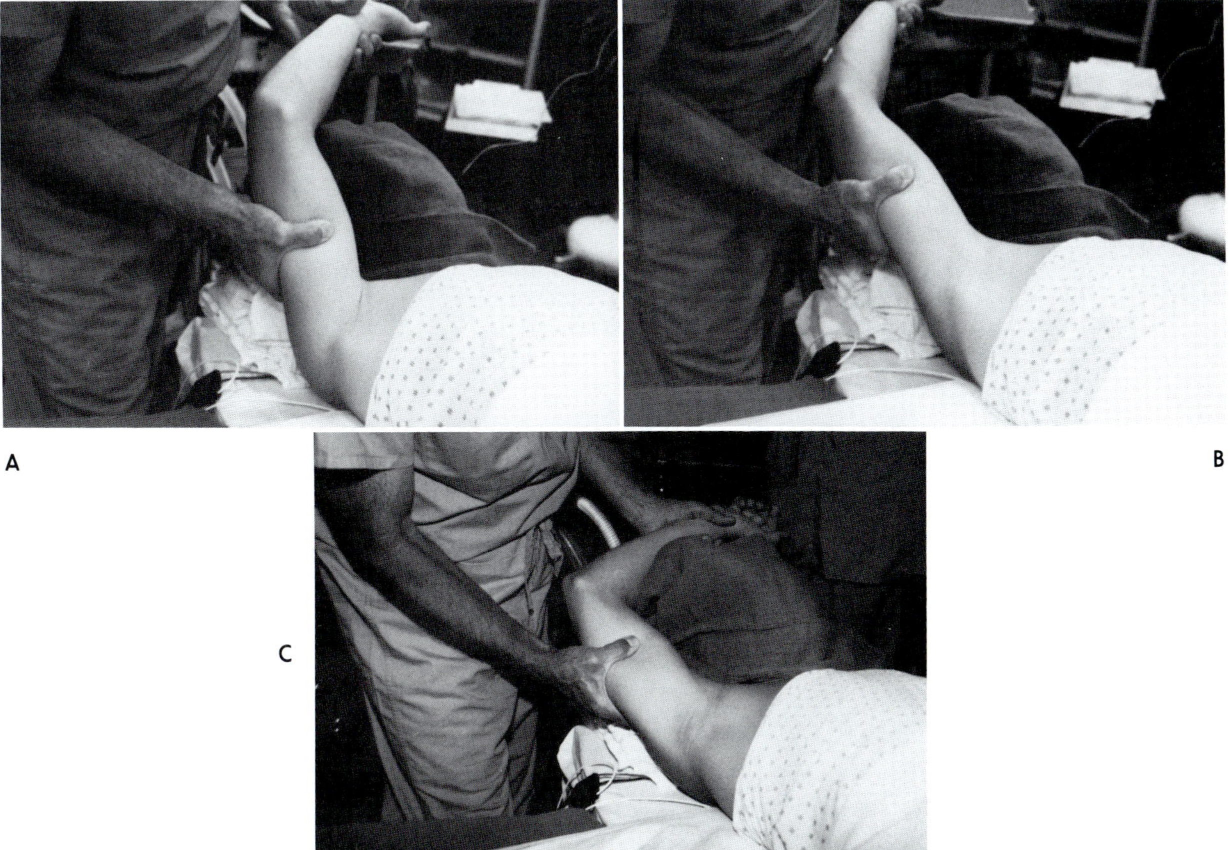

FIG. 8-39 Examination of stability under anesthesia.

A The arm is held in forward flexion. The examiner applies posterior force and assesses posterior instability.

B The humerus is held against the glenoid and the arm is slowly moved into elevated position with external rotation and medial force.

C The final move is continuance of the arm elevation, but with anterior force applied to the compressed joint. The compression creates the shift that is palpable. This movement is repeated several times with slight variations in humeral positioning. A rocking motion can be effective at the end point, similar to testing for rocking at the end point of a pivot shift in the unstable knee joint.

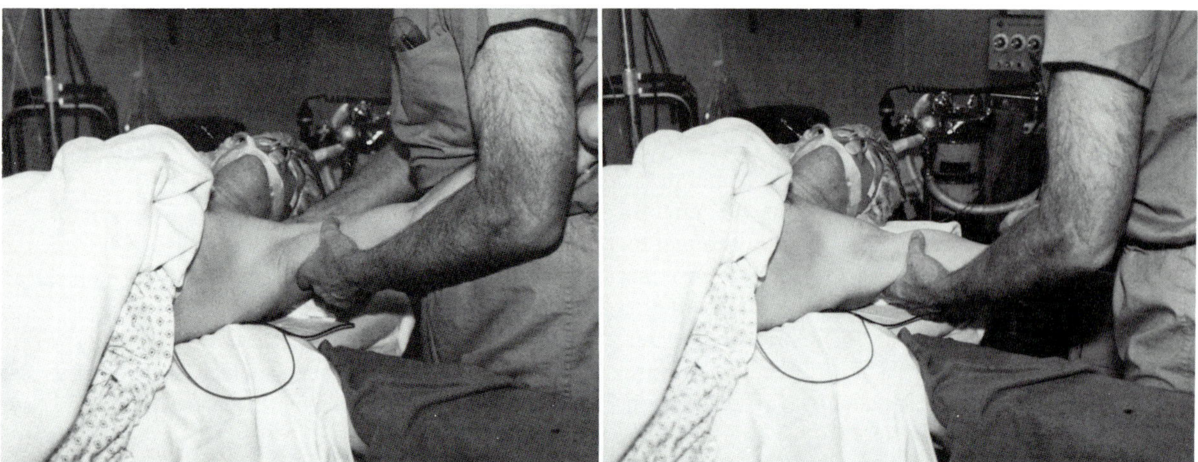

A B

FIG. 8-40 Second test for stability under anesthesia: The patient's arm is taken to the side and the forearm is captured by the examiner's arm. The scapula is stabilized with the examiner's one hand. The other hand moves the humeral head in various directions.

A The first step is to "load" humeral head in the glenoid. The arm is taken into 15 degrees flexion and the humerus is gently pushed against the glenoid.

B The arm is moved anterior from the starting position to extension with application of anterior force. The examiner must be alert to shifting motion of the humeral head over the anterior glenoid. Manipulation in other directions (posterior and inferior) is also possible.

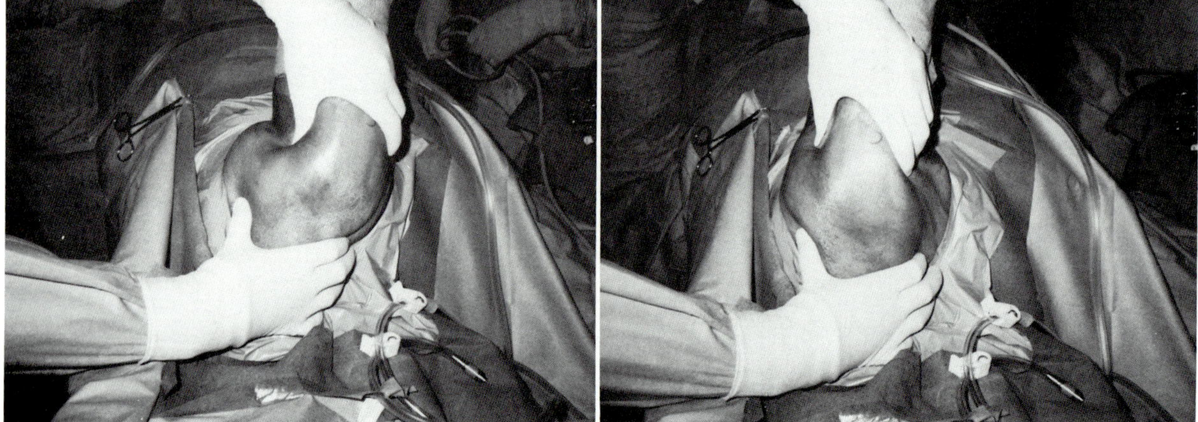

A B

FIG. 8-41 Examination under anesthesia in suspension: Another opportunity for examination under anesthesia is when the patient's arm is suspended.

A The left scapula is stabilized by one hand and the humeral head is displaced anterior with the other. A positive sign is demonstrated.

B The opposite force on this left shoulder shows no posterior instability.

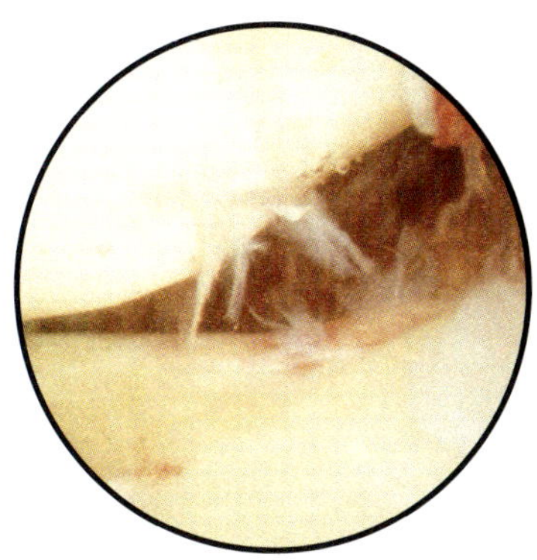

FIG. 8-42 DO NOT ADD FURTHER TRAUMA TO THE JOINT. Arthroscopic view after manipulation that caused further anterior joint disruption. If shoulder is re-dislocated with force under anesthesia, joint hemorrhage is produced that makes subsequent poor viewing during arthroscopy.

matic side may provide additional insight into the nature of the involved side as directional instability may be evident.

The tests are performed at various positions—abduction, external rotation, and anterior displacement—with the humerus used as a lever arm (Fig. 8-39). For the second test, I stabilize the scapula, control the upper extremity and manipulate the humeral head (Fig. 8-40). Both tests use a rocking motion to perceive subtle instability.

After the patient's upper extremity is suspended for the arthroscopy, I perform another instability test (Fig. 8-41). With one hand I capture the clavicle and scapula, and with the other hand I produce first an anterior force, then a posterior force. The surgeon should perform this examination on shoulder patients with different diagnoses to gain a feel of normal stability. Such testing will confirm the clinical impression or may be the only test showing an unsuspected multidirectional instability.

Although these tests are valuable in assessing glenohumeral instability, they are not the sole criteria to determine operative intervention. A false negative stable shoulder exam may be found with the patient under anesthesia. Surgery should not be based solely on the surgeon's ability to dislocate the shoulder under anesthesia. Also, an aggressive manipulative dislocation immediately before surgery will produce further trauma and sometimes bleeding that interferes with arthroscopic visualization (Fig. 8-42).

Treatment Alternatives

Treatment alternatives are based on clinical presentation and the patient's needs. A treatment program may be initiated before a definitive diagnosis has been established.

Exercise Program. An exercise program is used in a patient with instability findings unsubstantiated by imaging or examination under anesthesia and/or arthroscopy. Exercise is also used in a patient with initial episodes of unilateral or bilateral instability under anesthesia and no Bankart or Hill-Sachs lesion.[23]

Exercise programs have been advocated for traumatic dislocation in military personnel.[6] In my experience the nonoperative treatment in traumatic dislocation will decrease the frequency of repeat dislocation but will not remove the inevitability of another occurrence in a young person.

Surgery. Surgical consideration is given to the following situations[45,71,88,89]:

A. Failure on previous well-controlled exercise program.
B. Shoulder goes out with everyday activity.
C. Shoulder goes out with desired stressful activity.
D. Patient desires to reduce incidence or inconvenience of repeat dislocation.
E. Patient desires safety of joint stability (e.g., job, sports).
F. Imaging or arthroscopy indicates Bankart or Hill-Sachs lesion.

ROLE OF ARTHROSCOPY IN TRAUMATIC ANTERIOR DISLOCATION

Arthroscopy has three roles in the treatment of anterior traumatic dislocation of the glenohumeral joint. They are diagnostic, therapeutic, and investigational.

The greatest present value of arthroscopy is diagnostic. Arthroscopic debridement carries a surgical therapeutic benefit. Arthroscopic surgical repair is performed in selected cases. The investigational and research value of arthroscopy has been under used. Arthroscopy has provided further descriptions of the glenohumeral ligamentous anatomy and clarified some previous misunderstandings.* The value of arthroscopic second look inspections heretofore not possible should provide more knowledge of anatomy, pathology, and results of surgical repair. The global nature of the intraarticular injury was apparent on my diagnostic findings in anterior traumatic dislocation of the shoulder.

This procedural discussion is directed toward the traumatic anterior dislocation. Broader discussions of preparation, environment, instrumentation, and surgical techniques were presented in previous chapters.

Other instability diagnoses have been eliminated clinically but not forgotten, in that the arthroscopic inspection may reveal a previously undetected type of problem.

The patient is positioned in the opposite lateral decubitus. The arm is suspended with a balanced weight over pulleys (10 to 16 pounds). Traction is avoided because neurovascular injury may occur.[3,5,55]

*2, 18, 26, 48, 77, 109

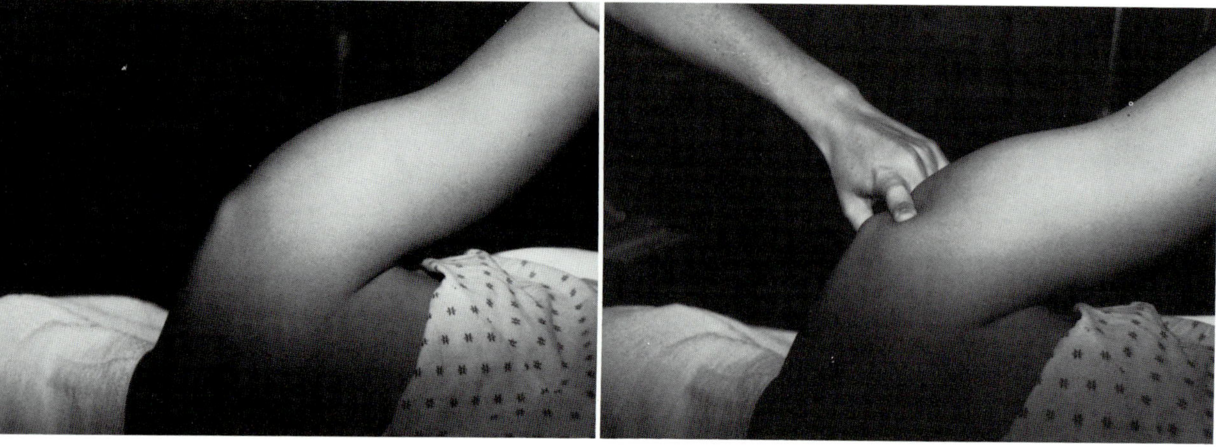

FIG. 8-43 The Sulcus sign.

A This topographical sign is seen with patient in suspended position. Sign indicates existence of significant inferior laxity and need for capsular shift.

B The examiner illustrates this sign with placement of finger under acromion and on the displaced humeral head.

The suspended upper extremity provides yet another opportunity for evaluation (see Fig. 8-41). Inspection may show the arm subluxed in external rotation with passive traction. This finding may indicate complete loss of anterior and inferior capsular ligamentous integrity.

A topographical depression may be noticed between the acromion and humerus (Fig. 8-43). This depression represents an inferior instability and is a reason to include capsular shift in a surgical procedure, perhaps by open surgery.

The passive subluxation should be reduced at the time of arthroscope cannula insertion by internal rotation of the humerus to facilitate joint entry (see Chapter 5).

Diagnostic Arthroscopy

The arthroscopic findings that accompany subluxation show no evidence of a Hill-Sachs lesion. This can occur only if the humerus completely disengages in front of the glenoid. The mere presence of an enlarged anterior sulcus is not by itself an indication of subluxation or dislocation (Fig. 8-44). The labral findings of subluxation show tissue disruption with an area of blood products (Fig. 8-45, *A*). Only elevation of the labrum with synovial reaction may be present, as seen in a swimmer with overuse syndrome (8-45, *B*). Often the anterior glenohumeral ligaments will be thinned and the anterior space enlarged (Fig. 8-46). The humerus will easily distract from the glenoid with increased intraarticular pressure. Minimal arthroscopic anterior labral debridement and rehabilitation may be adequate initial treatment (Fig. 8-47).

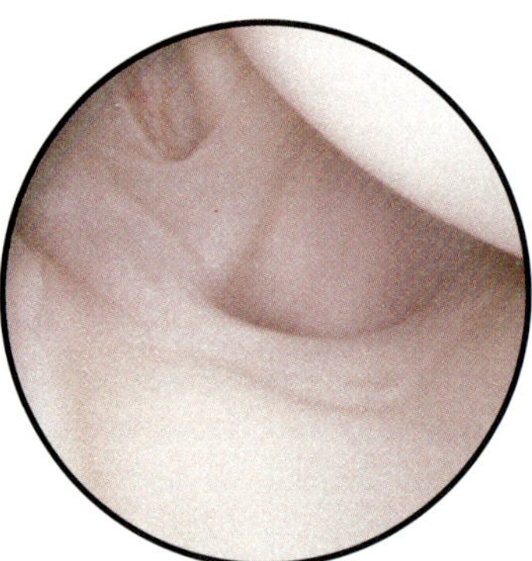

FIG. 8-44 Arthroscopic view of anatomical variation of prominent anterior sulcus. Variation is not pathological in itself, unless associated fragmentation or hemorrhage is present. The labrum is intact and the ligaments are normal in this case.

In dislocation, the arthroscopic pathologic findings are those related to trauma and the anterior positional change of humerus (Fig. 8-48, *B* and *C*; see also Fig. 8-52). The evidence of trauma is blood, blood products, and tissue disruption supporting the anterior translation. This statement might seem unnecessary but must be said to rule out the anatomical variations and other instabilities that might be confused with traumatic anterior dislocation (see Chapters 1 and 7).

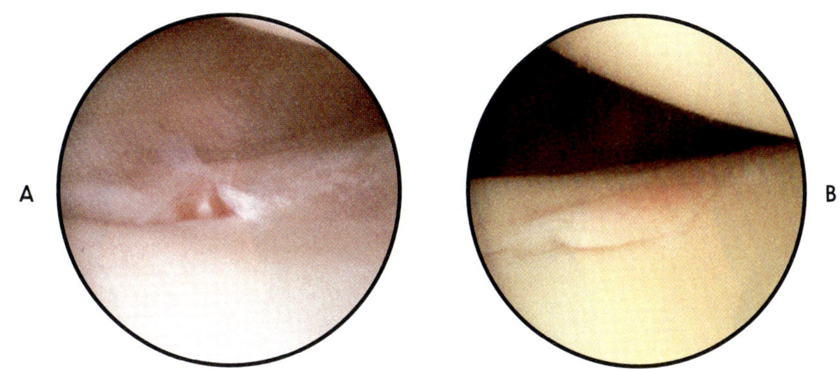

FIG. 8-45 Arthroscopic evidence of subluxation.

A Tearing and hemorrhage of the anterior labrum correlates with clinical findings.

B Labral separation and inflammation of the anterior labrum correlates with clinical suspicion in this swimmer.

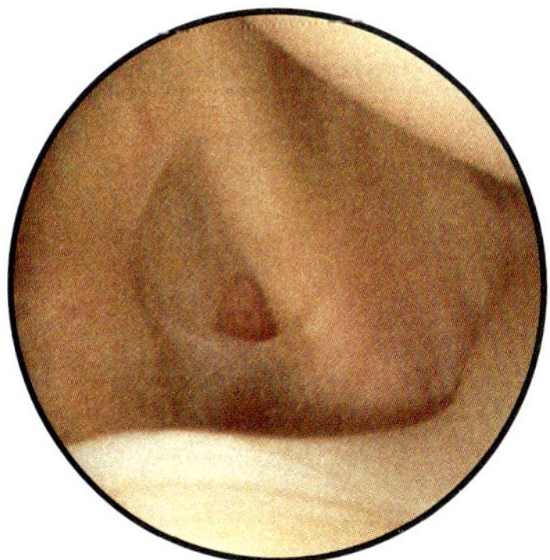

FIG. 8-46 Subluxation: In another variation, the arthroscopic findings show labrum intact, but enlarged anterior space with anterior displacement of the attenuated ligaments. This enlarged space is not a large bursa, but is created by ligamentous incompetency and stretching. The bursal opening is seen next to the subscapularis tendon.

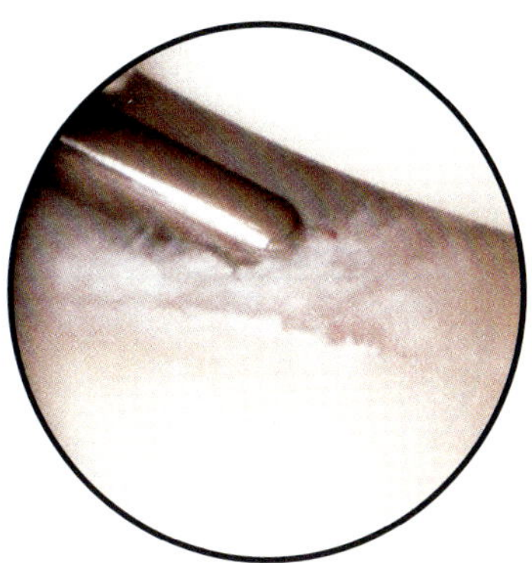

FIG. 8-47 Subluxation treatment alternative: A treatment alternative for subluxation may be arthroscopic labral debridement and vigorous rehabilitation.

Glenohumeral hemarthrosis occurs following an initial acute dislocation. It also occurs with a recurrent dislocation, even following manipulation with the patient under anesthesia (Fig 8-42). Later, blood staining occurs. Hemorrhage and blood-stained tissues may exist anterior and inferior in the capsule or posterior on the humerus. Hemorrhage on the posterior-inferior labrum and superior in the rotator cuff may be evident.

The arthroscopic pathological findings that accompany traumatic anterior dislocation are global in location (Fig. 8-49).

The primary lesion of dislocation is the Perthes/Bankart lesion (Fig. 8-50). Various types of this lesion exist; see my classification in the box on p. 308.

Tissue disruption is seen at the anterior glenoid sulcus and posterior inferior glenoid rim (labrum). This area can be visualized from posterior with a 90-degree inclined arthroscope (Fig. 8-51). The posterior tissue tearing demon-

tire area superior to inferior, and others extend posterior to central. The largest lesions include all these areas. The size varies from 1.0 cm diameter to 5.0 by 4.0 cm.

In the very loose shoulder, the dislocation may occur with ease and little compression of the bony tissues. The depth of the lesion may only be a partial-thickness articular cartilage abrasion. In the structurally tight shoulder or with the most forceful injury the depth of the Hill-Sachs lesion may be greater than 1 centimeter. Less common sites of soft tissue disruption are the rotator cuff and subscapularis tendon (Fig. 8-55).

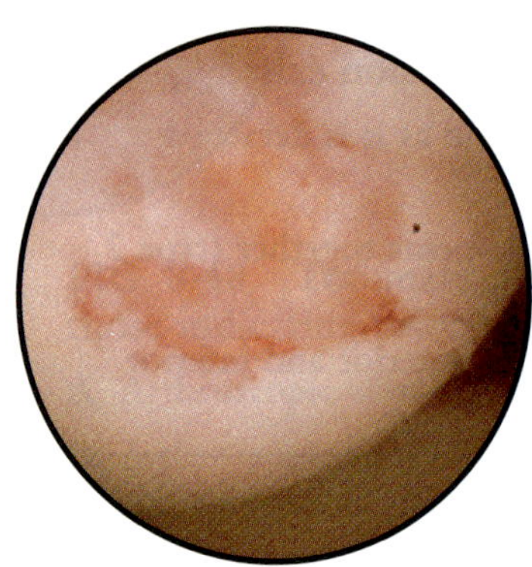

FIG. 8-53 Hill-Sachs lesion (left): This is the sine qua non for dislocation. Arthroscopic view of lesion that is superficial in depth. Only the articular cartilage has been avulsed. The x-ray film would be negative, since there is no bone fracture or compression.

The articular cartilage may be disrupted on either the glenoid or humeral surface (Figs. 8-56 and 8-57). A humeral lesion on the opposing surface from the glenoid does not represent the classic Hill-Sachs lesion, which is located more posterior. Injury to the joint surface potentially adversely affects the prognosis. Postoperatively the patient may have catching in the joint because of the incongruous surfaces. Degenerative arthritis may develop. Samilson and Prieto[95] reported 29 cases of degenerative arthritis occurring in nonoperative traumatic anterior glenohumeral dislocation. The unaffected opposite side was without x-ray changes. Posterior dislocations and operative cases with internal fixation had a higher incidence of moderate and severe degenerative changes.

Bony fracture may occur on the anterior glenoid (see Figs. 8-7, *A* and *B* and 8-8). The fracture of glenoid varies from osteochondral avulsion to a larger portion of glenoid. Loose bodies may be produced by either lesion (Fig. 8-57, *B*).

The natural healing process results in anterior capsular ligament fibrosis and intraarticular fibrosis. Articular cartilage defects can be in various stages of repair (Figs. 8-57, *A* and 8-58).

Illustrative Diagnostic Arthroscopy in Chronic Case Series. In order to characterize the arthroscopic diagnostic findings, a computer search was made on the diagnostic arthroscopic findings in patients with traumatic anterior dislocation of the glenohumeral joint between August 1982 and December 1988. There were 117 patients in the data base with this condition (98 men and 19 women) with 121 shoulders inspected. The chronic nature of this group was evident by the time of onset to the arthroscopic

A

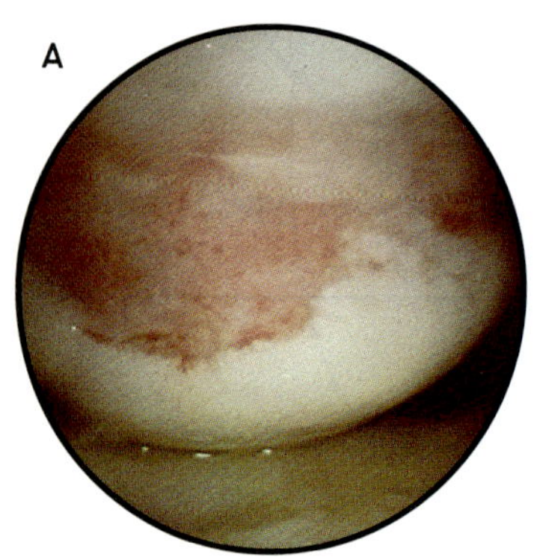

B

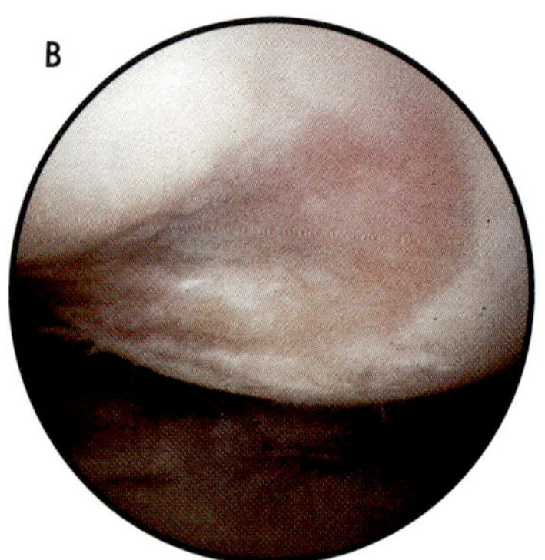

C

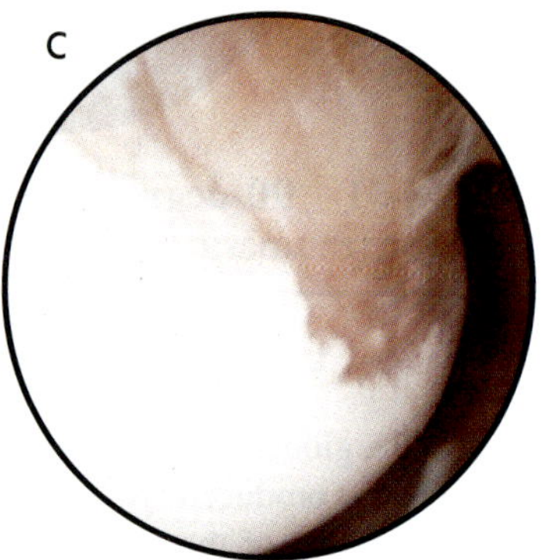

FIG. 8-54 Hill-Sachs lesions vary in position and size.

A Arthroscopic view of large lesion extending entire length of posterior humerus. X-ray film would be positive.

B Arthroscopic view of large lesion that is in oblique direction from central area to anterior and inferior on the humerus. X-ray film would be positive.

C Small posterior and laterally positioned lesion. It is superficial. X-ray film may be positive.

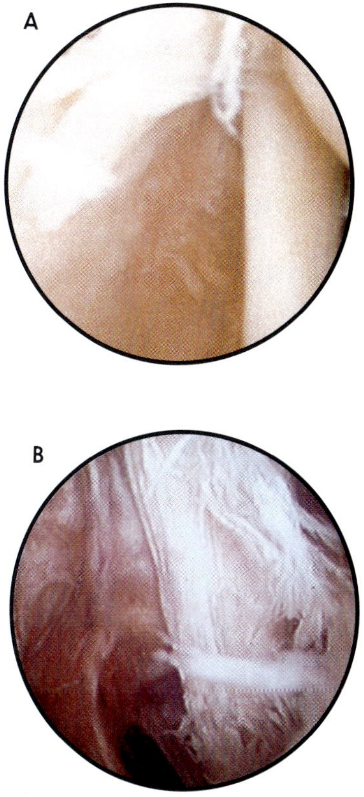

FIG. 8-55 Soft tissue disruption.

A Arthroscopic view of partial-thickness rotator cuff tear. Notice the suggestion of undermining in the capsular area.

B Fragmentation of the subscapularis tendon in chronic recurrent traumatic dislocation.

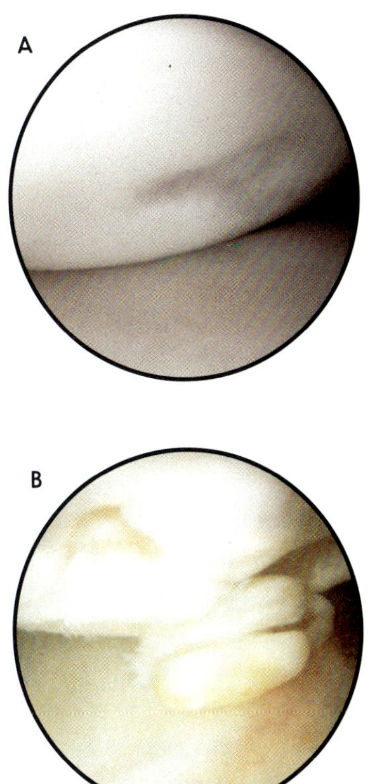

FIG. 8-57 Humeral articular cartilage damage.

A Superficial healing lesion on juxtaarticular surface of humerus.

B Deep articular cartilage injury with adjacent loose bodies.

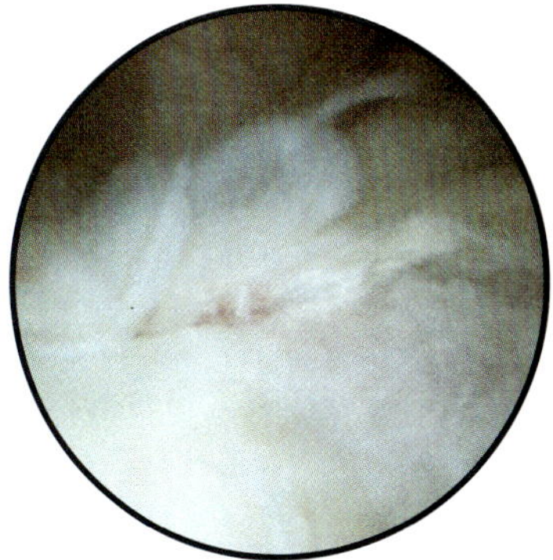

FIG. 8-56 Glenoid articular cartilage damage. Articular cartilage is disrupted anterior with fragmentation of labrum in chronic case.

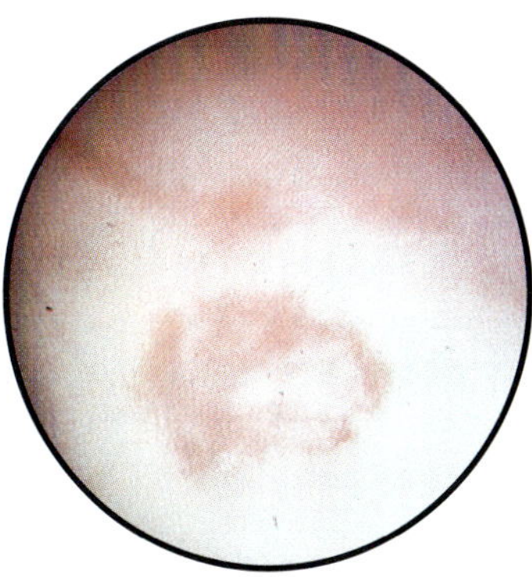

FIG. 8-58 Natural healing of articular cartilage injury: Arthroscopic view of articular cartilage injury with central area of repair.

inspection (3½ years) and the average number of dislocations (10). The incidence of redislocation was between 1 and 100.

Average patient age was 26 years with a range of 14 to 54 years. The right hand was dominant in 84, the left in 9, and 1 patient was truly ambidextrous; 27 patients did not respond to the question. The problematic side was the right in 64 and the left in 57.

The examination with the patient under anesthesia showed a decreased range of external rotation motion when compared to the opposite unaffected shoulder. The examination was performed with the arm at the side and with the starting position at 90 degrees abduction. Restriction averaged 15 degrees with the arm at the side and 5 degrees with the arm abducted (Table 8-1). This static restriction reflects the chronic nature of these patients' conditions and the anterior fibrosis.

Findings and descriptions of lesions in this series follow.

Synovitis. Synovitis existed in 37% of these patients. The nature was reactive. It was often villous and vascular. The most common location was in the anterior-superior wall.

Fibrosis. Fibrous bands spanned the joint or synovium in 23% of patients. This finding is representative of the repeated trauma over time in this series.

Loose bodies. Loose bodies were observed in 19% of these patients. When loose bodies existed, they were multiple in 11 patients. The frequency was one loose body in 13 patients, two in 4 patients, three in 3 patients, four in 1, and 2 patients had many loose bodies.

The nature of the loose bodies were cartilaginous (54%), bony (29%), synovial (13%), and varied (4%).

Articular cartilage injury. The juxtaarticular surfaces of the glenohumeral joint was traumatically disrupted in many of these patients. Injury was observed on the humerus (36%) and the glenoid (15%).

Degenerative arthritis. Degenerative changes were observed in 21% of patients. Changes were seen on the humerus (10%) and the glenoid (11%).

Bone injury. The bone was injured in many patients. This injury was separate from articular cartilage trauma and degenerative lesions. Bone was injured on the glenoid in 22%. The humerus was injured in 86%. Bone was fractured in both the humerus and glenoid in 21% of patients.

Hill-Sachs lesion. A posterior defect in the Hill-Sachs area was observed in 104 of the 121 patients (86%). The incidence has been reported as 47% in first time dislocation.[16] Comparison of these two observations would suggest that the Hill-Sachs lesion increases with chronicity.

Glenoid labrum. The labrum was described as abnormal in 72% of these patients. It was further described as torn in 52%, separated from the glenoid in 54%, and absent in 2%.

The location of labrum tears was global and circumferential. The tear was observed anterior in 94 (78%); inferior in 54 (45%); posterior in 47 (39%); and superior in 12 (10%).

The chronicity of the condition in this patient group was reflected in the labrum tear being described as old in 90%. The 10% of tears that were acute were the result of recent redislocation.

Glenohumeral ligaments. The glenohumeral ligaments were documented as abnormal in 69%. They were torn in 54% and were separated from the glenoid in 50%. The ligaments were separated, contracted, fibrotic, and fixed in 20%. No anterior glenohumeral ligaments were observed in 2%.

Rotator cuff tears. A partial rotator cuff tear was seen on the glenohumeral side in 13% of patients. It was not full thickness in any of these cases. The tear involved the synovial and capsular layers.

Global nature of condition. All quadrants were observed to have lesions. The anterior quadrant had synovitis, labrum tears, and ligament tears. This is consistent with Calandra's observations in acute first time dislocations, which showed anterior tissue tearing in all patients in that series. Only two of their patients did not have classic Bankart lesions.

The superior quadrant had rotator cuff tears, labrum tears, and fibrosis.

The posterior quadrant had abnormalities in 32% of patients and the inferior quadrant was abnormal in 36%. The lesions in these locations were usually labrum tears or loose bodies. The posterior labrum tears were probably caused by traction from the anterior displacement.

Ideal Circumstances for Arthroscopic Reconstruction. After reviewing the above-mentioned illustrative diagnostic series, I arbitrarily decided what circumstances constitute an ideal situation for arthroscopic repair of traumatic anterior dislocation. This analysis did not include the important patient requirements, like cosmesis, return to work, sports, and so forth.

It seemed the ideal circumstance should involve few dislocations, with good range of motion, but not excessive. The physical examination should show no sulcus sign. No external rotation or subluxation should occur during arthroscopic suspension. A simple Bankart lesion (Type 1 or 2; see the box on p. 308) should be present at arthroscopy. Integrity to the anterior glenohumeral ligaments should be normal. The labrum should be restorable. No significant cartilage and bone injury should be present. There should be no degenerative arthritis so that the prognosis is good.

When I applied these ideal criteria to my diagnostic series, only 31% of my patients in this series fit this *ideal* repair category. It should not be suprising that my results showed 21% recurrence after metal staple capsulorrhaphy in series I and 13% in series II (see below), when the patient population was chronic in nature and labral ligamentous complex was absent or contracted in so many patients.

One third of my patients had pain after surgery. This postoperative result could be due to the presence of the metal staple, but it must be realized 50% of patients had degenerative or articular trauma identified at time of surgery. Degenerative arthritis is a common x-ray finding in nonoperative patients and following open surgical reconstruction, even without metal internal fixation.[95]

Influence of Diagnostic Findings on Surgical Treatment and Results

Diagnostic arthroscopy provides information that is not available by any other method. A review of the various components of traumatic anterior dislocation showed them to be varied in presence, magnitude, and location. Thus all dislocations are NOT created equal, and therefore they are not going to be treated the same. Let's review each component lesion and discuss the influence of the diagnostic findings on the selection of the surgical treatment and the subsequent results.

NOT ALL INSTABILITIES ARE CREATED EQUAL, NOR ARE THEY TREATED THE SAME

Labrum Tear

Description. The site of the labral tear may be anywhere on the circumference of the glenoid (see Fig. 8-10).

Since the labrum configuration and tissue make-up varies with the patient and the location on the glenoid, the variety of tears also varies. A well-defined mobile labrum of fibrocartilage may produce a bucket handle-like tear. Also, a flap tear may occur when the labrum is well defined.

A labrum tear is not synonymous with a coexistent dislocation. It may occur with subluxation or with a throwing athlete's instability.[4] Yet a labrum tear often accompanies a traumatic anterior dislocation. The normal, anatomically well-defined labral lip may tear similar to the meniscus in the knee. In this case there need not be any disruption of the glenohumeral ligaments. A labral resection is therapeutic when followed by rehabilitation.

A labrum tear must be differentiated from normal anatomical variations, especially the normal anterior glenoid sulcus and the anterior-superior foramen (see Chapter 6). The latter anatomical variant communicates with the subscapularis bursa.

Surgical treatment decisions. Many of the lesions associated with traumatic anterior dislocation are small, partial thickness, flap shaped, and irreparable. They are located in all quadrants of the joint. These lesions are more easily assessable and more effectively debrided by arthroscopy than by open arthrotomy. Some lesions are amenable to restoration by arthroscopy or open surgery.

Perthes/Bankart Lesion

Description. The classic Bankart lesion placed emphasis on the separation of the labrum from the anterior glenoid. These observations, made at time of open surgery, did not place emphasis on the status of the glenohumeral ligaments (Fig. 8-59).

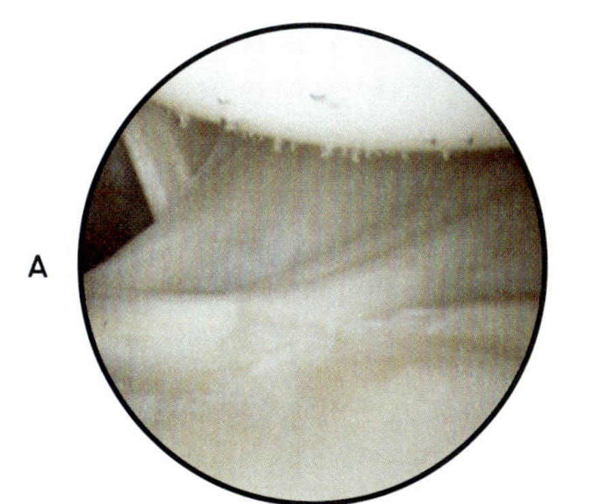

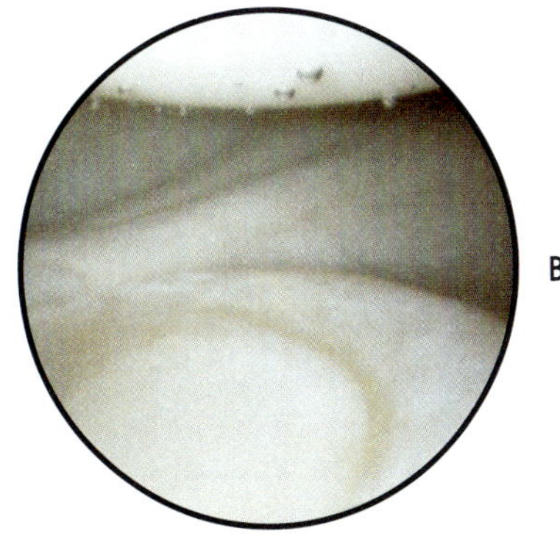

FIG. 8-59 Normal glenohumeral ligaments status is benchmark for comparison. The configuration can be used to judge pathological changes, although many normal variations of the labrum and ligament configurations exist.

A Arthroscopic view of confluent middle and inferior glenohumeral ligaments. Notice superior extension of both middle and inferior ligaments.

B Arthroscopic view of anterior and inferior shows the superior band of the inferior ligament and the inferior glenoid rim.

It would be nice if all anterior structural lesions were of this type. Unfortunately, not all dislocations are created equal nor are they treated the same. Many varieties of this anterior labral and ligamentous injury exist.

Since considerable variation occurs in the normal anatomical structures of the anterior glenohumeral ligaments, subsequent trauma with disruption creates further difficulty in determining prior integrity and repair methods.

The superior glenohumeral ligament is not involved in clinical anterior-inferior dislocation. This ligament is rarely seen during arthroscopic inspection and is poorly developed when anatomically dissected. This ligament has been selectively sectioned in experiments and shown to play a minor role in typical clinical anterior-inferior dislocations.[64,114]

The middle glenohumeral ligament identified by arthroscopy is the capsular ligament of open shoulder surgical approaches.[26] Its size and shape vary greatly in normal anatomy. Its structure has two aspects (Fig. 8-59). One is the superior band, which crosses the superior tendon of the subscapularis. It may have two strands that cross the tendon. The other and structurally larger is the inferior portion. The thicker inferior portion of the middle glenohumeral ligament is continuous with the inferior glenohumeral ligament superior band (Fig. 8-59, *A*).

The classical traumatic disruption occurs within the lower portion of the superior extension of the inferior glenohumeral ligament.[64,114] This is an important distinction because both the lesion and the repair are inferior on the anterior glenoid. A distinct bony attachment of the inferior glenohumeral ligament has been seen following acute dislocation with small bony wafer avulsion on the inferior glenohumeral ligament. The site of origin was anterior and inferior on the glenoid. These clinical observations suggest the inferior glenohumeral ligament has two attachments: superior to the glenoid and inferior to the bone of anterior glenoid.

Diagnostic classification. A closer look at the anterior structures via diagnostic arthroscopy provides for a classification of the various types of Bankart lesions. The first observation to be made is whether both labrum and the ligaments have maintained structural integrity. If they are uninjured, then did they stay as a unit or have they separated one from the other? If they separated from each other, did one or the other maintain structural integrity? Are they both damaged and separated from the glenoid? Is evidence of both separation and contraction present? Is either structure missing?

With those considerations, the following grouping is suggested (see the box). This classification reflects the type and magnitude of injury as well as affecting surgical considerations. Subtypes could be created, especially in Type 5, where labrum and ligament combinations could be more extensive. Also in Type 6, either the labrum or ligaments could be absent, not just both. The purpose of the classification is to draw attention to the many variables and their treatment implications.

CLASSIFICATION OF BANKART LESIONS

Type 1: Labrum and ligaments are together and in juxtaposition to the glenoid (Fig. 8-60, *A*)

Type 2: Labrum and ligaments are together, but separated from the bony glenoid (Fig. 8-60, *B*)

Type 3: Labrum and ligaments are NOT together; labrum is in juxtaposition, but the ligaments are separated (Fig. 8-60, *C*)

Type 4: Labrum and ligaments NOT together; labrum is separated from the glenoid, but the ligaments are intact and in juxtaposition (Fig. 8-60, *D*)

Type 5: Labrum and ligaments NOT together; labrum torn and separated, plus ligaments are torn and separated (Fig. 8-60, *E*)

Type 6: Both labrum and ligaments ABSENT (Fig. 8-60, *F*)

Surgical treatment decisions. The type 1 lesion may not require any surgical treatment. Simple debridement and approximation should suffice.[30] A good outcome should be expected.

A type 2 lesion requires removal of the interposing tissue and reapproximation and fixation. The outcome should be good with any arthroscopic or open method.

A type 3 lesion requires reattachment of ligaments. This problem requires mobilization or even imbrication of the ligaments. The outcome expectation would not be as good as types 1 and 2.

The type 4 lesion may require resection of the labral fragments with capsular shift of the intact ligaments to recreate labral butyrous. The outcome depends on restoration of the labral ligamentous complex, which may be difficult by arthroscopic surgery.

The type 5 lesion requires debridement of both torn tissues and capsular ligament restoration to butyrous labrum. If the capsule is patulous, a localized arthroscopic resection and advancement may be indicated. An open capsular shift and imbrication may be the treatment of choice. The outcome in this severe problem would be poorer than with types 1 and 2 lesions.

The type 6 lesion requires arthroscopic substitution of anterior structures with subscapularis tendon slip or a similar open procedure. The outcome depends on recognition and proper substitution whether by arthroscopy or open surgery.

Hill-Sachs Lesion

Description. As with the Perthes lesion, there are several types of Hill-Sachs lesions. This lesion varies consid-

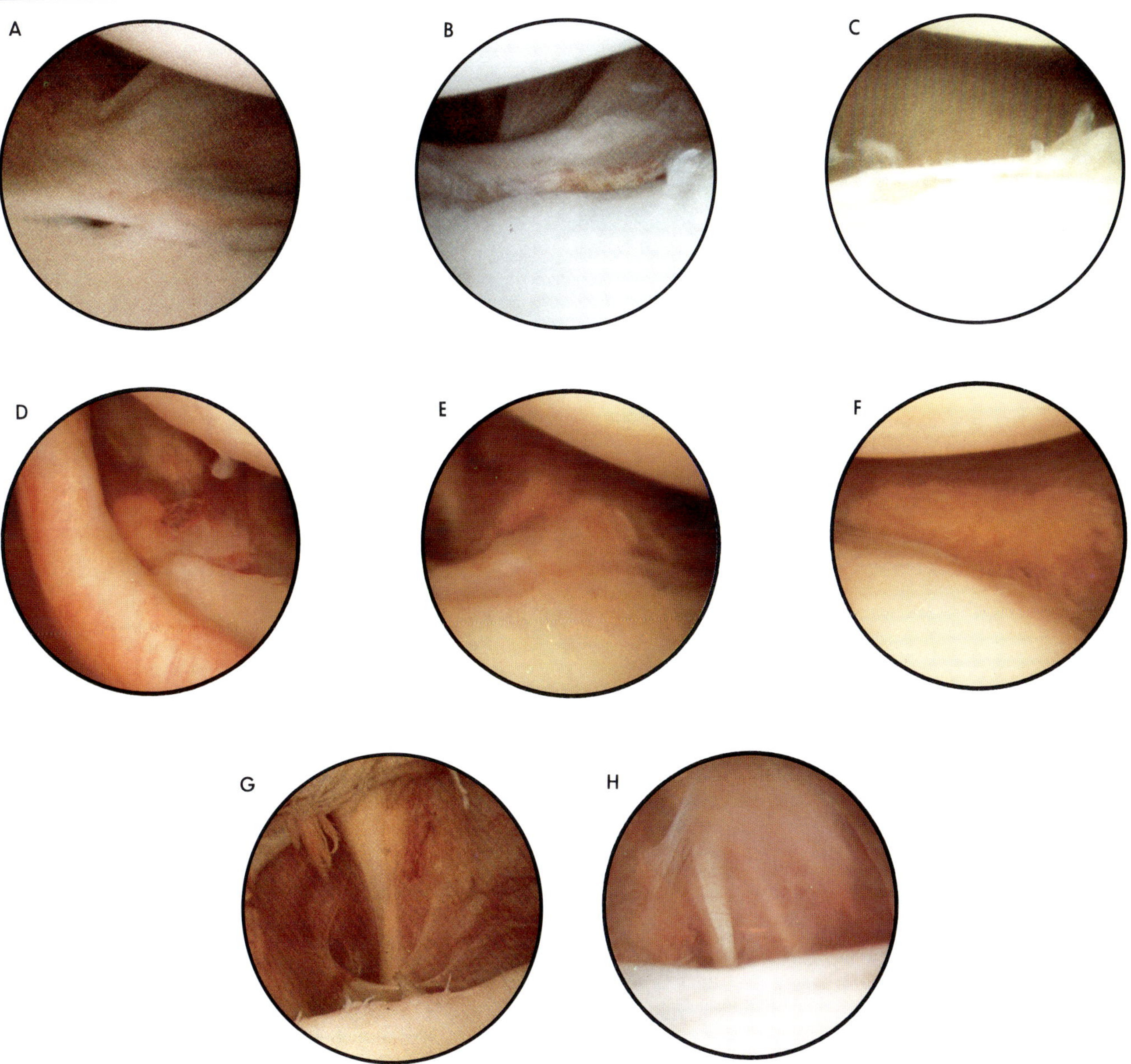

FIG. 8-60 Classification of bankart lesions.

A Type 1: Labrum and ligaments are together and in juxtaposition to the glenoid.

B Type 2: Labrum and ligaments are together but separated from the bony glenoid.

C Type 3: Labrum and ligaments are *not* together: labrum is in juxtaposition, but ligaments are separated.

D, E, AND F Type 4: Labrum and ligaments are *not* together; labrum is separated from glenoid, but the ligaments are intact and in juxtaposition to the glenoid.

G Type 5: Labrum and ligaments are *not* together; labrum is torn and separated; ligaments are torn and separated.

H Type 6: Both labrum and ligaments absent.

erably in location, size, depth, and configuration (Figs. 8-53 and 8-54). The large lesions are easily seen on Stryker view x-ray films (Figs. 8-35 and 8-36). However, a negative Stryker x-ray does not rule out the prior existence of a dislocation. The injury may be only articular cartilagenous in depth and therefore not show on plain film x-ray.

Fragmentation of the edges is common with a Hill-Sachs lesion. "Loose bodies" may be hanging from the lesion.

Surgical treatment decisions. Arthroscopic debridement may be indicated for fragmentation or impending loose bodies. A large compression fracture of the Hill-Sachs lesion may extend toward the central articular surface such that restriction of external rotation would be necessary to avoid the margin of defect catching on the anterior glenoid margin. Anterior ligamentous reattachment alone may not suffice, and open surgery may be necessary. In some cases a Connolly procedure is necessary, filling the large defect with a transferred infraspinatus tendon inserted into the large defect.[22] In the most severe cases rotational osteotomies have been performed of the humeral head.[117]

Rotator Cuff Tear

Description. The rotator cuff tear may occur secondary to the traumatic dislocation. They are of varying size and depth.

Surgical treatment decisions. A small partial-thickness lesion on the underside involving capsule and synovium, but not the tendons, is amenable to localized debridement. The full-thickness tear requires tendon repair by arthroscopy or open surgery.

Subscapularis Tendon Tear

Description. The tearing of the superior margin of the subscapularis tendon accompanies dislocations with inferior displacement or repeated episodes.

Surgical treatment decisions. If no separation from the rotator cuff has occurred, then surgical treatment need only be localized debridement. If major separation occurs at this interval, then open suture closure may be indicated.

Fracture

Description. An osteochondral fracture may occur without tearing of labrum or glenohumeral ligaments. This usually occurs with a violent direct blow to the posterior and lateral shoulder. The bony glenoid defect permits the humeral translation. A larger bony glenoid avulsion fracture often is healed anterior and inferior on the glenoid neck following traumatic dislocation.

Surgical treatment decisions. This fracture requires reduction and internal fixation. If a malunion is present, surgical separation and reattachment are indicated and open surgery may be required. If the bone defect is great, either a bone graft or Bristow procedure may be required to fill the defect.

Articular Cartilage Injury/Degenerative Arthritis

Description. My diagnostic arthroscopy series in chronic cases showed a high incidence of articular cartilage injury or degeneration. The preoperative presence of articular cartilage injury and degenerative arthritis would adversely affect the prognosis.[95] The articular cartilage injury is not as easily identified, appreciated, or described by the limited exposure that open anterior arthrotomy provides.

Surgical treatment decisions. An arthroscopic debridement is performed in cases of articular injury or degeneration to remove flaps, fragments, and potential loose bodies even if open surgical repair is anticipated. The degenerative joint has less potential for a satisfactory outcome concerning the symptom of pain.

THE BENEFITS OF DIAGNOSTIC ARTHROSCOPY ARE SO GREAT THAT THIS PROCEDURE SHOULD PRECEDE OR ACCOMPANY MOST SHOULDER SURGERY

Arthroscopic Technical Considerations Based on Specific Diagnostic Findings

Position Assessment. The initial puncture of the glenohumeral joint causes decompression of negative joint presssure. The humeral head moves into the anterior-inferior position with the introduction of air. The suspension device creates an additional distraction force. The instillation of fluid causes further displacement of the humerus toward the subluxed position. The normal shoulder should not be dislocated under these normal arthroscopic environmental circumstances.

If during arthroscopic distention the humerus is easily distracted from the glenoid, capsular laxity exists (Fig. 8-61). This finding may represent multidirectional instability even if signs of anterior trauma are present. Open capsular shift may be indicated.

A glenohumeral dislocation will often correlate with sulcus sign (Fig. 8-43). If so, then capsular shift, perhaps by open surgery, is indicated.

Ligament Assessment. Pathologically the middle glenohumeral ligament may be atrophied or absent. It may be congenitally elongated and lax, creating a large anterior pouch. The same situation may occur by repeated trauma. In either case no evidence of acute tearing is present. The glenohumeral ligaments are torn or stretched in my type 3 or 5 Bankart lesion. The inferior glenohumeral ligament may appear intact, with no labral tear (Perthes lesion). The repair in this situation requires resection or shortening of the middle glenohumeral ligament. Repair may have to be performed by open surgery.[4]

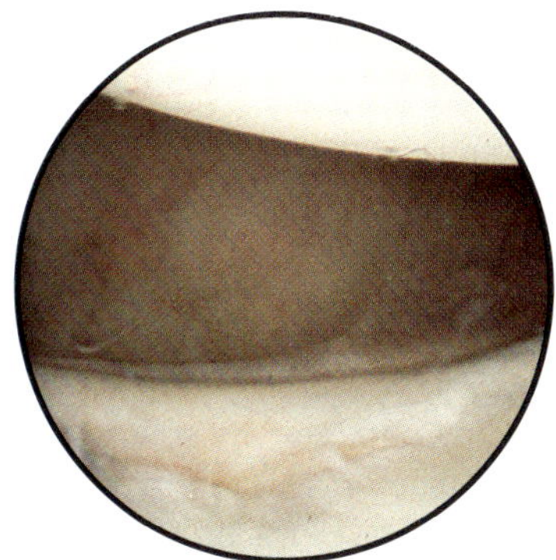

FIG. 8-61 Arthroscopic view of marked distraction of the humerus from the glenoid. This situation is created only by intraarticular pressure and not by external traction. Distraction is a sign of marked capsular laxity. Findings are just the opposite of those seen in frozen shoulder.

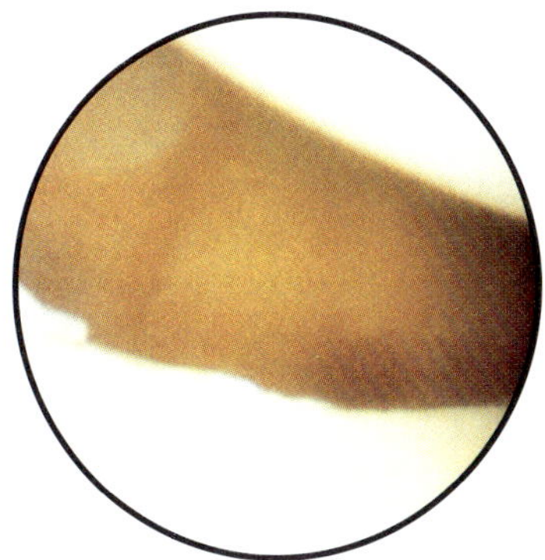

FIG. 8-62 Arthroscopic view of absent labrum and inferior glenohumeral ligament. Only the middle glenohumeral ligament is seen on the anterior wall. It is of sufficient thickness that one can not see the subscapularis beneath. The middle glenohumeral ligament is used for the repair.

In some of these cases, an advancement of the inferior ligament can be attempted by arthroscopy. Unfortunately this ligament is often contracted and not mobile in this situation. In this case an arthroscopic subscapularis substitution, or open surgery with capsular shift or subscapularis substitution, is indicated.

Some patients have no inferior glenohumeral ligament superior extension and no tissue to grasp or advance. In this case the middle glenohumeral ligament is grasped near its humeral (inferior) portion and advanced to the glenoid (Fig. 8-62). The normal anatomical connection to the inferior ligament cause it to be advanced to the anterior and inferior glenoid as the middle is secured to the superior-anterior glenoid surface (Fig. 8-59).

The chronically torn and contracted middle and inferior glenohumeral ligaments may be thickened with fibrosis. This contracture may preclude ligament advancement by either arthroscopic or open surgery and substitution is required. If bone has formed in this thickened ligament, resection of bone is indicated to mobilize the ligaments for capsular shift.

Mobilization of the inferior capsular ligament (arcuate or axillary pouch portion) off the glenoid neck by knife blade or arthroscopic motorized instrumentation extends the operative site around the anterior-inferior corner (Fig. 8-64). This maneuver will detach the ligament and labrum from that area, so that subsequent rotational advancement is possible.

MY PRESENT SURGICAL APPROACH TO ANTERIOR SHOULDER INSTABILITY

I am often asked, "What are you doing now?" The following is an outline of my approach to the patient with shoulder instability. This outline varies from other procedures only in the final method of fixation, so it can be used as a guide for surgeons no matter what method of fixation they use—staple, screw, suture, or biodegradable tac.

Documentation of the Type of Instability

Although this text is written primarily about a surgical technique, a perfect operation based on an imperfect diagnosis yields an imperfect result.

Medical History and Patient Assessment. I consider it a luxury when the exact diagnosis can be established from the medical history. Extracting an exact description of the mechanism of injury is important. I encourage the patient to demonstrate what happened. Is he or she able to reproduce the injury? This is the best opportunity to assess direction of the instability. Was the condition voluntary before the traumatic episode? Is the condition voluntary now? Having the patient demonstrate the present instability is especially important (see Figs. 8-31 and 8-32).

Physical Examination. The most reliable evidence of the type of instability is the correlation of the medical history with the patient assessment during the interview that is confirmed by the physical examination. I want to know that I understand what the patient is talking about and that I can reproduce the symptoms. Often the medical history is vague, but its clarification is the purpose of the interview, assessment, and correlative physical examination.

The various physical examination tests are outlined in Chapter 1 and more extensively in the writings of others.[38,71,88,89] Rockwood's method of grasping and securing the scapula with the examiner's forearm and moving the humeral head with the other hand is a valuable and sensitive method of testing. The supine position often relaxes the patient for more sensitive testing. Jobe's method of anterior humeral head pressure, followed by external rotation, and sudden release demonstrates the anterior instability.

Voluntary guarding by the patient not only may restrict motion, yielding a false negative examination, but guarding with sudden relaxation may lead the examiner to a false-positive evaluation of instability. At the end of the physical examination I always give the patient another chance to voluntarily reproduce the instability. For some unknown reason, this type of patient wants to withhold this information. Perhaps they believe they may be prejudicing the surgeon's judgement.

Imaging. A plain film x-ray taken during the pre-reduction position may confirm a dislocation, including the direction if an axillary view was obtained (Fig. 8-36).

Plain film x-rays should include West Point or Stryker views.[84] The presence of a bony defect on the posterior humeral head confirms glenohumeral dislocation (Fig. 8-35).

X-ray films can be obtained with the shoulder in the voluntary unstable position. An anterior-posterior and axillary view confirms the direction of the instability (Fig. 8-33).

I rarely request CAT scans or MRI, but many patients bring these with them. Computed arthrotomography will show the large labrum tears and ones that might be amenable to arthroscopic repair.[76] Gross reported high levels of sensitivity, specificity, and positive and negative predictive values with MRI for imaging the glenoid labrum in athletes.[4] High-resolution magnetic resonance imaging has been reported as 88% sensitive and 93% specific.[46] These modalities may show a labrum tear, but I still consider this circumstantial evidence of the diagnosis. I rely more on the patient assessment and physical examination because of lack of personal expertise or community availability of these technologies.

Examination with Anesthesia. Years ago, the old adage was "if you cannot dislocate the shoulder under anesthesia, then you should not perform an open reconstruction." Manual dislocation of the glenohumeral joint with the patient under anesthesia will confirm the diagnosis.[20] However, not only is this maneuver unnecessary to confirm the diagnosis, but it is another traumatic episode that produces bleeding and can obscure arthroscopic viewing. Therefore I do not attempt to dislocate the involved shoulder during anesthesia. Instead, I try to perform gentle manipulation to obtain a sense of instability short of dislocation in the patient in whom the diagnosis is still not clear at this juncture.

Some shoulder experts suggest that the examination during anesthesia is not an important part of their assessment and may even be misleading.[88] I believe just the opposite. It is another opportunity to evaluate the shoulder. The very act of the examination increases my experience. Additional information may be gained that otherwise would not be obtained. This examination may not change my ultimate surgical treatment, but it does provide another check and balance during the patient's care so that I am not overlooking other types of instability.

My method of examination during anesthesia is to gently confirm the direction of suspected instability without manual dislocation (see Figs. 8-39 and 8-40). More importantly, I want to use this opportunity to test for other directional instabilities that may have been overlooked. Another valuable aspect of examination with the patient under anesthesia is the opportunity to examine the opposite shoulder. I find more subtle opposite shoulder instabilities with the use of anesthesia than had been uncovered during the prior routine office examination. In fact, anterior glenohumeral instability is common on the uninvolved asymptomatic opposite side. This finding indicates a predisposition to dislocation that is not merely traumatic in etiology. The predisposition may affect the subsequent outcome of the treated shoulder.

The positioning for arthroscopy provides yet another opportunity for examining the glenohumeral joint for instability. A sulcus sign may be apparent for the first time (Fig. 8-43). With the suspension force, the humerus may externally rotate and even be subluxated in the very lax shoulder. When the upper extremity is mechanically suspended, the weight of the arm is controlled and not held by the examiner. The examiner can focus all the sensory attention on the instability without diverting energy to positioning the patient's arm. This provides yet another test for direction and magnitude of glenohumeral instability.

You may wonder why I take so many opportunities to check direction and magnitude of instability. The answer is simple. I have missed various types of instabilities in the past. I also believe that taking advantage of every opportunity improves my skill and avoids missing a diagnosis.

Operating Room Environment. If this is the reader's first topic or page in this text, I refer you to Chapter 2 for a complete review of this important topic.

Instrumentation. Again, I refer you to Chapter 3 for a thorough discussion of the instrumentation.

Diagnostic Arthroscopy. The reader is referred to chapter 5 for general techniques of diagnostic arthroscopy. Those diagnostic techniques specific for evaluation of glenohumeral instability are emphasized. One very important point concerns joint penetration. The instable shoulder has a propensity for subluxation and external rotation when suspended during arthroscopy. Therefore the shoulder should be reduced with internal rotation of the humerus to facilitate the arthroscope cannula and obturator penetration into the joint.

The diagnostic decision process is directed to clearly defining the shoulder lesions and directing the method of treatment: arthroscopic or open. A step by step assessment is outlined above (see page 311).

If at any stage the criteria for an arthroscopic repair are not met, then an open procedure is performed. For instance, if the humerus rests in the subluxed, external rotation position and arthroscopic assessment shows intrasubstance stretching of thinned glenohumeral ligaments, an open procedure is performed.

Maximal distention of the glenohumeral joint with a closed irrigation system demonstrates the general capsular laxity. The lax shoulder will hold a greater amount of fluid. The humerus is displaced off the glenoid to such an extent that the anterior wall is easily visible, even in its entirety in some cases (Figs. 8-60, 8-61, and 8-62). This amount of laxity may be an indication for open capsular shift.

A complete diagnostic arthroscopy is necessary, including looking for lesions in all quadrants. The global nature of traumatic anterior dislocation is illustrated earlier in this chapter (Fig. 8-49). An anterior portal may be necessary to see the posterior wall in its entirety.

Glenohumeral joint stability assessment. The stability of the glenohumeral joint is again assessed while looking with the arthroscope. The humerus is manually reduced and then released to assess the passive forces of instability. The humerus is moved in various directions (anterior, inferior, and posterior) while observing the amount of motion and the areas of contact correlated with points of tissue disruption.

Labrum assessment. The anterior margin of the glenoid is inspected for a labrum, as it is not present in some normal patients (Chapter 6). Evidence of injury is sought, such as blood, blood products, and/or tissue disruption. Ideally the classic Bankart lesion exists and tissue can be simply reattached. Unfortunately, the situation is not always that simple. It may appear that the patient has a simple Bankart lesion for reattachment, but the lesion is in both labrum and ligaments (as in types 3, 4, and 5 lesions).

The surgeon must satisfy many questions concerning the labrum. If the labrum is intact and uninjured, did the humeral head go over the labrum and stretch or tear the glenohumeral ligaments? Is the labrum an integral extension of the glenohumeral ligaments? Is the labrum reattachable? If the labrum is absent or displaced, can it be reconstructed? If the labrum is fragmented, should it be resected and the ligaments advanced to create the anterior butyrous effect? If the labrum is resected, will the ligaments be released and difficult to grasp or advance? Should the advancement and attachment of the ligaments be performed, and then the redundant labrum removed? Does the labral separation extend to the inferior quadrant?

The labrum must be preserved because it contributes 50% to the depth of the glenoid.[43] The depth of the glenoid is an important fractor in providing stability to the glenohumeral joint.

Glenohumeral ligament assessment. The glenohumeral ligaments are inspected for their presence, anatomical configuration, and normal thickness. The anatomical variation of foramen superior on the glenoid and between the middle and inferior glenohumeral ligaments must not be mistaken for a tear (see Chapter 6). Another anatomical consideration is the physical connection between the middle and inferior glenohumeral ligaments (Fig. 8-59). This distinction is important to the subsequent assessment of mobilization.

The questions to be asked are many. Are the glenohumeral ligaments disrupted? Where is the disruption? Is it off with the labrum? Is it separate from the labrum? Is the injury within the substance of the ligament? Is the detachment from the humerus? Are the glenohumeral ligaments stretched or thinned? Can the ligaments be pulled superior? Is the axillary portion of the glenohumeral ligament involved, stretched, or torn?

Debridement to assist diagnosis. Surgical debridement may be necessary to better visualize a lesion or the extent of a lesion. This is especially true for shaggy tears of the undersurface of the rotator cuff.

Rotator cuff assessment. The usual situation accompanying anterior dislocation is a partial-thickness tear of the undersurface of the rotator cuff. A localized debridement suffices for confirming the status and no repair is necessary.

In cases of full-thickness rotator cuff tear, inspection into the subacromial bursa is indicated. This may be followed with arthroscopic acromioplasty. An open rotator cuff repair may be warranted. This factor may dictate a open repair of both cuff and glenohumeral ligaments. I have repaired both lesions arthroscopically with metallic staples, but this method required planned arthroscopic removal. Even though this approach is technically possible and has given good results, the finding of the combined lesion is usually repaired by open surgery.

Mobilization of Glenohumeral Ligaments

The anterior mobilization and subsequent anterior labral abrasion is facilitated by changing to a 90-degree arthroscope. The mobilization of the middle and inferior glenohumeral ligaments are tested by placing a grasper from an anterior superior portal (Fig. 8-63). The middle is grasped first near the glenoid and then at the opening of the subscapularis bursa. This test indicates the inherent laxity in the ligament.

Several questions are now asked. How much mobility exists in the middle glenohumeral ligament? Which anatomical site creates the most mobility—the labral attachment area or near the subscapularis bursa? Does an anatomical connection exist between the middle and the inferior glenohumeral ligaments? Does the inferior glenohumeral ligament advance with tension applied to the middle ligament? Will tension applied to the middle glenohumeral ligament pull the humeral head into a reduced position? If not, how much more distance must the humerus be moved

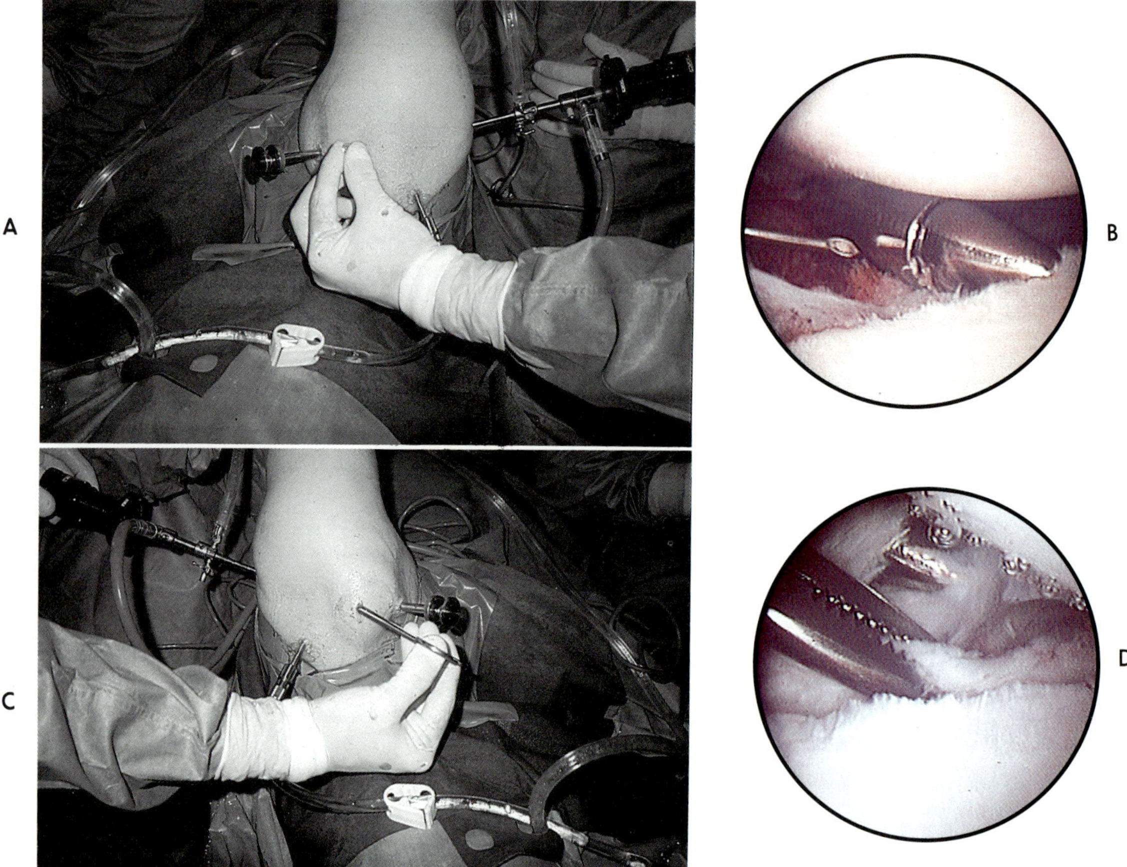

FIG. 8-63 Arthroscopic staple capsulorrhaphy.

A The scope is from posterior on the right shoulder. The large LCR cannula is in the anterior portal. A needle marker is placed from superior and anterior to identify the proper plane for transcutaneous forceps entry.

B Arthroscopic view of needle in joint from left (superior) and the LCR cannula in the joint.

C The forceps are placed transcutaneous from superior, while viewing from posterior.

D Arthroscopic view of grasping and mobilizing the labral/ligament complex in trial reduction.

Continued.

to be reduced? Answers to these questions assist the surgeon in deciding the amount of mobility necessary and the type of repair to be performed.

The inferior glenohumeral ligament is not as mobile as the middle glenohumeral ligament. The inferior ligament is grasped from the superior portal and tested in the same manner as the middle. Will tension applied to the inferior glenohumeral ligament pull the humeral head into a reduced position? If not, how much more distance must the humerus be moved to be reduced? If not, make sure the tear is not off the humeral side. Is the arcuate portion advanced with tension applied to the inferior ligament? Will further mobilization be necessary before repeating these tests?

Mobilization of the middle and inferior glenohumeral ligaments is accomplished in one of two ways, depending

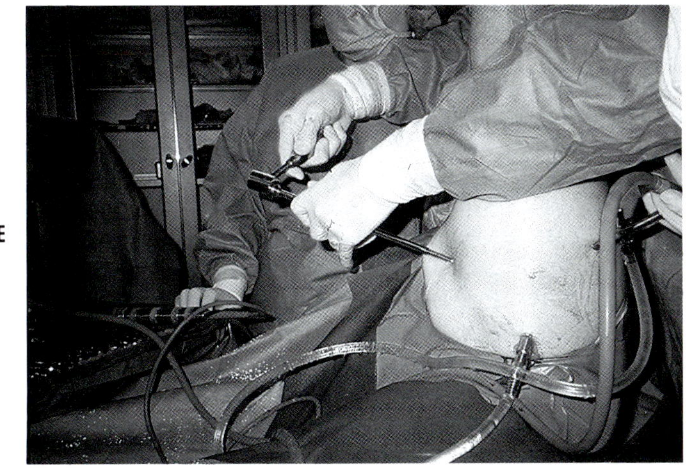

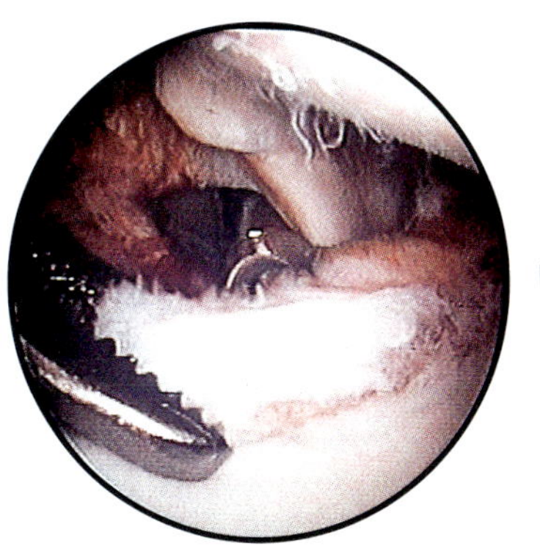

E

F

FIG. 8-63 *cont'd.* **Arthroscopic staple capsulorrhaphy.**

E Insertion of the staple with impaction with mallet.

F Arthroscopic view of capsular advancement into juxtaposition on the glenoid with staple insertion below the level of the joint. Notice the creation of a new butyrous labrum to the anterior joint with pushing up of the ligament.

on the anatomical structure and type of anterior injury. When the labrum and ligaments are pulled off together, the mobilization is completed with motorized instrumentation. The interval between the labral/ligament complex is developed with abrasion of the anterior glenoid. This step may cause fragmentation of the adjacent soft tissue, necessitating debridement of any loose tissue (Fig. 8-64, *A*). The labral/ligamentous complex may have to be reattached and dissection with motorized instruments will recreate the lesion (Fig. 8-64, *B*). This interval should be developed inferior, around the anterior inferior corner to free the arcuate ligament off the inferior glenoid (Fig. 8-64, *C*). This maneuver produces maximum mobilization.

Another diagnostic finding may show an absent labrum or destroyed integrity to the labrum. In the latter case, the labrum may be resected and the ligaments mobilized as described previously before reattachment.

Another diagnostic finding is a well-formed, intact labrum with intraligamentous tear or stretching of the glenohumeral ligaments. In this case I prefer to leave the labrum butyrous intact and create a defect in the glenohumeral ligaments next to the glenoid and under the labrum. The defect is extended to the anterior-inferior corner of the glenoid labrum. The defect is closed at capsulorrhaphy to shorten the previously stretched ligaments.

In all these mobilization techniques, the superior attachment of the middle and/or inferior glenohumeral ligaments must be left intact at the anterior-superior glenoid. Maintaining this normal anatomical connection prevents retraction of the ligaments and/or massive distention with fluid. Redundant tissue can be resected after advancement and fixation to the glenoid.

Another diagnostic finding is the detached labral/ligamentous complex with laxity. This condition is managed by developing the interval between the soft tissue and bone. If the labrum is anatomically absent or small, then the laxity is corrected by excision of the complex next to the glenoid, followed by reattachment. If the labrum is large and intact, an ellipse is excised out of the ligaments. In this case, the ligaments are advanced and secured separately from the labrum reattachment (Fig. 8-65). Another method of advancement that can be performed later in the procedure is to grasp the tissue with the staple and rotate the insertion device. This maneuver winds the tissue up, before insertion of the staple into the glenoid.

Glenoid Bony Abrasion

A superficial abrasion is performed on the anterior glenoid (Fig. 8-66). This step may be accomplished during the mobilization of the labrum or glenohumeral ligaments using a 90-degree arthroscope. The decortication of the bone creates a biological environment for bleeding and removes the barrier of interposing soft tissue to the subsequent adhesion. This dissection may also continue around the anterior-inferior corner of the glenoid. Care is taken to remove the cortex superior on the glenoid at the anticipated site of staple fixation. Exposure of cancellous bone facilitates staple insertion.

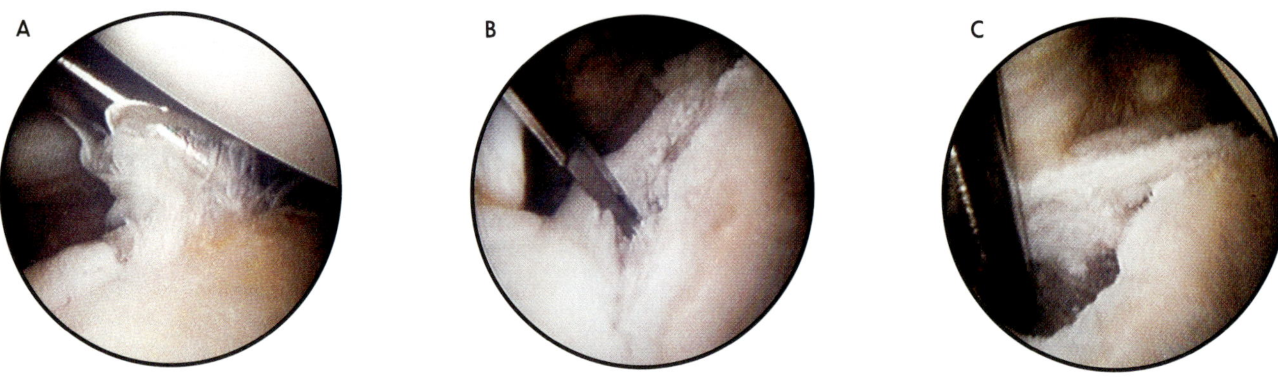

FIG. 8-64 Debridement and mobilization of Bankart lesion.

A Arthroscopic debridement with motorized instrumentation permits assessment of lesion.

B Knife blade incision is made to recreate the Bankart defect that has reattached to the glenoid.

C Mobilization of the labrum/ligament complex is demonstrated with motorized instrumentation in defect.

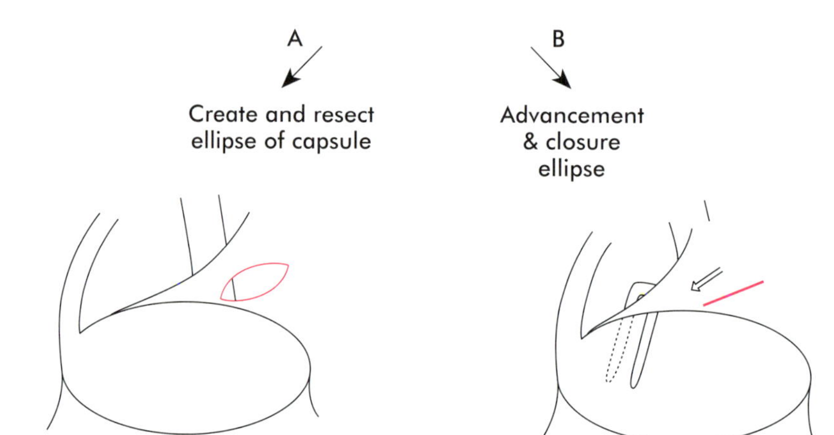

FIG. 8-65 Type 3 Bankart lesion with the labrum intact and the ligaments stretched. The area of ligamentous resection is shown. The middle glenohumeral ligaments remain intact. The capsular advancement closes the defect and places it in juxtaposition to the glenoid.

A Area of elliptical resection.

B Middle ligament advancement and resultant closure and advancement of the previously excised area.

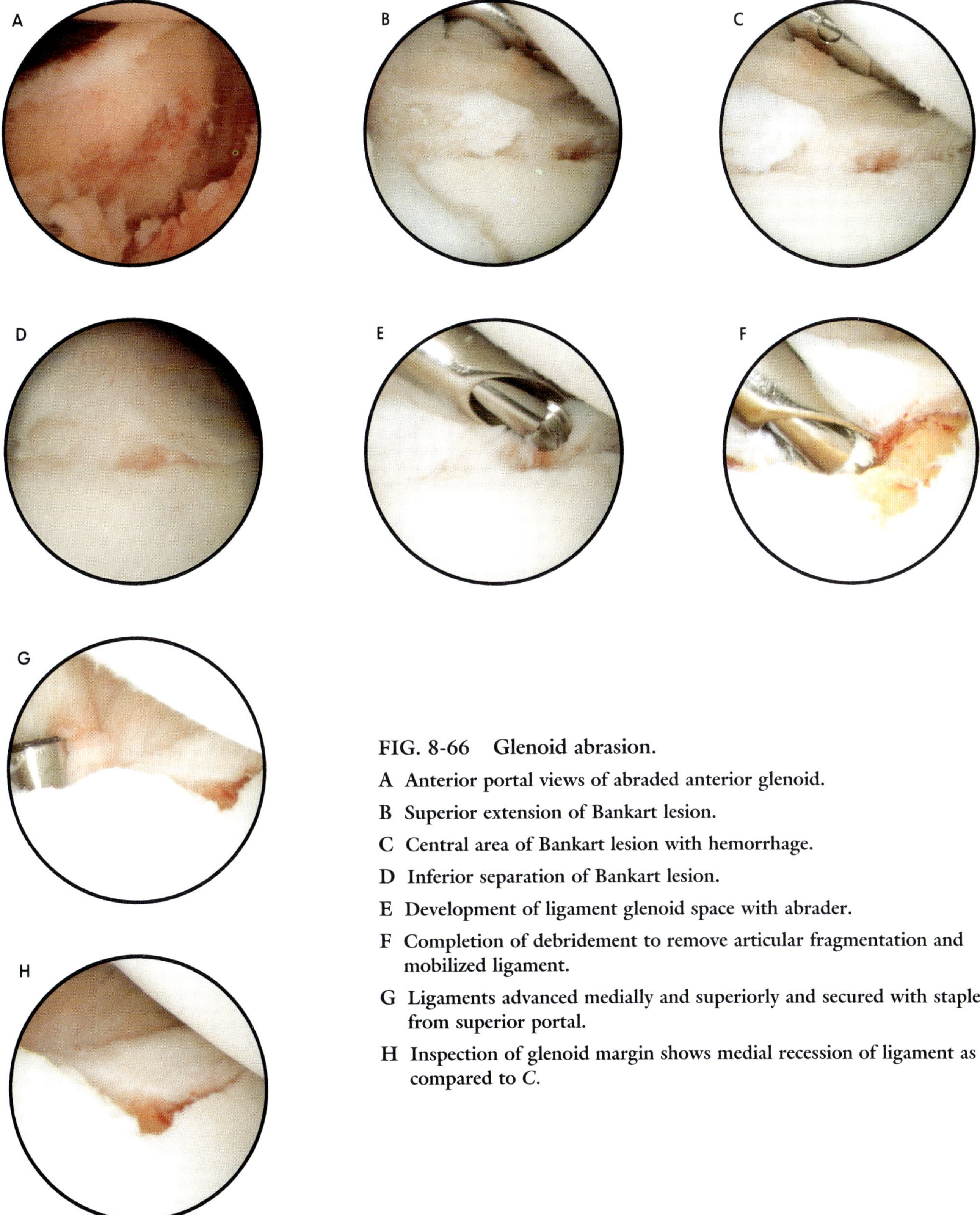

FIG. 8-66 Glenoid abrasion.

A Anterior portal views of abraded anterior glenoid.

B Superior extension of Bankart lesion.

C Central area of Bankart lesion with hemorrhage.

D Inferior separation of Bankart lesion.

E Development of ligament glenoid space with abrader.

F Completion of debridement to remove articular fragmentation and mobilized ligament.

G Ligaments advanced medially and superiorly and secured with staple from superior portal.

H Inspection of glenoid margin shows medial recession of ligament as compared to *C*.

Combined Joint Reduction and Ligament Mobilization

At the moment the ligament and/or labrum has been mobilized, I switch back to a 30-degree inclined arthroscope for the reduction and fixation. Traction is applied with a grasper to the anterior complex (Fig. 8-63 *E* and *F*). Several tests are now performed. Will advancement of the anterior capsular ligaments reduce the shoulder? If so, this is an ideal circumstance for proceeding arthroscopically. If the anterior capsular ligaments are maximally advanced and the humerus is not reduced, how much more distance is necessary to reduce the joint? A decision may be made that even maximal capsular advancement does not reduce the joint. In that case, an open capsular shift and imbrication operation would be indicated.

Reduction of the humeral head with direct posterior pull provides good exposure of the anterior and inferior ligaments (Fig. 8-67). With reduction of the joint, the status of the ligaments is again assessed with grasper.

Position of Reduction

Originally, I removed the suspension and placed the arm in flexion and adduction immediately before staple insertion. This maneuver relaxed the anterior capsular structures but obscured vision.

Presently, I prefer to leave the shoulder in the suspended position and reduce the humerus with external pressure anteriorly by the assistant on the arm and the humeral head posterior and superior (Fig. 8-67). This method provides reduction of the joint, excellent visualization, and an opportunity for assessing ligamentous tightening and security of staple fixation.

In summary, three methods of reattachment are presented: simple reattachment of types 1 and 2 lesions; capsular shift or resection and shift for types 3 and 5 lesions; and ligamentous shift to butyrous labrum in types 4 and 5 lesions.

FIXATION DEVICES

Arthroscopic Staple Capsulorrhaphy

Arthroscopic stapling capsulorrhaphy was proposed in 1982 by Donald G. Paish, Jr, M.D. of Glens Falls, New York. I had developed a metallic arthroscopic staple that could be passed through a cannula for anterior cruciate ligament surgery. After two long discussions he convinced me that it was reasonable to consider using this staple for arthroscopic staple capsulorrhaphy. Like most arthroscopic procedures, the rationale was the application of arthroscopic techniques to an established open surgical procedure. Staple capsulorrhaphy of the glenohumeral joint in the treatment of anterior traumatic instability had been reported.[29,101] Subsequent to that report a long term follow-up of DuToit staple capsulorrhaphy was reported by O'Driscoll.[79]

I performed the first such procedure by arthroscopy on August 12, 1982. Dr. Paish was the first patient. He had a traumatic dislocation 6 months before surgery and 100 subsequent instability episodes. The inflammatory response was great. The visualization was poor. My understanding of the capsular lesion was primitive. Three staples were used to reattach the glenohumeral ligaments. Two staples were inserted; one staple was lost in the joint and never retrieved. Stability was restored and the initial result was good. The loose staple has remained in the inferior capsule without migration.

One month later, a second patient who heard from a nurse about the technique requested the same procedure. I performed the second procedure with much better visualization and without technical problems. I waited several months to determine the early outcome of these two patients before considering another candidate. Both of these patients had good early results. Furthermore, no recurrence has occurred in either patient, now 9 years later. I performed this operation regularly for the next 8 years, until 1990 when I started a modified sabbatical leave for research purposes. The frequency of procedures is listed below by year.

Patient follow-up continues to this day. It has included routine postoperative office examination through 1 year. Thereafter annual contact is made by telephone and mailings. Reply is by self-addressed, postage-paid postcard questionnaire. Subsequent evaluations have included formal questionnaires, physical examinations, and x-ray examinations.

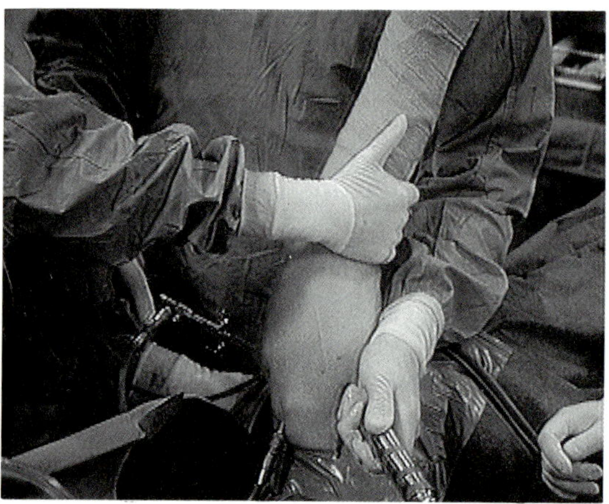

FIG. 8-67 The humerus is reduced with external pull by assistant. This facilitates exposure of anterior-inferior glenoid as well as positions the joint for reduction and internal fixation (left shoulder).

Clinical Studies of Staple Capsulorrhaphy

Series I. 77 cases involving arthroscopic staple capsulorrhaphy were performed from August 12, 1982, through December 31, 1984.

YEAR	NUMBER OF CASES
1982	2
1983	18
1984	57
Total	77

The patient selection, surgical procedure, and postoperative management were as outlined previously.

A 21% recurrent dislocation rate occurred in the initial series with a minimum 2 years follow-up. The initial series provided insight into the anatomy of the glenohumeral ligaments and experience with the surgical technique. The minimal morbidity of the arthroscopy surgical approach resulted in two deleterious factors affecting redislocation. First, few patients immobilized the shoulder for 3 weeks, the minimum time necessary for healing of the ligament to glenoid bone. Furthermore, an early return to sports and a subsequent collision was a major factor in redislocation.

Series II. In 1989 the results obtained after the first 77 cases (Series I) were reviewed. Modifications were made in the patient selection, surgical technique, and postoperative management. This series included the next 124 arthroscopic stapling capsulorrhaphy procedures. They were performed in the calendar years of 1985 (36), 1986 (45), and 1987 (43).

The series included 124 patients with traumatic anterior glenohumeral dislocation who underwent arthroscopic stapling capsulorrhaphy between January 1, 1985, and December 31, 1987. The operations were performed at the Ingham Medical Center, Lansing, Michigan, by one surgeon (myself). There were 101 males and 23 females. The average age was 26 years (range 11 to 57 years).

The series consisted of unselected consecutive cases. The medical history, physical examination, x-ray reports, surgical report, progress notes, and follow-up evaluations were entered into a computerized medical record. Each surgical case was recorded on videotape and stored for future viewing.

No case was aborted regardless of the diagnostic findings or for technical reasons during the capsulorrhaphy. The postoperative management included 1 month in an immobilizer, followed by range of motion exercises. At 3 months muscle strengthening exercises were initiated. The return to sports activity was restricted until 6 months following surgery.

The follow-up was a minimum of 2 years, and a maximum of 4 years, with an average of 3 years. After the initial postoperative care, an annual follow-up was achieved by correspondence and questionnaire response. Although physical examinations and x-ray films were obtained on this group at this time, they are not included here.

Table 8-2 Summary of 1989 Questionnaire Results (Series II)

	1985	1986	1987	Total	Percent
Number of cases	34	43	42	119	
Pain:	14	21	22	57	47%
activity	7	6	19	32	27%
rest	4	6	5	15	13%
night	5	8	11	24	20%
Pain medication	0	5	4	9	8%
Loss of motion	11	12	16	39	33%
Doctor's care	4	3	5	12	10%
Redislocation	3	9	5	17	14%
time interval	11 mos	23 mos	11 mos		
number of times	6	2	3		
Subsequent Surgery	5	3	2	10	8%

Of the 124 patients, 119 were available for follow-up. The 1989 questionnaire results are listed in Table 8-2. Of these patients, 47% said they had pain in the shoulder. In 27% the pain occurred with activity, 13% had pain at rest, and 20% had pain at night; 8% took medication for the pain.

Thirty-three percent said they experienced a loss of shoulder motion. Ten percent were under a doctor's care for the shoulder at the time of the follow up.

Fourteen percent had a postoperative recurrent dislocation of the shoulder. This problem occurred an average of 15 months after surgery, with an average incidence of three times. The initial recurrence was associated with significant trauma, usually in sports in 13 patients. Recurrence occurred with daily activities in four patients.

Repeat surgery was performed in 8% of Series II. Eight patients underwent open surgical procedures, three had repeat arthroscopic staple capsulorrhaphy, and one patient had staple removal. The incidence of this type of arthroscopic repair by year performed is as follows:

YEAR	NUMBER OF CASES
1982	2
1983	18
1984	57
1985	36
1986	45
1987	43
Total	201

Series III. The last time for routine follow-up was in December 1990. Therefore the 1988 cases that had not been evaluated with a minimum 2-year follow-up were not included in Series II.

Twenty-five patients underwent arthroscopic staple capsulorrhaphy in 1988, 19 males and 6 females. The average age was 26 years and the range was 15 to 48 years.

Only 15 of these 25 patients replied to the questionnaire in December of 1990. The questionnaire results were tabulated (see the box). This review shows 60% of respondents had pain. The two patients (13%) with redislocation underwent reoperation.

SUMMARY OF 1990 QUESTIONNAIRE RESULTS (SERIES III)

Pain:	9
with activity	5
at rest	2
night	6
Uses pain medication	2
Loss of motion	6
Doctor's care	2
Redislocation	2
time interval	1.7 years
number times	average of 6
Subsequent surgery	2

Perspective: on the Job Training. This operation must be placed in a historical perspective to allow the reader an understanding of the review of these series.

My practice profile. I was not trained in shoulder surgery. I was not adept at recognizing functional or multidirectional instability at the time. Before this time, my shoulder practice profile included only a few referral patients, usually for diagnostic shoulder arthroscopy. As a result, some of the patients with traumatic dislocation had underlying other instability problems. I had little fundamental knowledge of open surgical reconstruction for shoulder dislocation. I had seen Bankart, Putti-Platt, Nicola, Magnuson, and Bristow procedures in my residency.[108] I usually performed a modified Bristow procedure in my practice.

Anatomical understanding. There was little knowledge of arthroscopic shoulder anatomy by me or others. Often the identity of the various glenohumeral ligaments was confusing. For example, it was not generally know that the subscapularis tendon had an intraarticular portion.

Pathologic understanding. The understanding of the fundamental defect was of the Perthes/Bankart lesion.[8,9,83] The Bankart lesion was recognized as a tearing of the labrum/ligament complex, but without the arthroscopic perspective that permitted recognition of the various types previously described in this text. Another common denominator of dislocation was the Hill-Sachs lesion, but never so clearly visualized as during arthroscopy. The global nature of the problem was not recognized, at least by me.

Initial surgical repair concept. The arthroscopic surgical repair was based on the Bankart concept from open surgery. That approach was to suture the anterior capsule (middle glenohumeral ligament) to the anterior glenoid with drill holes placed into the articular cartilage. This arthroscopic repair was a modification of open staple capsulorrhaphy.

Initial patient selection. These patients first selected a doctor who might be able to perform their surgery by arthroscopy. It must be recognized that patients selecting me for an evaluation are usually inquiring if an arthroscopic application is possible for their condition. This eschews my patient population.

Then, my selection was limited to those who had evidence of a traumatic anterior dislocation. The development of my ability to adequately and completely examine a patient lagged behind the development of the surgical technique. For instance, I did not realize the significance of the sulcus sign that was manifest when the patient was in suspension before arthroscopy (see Fig. 8-43). Only now am I able to appreciate subtle glenohumeral instabilities and I am still not an expert.

As a result, the preoperative selection process included patients who had other conditions, including the traumatic anterior dislocation. No consideration was given to the patient's desire to return to collision athletics, including basketball and water skiing.

Subsequently, a retrospective evaluation of one group of my patients' arthroscopic findings indicated only 31% would have been ideal surgical candidates.

Initial surgical procedure. The surgical approach was to identify the Bankart lesion, or what was left of the ligaments, and perform direct attachment to the glenoid with a metallic staple. I was 1 year into the procedure experience before I thought to perform a glenoid abrasion. This step became an important part of the procedure.

I first used simple reattachment, then capsular shift medial to take up the slack. Eventually the shift went superior as well. Finally, I recognized the importance of buttressing or restoring labrum.

Initially the reattachment advanced the tissue medial on the glenoid neck for tightening. Subsequently, the tissue was moved medial and superior. Only in recent years has the concept of capsular shifting been introduced with an attempt to reconstruct the butyrous labrum.

I experienced metal staple implant problems. The original staple was malleable and bent. First one and then multiple staples were used. Subsequently, only one properly placed and secured staple was used. I originally experienced "loose staples," but review of my original videotapes showed they were not implanted in the first place. In one case I placed the staple near the anterior labrum, which required a planned removal (see Fig. 8-79, *C*). The ligaments were cut during metal staple placement, but subsequent replacement solved the problem.

Postoperative management. The initial postoperative

management initially consisted of sling immobilization until the patient was comfortable. The shoulder was mobilized as a matter of patient comfort and initiative. The immobilization following surgery was usually less than 3 weeks because of the minimal morbidity of the procedure. In series I, a young man redislocated 3 weeks postoperatively while hitting an overhand smash in racquetball.

After a near normal range of motion was restored, strengthening exercises were begun. Return to sports was either at the patient's discretion or 6 months, whichever came first.

Subsequently, the necessity for postoperative immobilization was recognized, as well as a delay in return to activity.

These and other observations have helped me improve patient selection, examination and surgical techniques, and postoperative management. My frequent presentations of results at continuing education courses have allowed others to better select patients for their practice, design new techniques, and provide better postoperative management and, hopefully, improved results (see Fig. 8-63).

Metal Staple Fixation

I still use the metallic staple for fixation. I like the configuration of the device for this use, so I anticipate only a change to a bioabsorbable staple (see Chapter 11). The configuration of the staple design allows independent grasping of the ligamentous tissue in the crotch of the device, if necessary (Fig. 8-68). All of the above criteria (pages 311-318) must be met for suitability for completion by arthroscopy.

Advantages. This method has several advantages. First and foremost, the device has a simple design and is strong. Its double tine configuration grasps and holds the tissue well. The exposure is limited to the joint. The method of device insertion is through a cannula. The technique of fixation is simple impaction. The ligament is securely fixed in juxtaposition to the bone. The operative time is short (under 1 hour). Lastly, I am experienced with this method and have had good results in properly selected cases with this method at this stage of its development.

Disadvantages. The present disadvantages are all related to the metallic material of the staple (see Fig. 8-79). A second operation may be necessary to remove the staple. A planned staple removal is necessary if it was improperly placed or if the patient is a throwing athlete. An unplanned removal is necessary if subsequent malposition occurs by failure to implant in bone, improper positioning, or subsequent loosening. Postoperative pain is another reason for a second procedure to remove an implant. My patients have experienced all of these reasons for removal. Careful postoperative follow-up provides ample time for safe removal if one of these problems occurs.

Technique. The anterior portal cannula is interchanged via switching sticks with a larger one that accommodates the staple (LCR cannula). I rarely use an auxiliary anterior-inferior portal. For this inferior approach to be safe, the arm must be taken into the adducted position as described by Michael Gross.[34]

The surgical team is alerted to the upcoming moment of fixation. The circulating nurse attends to the suspension weight. It may be removed during the fixation, especially

A

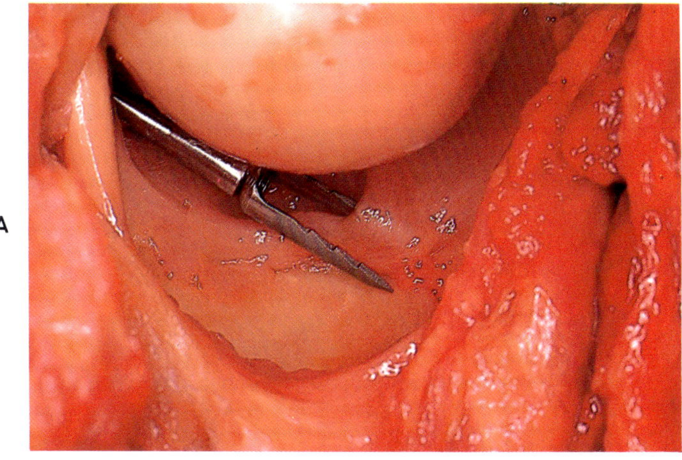

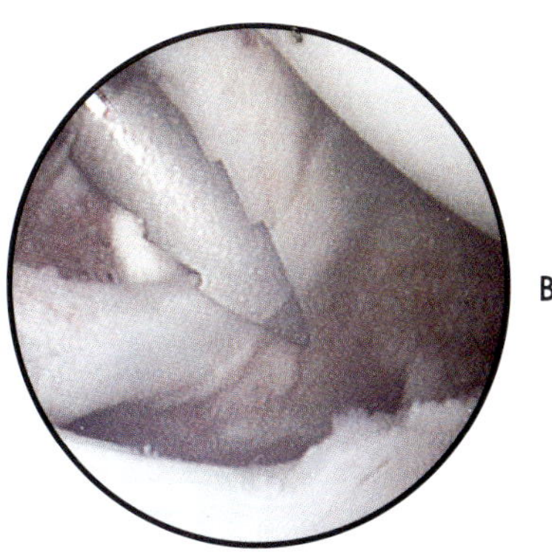

B

FIG. 8-68 Staple configuration facilitates grasping and advancing the ligament.

A Demonstration on a cadaver specimen.

B Arthroscopic view of same maneuver on middle glenohumeral ligament.

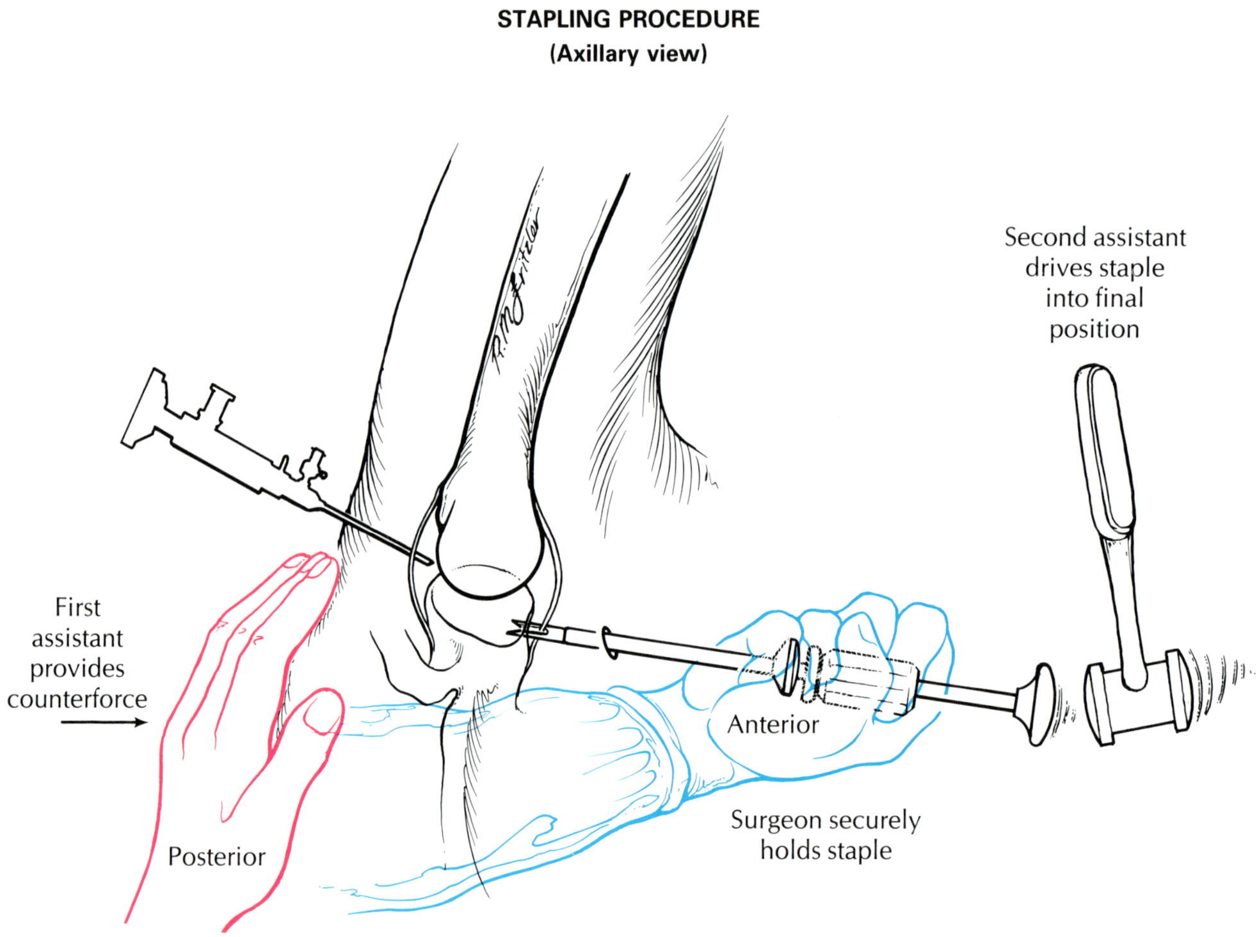

STAPLING PROCEDURE
(Axillary view)

FIG. 8-69 Driving of staple into glenoid neck. Separate hammer is used for staple driving in shoulder. Sliding hammer offers less mechanical advantage with opposite side driving. Axillary view showing arthroscope posterior, staple anterior *(red)*. Hand of assistant secures scapula for countertraction *(blue)*. Hand of surgcon controls insertion.

if adduction and internal rotation are necessary for approximation of the ligaments. Otherwise the weights are removed after the fixation of the ligaments.

The first assistant reduces the shoulder with posterior and superior traction on the humerus with one hand and holds the arthroscope with the other. Since the scapula is floating on the chest wall, the scapula must be stabilized for impact (Fig. 8-69).

The simple Bankart lesion (types 1 and 2) may not require mobilization and therefore only direct reattachment is indicated. Care must be taken not to overlook concomitant stretching of the glenohumeral ligaments, which simple reattachment of the Bankart lesion would not address (type 4 lesion).

The surgeon grasps the anterior structures previously mobilized with a forceps from the anterior and superior portal.

Choice of Staple. These staples come in two configurations: multi-barbed (Original) and single barbed (Profile '90) (see Chapter 3). The Original comes in three sizes:

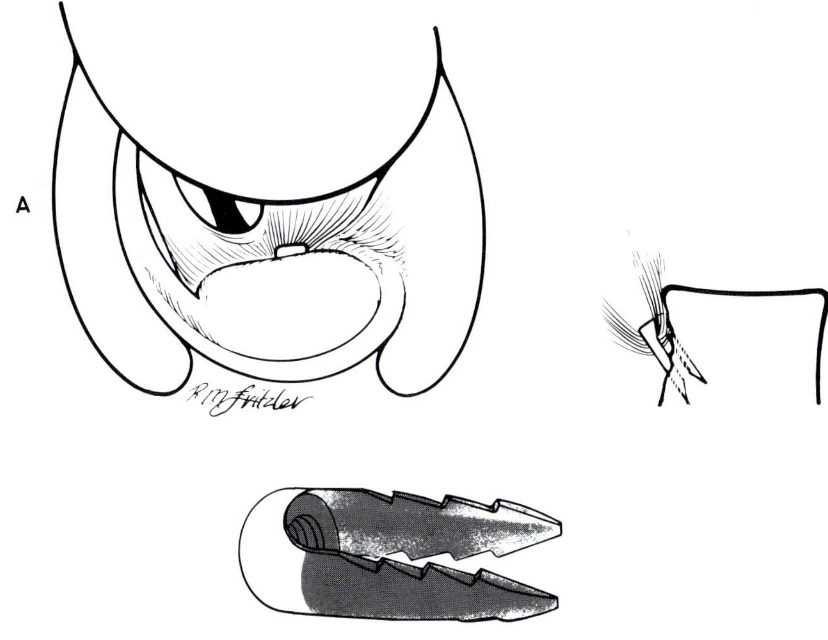

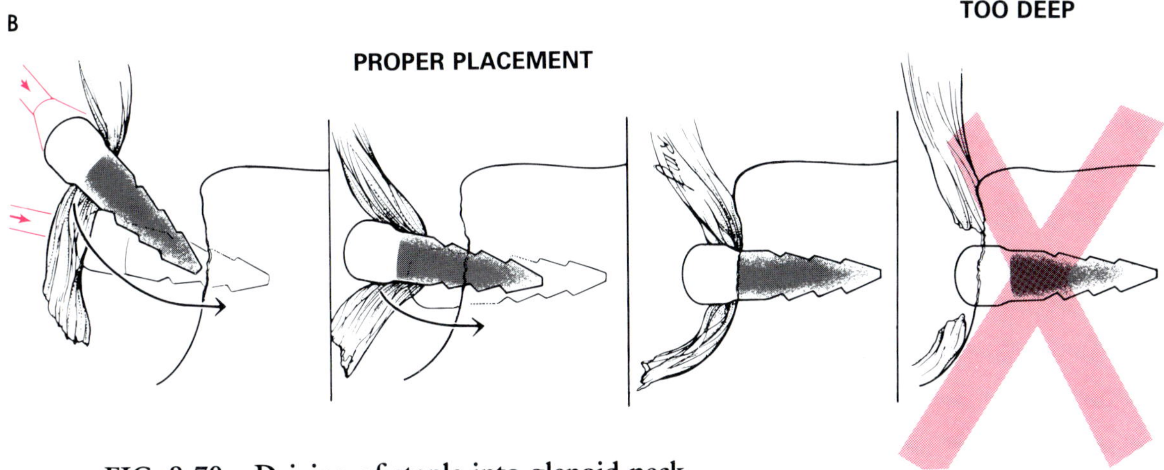

FIG. 8-70 Driving of staple into glenoid neck.

A Vertical placement of staple in ligament. Staple secured into bone away from joint line.

B Proper staple insertion—or too deep.

small, regular, and large. The Profile '90 comes in medium and large sizes.

Staple selection is based on general patient size, the thickness of the ligament, and the size of the bony glenoid site. The staple selected must be of such a size to capture and house the ligament with enough tine length to fix well in bone without subsequent amputation of the ligament (Fig. 8-70).

The Original staple has many barbs and thin tines (see Fig. 8-68, *B*). Although the crotch of the original staple design has been smoothed, the barbs and numerous tines tend to cut the tissue or may result in subsequent tissue tearing or loosening. The Profile '90 staple was developed to overcome these objections. The crotch is smooth, the tine shaft is round, and there is only one tine (see Chapter 3). At present I usually use the Profile '90 staple, most often in the medium size. The small Original staple is used in smaller patients; otherwise I do not use the Original design. Pretapping of bone may be helpful in hard bone or if a bioabsorbable staple device is contemplated.

The second assistant attaches the selected staple to the driver/extractor. The staple is screwed on the insertion device. Grasping the staple with a sponge or towel provides a method of maximal tightening without tearing surgical gloves. It should be noted that the male part screw mechanism protrudes into the crotch area of the staple as a safety factor (see Fig. 8-68, *A*). This protruding part acts as a bumper to prevent cutting through the ligamentous tissue at impaction.

The second assistant removes the obturator and places the insertion device and staple into the cannula. The cannula is removed in retrograde fashion. The insertion device has a proximal screw mechanism on the shaft that provides for attachment of the cannula. The cannula will not move back and forth during impaction.

Although the insertion device has a sliding hammer, it should not be used in shoulder surgery impaction. This device is best reserved for staple removal. The use of a sliding hammer for insertion results in side to side motion of the insertion device as this hammer is activated. The preferred method is impaction of the end of the device with a hammer (see Fig. 8-63, *E*). The rapid impact of the hammer removes angulatory force and provides a straighter, measured depth of insertion.

At this moment, the joint is reduced, and the ligament is approximated and/or advanced with the grasper from the superior portal (see Fig. 8-63, *F*). The staple is brought into position to secure the capsular ligaments on the anterior-superior face of the glenoid. Perspective can be difficult to obtain at this moment. A look at the outside position of the insertion device, coupled with palpation and the arthroscopic perspective, are necessary for proper placement. This outside position of the insertion device will appear to be aiming superior and medial (Fig. 8-71). If the angulation is toward inferior, then the staple may miss the glenoid on the inferior aspect. If angulation is too superior, the staple tines may be exposed above the coracoid process (see Fig. 8-80).

The surgeon must be careful, using palpation, to have the staple alignment at right angles to the glenoid face (see Fig. 8-70). Care must be taken not to amputate the ligament. If angulation is too medial, the staple will slide along and not into the glenoid bone.

Finally, the arthroscopic view must be maintained. This may require scope rotation and increased intraarticular fluid pressure. A 90-degree scope may be used during this inspection.

When all systems have been checked and are satisfactory, the staple is inserted with impaction. A separate hammer is used for this maneuver. The first assistant stabilizes the scapula with his or her hand (see Fig. 8-69). The surgeon holds the insertion device in place, with the staple impaling the ligament and flush against bone. The second assistant makes the initial impact with the hammer. After the staple engages the bone, careful lesser impacts are applied until the staple is secured.

The selection of proper depth of staple insertion is assisted by the design of the staple. The limbs of the tines are sand blasted during manufacture and the proximal portion of the head is smooth and shiny, including a portion of the crotch (see Fig. 8-68, *B*). The proper level of insertion should leave all the shiny head of the staple exposed,

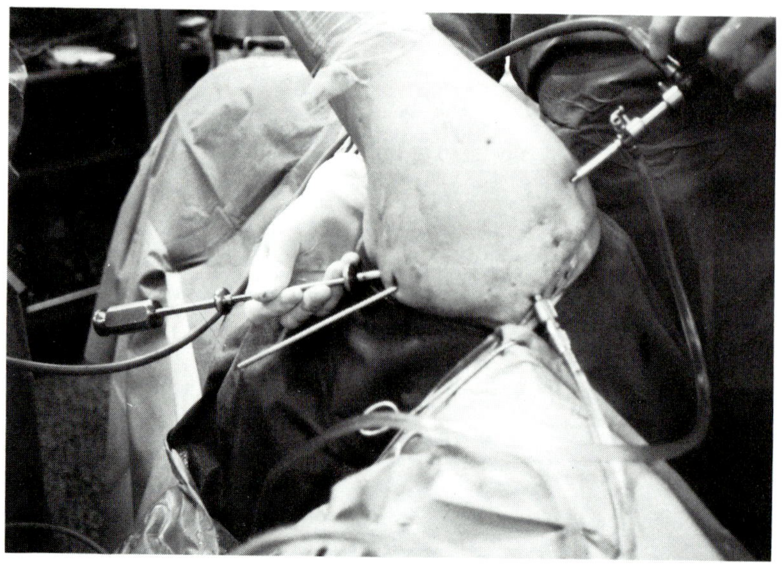

FIG. 8-71 Technique of staple insertion.

otherwise the ligament will be cut through.

The attachment concept can be visualized on a gross anatomical specimen (Fig. 8-72).

The staple placement is usually medial to the glenoid surface and superior on the glenoid (Fig. 8-73). Placement is visualized best with a 90-degree arthroscope.

The staple position on x-ray view will often be a false-positive superior position. This position is best demonstrated by placement of a staple in a gross specimen and then x-ray of the specimen. Notice the superior position on x-ray film (Fig. 8-74). A proper position is illustrated by arthroscopy and correlative x-ray view (Fig. 8-75).

After insertion of the first staple, the surgeon tests the security of fixation with force applied to the insertion device. A back and forth motion should move the impaled scapula. If it seems secure, then the insertion device is rotated and partially removed from the staple. Another check is made for motion of the staple. If none is seen, the insertion device is removed over the reinserted cannula.

If the insertion was made with the arm in the adducted internally rotated position, then manual repositioning and distention may be necessary to continue checking the security of the staple and the reattached ligament.

A probe is used to palpate the head of the staple for security. The ligament attachment is also probed for security of attachment. If the shoulder is reduced, and the ligament and staple secure, then the arm is taken across the chest for immobilization.

Staple Removal. If the staple is loose, it should be removed. The LCR cannula is reinserted for this maneuver.

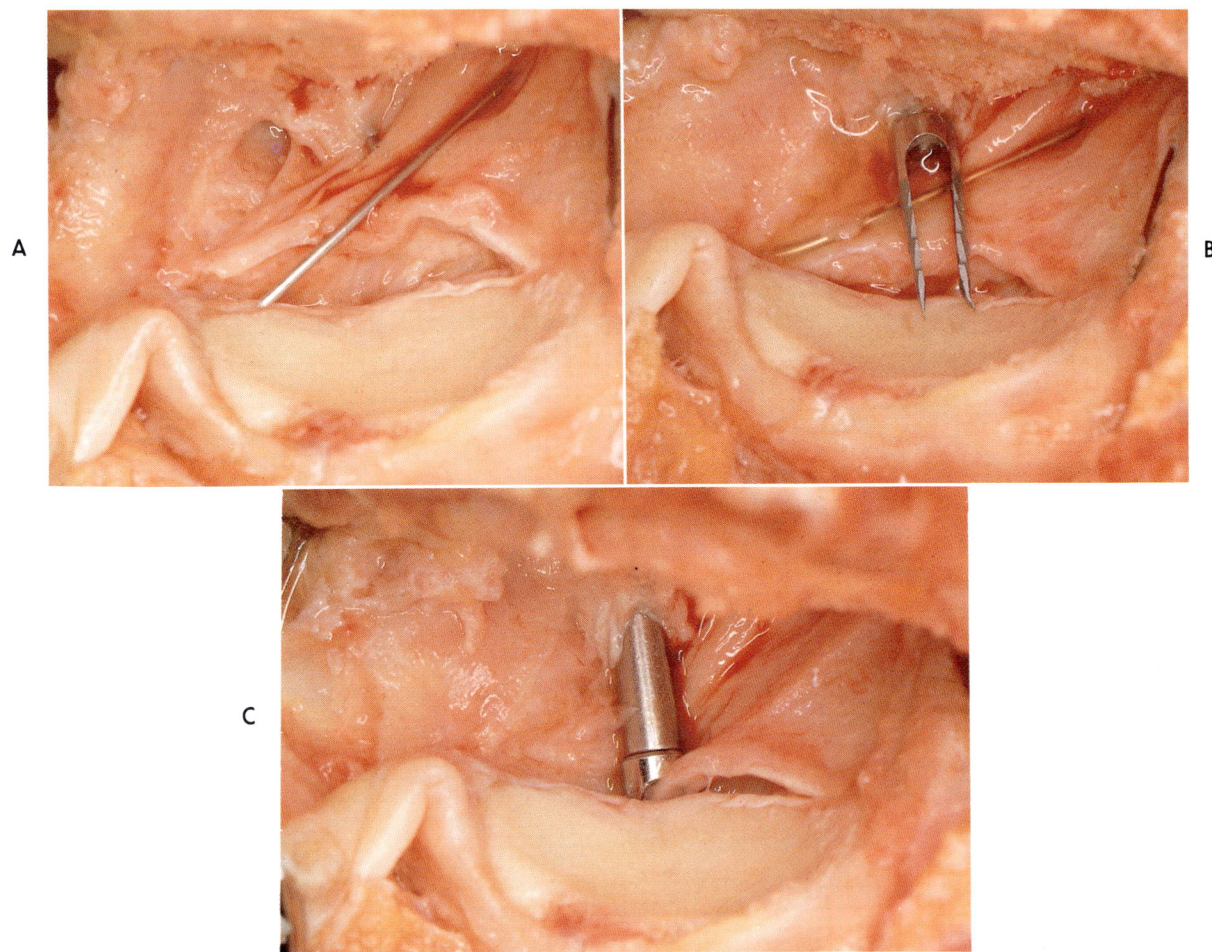

FIG. 8-72 Staple placement in gross cadaver specimen.

A Bankart lesion created on length of anterior glenoid.

B Staple approach above subscapularis tendon.

C Staple inserted in center of glenoid neck.

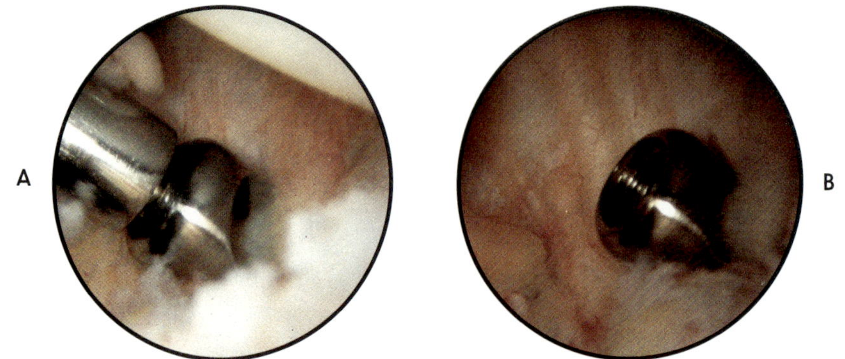

FIG. 8-73 Arthroscopic view with 90-degree scope shows staple placement.

A At time of insertion.

B After insertion device removal.

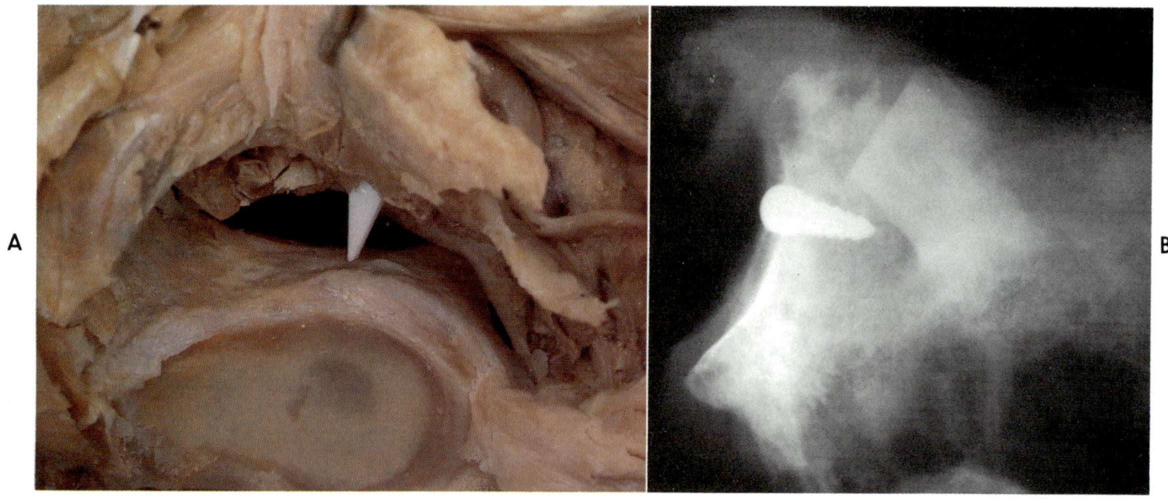

FIG. 8-74 Staple position on scapular neck.

A Placement site in central portion of neck dissected in gross specimen to see bony contour.

B X-ray film of scapular specimen of Fig. 8-72, *C*, shows position of staple to appear superior on glenoid. This results from scapular position and contour.

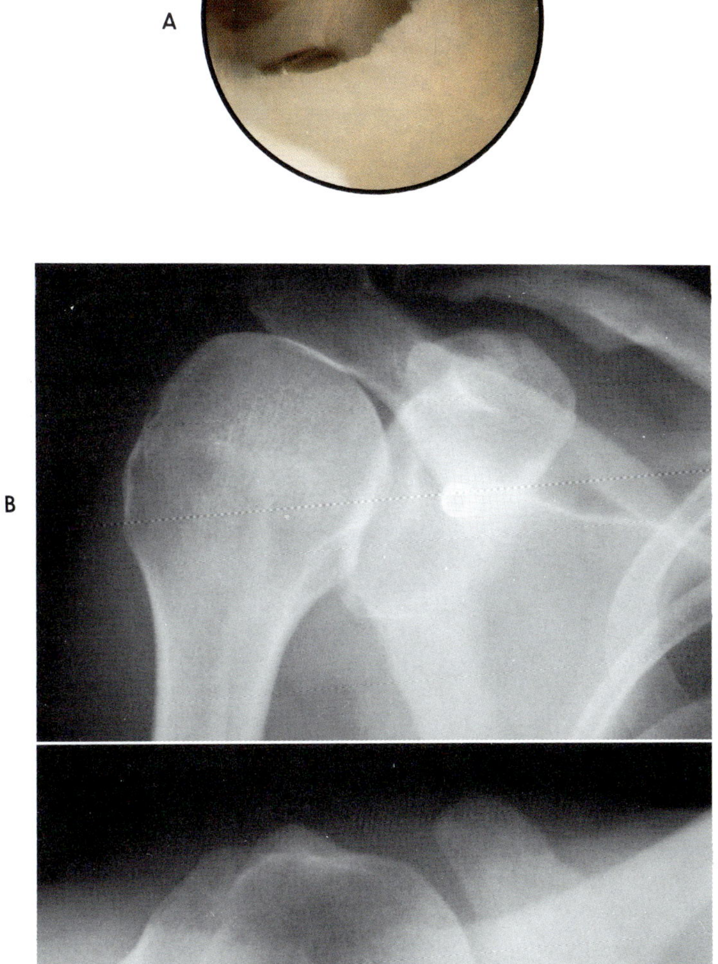

FIG. 8-75 **Proper clinical position of staple in scapula.**

A Arthroscopic view showing staple well displaced from joint line.

B Anterior-posterior x-ray film of same patient showing staple location.

C Axillary x-ray film shows proper position of staple.

A gold-colored, extractor Bullet Nosed Tip is designed for this purpose (Fig. 8-76). It is attached tightly to the extractor device and provides for entry into the female part screw mechanism of the staple. The bullet nose allows angled approach to the staple head. The metal of the bullet is gold so it can be easily differentiated from the silver-colored staple during arthroscopy. The metal of the Bullet Nose Tip is softer than that of the staple, so that stripping of the threads will not occur and prevent subsequent staple removal. The extractor can be used with its own threads if the direct approach can be used. When the staple to be removed is secured, the cannula should be replaced into the joint to provide a conduit for safe and complete removal of the staple. The attached sliding hammer is used to remove the staple by repetitive motion.

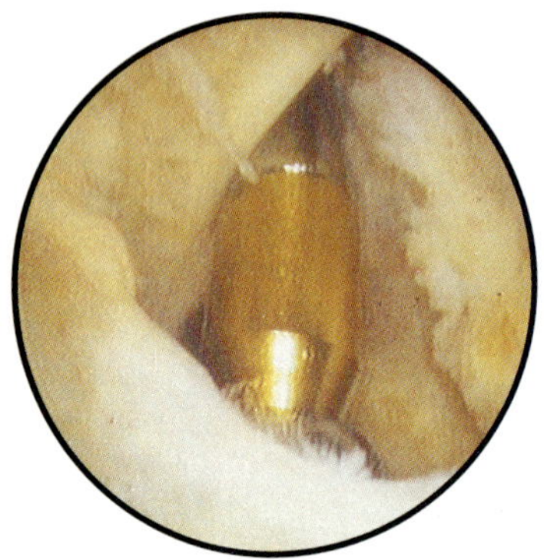

FIG. 8-76 Arthroscopic view of Bullet Nosed Golden Extractor tip in the end of the staple. This maneuver facilitates removal of the staple.

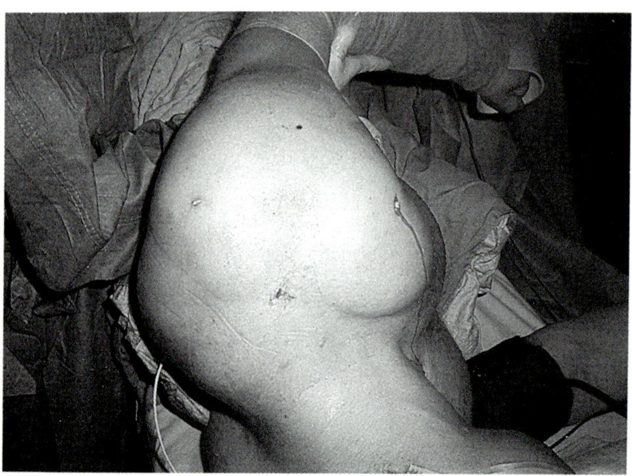

FIG. 8-77 Complications: Fluid extravasation. The swelling increases the depth to the shoulder joint and makes instrument manipulation difficult.

In some cases of late removal, greater force must be applied with a hammer. In this case the shaft of the extractor is grasped with a vise grip. The impacts are placed against the vise grip. The knob at the end of the extractor prevents the vise grip from sliding during hammering.

The operative procedure is repeated if the integrity of the ligamentous tissue has not been jeopardized and reattachment is possible.

Intraoperative Complications. The most common intraoperative complication is extravasation of the fluids used for distention (Fig. 8-77). The risk of this complication increases with the length of the operation.

Complications do occur with the staple device. The earliest staples were purposely malleable so that they would bend and not break (Fig. 8-78). The second generation devices were less malleable. Breakage is a possibility, but infrequent (Fig. 8- 79, *A*).

Placement of the staple is a potential problem. Orientation is difficult when looking from posterior and operating toward oneself. This is similar to working with a mirror image. As a result, the staple orientation may not be perpendicular to the anterior glenoid. To pass inferior to the glenoid or parallel and medial is most common. In some cases the staple is placed too superior or even in the coracoid process (Fig. 8-80). In another situation, one time may be in bone and the other out (Fig. 8-81).

A properly placed staple may be driven into bone so far as to amputate the glenohumeral ligaments, acting as a "cookie-cutter" through the ligaments or labrum.

Postoperative Complications. I have seen no infections, hemorrhage, neurovascular injury, or thromboembolic phenomena. The redislocation incidence is recorded on p. 319-320.

The common reasons for reoperation are related to a loose staple, pain with staple as a suspected cause, and redislocation.

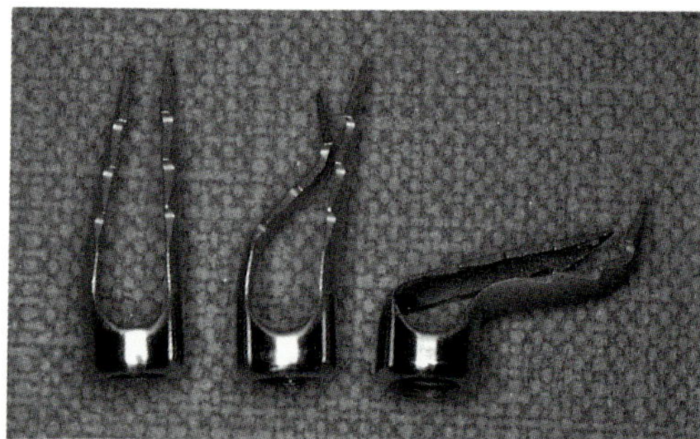

FIG. 8-78 Problem with original staple implantation: Bent staples result from forceful direction change after initiating insertion.

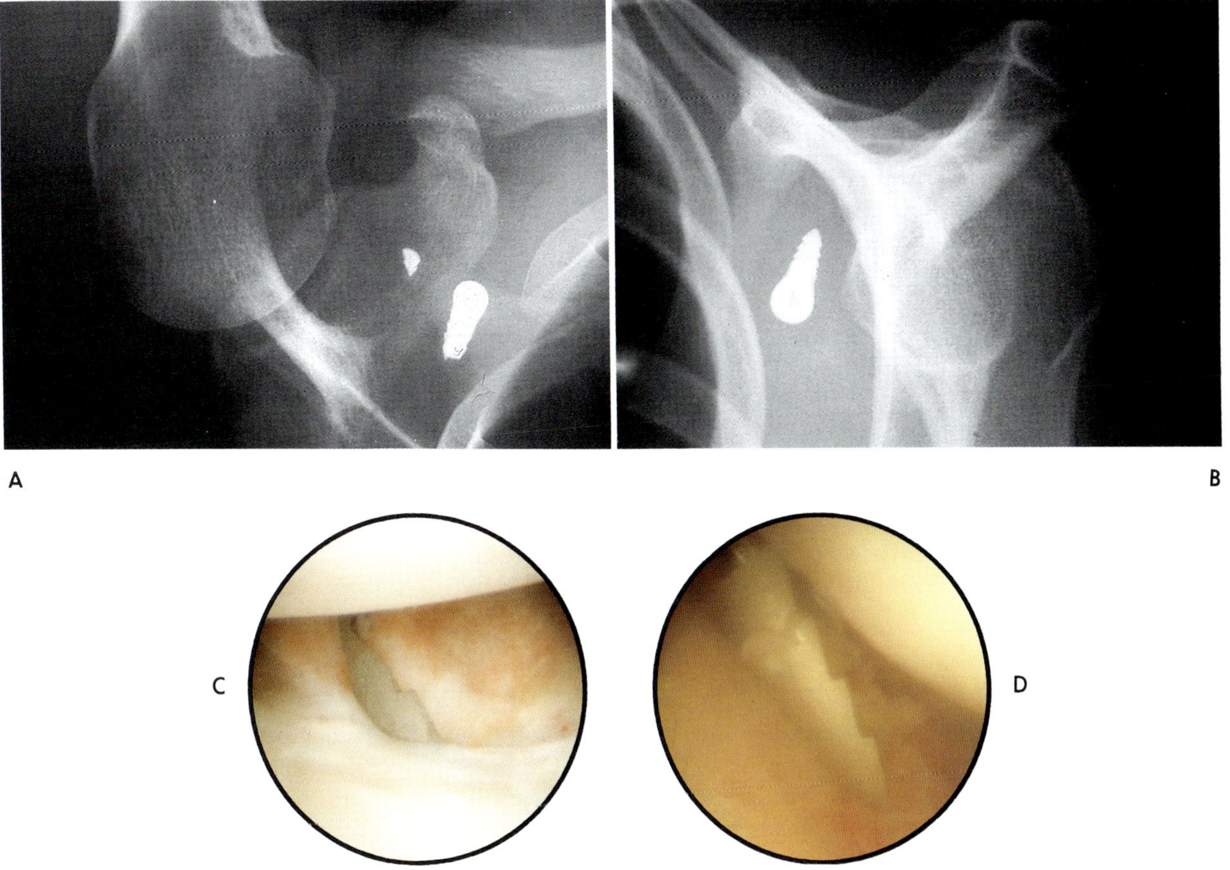

FIG. 8-79 Staple complications.

A X-ray film showing breakage.

B X-ray film showing loosening.

C Arthroscopic view of improper staple placement 5 months after reconstruction.

D Free staple in joint of patient who returned to competitive skiing 3 weeks after surgery. No repeat dislocation occurred.

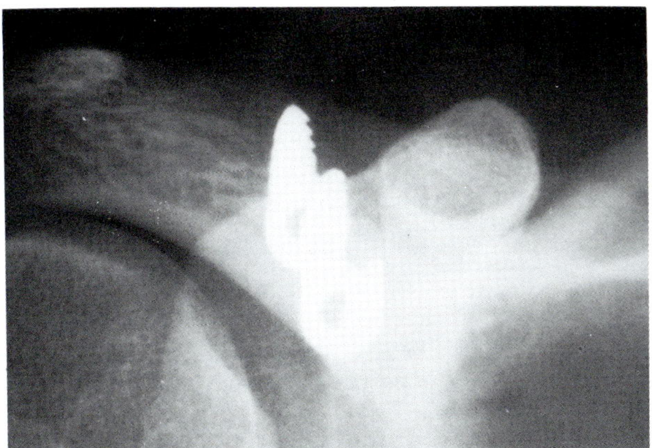

FIG. 8-80 X-ray view of superior staple placed out of bone. Removal reduced symptoms of pain.

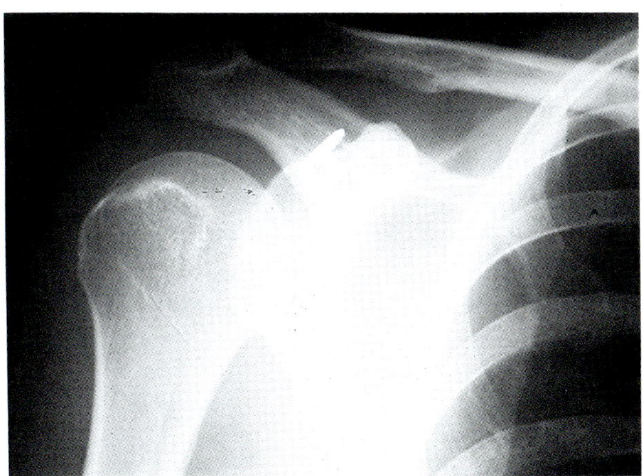

FIG. 8-81 Only one tine in bone.

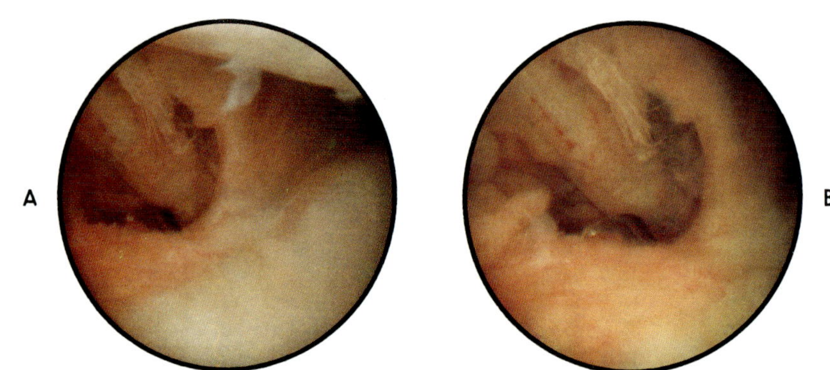

FIG. 8-82 Shoulder joint irritation 1 year postoperatively in competitive athlete.

A Note superficial disruption of subscapularis tendon, even though staple is properly placed on glenoid. Routine staple removal is indicated in this patient.

B Close-up of subscapularis fraying. (Note healed surface of glenoid to ligaments.)

Loose staple. I reiterate that a properly placed staple will not migrate out of bone (Fig. 8-79). In fact, it takes a great force to remove the staple immediately after insertion and even years after implantation. Most reports of staple loosening are illegitimate; by this I mean they were probably never inserted in the first place. The rare legitimate loosening usually follows reinjury or redislocation. Any surgeon who has experienced the difficultly of dislodging a properly placed staple in bone will not easily believe those who say this type of staple routinely loosens and migrates.

A loose staple is a reason for reoperation. Although I have not seen a staple migrate out of the immediate glenohumeral joint area, others have reported significant migration.[94] The loose staple is usually within the joint, often with one tine out and the staple straddling the capsule with its crotch.

Visualization is best attempted by arthroscopy. Removal is also easier by arthroscopy if a portion of the staple is within the joint. Use of tissue debridement, the magnetic suction Golden Retriever, and the Bullet Nosed attachment are necessary. The first step is to determine if the staple can be rethreaded where it rests. If so, the tissue holding the staple will provide enough stability to rethread it. Tissue must be debrided from the head and threaded area. Attention should be given to the angle of approach by the extractor. If the approach is head on, then the gold Bullet Nosed attachment is unnecessary. If an angle is used, then rethreading is assisted by the Bullet Nosed attachment.

In some cases the staple cannot be properly approached by the extractor device. In this case, every attempt should be made to free the staple into the joint. The free staple is movable and difficult to rethread with the extractor. The free staple is best removed by cannula, so it is not lost in the soft tissues. I use a transcutaneous forceps for removal only as a last resort. The cannula system may be a conduit for a small jaws forceps, but is not usually large enough for staple and forceps passage. Both must be removed together.

The cannula system creates a flow of fluids out of the joint. That force, coupled with the Golden Retriever magnetic suction, may remove the loose staple.

The simplest method to remove a free staple is to place a probe through an LCR cannula to manipulate the staple so the head approaches the cannula. The hook of the probe is placed into the head via the hole for the threads and pulls the staple out of the joint.

In my experience, the staple has always been visible within the joint, even if attached to the capsule. Open surgery removal may be necessary for those staples not accessible to arthroscopic removal. X-ray–guided control may be necessary. A loose staple inaccessible to arthroscopy and requiring major anatomical dissection will require x-ray control to locate.

Pain. Although other causes of postoperative pain exist, any patient experiencing pain should consider staple removal because it may be the cause (Fig. 8-82). Although a third of the patients say they experience pain on our routine questionnaires, very few decide to have staple removal.

Redislocation. In that the metal staple is placed superior on the glenoid, any subsequent anterior-inferior dislocation will not impinge the staple and the humeral head (Fig. 8-83). I routinely recommend that open surgery be performed when repeat dislocation occurs after arthroscopic staple capsulorrhaphy.

Reoperation. A review of my series shows that reoperation was performed for persistent instability in 21%.

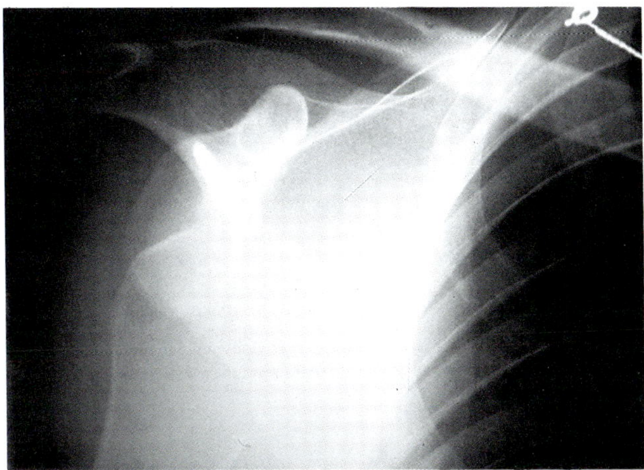

FIG. 8-83 X-ray film shows repeat dislocation after staple placement. The properly placed staple is superior on the glenoid and will not impinge on the dislocated humeral head.

Twenty-six of my patients had a subsequent open surgery by another surgeon; 4 patients had an open reconstruction performed by me. Eighteen patients with recurrence choose a repeat arthroscopic stapling capsulorrhaphy that I performed. One patient had another arthroscopic procedure by another doctor.

In sum, 11% of the patients with shoulder reconstructions had an open procedure by another surgeon; 2% had an open procedure performed by me. I performed 10% reoperations by arthroscopy; 0.4% had arthroscopic repeat reconstruction by another physician.

Of the 18 patients who had subsequent arthroscopic surgery by me, 6 continued to have shoulder problems while 9 patients said they had no problems. Two went on to subsequent open surgery. Three did not reply to the questionnaire or telephone attempts to contact. Three patients in whom I performed elective metal staple removal had subsequent surgery.

My reoperation rate is too high. The main reason is an unselected patient group. Other reasons are that I missed multidirectional instabilities. I performed the operation on patients who had sulcus signs. Both groups I now consider to be better treated by open capsular shift. I gave no consideration to the status of labrum or glenohumeral ligament integrity. Some of the reoperations were due to the presence of a metal staple near the joint. This implant problem can be corrected by bioabsorbable material.

Subscapularis Tendon Grafting

In 1983 I recognized that some patients had decompensated capsular ligamentous tissue, and I first used the superior slip of the subscapularis tendon to substitute for poor ligamentous tissue. As with most arthroscopic procedures, the use of the subscapularis tendon graft had previously been reported by open surgery. Neer[71] has suggested using a portion of this tendon as a substitute for capsular tissue in selected cases.

I recently reviewed the videotapes of the surgical procedures that used the subscapularis tendon in the repair. These cases had an absence of the labrum and middle glenohumeral ligament resulting in an enlarged subscapularis bursal space and easily visualized subscapularis tendon. Often the inferior glenohumeral ligaments were absent down to the inferior glenoid and were contracted. In this circumstance no other tissue was present to create an anterior butyrous to the joint. I then used the superior tendon slip of the subscapularis tendon as a support or substitute for compromised or absent capsular ligaments.

The anatomical structure of the musculotendinous junction lends itself to this alternative (Fig. 8-84). The subscapularis muscle comes off the underside of the scapula. As it approaches the humeral neck, several tendinous slips arise to compose the broad-based junction with the humerus. The superior slip is intraarticular. It attaches to the humerus, but not to the scapula. The slip can be mobilized from the subscapularis muscle and transferred to the underside of the scapula near the glenoid neck.

The surgical procedure isolates the superior slip of the subscapularis by capturing this tendon in the crotch of the staple (Fig. 8-85). Manipulation with the implantation device mobilizes the tendon. Further manipulation moves this slip to the anterior surface of the scapula, near the glenoid neck. No attempt is made to completely separate the tendon from the muscle. If thinned capsular ligaments are

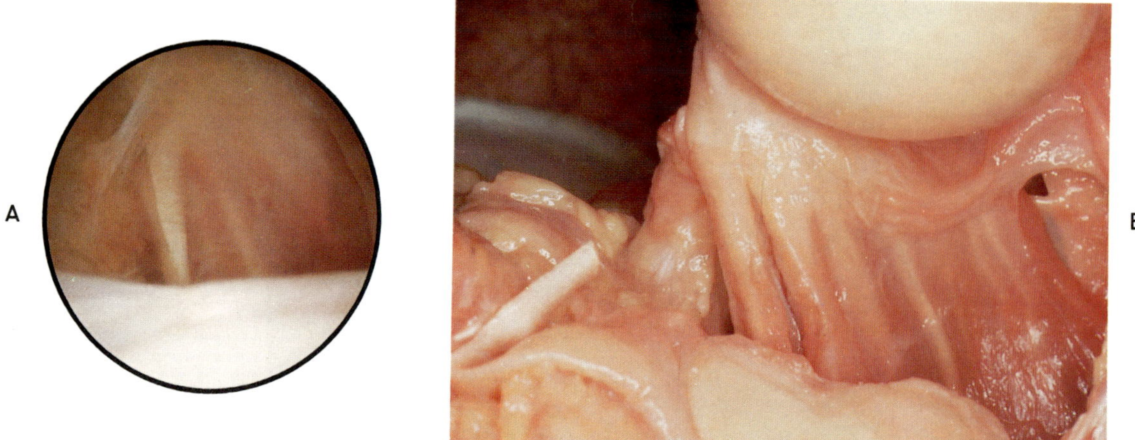

FIG. 8-84 Absence of glenohumeral ligaments requires repair to include superior tendon slip of subscapularis tendon.

A Arthroscopic view of subscapularis muscle-tendon junction in absence of glenohumeral ligaments.

B Gross dissection of subscapularis muscle-tendon junction correlates with arthroscopic photograph.

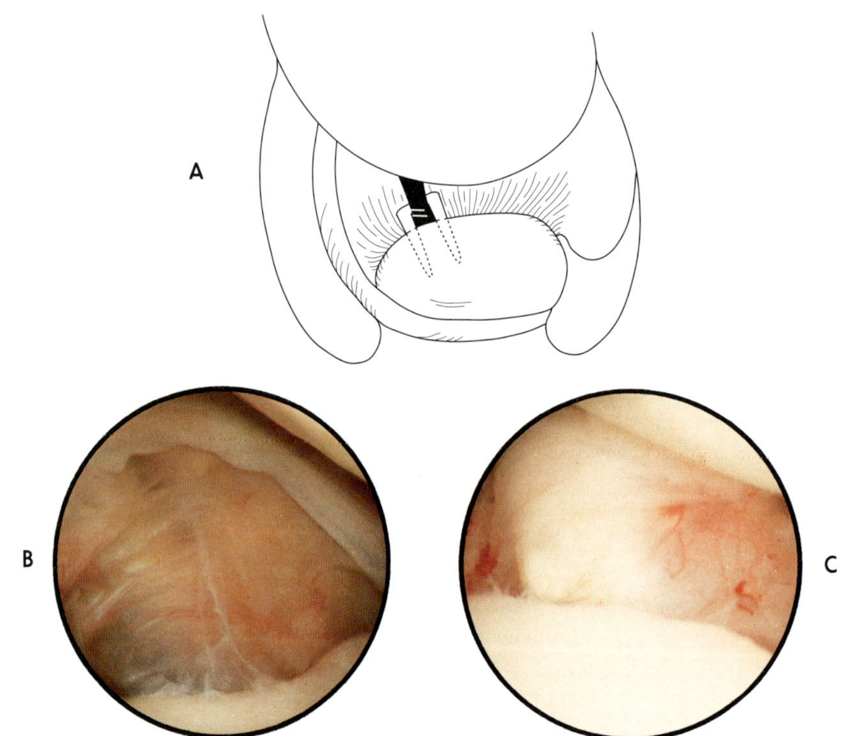

FIG. 8-85 Arthroscopic repair in absence of glenohumeral ligaments.

A Drawing of horizontal placement of staple in superior tendon slip.

B Arthroscopic view in patient with absence of glenohumeral ligaments.

C Immediate postoperative view of superior tendon slip of subscapularis attached to glenoid.

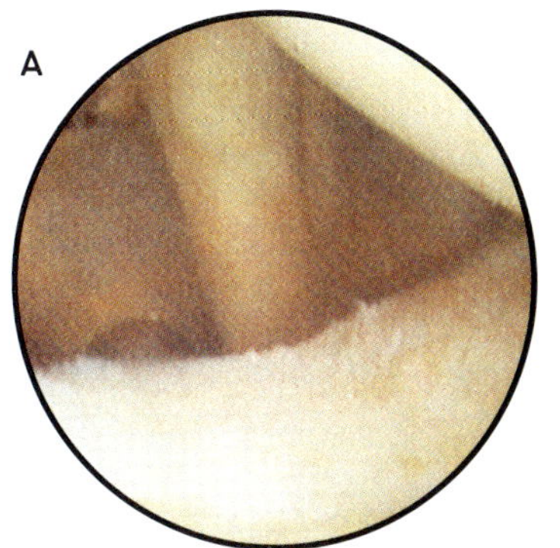

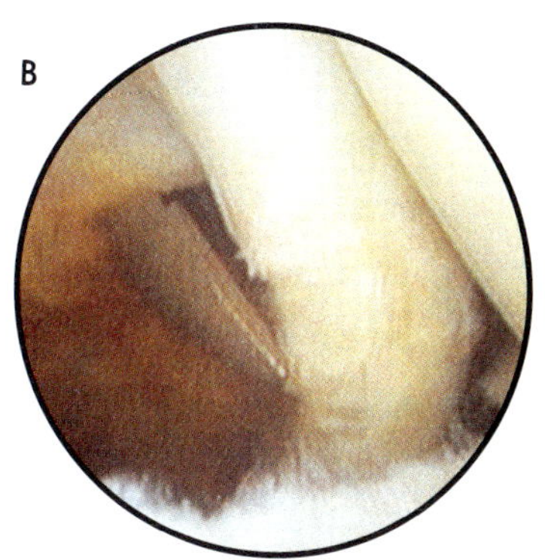

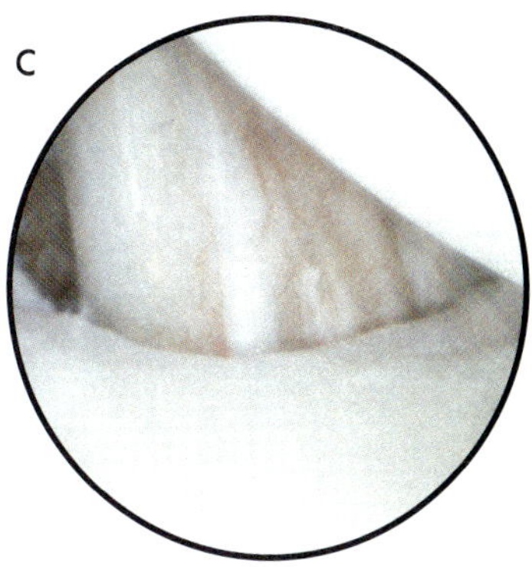

FIG. 8-86 Subscapularis tendon augmentation.

A Arthroscopic view shows thin tissue in front of the subscapularis and no ligament to reattach.

B This view shows the staple grasping the superior aspect of the tendon and moving it toward the glenoid for transfer.

C Arthroscopic second look after healing of subscapularis grafting substitute for glenohumeral ligaments.

present, then they are included with the staple or by pulling into place with a grasper from above (Fig. 8-86).

Subscapularis tendon grafting has been performed on 20 occasions:

YEAR	NUMBER OF CASES
1982	0
1983	1
1984	11
1985	0
1986	1
1987	0
1988	1
1989	6
Total	20

The demographics of this group of patients showed 10 men and 10 women. The average age was 30 years (range 18 to 73 years). There were 18 Caucasians and 2 whose race was not recorded. The dominant hand was left in 4 and right in 16. The dominant extremity was involved with the dislocation in 10 of the 20.

A second look showed a prominent vertical anterior wall of the anterior butyrous (Fig. 8-86, *C*).

The average number of prior dislocations was six. The average time from first dislocation to surgery was 4 years. Two patients had had previous surgery; one had closed manipulation, the other had a Bristow procedure.

Arthroscopic findings on the 20 patients showed that four patients had loose bodies. Fibrosis existed in one patient, the one with previous open surgery.

Three cases showed partial rotator cuff tear on the undersurface.

Nineteen patients had an abnormal labrum. The glenohumeral ligaments were described as torn in 11 patients, recessed in 14 cases, and contracted in 9. Four showed a pathological absence of these ligaments.

The anterior glenoid sulcus was abnormal in 15 patients. The glenoid surface was normal in 12 patients and abnormal in 8, of which 6 had a degenerative surface.

The humeral head was traumatized (4) or degenerative (1) in 5 patients. The Hill-Sachs lesion was seen in 16 patients, not present in 2 and not seen in 2.

Results of subscapularis reconstruction: 18 of the 20 patients responded to minimum 2-year follow-up. Seventeen of the 18 had neither subluxation or dislocation at minimum 2-year follow-up. I reoperated on 4 of the 18 patients. Three had planned staple removal. One had reoperation because of redislocation. A repeat arthroscopic stapling was performed with good results. The average time of reoperation was 18 months. Two patients were lost to follow-up.

Critique of Various Methods of Fixation

The basic principles of the various arthroscopic procedures differ only in the method of fixation.[62] All procedures include examination under anesthesia, diagnostic arthroscopy, arthroscopic debridement, anterior glenoid abrasion, and labral/ligament mobilization as outlined previously.

The variability in arthroscopic techniques involves the method of fixation. The fixation technique influences to

COMMON DENOMINATORS OF SUCCESSFUL OUTCOME BY ANY METHOD

Patient selection
- Few dislocations
- Recent onset

Integrity of Labrum and Ligament Maintained Together
- Type 1 and 2 Bankart lesions

Ease of Approximation of Original Anatomy
Normal Articular Surfaces
Postoperative Immobilization of Three Weeks
Postoperative Activity Modification
- Collision sports avoided

some extent the type of ligament disruption that is adaptable and the ligament mobilization.

Each of the various techniques has generated thought on this issue. Each one has advantages and some disadvantages. A critique of each will increase our learning and contribute to fundamentals of treating this disorder.

The ideal method of fixation is simple in technique and design. The technique should restrict the surgery to the area of the lesion, or in this case, the glenohumeral joint. The fixation device's configuration should provide an effective method of grasping and holding the glenohumeral ligament and/or labral tissue. It should provide for firm and continued approximation of the ligaments/labrum to bone. It should be strong enough not to break during insertion, shaped in such a way as to maintain fixation and durable enough to outlast the biological repair. Neither the technique nor the device should be potentially injurious to the patient.

The No Internal Fixation Technique

Description. The idea of performing the operation without the use of internal fixation is intriguing. Such an approach simplifies the technique and removes any potential complication of fixation of any type. At its foundation is the recognition that redislocation incidence has been minimized by exercise programs only.[6,23] Also, arthroscopic observations show the approximation of glenohumeral ligaments with joint decompression.

Incidental reports are documented in the literature. Wheeler et al[119] mention three such cases in their series, one of which recurred. Hawkins[37] reported one such case in his series, in which he was unable to achieve metallic staple fixation. No recurrence was evident at the seventh month.

Joel H. Eisenberg of Connecticut reported results of arthroscopic anterior debridement and abrasion without fixation at the 1991 ANNA annual meeting.[30] The exact classification of the lesions in his cases was not clear to me. He included recurrent dislocation and subluxing shoulders, without further identification. The cases were those with multiple "instabilities." The cases were typically young patients. The report was lacking in details of the arthroscopic diagnostic findings, especially the status of the Perthes lesion and the glenohumeral ligaments in regard to the complexity of the lesions.

The videotape that accompanied the presentation showed excision of the synovium of the subscapularis bursa. Emphasis was placed on an extensive decortication of the anterior glenoid. The patients were immobilized for 4 weeks and allowed limited motion in a sling for 2 additional weeks.

The length of follow-up averaged 18 months (range 6 to 38 months). Eisenberg's results showed a 95 point average on the Rowe 100 Point Rating System (see Table 8-3). One recurrence with significant trauma was reported.

Common denominators. Although Eisenberg's report was lacking in some detail and time of follow-up, it did include some important common denominators.

Extensive abrasion of glenoid. The arthroscopic debridement of the anterior soft tissues was more extensive than I have performed and that which I have seen on videotape presentation of other surgeons. The extensive abrasion broadens the area of attachment and produces an environment conducive to fibrosis.

Obliteration of subscapularis bursa. The subscapularis bursa was resected. Obliteration of this bursae provides reduction of space in the anterior pouch and juxtaposition of the subscapularis tendon to the anterior glenoid.

Postoperative immobilization of 1 month. The postoperative period exceeded 1 month. This period is consistent with my early observations of the necessity for greater than 3 weeks of immobilization.

Critique. Debridement, bursal resection, and immobilization without internal fixation may be adequate for first-time traumatic cases or subluxation. It is probably not treatment enough in complex tears or retracted or contracted ligaments. I doubt if it would be adequate for a pathological state without labrum or ligaments.

If this method were adequate, then all methods performed in a similar manner with the addition of internal fixation would be equally successful. They are not. This method without internal fixation is very dependent on case selection and probably not widely applicable.

Metal Staple

Description. This method was the arthroscopic adaptation of previously reported open staple capsulorrhaphy.[29,116] Stapling was the first of the arthroscopic techniques to be performed (August 1982). Many surgeons have used the procedure with success.[37,119]

Gross[34] showed a method of metal staple capsulorrhaphy with a wire staple. The device and technique were included in an article about extremity positioning. There have been no subsequent reports on this device or method.

Some surgeons have reported unsuccessful use of this means of fixation. Richardson[85] reported a 45% failure rate. Sachs et al[94] reported repeat of at least one dislocation. Matthews et al[63] reported 67% excellent to good results on the Rowe Rating Scale. Five patients underwent a repeat surgical procedure. One experienced a metal staple–related problem with excoriation of the humeral head (I assume with staple malplacement).

Common denominators. Arthroscopic metal staple capsulorrhaphy includes all the common denomimators listed previously. The device configuration is ideal for arthroscopic placement, grasping, and holding the labral/ligamentous complex for reattachment. During the development of this procedure I introduced the concept of glenoid abrasion. Next was the observation that the failure rate increased with less than 3 weeks immobilization. I reported the higher failure rate in collision athletes. As the technique evolved, the mobilization of the labral/ligamentous complex was introduced with the capsular shift concept.

Critique. The metallic material of the staple is its sole disadvantage. Improperly placed metal is a legitimate concern.[125] Its main disadvantage for many surgeons is the medical-legal risk incurred when an x-ray film is taken by another surgeon who is unfriendly to the original surgeon and/or the procedure. Many surgeons have abandoned the metal staple method because of x-ray film identification. This "fault" in material results in a passive restraint for those who are technically unable to safely perform the procedure. They have switched to a fixation device that does not show on plain film x-rays. The procedure is still popular with surgeons who have the technical ability to properly insert the staple.

A high percentage of my patients report pain at two-year follow-up.

Another problem is that the use of metal requires a planned or unplanned removal. Fifty-three of 225 patients underwent staple(s) removal by me. Seventeen of the 53 patients had staple(s) removed at time or repeat surgery. Three additional patients had staple removal by another surgeon and subsequent open reconstruction. Thirty-five of the entire group had only staple removal and no subsequent surgery.

The configuration of the staple device is ideal for grasping tissue and fixation into decorticated anterior glenoid. Introduction of a bioabsorbable staple will refocus attention to the original method (see Chapters 3 and 11).

Metal Rivet (Wiley)

Description. Wiley[121] developed a metallic rivet with a protruding stem. This method requires a planned removal by second procedure in all patients. This method never gained popularity.

Common denominators. These were never clearly listed.

Critique. The device had a protruding spike that required planned removal, which was the purpose of the spike. Furthermore, the device was metallic.

Fascial Allograft (Caspari)

Description. This was an adaptation of the open surgical method of Gallie.[17,60] Richard Caspari was the first to report this adaptation to arthroscopic surgery. Garret J. Lynch[59] reported 16 patients with this same operation in "anterior recurrent instability." He reported prevention of recurrence in 85% of patients followed for a mean of 37 months.

Common denominators. The debridement and glenoid abrasion was reported as part of the procedure. The graft provided a thick anterior tissue butyrous.

Critique. The expense and biocompatibilty issue of allografts is unnecessary. The operation was not limited to the shoulder joint. In fact, it was accompanied by open incision at least 1 inch in length –hardly an arthroscopic procedure. Drill holes through the glenoid and into the humerus were necessary for fixation. The procedure was technically difficult.

The fascial allograft method of Caspari has been abandoned by everyone, including Dr. Caspari.

Metal Screw and Washer (Wolf)

Description. It was thought that a screw and washer would be a better means of fixation. Such a system was introduced by several companies and popularized by Eugene Wolf.[122,123]

Common denominators. The basic common denominators were included.

Critique. The procedure was technically difficult. Tissue wrapped up on the screw during insertion. The drill hole through the scapula placed the suprascapular nerve at risk if the surgeon drilled too deep.

The screw and washer method has been abandoned.

Suture Techniques

Morgan

Description. Morgan[67,68] introduced an arthroscopic adaptation of the open transscapular suture method of Luckey-Viek-Reider. He proposed that two Beaff needles could be passed anterior to posterior on the scapular glenoid with multiple knots tied anterior and posterior for fixation. The recurrence rate was 1.5% on non-collision athletes and 16% on collision athletes. No complications were directly related to the surgery. The potential of injury to the suprascapular nerve was avoided by an oblique inferior course of the needle placement. His second series has a

5.8% recurrence rate. Morgan originally reported a very low recurrence rate and results with normal restoration of motion. The paper did not record any range of motion measurement, however, nor was this included in the method of assessment.

A recent communication from Dr. Morgan (June 17, 1991) brings his present series up to date. He used the Rowe system of grading. He had 161 original cases with 1- to 6-year follow-up. The failure rate was 5.2% in the entire group. These patients' problems included both subluxation and dislocation (without an indication of numbers in each group).

His experience with 42 collision athletes is similar to what I reported several years ago. His recurrence rate in the collision athlete population is 16.7%. In other words, 7 of the 9 failures in his entire group of 161 patients were in the collision athlete. He was kind enough to supply his personal recurrence rate for collision athletes treated by open reconstruction. It was not much different: 15% in the years before he started arthroscopic repairs.

Common denominators. Most common denominators are present. There is no emphasis on ligament mobilization; this may be due to case selection, which were simple detachments and did not require such. Internal fixation is with suture.

Critique. It appears that case selection was excellent. This is only a point of criticism because more complex labral/ligamentous injuries are not suitable for this method. The drilling of Kirschner wire through the scapula carries a potential risk. The suture material cannot be maximally secured and has a shorter life in the joint than more permanent materials. It has turned out that this method is no better in collision athletes.

Caspari (suture method)

Description. The Caspari suture technique included many common denominators. The surgical suture punch instrument allows multiple placement of sutures in order to gather the capsule. This is an advantage. A ¼-inch diameter drill hole is placed through the scapular neck and out posterior. The sutures are gathered together and taken through the drill hole from anterior to posterior. The multiple sutures are tied over the infraspinatus muscle.

Common denominators. This technique has all common denominators.

Critique. The multiple instrument passages and organization of the many sutures, plus fluid leakage out of the large cannula, are technically challenging. Recently the developer of this procedure has demonstrated the technical difficulties at continuing education courses. The knot tied over the posterior infraspinatus muscle belly cannot remain tight. There will be either necrosis of the muscle or a resultant loose fixation. Caspari has reported one synovial cyst in the area of the drill hole that required open surgical correction.

The transcutaneous ¼-inch drill hole is potentially injurious to the suprascapular nerve, even be it its branches. Although complete disruption has not been reported, I suspect injury to the branches could be common with some of these techniques. Partial injury could go unnoticed. I await CAT scan or MRI reports on focal infraspinatus muscle atrophy in patients treated by this method.

Maki/Wolf/Barrett

Description. Neil Maki of Thibodaux, Louisiana, has introduced several modifications of the suture techniques. Eugene Wolf of San Francisco and Ed Barrett of North Carolina also developed these technique concepts.[61] One method ties the knots posteriorly on the posterior glenoid, followed by anterior knot tying (Fig. 8-87). A second technique places a loop anterior and ties the knot over posterior glenoid (Fig. 8-87).

When we are discussing arthroscopic methods, we think in terms of short length incisions, but the depth of the incision is the same as in open surgery. If an arthroscopic method requires a 2- to 3-inch incision on the back of the shoulder to tie suture to bone, then I call that anterior arthroscopy and posterior open surgery. This incision is just about as long as if open surgery were done from anterior. It is hard to see an incision on one's own back, so maybe "out of sight, out of mind."

Common denominators. This method has all the common denominators, plus 4 weeks of immobilization.

Critique. The Maki method removes the potentially hazardous procedure of drilling through the scapula. It also removes the potential laxity of tying posterior over muscle or the technically difficult tying on the back of the scapula or glenoid neck.

Richmond

Description. Richmond et al[86] reported the use of Mitek metal sutures and intraarticular knot typing. He argues for simplification of the suture technique. This has the advantage of surgery being limited to the joint. Multiple points of fixation are possible. The knot is tied anterior. He reported 94% excellent to good results on the Rowe Rating Scale (see Table 8-3).

Common denominators. The common denominators of success are present in this method. The metal device should produce secure fixation of sutured labral/ligamentous complex to bone.

Critique. Although the Mitek metallic device is small and completely buried into bone, this procedure returns to the original objection of metal placed around a joint. Tying of intraarticular knots presents some technical difficulty.

The case numbers are small (17) and the follow-up is short (minimum 1 year).

These disadvantages, added to the technical difficulty, will make this method obsolete when bioabsorbable implantation devices are available.

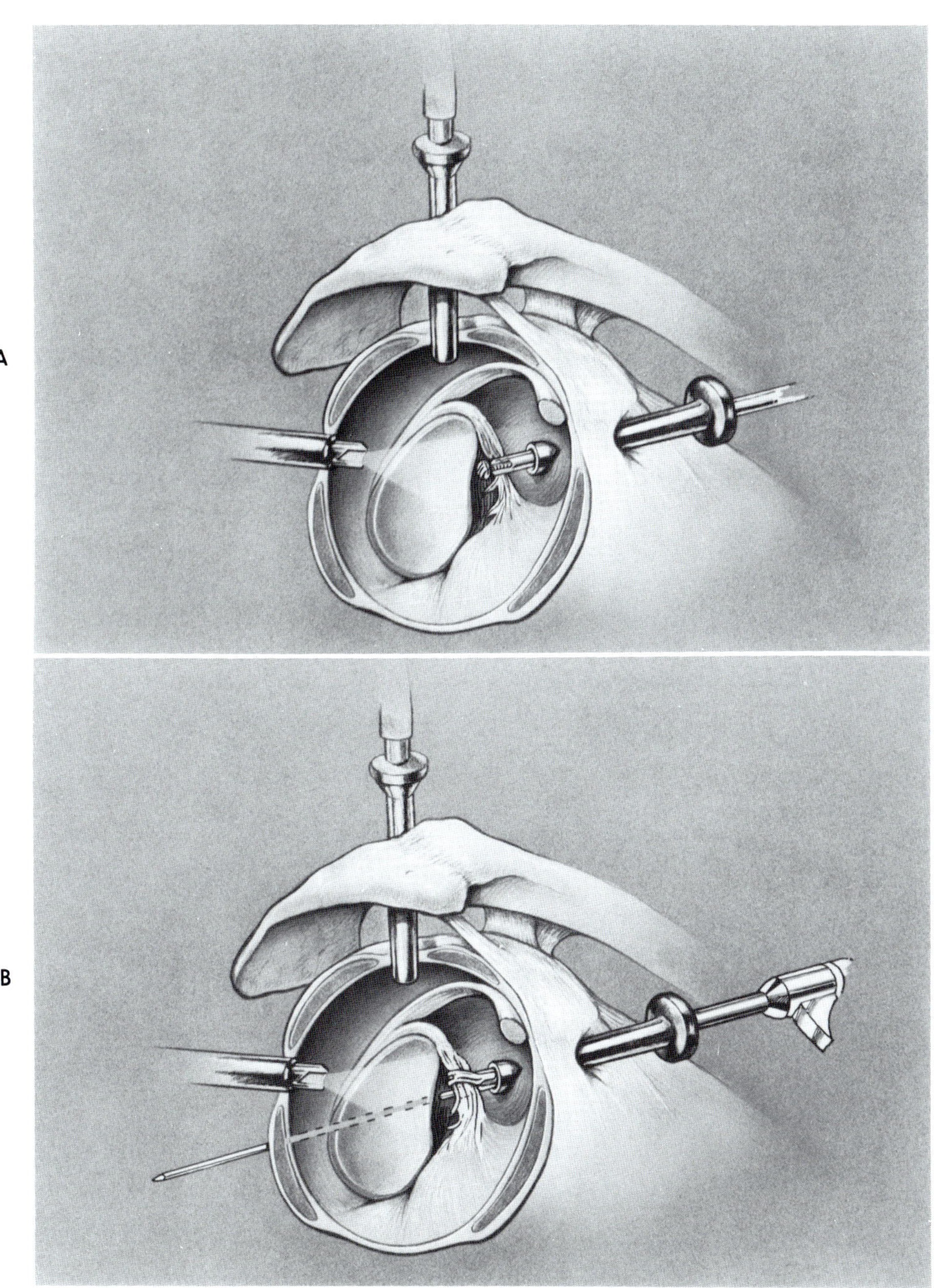

FIG. 8-87 Suture method (courtesy Neil J. Maki, Thibodaux, Louisiana).
A Abrasion and debridement.
B Suture pin and tissue grasper.

Continued.

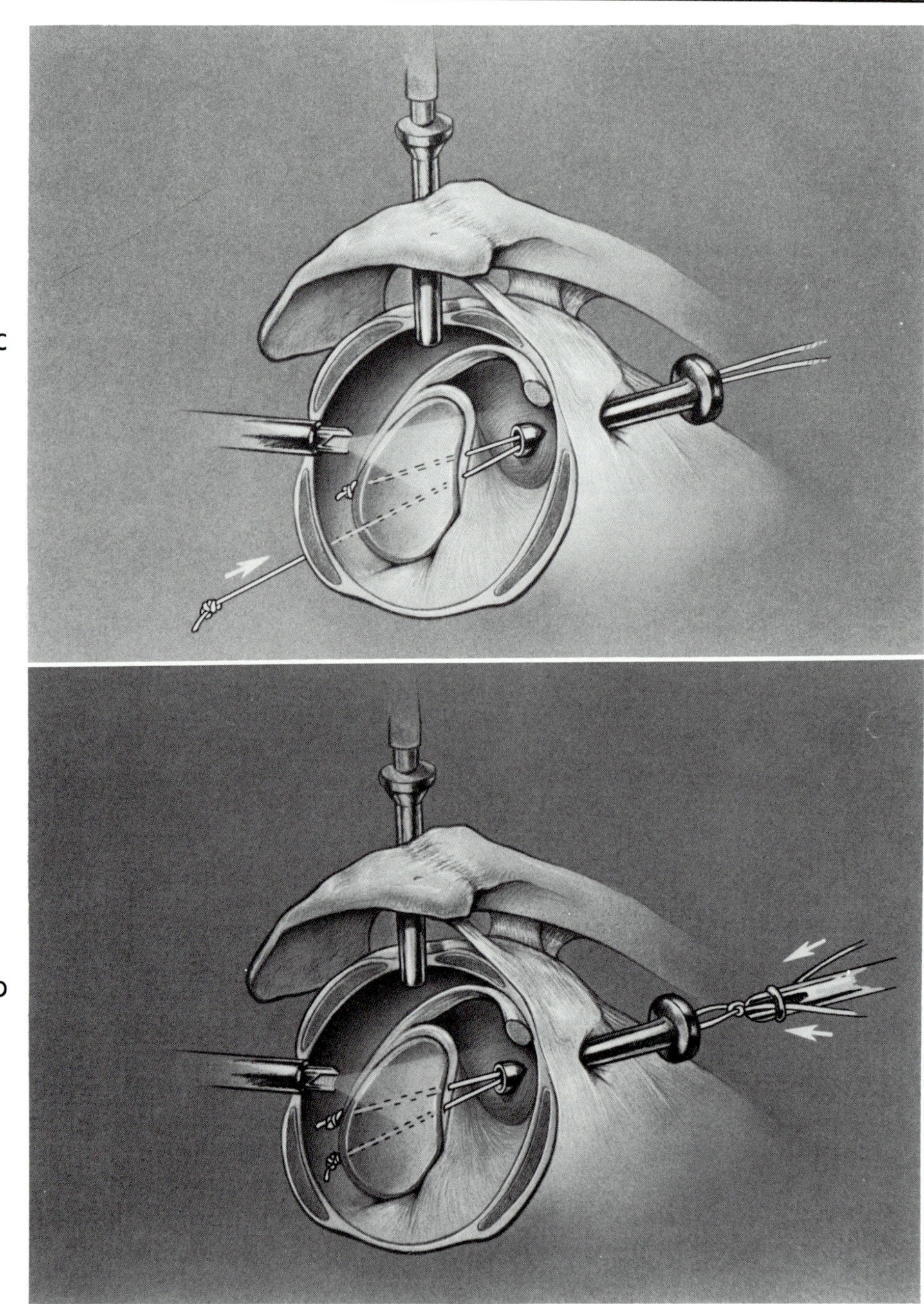

FIG. 8-87 *cont'd.* **Suture method.**

C **Mullbuerry Knots tied posteriorly.**

D **Knot outside cannula with knot pusher.**

Continued.

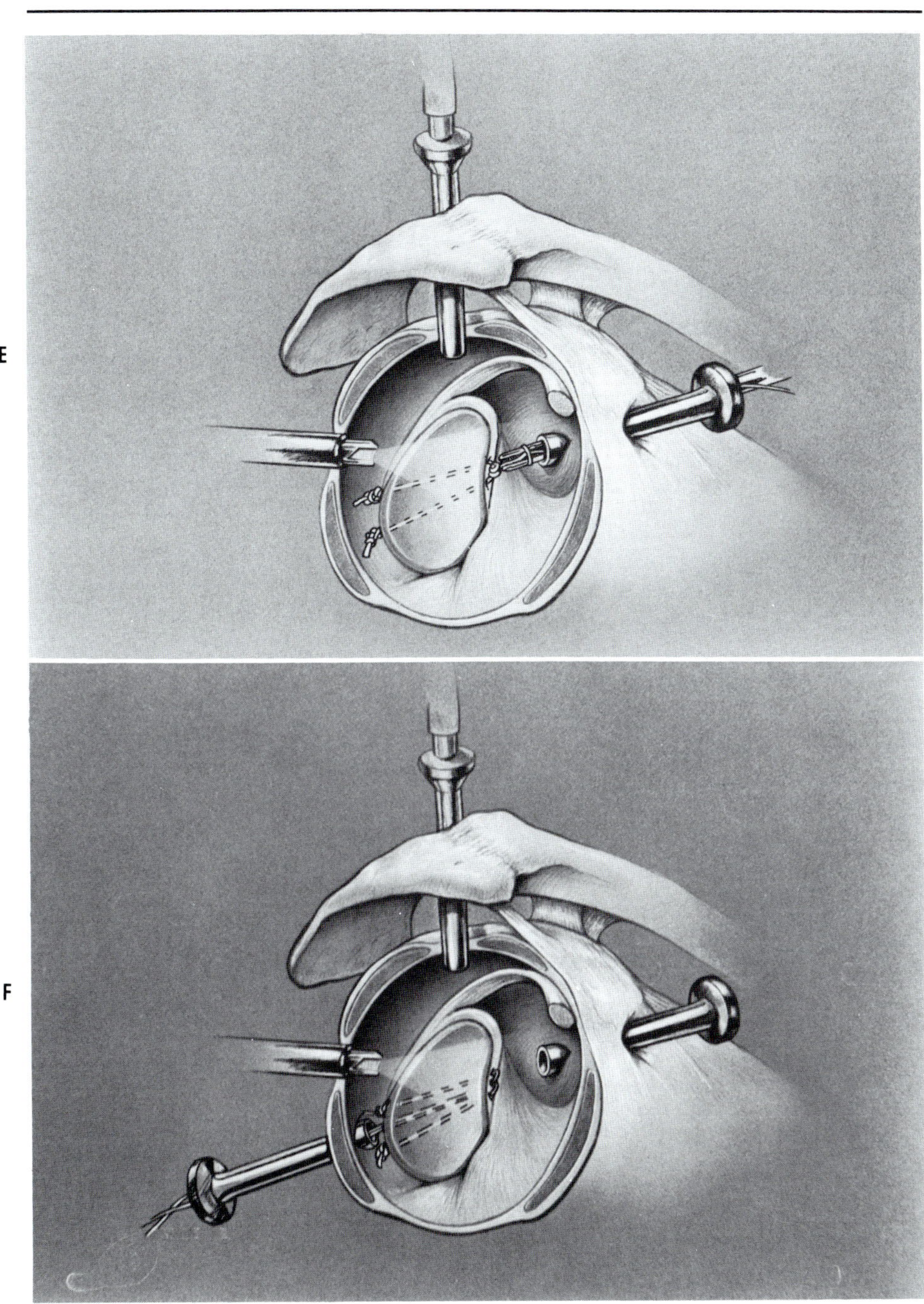

FIG. 8-87 *cont'd.* **Suture method.**

E Knot tied anteriorly.

F Sutures passed posteriorly (alternative).

Continued.

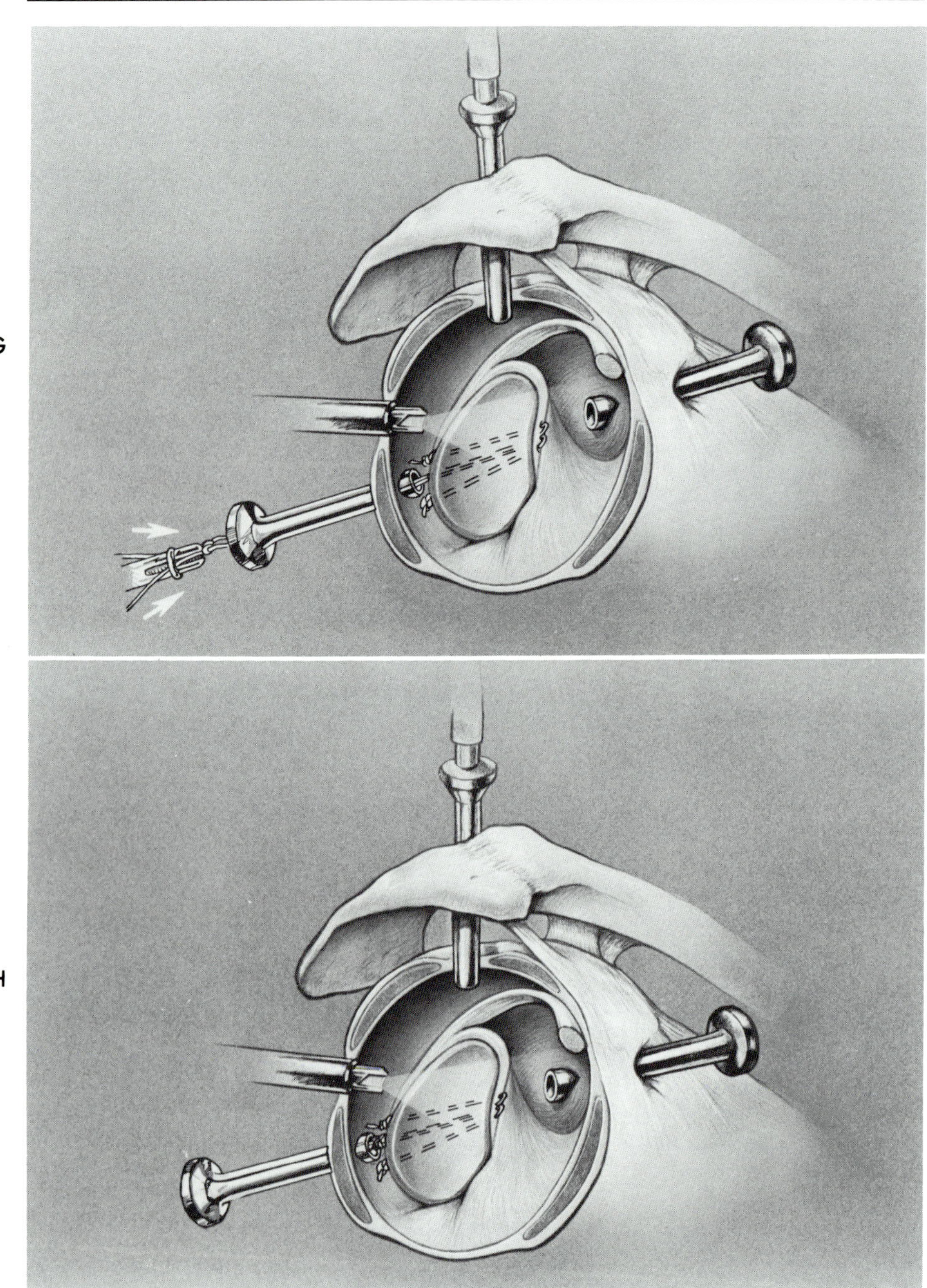

FIG. 8-87 *cont'd.* **Suture method.**

G Knot advanced posteriorly.

H Knot tied posteriorly.

Bioabsorbable Devices

Description. The first report on the use of biodegradable fixation device was at the 1991 annual meeting of the American Academy of Orthopedic Surgeons. The authors were Jon J.P Warner, Michael Pagnani, Russell F. Warren, John Cavanaugh, and William Montgomery.[116]

They used a cannulated cylindrical device with a head and series of circumferential protruding ribs down the shaft. The material was polygluconate (this is the same material as Dexon) and is completely reabsorbed in 6 weeks. Its effective mechanical holding strength was not mentioned. The immobilization period was 4 weeks. Twenty-three patients were available with a minimum of 2 years of follow-up.

Several different diagnoses were included in their series. Nineteen patients had anterior instability, without definition of dislocation or subluxation. This eliminated patients with inferior instability as a component of the anterior problem. The results of this group were 8 excellent; 8 good; 2 fair; and 1 poor. They presented two cases of anterior subluxation; both had postoperative pain, one had restriction of motion.

Common denominators. The common denominators can be instituted by this method.

Critique. The design of the device is cylindrical and cannulated, with transverse fins and a head for holding tissue. The design is not ideal in my opinion. The technique for this design requires transcutaneous Kirschner wire placement. The device shape does not grasp tissue well. The holding potential is limited to the circular head, which is not much larger than the cylindral shaft. If tissue tearing occurred during insertion of the shaft, then the capsule would not be held by a slightly larger diameter head.

The design does not provide an effective method of capturing labrum as with a staple. Hence this device must pierce the small labrum, resulting in tissue tearing during reattachment.

The material of polygluconate is very short lasting, especially so in the fluid medium of the joint. I doubt if the device had effective longevity in the joint;[10] no evidence is given to that point. It should be noted that these investigators have subsequently changed the device material to longer lasting polylactate. Their early experience with the longer lasting material has presented problems with fragmentation of the more brittle plastic. This has resulted in separation of the device head and the symptomatic patient requiring a second operation to remove the loose body.

OPEN VS ARTHROSCOPIC SURGERY

The issue is not open versus arthroscopic surgery. It is not just one or the other. It is not an either/or decision. The decision concerning the method of treatment is based on patient history, patient selection, physical and x-ray examination, MRI, examination of the other shoulder, family history, arthroscopic findings and status of ligaments.[100]

The arthroscopic approach can *not* do some things at this time.

Advantages of open reconstructive surgery.

1. Imbrication of capsule.
   - A. Surgical exposure adequate to develop two capsular flaps.
   - B. Decreases anterior joint volume by imbrication alone.
   - C. Shifts capsule extensively, effectively, and accurately.
2. Augmentation of repair.
   - A. Possible with broad expanse of subscapular tendon, as with Neer open method.
   - B. Fibrosis produced at every layer of dissection: capsule to skin.
3. Advancement or tightening of connective tissue layers, including subscapularis tendon insertion at time of closure.

Open repair does have some disadvantages.

Disadvantages of open reconstructive surgery

1. Conventional suture placement penetrates ¼ inch onto articular surface of the glenoid.
2. If sutures are replaced on anterior glenoid by a Mitek device, then metal is next to joint.
   - A. Problem with any future surgery for removal.
   - B. Interferes with future MRI evaluation.

Arthroscopy has some benefits in glenohumeral problems.

Advantages of arthroscopy

1. Diagnosis.
   - A. Identifying lesions.
   - B. Visualizing all compartments.
   - C. Evaluating articular surfaces for prognosis.
2. Debridement potential.
   - A. Accurate and minimal.
   - B. Tears, loose bodies, vacuuming/lavage mobility.
3. Important role in selection of method of treatment.
   - A. Arthroscopic/open approach.
   - B. Sites of lesions.
   - C. Magnitude of lesions.
   - D. Simulate repair with apposition of tissue and shoulder pulled into reduced position posterior.
4. Minimal invasion/decreased morbidity.
5. Cosmetic.
6. Outpatient surgery possible.
7. Potential for reduced cost.

On some factors, the two methods are basically equal.

Comparable benefits of open and arthroscopic surgeries

1. Cosmesis: The anterior axillary incision of open surgery is cosmetically acceptable (Fig. 8-88).
2. Rehabilitation time might be started sooner in open surgery.
3. Time to heal tissues is same in each.
4. Time to resuming sports is the same and is dependent on healing.

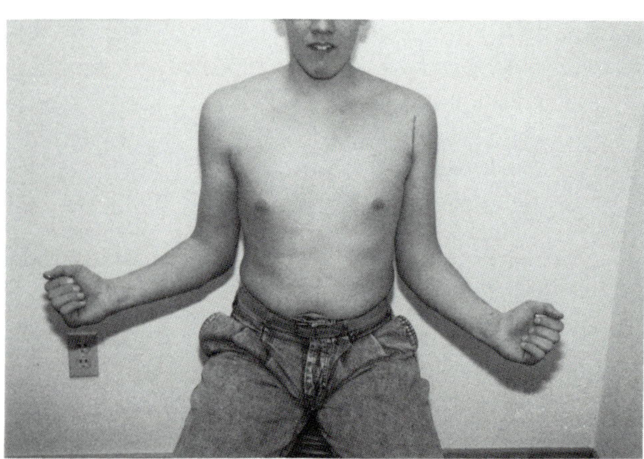

FIG. 8-88 Open surgical incision may be cosmetically pleasing as well.

5. Hospitalization is required for some of the arthroscopic cases. Next-day discharge is standard for my open reconstructions.
6. The surgical objective is to restore the labrum, to restore the continuity of the glenohumeral ligaments while obliterating the anterior pouch. Both methods may be used to achieve this end.

To think "one size fits all" is a mistake. Equally wrong is to think *only* arthroscopy, just as it would be to think *only* open surgery.

Even today after 10 years, the arthroscopic approach to the shoulder is just the beginning, not the end of this application.

Critique of Reported Open and Arthroscopic Results

To date, reports of results of these types of surgery have been confused by the use of the word instability. Most series combine dislocations and subluxations without regard to definition or result of each group. If the preoperative condition were "instability," then the postoperative measurement of result would be a failure if the patient had any symptom or sign of "instability." If the diagnosis were subluxation, then any repeat episode of subluxation would be a failure, as would a subsequent frank dislocation. If the preoperative condition were dislocation of the glenohumeral joint then the results should be evaluated on the recurrence of frank dislocation. A symptom of "instability" or "subluxation" would be a less-than-optimal result when treating dislocation.

The direction of the instability should be reported separately. I realize that case numbers may be small, but similar standards of preoperative and postoperative assessment allow combining of various surgeons' case experience. At present that is not possible, we are always comparing "apples and oranges". Presently, the American Shoulder and Elbow Society is establishing a minimum standard for patient assessment (see Appendix B). This is a positive initiative.

The benchmark condition should be better described in terms of the number or dislocations, and the duration of the condition is important in describing chronicity.

The attention to range of motion evaluations has been usually without measurement, but reported as normal.[68] Careful analysis of the labrum and ligamentous status is not clear. The results or recurrences confuse instability and frank dislocations. A rating system may combine the two factors (Table 8-3).[89,90]

I would make the following suggestions for minimal standards of reporting.

1. Dislocations and subluxations should be defined. Separate findings and results should be reported for each group.
2. The primary treatment objective is to eliminate the dislocations. To eliminate "fudging" on results, any instability episode is the common denominator of failure.
3. The magnitude and frequency can be further clarified.
4. The patient's modification of activity can reduce the incidence of dislocation, so an attempt should be made to qualify this factor.
5. Since most recurrences occur within the first 2 years, a minimum follow-up of 2 years seems proper.
6. Other conditions such as pain are important and should be compared to the operative incidence of degenerative arthritis or articular traumatic lesions. Comparison to previous rating scales like that of Rowe provides only a rough comparison of one series to another, but is some measure with the past.
7. Preoperative range of motion should be measured at both clinical presentation and with the patient under anesthesia for postoperative comparisons.

Arthroscopy Combined with Open Procedures

Arthroscopy can be easily combined with open procedures. Arthroscopy is performed with minimal puncture wounds that do not encroach any subsequent open incision. Arthroscopic diagnostic exposure cannot be duplicated by open surgical inspection. Once the joint is opened, normal anatomical relationships are distorted. The visualization by open surgery is less than by arthroscopy and its inherent magnification. A variety of intraarticular lesions are amenable to arthroscopic debridement that otherwise would not be seen or appreciated by open technique, let alone be removed.

Arthroscopic Facilitating Techniques. Certain preparatory procedures can be performed by arthroscopy that

Table 8-3 Rating Sheet for Bankart Repair

Scoring system	Units	Excellent	Good	Fair	Poor
Stability					
No recurrence, subluxation, or apprehension	50	No recurrences	No recurrences	No recurrences	Recurrence of dislocation
Apprehension when placing arm in certain positions	30	No apprehension when placing arm in complete elevation and external rotation	Mild apprehension when placing arm in elevation and external rotation	Moderate apprehension during elevation and external rotation	Marked apprehension during elevation or extension
Subluxation (not requiring reduction)	10	No subluxations	No subluxations	No subluxations	
Recurrent dislocation	0				
Motion					
100% of normal external rotation, internal rotation, and elevation	20	100% of normal external rotation; complete elevation and internal rotation	75% of normal external rotation; complete elevation and internal rotation	50% of normal external rotation; 75% of elevation and internal rotation	No external rotation 50% of elevation (can get hand only to face) and 50% of internal rotation
75% of normal external rotation, and normal elevation and internal rotation	15				
50% of normal external rotation and 75% of normal elevation and internal rotation	10				
50% of normal elevation and internal rotation; no external rotation	5				
Function					
No limitation in work or sports; little or no discomfort	30	Performs all work and sports; no limitation in overhead activities; shoulder strong in lifting, swimming, tennis, throwing, no discomfort	Mild limitation in work and sports; shoulder strong; minimum discomfort	Moderate limitation doing overhead work and heavy lifting, unable to throw, serve hard in tennis, or swim; moderate disabling pain	Marked limitation unable to perform overhead work and lifting; cannot throw, play tennis, or swim; chronic discomfort
Mild limitation and minimum discomfort	25				
Moderate limitation and discomfort	10				
Marked limitation and pain	0				
Total units possible	100				

(From Rowe CR, Patel D, Southmayd WW: Method of results evaluation for Bankart repair of recurrent anterior dislocation of the shoulder. Reprinted from *J Bone Joint Surg* 60A (1), 1978.)

will facilitate a planned open surgical repair in the glenohumeral joint.

The routine removal of smaller loose bodies and debridement procedures for soft tissue tears and degenerative tissue should accompany all planned open glenohumeral surgery. A large loose body should be reserved for removal at open surgery.

An arthroscopic assessement is made of the labral/ligamentous complex for integrity and mobility. A preliminary incision may be made in the labrum or ligaments at the position of the anticipated site for open surgery. If a resection of labrum or ligamentous tissue is required, this could be performed arthroscopically. Either of these techniques would minimize the open procedure to suturing. With this method the surgeon must be careful not to create an incisional passage for extravasation of fluids, which makes an open procedure more difficult.

Glenoid labrum drill holes can be placed before opening the joint. A plain Kirschner wire can be placed transcutaneously from posterior and superior. The anterior glenoid is carefully penetrated from the posterior approach. This same angle is not possible from an open anterior exposure. This posterior drill hole on the glenoid surface may be joined by the same transcutaneous Kirshner wire technique from anterior portal. This maneuver provides a careful connecting of these holes for the ensuing open Bankart repair.

Debridement. Fragmentation of the torn anterior glenohumeral ligaments can be trimmed via arthroscopy, providing a clean smooth margin for open suturing (Fig. 8-89, *A*).

Glenoid preparation. The anterior glenoid bone can be carefully debrided and prepared via arthroscopy with better vision than is possible at the bottom of the anterior open surgical exposure.

Hemostasis. Hemostasis can be performed arthroscopically, thereby presenting a clean, dry, and surgically prepared field for the open surgery (Fig. 8-89, *B*).

Change of Patient Position. I routinely perform shoulder arthroscopy with the patient in the opposite lateral decubitus position (see Chapter 5). The upper extremity is suspended. The change of patient position for arthroscopy to open surgery is accomplished with a minimum of time and risk.

At the conclusion of the arthroscopy, the suspension apparatus is released. The hand is covered with a sterile drape. Coban is used to wrap the sterile cover in place and connect it to the existing sterile field.

The patient is secured with an Olympus Vac Pac. The valve of this holding device is released, letting air into the bag. This softening of the bag allows the patient to roll into the supine position. The bag is firmed again with application of suction to the valve. The head of the table is elevated to provide a semi-sitting position for the patient. The arm is draped free for manipulation. This positional change takes but a few minutes. The open operative position is uncompromised. Another skin antiseptic preparation is applied. Repeat draping is not necessary in most cases, and is reserved for compromise of drape during arthroscopy by tearing or contamination.

Some surgeons have advocated the beach chair position for planned combined arthroscopy and open surgery.[102,103] This position compromises the arthroscopy in several ways. The orientation for entry is difficult since the direction is not parallel to the floor. In an obese patient, the subcutaneous fat hangs down by gravity to distort and deepen the entry site. The orientation of the arthroscopic picture is anatomical, but complicated by failure to be orientated to the horizonal of the floor. Subsequent fluid leakage from the various wounds comes over the arthroscope

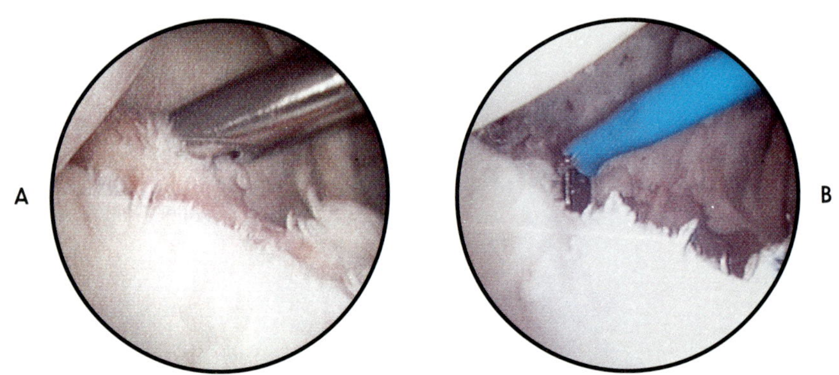

FIG. 8-89 Arthroscopic facilitating techniques (left shoulder).

A Debridement and mobilization of anterior labrum.

B Electrocautery provides subsequent hemostasis for open procedure.

by gravity. The beach chair position requires an assistant to control the arm rather than suspension.

Open Surgical Procedures after Arthroscopy. This method accounts for approximately two thirds of my cases. I perform a Bankart type of repair, often with a capsular shift, since one of my indications for a nonarthroscopic approach is an enlarged, thinned capsule that requires imbrication to increase thickness. I have used the Bristow procedure over the years without complication with the metal screw, but my patients do have a significant loss of range of external rotation. I now reserve the Bristow procedure for those patients who have loss of anterior-inferior glenoid bone caused by fracture or failure of previous open surgical repairs.

In an occasional patient with a large Hill-Sachs lesion, I have combined arthroscopic capsulorrhaphy with open posterior transfer of the infraspinatus tendon into the defect. This procedure was described by Connolly.[22] The posterior shoulder approach described by Brodsy, Tullos, and Gardsman[13] is helpful for this operation.

SPECIAL SITUATIONS

Posterior Glenohumeral Instability

True posterior instabilities of the glenohumeral joint are not as common clinically as anterior instabilities.[75,118] In spite of its infrequency, the surgeon must still be alert to its existence. Often the posterior instability is a component of a multidirectional instability that is equally as important of a diagnosis.[39] The single posterior instabilities can be divided into subluxation and dislocation.

Open Surgery. Open surgical repair has high failure rates. Recently, Tibone and Ting[111] reported on 20 cases of recurrent posterior subluxation of the shoulder treated with *open* conventional staple capsulorrhaphy, with 9 unsatisfactory results. Six had recurrence of the instability. Often the posterior instability was associated with anterior instability.[112]

Arthroscopic Diagnosis. The arthroscopic presence of a posterior labrum tear is not pathognomonic of a posterior instability. This tear must be differentiated from those findings associated with anterior instability. In fact, the most common cause of this location of labrum tear is an anterior instability. The anterior instability posterior lesion is located inferior. The posterior labrum tear location associated with a posterior instability involves the superior aspect or extends superior (Fig. 8-90).

In my practice, the voluntary posterior subluxator is the most common of these entities (Fig. 8-91). I have successfully used arthroscopic debridement of the posterior labral lesion, combined with a postoperative exercise rehabilitation program (Fig. 8-92). The surgical technique uses the superior portal to approach the posterior lesion (Fig. 8-93). Another method would be to place the scope anterior and the instrument portal posterior.

Arthroscopic Treatment. If the posterior subluxation contains a traumatic component and the patient is emotionally stable, I have used posterior staple capsulorrhaphy (Fig. 8-94). The patient is held in a sling, not an external rotation orthotic device. Arthroscopic inspection shows that this position is not placing undue tension on the repair. A planned staple removal is performed at 1 month after the operation, before mobilization of the shoulder. Not as much room posteriorly for staple placement is available and the head can injure the humeral head (Fig. 8-95). Other second looks have showed good repair at the time of staple removal at 6 weeks (Fig. 8-96). The opportunity for this procedure is infrequent and its stage of use should be considered developmental.

Russ Warren reported the use of a bioabsorbable polyglycolic acid tac for treatment of posterior subluxation in three patients, with good results in two and poor in one.[116a] One patient with combined anterior and posterior instability had both areas secured with tac with good results.

Posterior Dislocation. Posterior dislocation is rare.

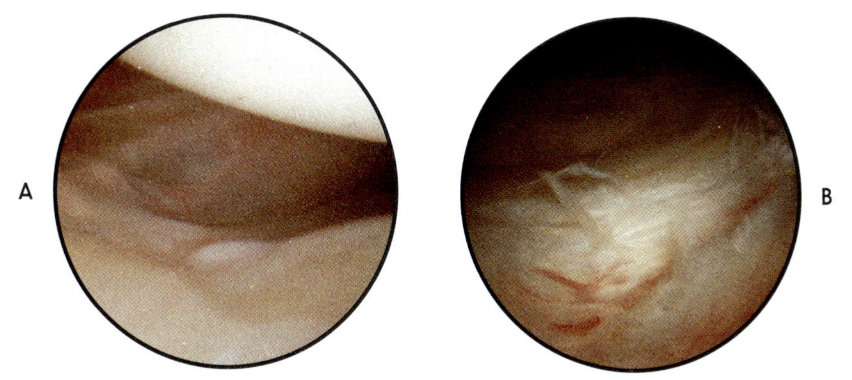

FIG. 8-90 Posterior glenohumeral instability.

A Arthroscopic view of anterior wall shows no abnormality.

B Arthroscopic view of posterior tear extending superior on glenoid.

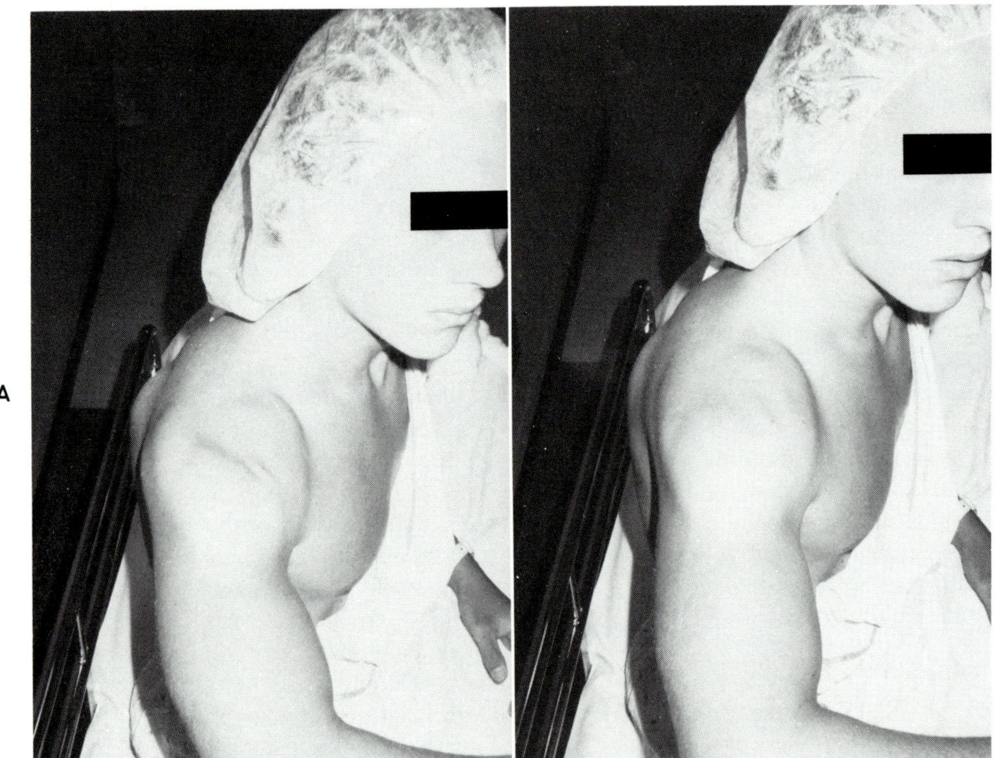

FIG. 8-91 Clinical photograph of voluntary posterior dislocator.

A Voluntary position of posterior dislocation with willful muscle contraction.

B Reduction is affected when elbow is moved posteriorly to neutral position.

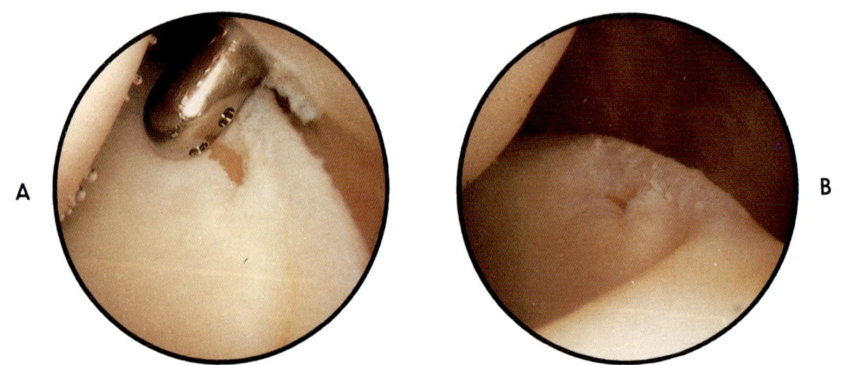

FIG. 8-92 Debridement of posterior labrum tear in voluntary posterior subluxation.

A Instrument placement is best done from superior for posterior labrum area.

B Postdebridement status shows resection into posterior wall for bony glenoid to create bleeding bed for healing.

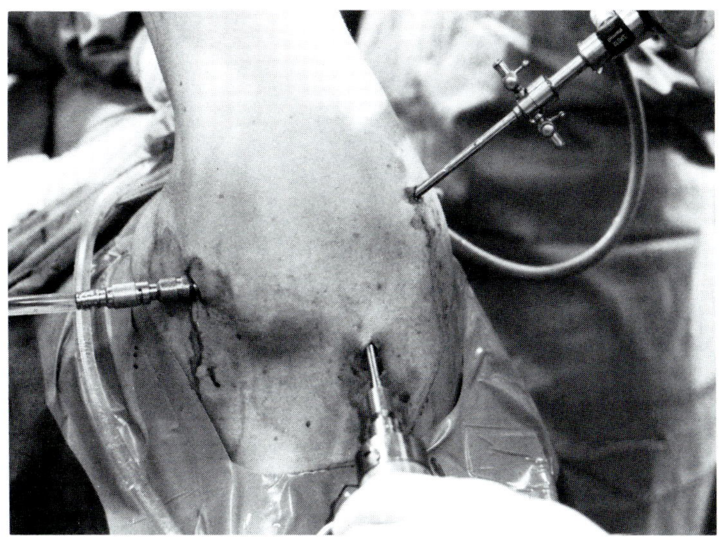

FIG. 8-93 In this case, scope is anterior and instrument superior for debridement of lesion.

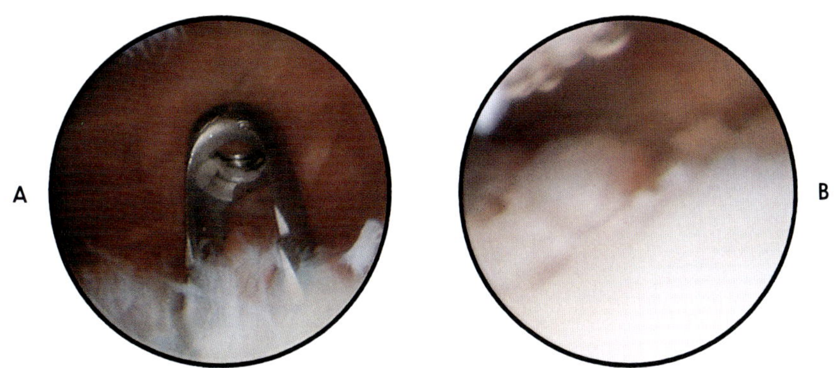

FIG. 8-94 Postoperative stapling of posterior capsule to glenoid.

A Arthroscopic view at 3 months. Staple is in bone, but no ligament or capsule is attached. It was removed.

B Fibrous tissue obliterates normal posterior sulcus after repair. Staple was removed.

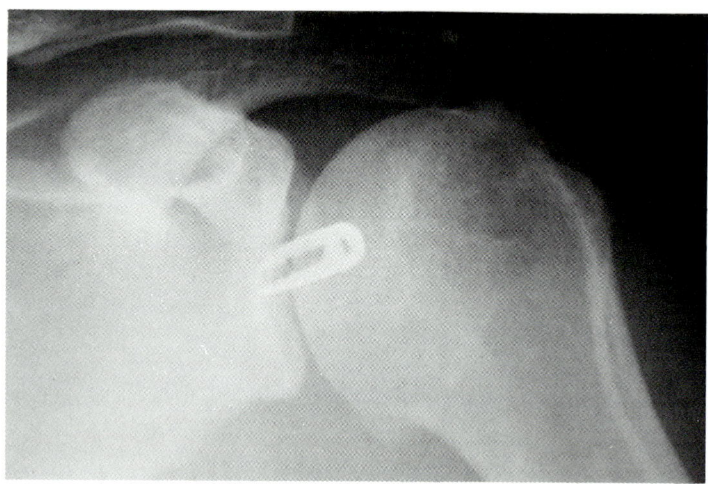

FIG. 8-95 Posterior position of staple on x-ray film. Tines are in bone.

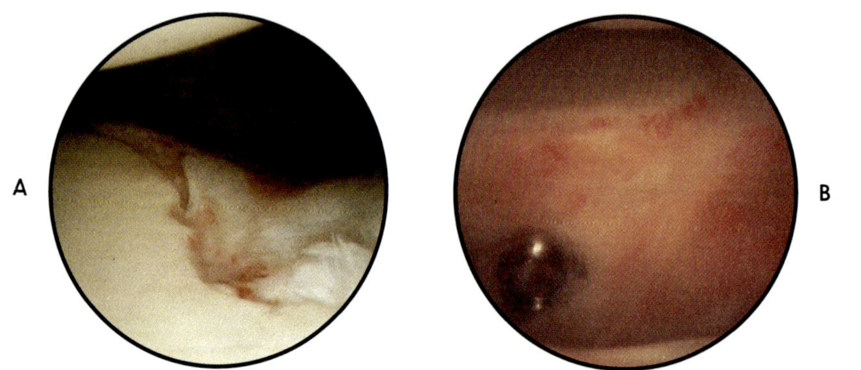

FIG. 8-96 Arthroscopic second looks at posterior repairs.
A View from anterior shows weld of ligaments into bony defect.
B View from posterior shows healing of posterior tear with staple in place.

The diagnosis is missed because of lack of clinical suspicion and failure to request a true axillary plain film x-ray (Fig. 8-97).

Because this diagnosis is often missed, the patient often presents with a fixed posterior humeral position (Fig. 8-98). The surgical treatment is open. McLaughlin described the anterior humeral head bony compression defect and the transfer of the subscapular tendon insertion into the defect as a means of treatment.[65]

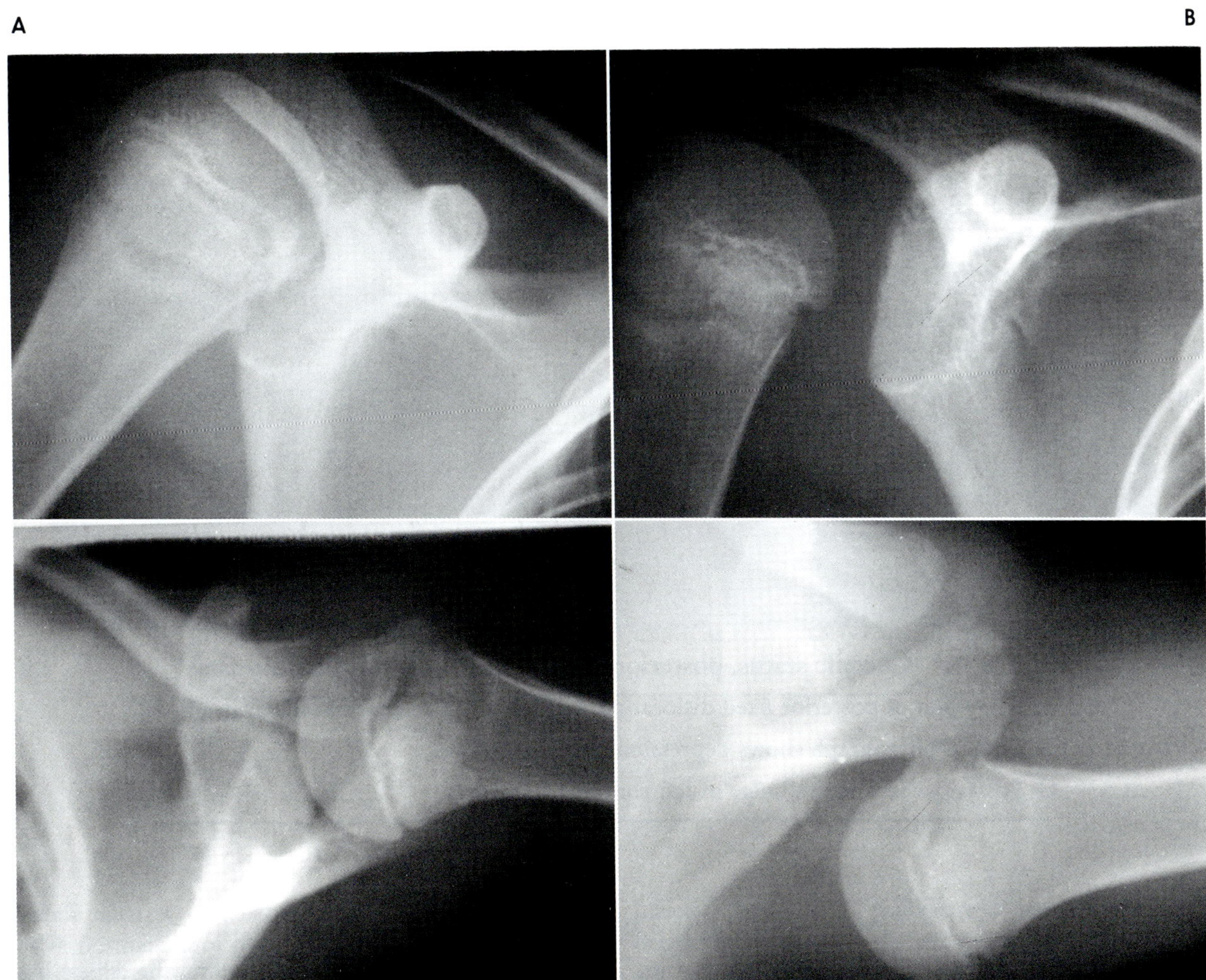

FIG. 8-97 X-ray views of posterior dislocation of shoulder.

A Anterior-posterior x-ray view shows reduced position.

B X-ray film showing dislocated position for comparison.

C Axillary view with shoulder in reduced position.

D Posterior dislocation identified in axillary x-ray film.

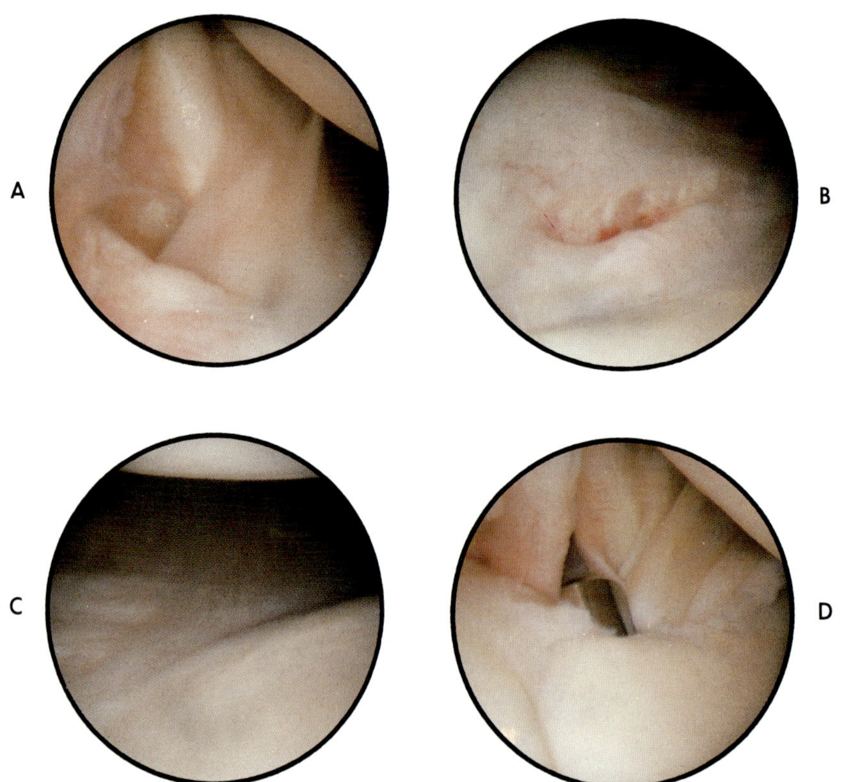

FIG. 8-100 Arthroscopic findings in subluxed shoulder.

A Intact middle glenohumeral ligaments.

B Small tear in conjoined ligaments. Blood in lesion differentiates it from normal sulcus.

C Intact inferior glenohumeral ligament.

D Postoperative repair with advancement of middle glenohumeral ligament and tear.

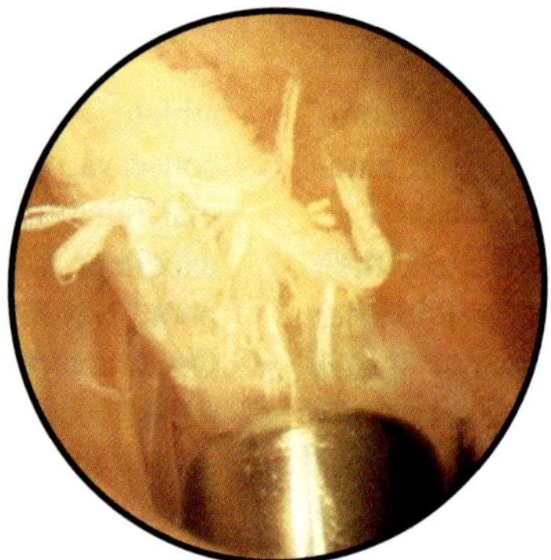

FIG. 8-101 Arthroscopic view of fraying of subscapularis tendon by the head of the staple in a throwing athlete. This is reason for prophylactic removal in this type of case, if the head is prominent or the patient experiences pain.

The Frozen Shoulder

"Frozen shoulder" or adhesive capsulitis is a common clinical problem.* This condition presents with spontaneous onset of pain in the shoulder, often without significant injury. There is pain and decreased range of motion of the glenohumeral joint.[25,70] Typically, the patient is a female over 40 years of age of sedentary lifestyle with the condition affecting the nondominant upper extremity. Pain onset is followed by a period of muscular inactivity and limb immobility. The condition often is associated with diabetes mellitus.[12] Recovery is spontaneous, even when untreated, but it may take up to 2 years.[33,113]

The etiology of adhesive capsulitis remains unknown.[25,70] A variety of structures have been implicated as the primary focus in this disorder. DuPlay,[28] who first described this condition, implicated the subacromial bursa. Pasteur,[81] Lippman,[58] and Turek[113] pointed to the biceps tendon. MacNab and Codman[60] implicated the rotator cuff. DePalma[19] singled out the fibrous capsule. Neviaser[72] suggested the axillary fold. These assumptions were largely based on cadaveric dissections, since the condition was usually self-limiting and surgical release was infrequent. Arthroscopic examination was not availablc to these investigators.

The nonoperative treatment includes use of local anesthetic, cortisone injections and physical therapy.[14,31,70,115] Brisement has also been advocated as a treatment method.[31,99] Manual manipulation under anesthesia has been reserved for failure of conservative treatment.[36,42]

Arthroscopic inspection in a frozen shoulder has been reported.[1,35,50,80,120] Diagnostic arthroscopy provides a means of intraarticular inspection not otherwise provided by noninvasive diagnostic techniques or by open surgery.[50]

Greg Uitvulgt and David Detrisac reviewed our clinical experience. Twenty patients (21 shoulders) underwent diagnostic glenohumeral joint arthroscopy prior to glenohumeral manipulation by three surgeons (Micheal D. Austin, David Detrisac, and myself) between July 7, 1976 and December 31, 1987. An immediate postmanipulation second-look arthroscopy was performed in 10 patients.

Six male and 14 female patients were studied, with an average age of 47 years (range 32 to 79 years). The average age of the female patients was 50 years, while that of the male patients was 40 years.

Thirteen left and 8 right shoulders were involved. The 21 shoulders were composed of 13 nondominant and 8 dominant limbs. Thirty percent of the patients had antecedent trauma and 70% had an insidious onset of symptoms. Of the males, 50% had a history of trauma, while only 21% of the females reported antecedent trauma. The duration of symptoms was greater than 6 months before treatment in all patients. Goniometric measurements were obtained for all patients as part of the physical examination. Preoperative plain film x-rays were also taken on all patients.

The operative procedure was performed with the patient under general anesthesia with endotracheal tube. The patient was placed in the opposite lateral decubitus position. The arm was held in abduction with skin traction and suspended by free weight countertraction of 10 to 16 pounds depending on the size of the patient. A Betadine skin preparation was applied. A sterile Johnson & Johnson plastic/paper shoulder drape was used to expose the area. The involved upper extremity was covered with sterile draping.

A posterior arthroscope portal was used.[50] Preliminary joint distention was not attempted. The skin was incised with a No. 11 blade. The arthroscope cannula and blunt obturator entered the joint in the direction of the coracoid process. Entry was confirmed by direct visualization. The joint was distended with 5 to 10 ml of normal saline. A 4.0 mm, 30-degree inclined arthroscope was used. After confirmation of entry, the joint was manually distended with fluid by maximal compression on a 60-ml syringe attached to the arthroscope spigot by a K-52 catheter. The small glenohumeral joint space, when fully distended, accommodated only 12 to 20 ml of fluid.

A systematic diagnostic arthroscopy was performed in the glenohumeral joint from the posterior portal. The anterior portal was established by placing the arthroscope against the anterior wall beneath the biceps tendon in a triangular space immediately superior to the scapularis tendon.[50] The arthroscope was removed and a semi-sharp Wissinger-type rod was passed through the cannula into subcutaneous tissue. An anterior skin incision was made over the protruding tip of the rod. The rod was advanced through the incision. A cannula was placed over the rod in a retrograde fashion before removal of the rod to establish the anterior portal for viewing, probing, or instrumentation.

The diagnostic arthroscopy was restricted to the glenohumeral joint. No arthroscopic surgery was performed. After the diagnostic arthroscopy, the arthroscope was removed and the portals were maintained using switching sticks (10 cases).

Shoulder Joint Manipulation. A closed manipulation was performed on the glenohumeral joint. This maneuver was facilitated by freeing the upper extremity from the suspension apparatus.

I perform what I call a "50% manipulation." What I mean by that is that the normal side range of motion is measured. The resultant manipulation under anesthesia on the affected side only approaches 50% of the normal side motion. This eliminates tissue tearing. Furthermore, the manipulation is performed slowly with accommodation of the tissue by stretching. The procedure is gentle, without

*12, 19, 25, 57, 70, 73

A
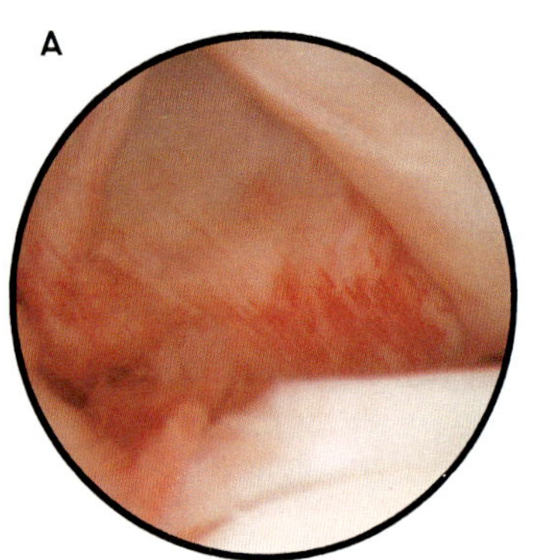
B
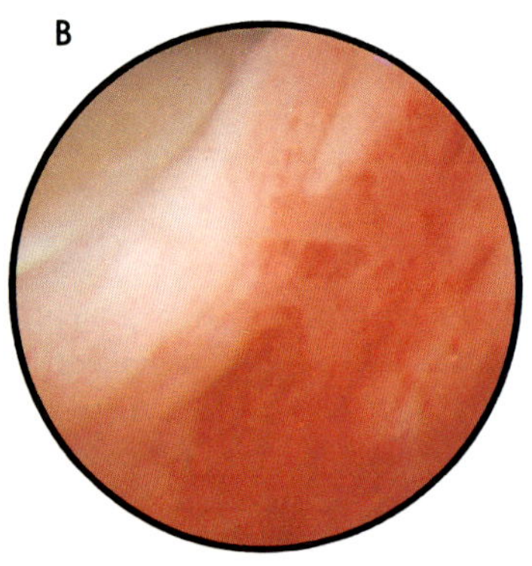
C
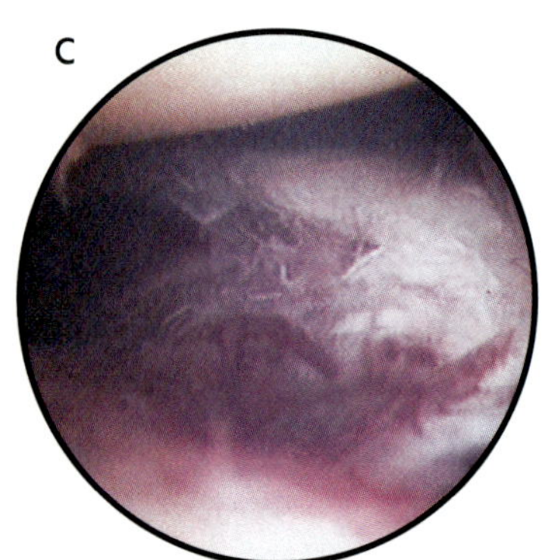

FIG. 8-102 Frozen shoulder manipulation.
A Anterior capsular hemorrhage after manipulation.
B Hemorrhage behind glenoid after manipulation.
C Tear in inferior glenohumeral ligament after manipulation.

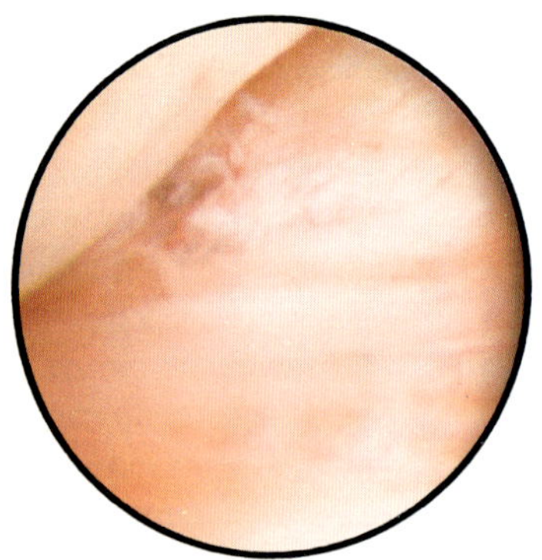

FIG. 8-103 Tear in inferior glenohumeral ligament after manipulation.

audible or palpable cracking or tearing. The objective is to gain at least 50% of the range of motion in all planes, using the opposite normal shoulder as the control. Although no attempt was made for a complete manipulation, minimal palpable and audible tearing sensations were nonetheless evident, especially during the combined abduction and external rotation maneuver.

The chance of subsequent dislocation or humeral fracture is reduced. Still, the postmanipulative inspection will show capsular hemorrhage (Fig. 8-102). Small tears have been seen in the anterior-inferior glenohumeral ligament (Fig. 8-103). A complete manipulation with audible tearing will show a complete glenohumeral ligament disruption.

Most importantly, the patient awakes with minimal discomfort, but a noticeable increase in motion. Because of this positive experience, formal physical therapy is unnecessary. The patient uses pendulum exercises, over-the-head arm lifts and butterfly motions (Fig. 8-104). Stretching with a broom stick and against a door jam can be helpful (Fig. 8-104).

A postmanipulation diagnostic arthroscopy was performed on 10 shoulders. The switching sticks were replaced with the arthroscope and cannulas. The entire procedure was recorded on videotape with sound. This included the inside arthroscopic views and outside documentation of the manipulation. The tapes were stored for subsequent review in constructing this report and for verification of the written medical record.

The patients were admitted as outpatients before surgery and admitted to the hospital after surgery for intensive physical therapy. The hospital stay averaged 2 days.

Observations. Several observations made at the time of arthroscopy were unique to the frozen shoulder condition. The capsular tissue was noticeably more difficult to penetrate than in shoulders with any other pathologic condition in our arthroscopic experience. Entry often required several attempts. The joint space contracture also hindered joint penetration.

The intraarticular volume capacity of the joint was diminished in all cases. The exact volume, however, was not recorded. The joint accepted only up to 20 ml of fluid, as compared to 90 to 120 ml in the average shoulder. No capsular disruption occurred in any case with maximal intraarticular distention applied with manual compression on a 60 ml syringe.

Diagnostic Findings. Premanipulation diagnostic shoulder arthroscopy showed the humeral head tightly against the scapular glenoid fossa in all patients (Fig. 8-105). The space between the rotator cuff and humeral

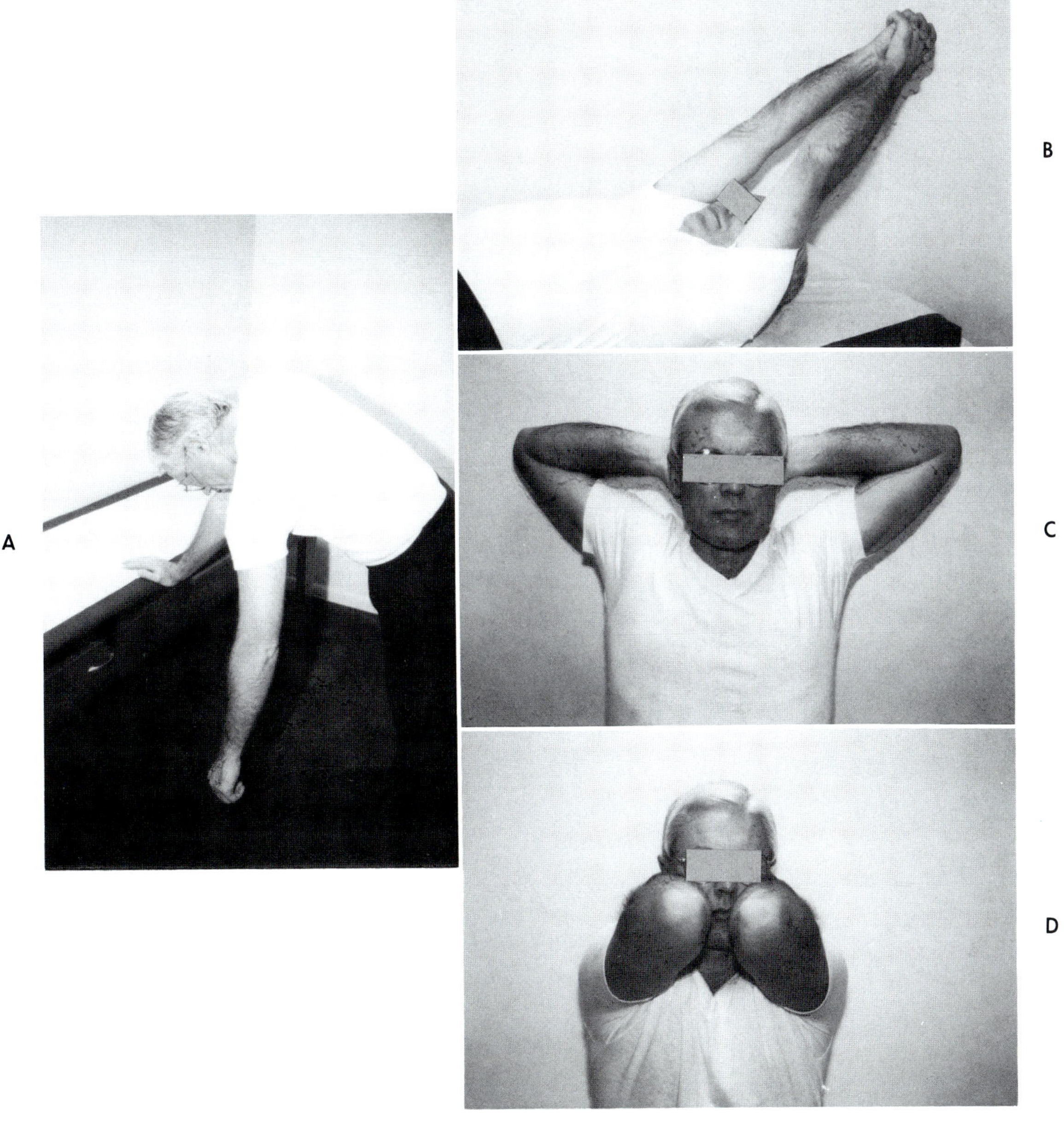

FIG. 8-104 Postmanipulation exercises.
A Pendulum exercises.
B Over-the-head exercises.
C, D Butterfly exercises.

Continued.

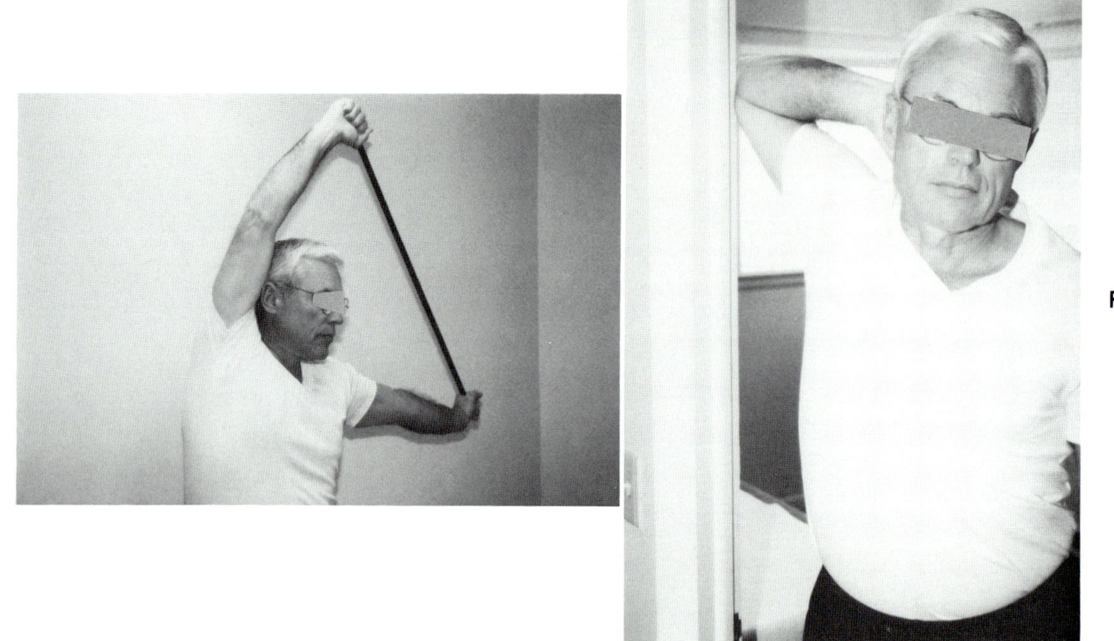

FIG. 8-104 *cont'd.* Postmanipulation exercises.
E Use of broom stick.
F Use of stretching on door jam.

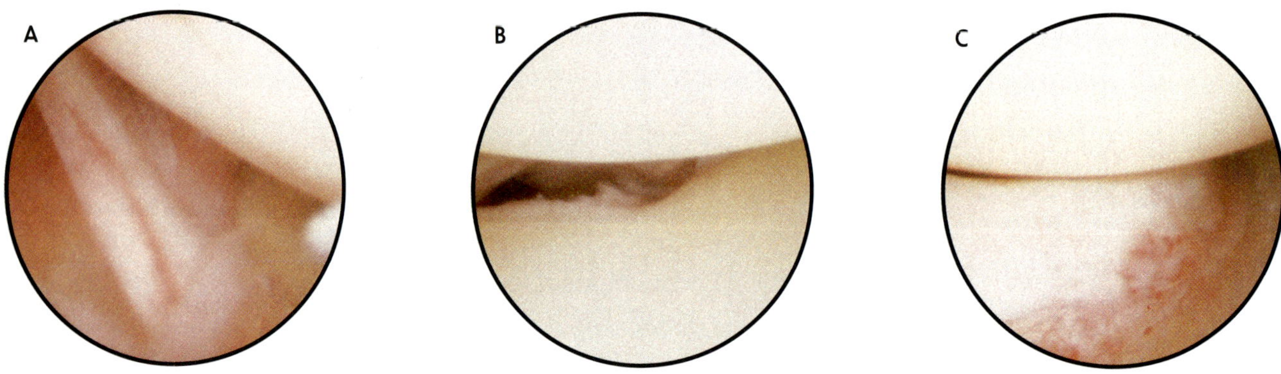

FIG. 8-105 Frozen shoulder: arthroscopic perspective.
A Inflammation seen on rotator cuff and biceps tendon.
B The humerus does not elevate off the glenoid even with much pressure.
C The humerus is on the inferior glenoid and synovitis is everywhere.

Table 8-4 Arthroscopic Findings in 21 Frozen Shoulders

Finding	No. of cases (%)
Anterior wall synovitis	19 (90%)
Subscapularis bursitis	12 (57%)
Middle glenohumeral ligament synovitis	3 (14%)
Axillary pouch synovitis	4 (19%)
Rotator cuff synovitis	12 (57%)
Rotator cuff tear	2 (10%)
Biceps tendon synovitis	11 (52%)
Posterior wall synovitis	5 (24%)
Labral tears	7 (33%)
Decreased distance between rotator cuff, biceps tendon, and glenohumeral head	5 (24%)
Intraarticular adhesions	0

Table 8-5 Postmanipulation Arthroscopic Findings in 10 Frozen Shoulders

Finding	No. of cases (%)
Anterior-inferior hemorrhage	7 (70%)
Subscapularis bursa hemorrhage	3 (30%)
Middle glenohumeral ligament hemorrhage	1 (10%)
Inferior glenohumeral ligament hemorrhage	6 (60%)
Axillary pouch hemorrhage	2 (20%)
Posterior wall hemorrhage	2 (20%)
Increased bicipital tendon-humeral head distance	2 (20%)

head was decreased in five patients. The joint was not distractable as is common in most shoulders with an increase of intraarticular fluid pressure manually applied with a 60-ml syringe. The lack of joint space and humeral distraction increased the technical difficulty of the diagnostic arthroscopy.

Synovitis existed in all cases (Fig. 8-105) and in different locations (Table 8-4). Synovitis was anterior, between the subscapularis and the biceps tendon, in 19 patients. In 12 patients the synovitis was observed to be in the subscapular bursa. Three patients exhibited synovitis over the middle glenohumeral ligament and four patients were noted to have synovitis involving the axillary pouch. In five patients, posterior wall synovitis was observed. Synovitis of the biceps tendon was seen in 11 patients, 6 at the origin of the tendon, 3 in its intraarticular expanse, and 2 at its point of exit. Synovitis was noted covering the rotator cuff in 12 patients. No intraarticular adhesions were visualized in any patient.

Two small undersurface incomplete rotator cuff tears were seen. Seven small anterior labral tears were noted, without intraarticular evidence of instability. No Bankart or Hill-Sachs lesions were observed. No significant degenerative changes were noted on either the humeral head or the glenoid fossa. Futhermore, in no case had the infraglenoid recess been obliterated.

Postmanipulation Findings. Following the manipulation, the joint accepted increased amounts of fluid. This occurred because increased joint space and capsular tears permitted extravasation of fluid. After the manipulation, the humeral head moved away from the glenoid with increasing joint distention in all patients. The distance between the biceps tendon and the head of the humerus increased in two patients.

The subsequent arthroscopic inspection showed bloody fluid related to tearing of the synovium or capsular ligaments (Fig. 8-102). Hemorrhage, indicative of tissue tearing, was noted in the anterior and inferior wall in 7 cases, subscapularis bursa in 3 cases, middle glenohumeral ligament in 1 case, inferior glenohumeral ligament in 6 cases, the axillary pouch in 2 cases, and in the posterior wall in 2 cases (Fig. 8-103) (Table 8-5).

The subacromial bursa was not inspected in this series. No arthroscopic surgical procedures were indicated. No intraoperative or perioperative complications occurred, including no rotator cuff or biceps tendon tears and no humeral fractures.

Our Present Understanding. The arthroscopic inspection in this series demonstrated the resultant pathological abnormalities accompanying adhesive capsulitis to be capsular contracture and vascular synovitis. Capsular thickening was demonstrated in this series by resistance to surgical penetration with the arthroscope cannula and obturator (posterior) and by cannula insertion (anterior). The capsular contracture was also evidenced by the minimal capacity of the joint space to accept fluid and the tight juxtaposition of the humerus to the glenoid (Fig. 8-105). Synovitis was documented in all cases, which is indicative of an inflammatory process.

The manual manipulation that increased the shoulder's range of motion was accompanied by audible and palpable tearing, which is indicative of capsular contracture. The subsequent arthroscopy showed the tearing and hemorrhage to be in the capsule and capsular ligaments. The postmanipulative change in position of the humerus, distracted away from the glenoid, supports the contractive nature of the capsular structures.

Although the capsular contracture and synovitis were seen with varying incidence around the joint, the primary involvement was anterior and inferior. This location of the main pathologic contracture was supported by the high incidence of anterior synovitis, the main resistance to passive range of motion being anterior and the subsequent anterior location of the capsular tearing following the manipulation. This location is supported by others.[28,81] Arthrogram studies of this condition have shown a contracted capsule, especially anteriorly, in the subscapularis bursa area.[31]

Our arthroscopic observations do not support the open surgical evidence of intraarticular adhesions or obliteration of the axillary or infraglenoid recess as reported by Neviaser. We do not have an explanation for the discrepancy. We did not see biceps tendon involvement as reported by others.[58,81,113] Although not a high incidence in this series, the relationship to rotator cuff disease should be considered in future cases. Attention should be given to the subacromial involvement as originally reported by DuPlay. Our present routine arthroscopy for this condition includes inspection of the subacromial space. Preliminary observations have shown fibrosis in the subacromial space plus erosion of the acromion, even in the absence of visible rotator cuff tears. This will be the subject of a subsequent report. Suspicion and existence of rotator cuff tear and impingement should be considered during diagnostic arthroscopy in this condition.

Our glenohumeral diagnostic arthroscopic findings were similar to previous reports.[1,35,50,80,120] on the presence of synovitis, capsular contracture, and no evidence of intraarticular adhesions. One report described accompanying complete rotator cuff tear and two cases with associated biceps tendon tears.[35] No previous report of the arthroscopic findings following manipulation exists. Etiological factors were not evident in this study.

The findings of synovitis in this series lend support to the use of antiinflammatory medication and intraarticular cortisone injections in the nonoperative treatment of this condition.[25,57,70,72]

We created maximal intraarticular pressure during arthroscopic observation. We saw no evidence in this series that increased intraarticular fluid pressure would cause stretching or tearing of the capsule. No secondary evidence was seen of capsular release with sudden increase in acceptance of fluid or of distraction of the humeral head from the glenoid. Range of motion was not improved at this point. Manipulation was necessary to affect any change in joint distraction or improved motion.

We have no explanation for the discrepancy between our experience and that reported by others concerning capsular rupture with maximal intraarticular pressure. The greater acceptance of fluid in their cases may have been due to fluid extravasation and not capsular disruption.[31] They showed extravasation of dye by x-ray examination in only one view. Two planes would be necessary to produce evidence of the exact location of capsular rupture. They presented no convincing evidence that distention alone was an effective method of treatment, since local anesthetics, cortisone, and immediate physical therapy with passive assistance was also used in their cases. No evidence was given concerning the immediate range of motion improvement. There was no arthroscopic confirmation of the capsular disruption with increased intraarticular pressure.

The use of arthroscopy in this series was investigative. However, the potential for additional accompanying pathological lesions, especially in rotator cuff disease, has caused us to consider arthroscopy an integral part of the frozen shoulder therapy. The risk of the procedure is minimal.[1,35,50,80,120] Few complications have been reported with arthroscopy for this condition.[104,105]

The potential for patient benefit exists with arthroscopic surgery in adhesive capsulitis, although it was not performed in this series. A surgical incision for release of the anterior capsule was considered, but the exact area of capsular involvement was determined only following manipulation. Therefore surgical release was not performed in this series. The labrum tears were so small that a debridement was not necessary. If a significant size tear of the labrum or rotator cuff existed, then a debridement would have been performed. The main potential for arthroscopic surgery would exist if an accompanying impingement lesion were identified. In this case, an arthroscopic subacromial bursectomy and acromioplasty would accompany the manual glenohumeral joint manipulation.

Similarly, closed manipulation has been reported to result in an 83% full range of motion without pain 8 weeks postmanipulation and without any reported complications.[99,110] Arthroscopic examination and manipulation fulfill the criteria of a low morbidity treatment regimen in compressing the period of disability in this self-limited disorder. Arthroscopic evaluation and manipulation is a safe and effective modality in the treatment of adhesive capsulitis and provides useful diagnostic information. It is a valuable adjunct to other conservative measures when symptoms persist for greater than 6 months and abduction is limited to less than 90 degrees.[25,70,99,110]

Shoulder Fusion

The indication for shoulder fusion is not frequent. The application of arthroscopic method to perform a shoulder fusion was attempted by my associate, David A. Detrisac, several years ago. The procedure failed because of osteoporotic bone and lack of mechanical ability to gain compression with lag screws and washers.

Craig D. Morgan has performed a successful shoulder fusion by arthroscopy (Fig. 8-106).[69] This case report has not been published, but Dr. Morgan has given me permission to share his experience. This patient was a 35-year-old woman with a 7-year history of traumatic true luxation that was chronic and disabling. He used the beach chair position and intraoperative imaging with a C-arm. He reports that she was pain free and functional at 3 months postoperation. At 6 months postoperation the fusion was united (Fig. 8-106, *C* and *D*).

Anyone attempting this adaption should contact Dr. Morgan for the details until he publishes his case.

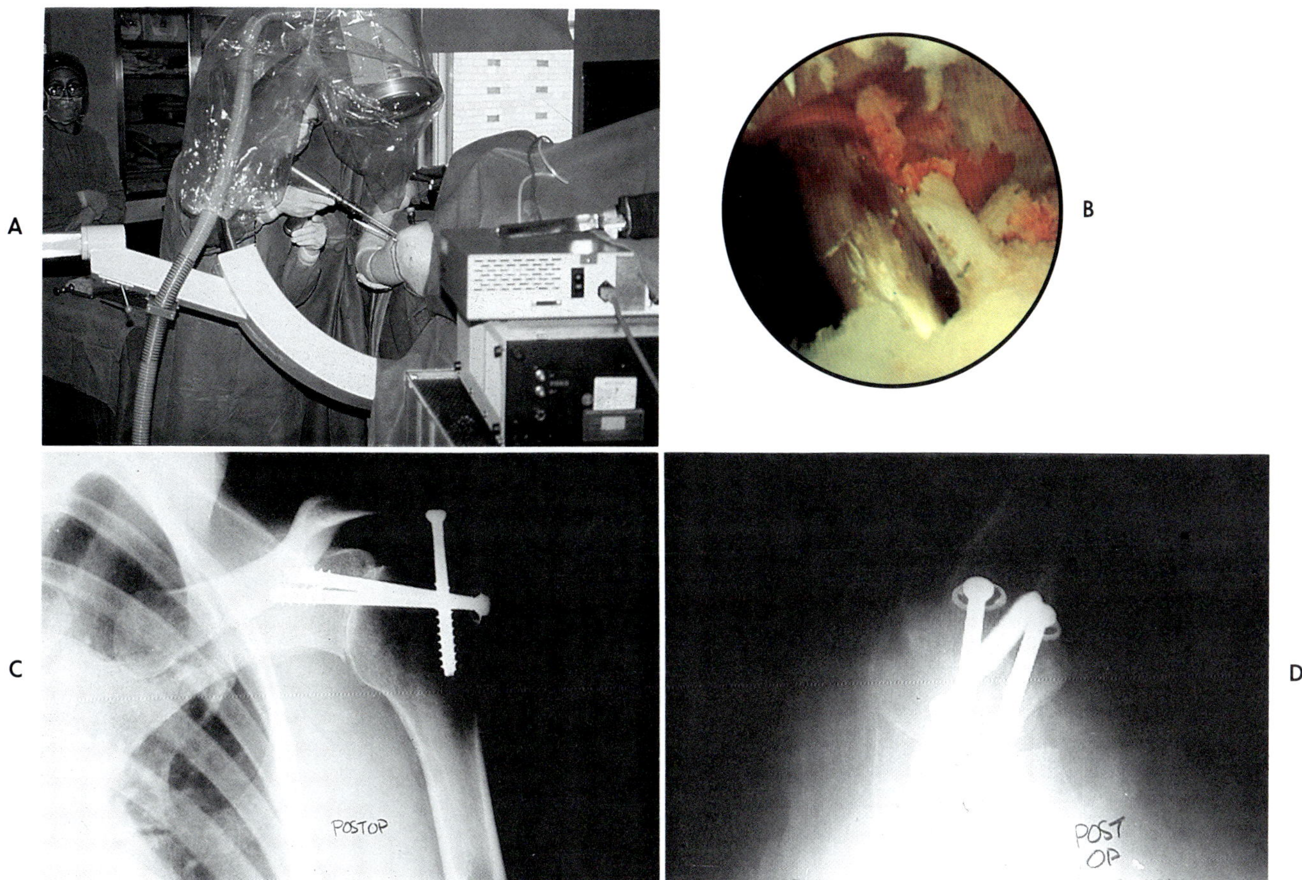

FIG. 8-106 Shoulder fusion. (Courtesy Craig D. Morgan, Wilmington, Delaware.)

A C-arm imaging is used for placement of internal fixation.

B Arthroscopic view of screw shaft crossing the glenohumeral joint.

C Postoperative anterior-posterior x-ray film.

D Postoperative axillary x-ray film.

ARTHROSCOPY AFTER PREVIOUS SURGERY

Arthroscopic Surgery

The most common repeat arthroscopy follows arthroscopic reconstructive procedures.

The most common internal fixation device to be removed in my practice is the metallic staple. It is removed in about 10% of cases. A planned removal is made in throwing athletes to avoid the irritation from the staple head on the subscapularis tendon (see Fig. 8-101). Removal is advised if the patient has persistent shoulder pain. Removal is necessary if the staple is not inserted or, in rare instances, loosens from bone.

Open Surgery

Failed surgical procedures are not limited to those performed by arthroscopy.[87,92,93] The stump of a biceps tendon may be left behind following open biceps tenodesis (Fig.8-16, *B*). To see large fragments of permanent suture material or fibrosis within the glenohumeral joint is not uncommon (Fig. 8-107). Loose bodies and degenerative fragments are often not visualized or debrided during open surgery and are the source of pain and/or catching. Arthroscopy provides a means of diagnosing the condition and treatment by debridement.

Suture material may be the source of postoperative joint irritation (Fig. 8-107, *C*). The suture material may be

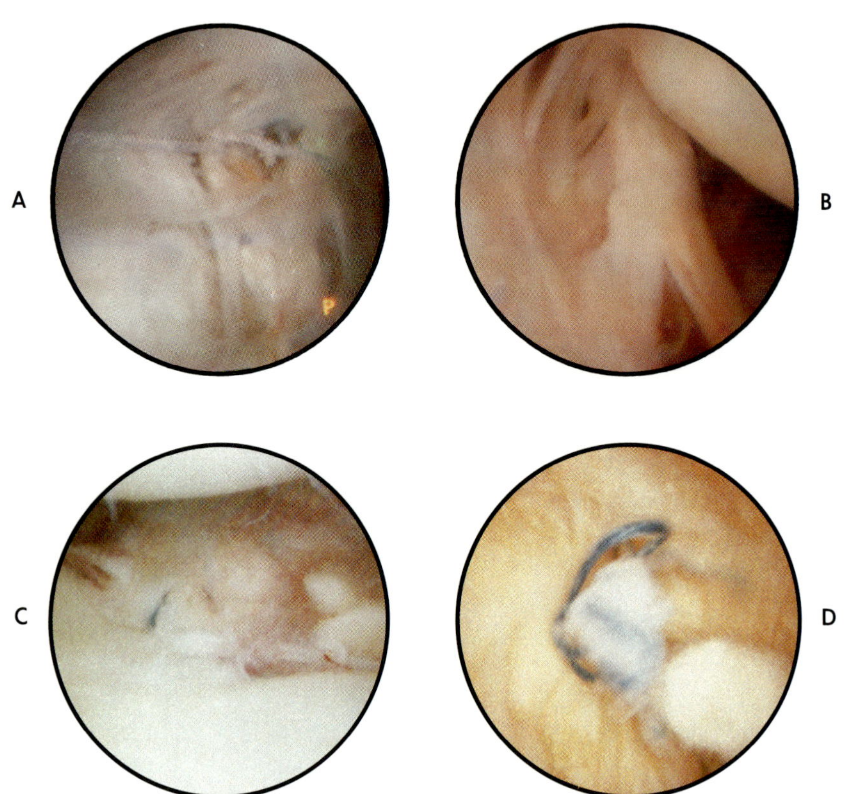

FIG. 8-107 Remnants of open surgery.

A **Suture material evident at intended insertion site.**

B **Intraarticular adhesions and lack of integrity of repair. Defect filled with scar tissue.**

C **Arthroscopic view of suture material exposed in glenoid in patient with marked restriction of motion after open surgery.**

D **Arthroscopic view of "bolus" of suture material causing inflammation in joint after failed attempt at open rotator cuff repair.**

removed by arthroscopy as well as by adjacent smoothing of irregular scar tissue.

Ankylosis may persist in spite of extensive physical therapy after open surgery. Arthroscopy provides a means of removing intraarticular suture material and measured incisional release of the anterior capsule (Fig. 8-107, *D*).

Various internal fixation devices placed by open surgery may be amenable to arthroscopic removal.[7] This method will reduce the surgical exposure of conventional open surgery. On one occasion I removed an intraarticular screw by the arthroscopic method. The screw had been placed by another surgeon during fixation of the coracoid process to the glenoid for dislocation. The patient redislocated and the bone fractured off the screw that remained in the glenoid neck. At arthroscopy a motorized instrument with an abrader burr attachment was placed anteriorly. The rotating burr was placed on the side of the screw and backed out the screw from bone. The loosened screw was removed with a forceps.

COMPLICATIONS

The old adage— "The only way to prevent complications, is to not perform surgery"—is still valid today.[97] Therefore, the surgeon's effort should be directed to minimize this risk. The importance of organization and planning has been emphasized throughout this text. The surgeon must prepare individually and be responsible for the arthroscopic team's preparation. Careful, deliberate, step-by-step operative protocol is necessary to avoid complications.

The risk of complication is greater with new surgical procedures with new equipment and previously unexplored anatomical regions.[24,104,105] Preparation with continuing education courses and motor skill laboratory experience is necessary. A staged progression, starting with diagnostic arthroscopy and progressing through the simpler to more complex procedures, will minimize arthroscopic complications.

Surgeons too often believe their knowledge of open surgery can be easily converted to arthroscopic methods. Arthroscopy requires a new set of skills, instrumentation, and surgical exposure. I have also observed that preconceived ideas result in complications. The most common one was to use the open surgical principle of placing sutures at the anterior glenoid margin during open Bankart repair with placement of a metallic staple at the same position by arthroscopy. It should not be surprising that erosion occurs to humeral head cartilage.

Small's first report on complications from arthroscopy[105] was a retrospective study from 299 surgeon questionnaires reporting 395,566 arthroscopic procedures. This report included 562 anterior shoulder stapling capsulorrhaphies. Thirty complications were reported for a 5.3% incidence: 19 loose staples, 6 impinging staples, 2 bent staples, 2 brachial plexus stretch injuries, and 1 unspecified equipment failure.

Small subsequently reported the incidence of complications from 21 experienced arthroscopic surgeons over a period of 19 months (August 1986 to February 1988).[105] A total of 10,262 procedures were performed: 1184 cases or 11.51% were performed in the shoulder region.

Anterior staple capsulorrhaphy had the highest complication rate at 3.3% (3 of 91 cases). Two of the complications were staple impingement on the humeral head. The other complication was a hemarthrosis (Table 8-6).

Table 8-6 Summary of Shoulder Complications

Complication	No. of procedures	No. of complications
Diagnostic only	204	1
Anterior staple capsulorrhaphy	91	3
Extraarticular capsular staple	4	0
Labrum debridement	206	1
Reconstruction with graft	35	0
Cuff debridement	138	0
Bankhart repair(suture)	18	0
Loose body removal	59	1
Synovectomy	51	0
Fracture fixation	2	0
TOTAL	808	6

From Small NC: Complications in arthroscopy: the knee and other joints, *Arthroscopy* 2:253-258, 1986.

Prevention

Preoperative. The best opportunity to prevent complications is before the surgical procedure begins. The surgeon prepares himself or herself and the surgical team for the procedure. The surgeon selects a surgical candidate for a procedure that is well within his or her technical capability. The instrumentation is carefully selected and in proper repair. The arm should be suspended, not placed under mechanical traction, to prevent neuropraxia.[5,55]

Intraoperative. Lack of surgical exposure will result in complications. Failure to visualize the surgical site or tips of instruments or devices will result in complications. Unwillingness to abort a long or frustrating case is potentially complicating. Failure to confirm device insertion by both visualization and palpation increases the risk of complication.

Puncture of the rotator cuff with instruments may produce permanent defects visible on arthrogram.[74]

Laceration of the cephalic vein may occur during anterior portal creation. Ligation is indicated to prevent postoperative bleeding. Intraarticular bleeding can be controlled with electrocautery. Instrument breakage management should be anticipated and magnetic instruments and devices should be used. A magnetized retrieval instrument should be available for such an occasion.

Extravasation of fluid may cause technical difficulty and increased compartment pressure.[21,82]

Postoperative. Postoperative complications are less within the control of the surgeon. The patient can be alerted to this potential by postoperative written instructions. Postoperative bleeding should be recognized at the conclusion of the operation. Continued postoperative puncture wound drainage may be a conduit for deep joint infection.

Deep venous thrombosis is a rare complication of shoulder arthroscopy.[15] In Burkhart's case it developed in the same extremity and was clinically manifest 3 days postoperative. A mediastinal tumor mass was the obstructing force in this case. Systemic causative and anatomic abnormalities should be considered in such a case.

Management

Infection. Infection is uncommon in arthroscopy.[52,53] I have not seen an infection following arthroscopy of the shoulder. This is probably due to the minimization of tissue injury with the small portal and the dilution of any bacteria with fluid irrigation. Prophylactic antibiotics have not been necessary. The surgeon may at his or her discretion use prophylactic antibiotics with placement of internal fixation.

Bleeding. Bleeding is minimized during arthroscopy because of increased hydrostatic pressure of the fluid medium. Potential postoperative bleeding is controlled by intraarticular electrocautery or ligation of small subcutaneous vessels.

Major Arterial Injury. Preoperative palpation of the

radial pulse of the involved extremity gives a baseline for recognition of this potential complication. I often palpate the pulse immediately before suspension of the arm when the patient is under anesthetic. (The pulse pressure is often diminished during anesthesia.) Careful attention to portal placement should avoid injury to a major artery.

Nerve Injury. Careful placement of the various portals should avoid this complication. A low posterior portal places the axillary nerve at risk. Transscapular drilling, Kirschner wire insertion, or screw placement potentially risk the suprascapular nerve.[11,27]

Thoracic Injury. Care should be taken in transscapular drilling with wires that might deviate. Shea[96] reported deviation of a guide wire short of the thorax but under the scapula that required open retrieval.

Instrument Malfunction or Breakage. Backup instrumentation solves the potential of instrument failure. Breakage should be anticipated, with magnetic instruments and retrievers kept close by.

REFERENCES

1. Andren L, Lundberg BJ: Treatment of rigid shoulders by joint distention during arthroscopy, *ACTA Orthop Scand* 36:45, 1965.
2. Andrews JR, Broussard TS, Carson WG: Arthroscopy of the shoulder in the management of partial tears of the rotator cuff: a preliminary report, *Arthroscopy* 1:117, 1985.
3. Andrews JR, Carson WG Jr: Shoulder joint arthroscopy, *Orthopaedics* 6:1157, 1983.
4. Andrews JR, Carson WG Jr, Mcleod WD: Glenoid labrum tears related to the long head of the biceps, *Am J Sports Med* 13(5):337-341, 1985.
5. Andrews JR, Carson WG Jr, Ortega K: Arthroscopy of the shoulder: techniques and normal anatomy, *Am J Sports Med* 12:1-7, 1984.
6. Aronen JG, Regan K: Decreasing the incidence of recurrence of first time anterior shoulder dislocations with rehabilitation, *Clin Orthop* 187 (Jul-Aug):150-153, 1984.
7. Bach BR: Arthroscopic removal of painful bristow hardware, *Arthroscopy* 6(4):324-326, 1990.
8. Bankart AB: The pathology and treatment of recurrent dislocation of the shoulder joint, *Br J Surg* 26:23-29, 1938.
9. Bankart AB: Recurrent or habitual dislocation of the shoulder joint, *Br Med J* 11:32, 1928.
10. Barber FA, Click JN: Long term strength of new slow absorption sutures, *Arthroscopy* 7:329, 1991.
11. Bigliani LU et al: An anatomical study of the suprascapular nerve, *Arthroscopy* 6(4):301-305, 1990.
12. Bridgman JF: Periarthritis of the shoulder and diabetes mellitus, *Ann Rheum Dis* 31:69-71, 1972.
13. Brodsky JW, Tullow HS, Gartsman GA: Simplified posterior approach to the shoulder joint, *J Bone Joint Surg* 69A(5):773-774, 1987.
14. Bulgen DY et al: Frozen shoulder: prospective clinical study with an evaluation of three treatment regimens, *Ann Rheum Dis* 43:353-360, 1984.
15. Burkhart SS: Deep venous thrombosis after shoulder arthroscopy, *J Arthroscopy Relat Surg* 6(1):61-63, 1990.
16. Calandra JJ, Baker CL, Uribe J: The incidence of Hill-Sachs lesions in initial anterior shoulder dislocations, *Arthroscopy* 5:254-257, 1989.
17. Caspari RB: Arthroscopic reconstruction for anterior shoulder instability, *Tech in Orthop* 3(1)59-66, 1988.
18. Clark J, Sidles JA, Matsen FA: The relationship of the glenohumeral joint capsule to the rotator cuff, *Clin Orthop* 254(5):29-34, 1990.
19. Codman EA: Stiff and painful shoulders. The anatomy of the subdeltoid subacromial bursa and its clinical importance: subdeltoid bursitis, *Boston Med Surg J* 154:613-620, 1906.
20. Cofield RH, Irving JF: Evaluation and classification of shoulder with special reference to examination under anesthesia, *Clin Orthop* 223(Oct):32-43, 1987.
21. Cohn L, Lee YF, Tooke SM: Intramuscular compartment pressures during shoulder arthroscopy, *Arthroscopy* 5(2):159, 1989.
22. Connolly JF: Humeral head defects associated with shoulder dislocations—their diagnostic and surgical significance, *AAOS Instructional Course Lectures,* St Louis, 1972, Mosby-Year Book.
23. Cronen JG, Regan K: Decreasing the incidence of recurrence of first time anterior shoulder dislocations with rehabilitation, *Am J Sports Med* 12:283, 1984.
24. DeLee JC: Complications of arthroscopy and arthroscopic surgery: results of a national survey, *Arthroscopy* 1:214, 1985.
25. DePalma AF: Loss of scapulohumeral motion (frozen shoulder), *Ann Surg* 135(2):193-204, 1952.
26. Detrisac DA, Johnson LL: Arthroscopic shoulder anatomy: pathological and surgical implications, Thoroughfare, New Jersey 1986, Slack.
27. Drez D, Proffer D: Suprascapular Nerve Anatomy and Relationship to the Glenoid. Presented at American Academy of Orthopedic Surgeons in Anaheim, California, March 1991.
28. DuPlay S: De la periarthrite scapulohumerale, *Rev Frat Med* 53:226, 1896.
29. duToit GT, Roux D: Recurrent dislocation of the shoulder: a twenty-four year study of the Johannesburg stapling operation, *J Bone Joint Surg* 38A:1, 1956.
30. Eisenberg JH, Fedler MR, Hecht PJ: Arthroscopic stabilization of the chronic subluxating or dislocating shoulder without the use of internal fixation, *Arthroscopy* 7(3):315, 1991.
31. Fareed DO, Gallivan WR Jr: Office management of frozen shoulder syndrome: treatment with hydraulic distension under local anesthesia, *Clin Orthop* 242(5):177-183, 1989.
32. Fowler P: Swimmer problems, *Am J Sports Med* 7:141-142, 1979.
33. Grey RG: The natural history of "idiopathic" frozen shoulder: brief note, *J Bone Joint Surg* 60A:564, 1978.
34. Gross M, Fitzgibbons TC: Shoulder arthroscopy: a modified approach, *Arthroscopy* 1(3):156-159, 1985.
35. Ha'eri GB, Maitland A: Arthroscopic findings in frozen shoulder, *J Rheumatol* 8:149-152, 1981.
36. Haines JF, Hargadon EJ: Manipulation as the primary treatment of the frozen shoulder, *J R Coll Surg Edinb* 27:5, 1982.
37. Hawkins RB: Arthroscopic stapling repair for shoulder instability: a retrospective study of 50 cases of arthroscopy 5(2):122-128, 1989.
38. Hawkins RJ, Hobeika P: Physical examination of the shoulder, *Orthopedics* 6(10):1270-1278, 1983.
39. Hawkins RJ, Koppert G, Johnston G: Recurrent posterior instability (subluxation) of the shoulder, *J Bone Joint Surg* 66A:169-174, 1984.
40. Hayes JM: Arthroscopic treatment of steroid-induced osteonecrosis of the humeral head, *Arthroscopy* 5(3):218-221, 1989.
41. Hill HA, Sachs MD: The grooved defect of the humeral head: a frequently unrecognized complication of dislocations of the shoulder joint, *Radiology* 35:690, 1940.
42. Hill JJ Jr, Bogumill H: Manipulation in the treatment of frozen shoulder, *Orthopedics* II 9:1255-1260, 1988.
43. Howell SM, Gilanat BJ: The glenoid-labral socket, *Clin Orth Rel Res* 243(6):122-125, 1989.

44. Hurley JA, Anderson TA: Shoulder arthroscopy: its role in evaluating shoulder disorders in the athlete, *Am J Sports Med* 18(5):480-483, 1990.
45. Hybbinette S: De la transplantation d'un fragment osseux pour remedier aux luxuations recidevantes de l'epaule: constatations et resultats operatoires, *Acta Chir Scand* 71:411, 1932.
46. Iannotti JP et al: Magnetic resonance imaging of the shoulder: sensitivity, specificity and predictive value, *J Bone Joint Surg* 73A:17-29, 1991.
47. Jobe FW et al: Anterior capsulolabral reconstruction of the shoulder in athletes in overhand sports, *Am J Sports Med* 19(5):428-434, 1991.
48. Johnson LL: The shoulder joint: an arthroscopist's perspective of anatomy and pathology, *Clin Orthop* 223:113-125, 1987.
49. Johnson LL: Arthroscopic abrasion arthroplasty historical and pathological perspective: present status, *Arthroscopy* 2(1):55-69, 1986.
50. Johnson LL: Arthroscopic surgery: principles and practice, ed 3, St Louis, 1986, Mosby–Year Book.
51. Johnson LL et al: Osteochondritis dissecans of the knee: arthroscopic compression screw fixation, *Arthroscopy* 6(3):179-189, 1990.
52. Johnson LL et al: Two percent glutaraldehyde: a disinfectant in arthroscopy and arthroscopic surgery, *J Bone Joint Surg* 64A:237, 1982.
53. Johnson LL et al: Cold sterilization method for arthroscopes using activated dialdehyde, *Orthop Rev* 6:75, 1977.
54. Kinnard P et al: Assessment of the unstable shoulder by computed arthrography, *Am J Sports Med* 11:157, 1983.
55. Klein AH et al: Measurement of brachial plexus strain in arthroscopy of the shoulder, *Arthroscopy* 3(1):45-52, 1987.
56. Kohn D: The clinical relevance of glenoid labrum lesions, *Arthroscopy* 3(4):223-230, 1987.
57. Leffert RD: The frozen shoulder, *Instr Course Lect* 34:199-203, 1985.
58. Lippman RK: Frozen shoulder, periarthritis, bicipital tenosynovitis, *Arch Surg* 47:283-296, 1943.
59. Lynch GJ: Arthroscopic substitution of the anterior inferior glenohumeral ligament, *Arthroscopy* 7(3):325, 1991.
60. MacNab I: Rotator cuff tendinitis, *Ann Royal College Surg Eng* 53:271, 1973.
61. Maki N: Personal communication, 1991.
62. Matthews LS, Oweida SJ: Glenohumeral instability in athletes: spectrum, diagnosis and treatment, *Adv Orthp Surg* 236-249, 1985.
63. Matthews LS et al: Arthroscopic staple capsulorrhaphy for recurrent anterior instability, *Arthroscopy* 4(2):106-111, 1988.
64. McGlynn FJ, Caspari RB. Arthroscopic findings in the subluxating shoulder, *Clin Orthop* 183:173, 1984.
65. McLaughlin H: Posterior dislocation of the shoulder, *J Bone Joint Surg* 34A:584-590, 1952.
66. McMaster WC: Anterior glenoid labrum damage: a painful lesion in swimmers, *Am J Sports Med* 14(5):383-387, 1986.
67. Morgan C: Arthroscopic transglenoid Bankart suture repair, *Operative Techniques in Orthopedics* 1(2) (April):171-179, 1991.
68. Morgan CD, Bodenstab AB: Arthroscopic suture repair: technique and early results, *Arthroscopy* 3(2):111-122, 1987.
69. Morgan CD: Personal communication, 1991.
70. Murnaghan JP: Adhesive capsulitis of the shoulder: current concepts and treatment, *Orthopedics* 11(1):153-158, 1988.
71. Neer CS II: *Shoulder Reconstruction,* Philadelphia, 1990, WB Saunders.
72. Neviaser JS: Adhesive capsulitis of the shoulder, *J Bone Joint Surg* 27:211-222, 1945.
73. Neviaser TJ: Adhesive capsulitis, *Orthop Clin North Am* 18(30): 439-443, 1987.
74. Norwood LA, Fowler HL: Rotator cuff tears, a shoulder arthroscopy complication, *Am J Sports Med* 17:837-841, 1989.
75. Norwood LA, Terry GC: Shoulder posterior subluxation, *Am J Sports Med* 12:25, 1984.
76. Nottage WM, Duge WD, Fields WA: Computed arthrotomography of the glenohumeral joint to evaluate anterior instability: correlation with the arthroscopic findings, *Arthroscopy* 3(4):273-276, 1987.
77. O'Brien SJ et al: The anatomy and histology of the inferior glenohumeral ligament complex of the shoulder, *Am J Sports Med* 18:449-456, 1990.
78. O'Driscoll SW: Contralateral shoulder instability following anterior repair, *JBJS* 73-B:941-946, 1991.
79. O'Driscoll SW, Evans DC: The DuToit staple capsulorrhaphy for recurrent anterior dislocation of the shoulder: twenty years of experience in six Toronto hospitals, American Shoulder and Elbow Surgeons 4th Open Meeting, Atlanta, 1988.
80. Ogilvie-Harris DJ, Wiley AM: Arthroscopic surgery of the shoulder: a general appraisial, *J Bone Joint Surg* 68B:201-207, 1986.
81. Patseur F: Sur une forme nouvelle de periarthralgie et d'ankylose de l'epaule, *J Radiol Eletrol* 18:327, 1934.
82. Peek R, Haynes DW: Compartment syndrome as a comlication of arthroscopy, *Am J Sports Med* 12:464, 1984.
83. Perthes G: Uber Operationen bei Habitueller Schulterluxation, *Deutsch Ztschr Chri* 85:199-227, 1906.
84. Resnick D, Niwayama G: *Diagnosis of Bone and Joint Disorders,* ed 2, Philadelphia, 1988, W.B. Saunders.
85. Richardson AB: *Arthroscopic stapling for treatment of anterior shoulder instability,* UCLA Arthroscopy Seminar, Maui, Hawaii, October 1989.
86. Richmond JC et al: Modification of the Bankart reconstruction with a suture anchor: report of a new technique, *Am J Sports Med* 19(4):343, 1991.
87. Rockwood CA Jr: Migration of pins used in operations on the shoulder, *J Bone Joint Surg (Am)* 72(8):1262-1267, 1990.
88. Rockwood CA Jr, Matsen FA III: *The shoulder,* Philadelphia, 1990, WB Saunders.
89. Rowe CR: The shoulder, New York, 1988, Churchill Livingstone.
90. Rowe CR, Patel D, Southmayd WW: The Bankart procedure: a long-term end result study, *J Bone Joint Surg* 60A:1-16, 1978.
91. Rowe CR, Pierce DS, Clark JG: Voluntary dislocation of the shoulder: a preliminary report on a clinical electromyographic and psychiatric study of twenty-six patients, *J Bone Joint Surg* 55A:445, 1973.
92. Rowe CR, Zarins B: Recurrent transient subluxation of the shoulder, *J Bone Joint Surg* 63A:863-871, 1981.
93. Rowe CR, Zarins B, Ciullo JV: Recurrent anterior dislocation of the shoulder after surgical repair: apparent causes of failure and treatment, *J Bone Joint Surg* 66A:159, 1984.
94. Sachs RA, Riehl B, Lane JA: Arthroscopic staple capsulorrhaphy: a long term followup, *Arthroscopy* 7 (3): 324, 1991.
95. Samilson RL, Prieto V: Dislocation arthropathy of the shoulder, *J Bone Joint Surg* 65A:456, 1983.
96. Shea KP, Lovallo JL: Scapulothoracic penetration of the beath pin: an unusual complication of arthroscopic bankart suture repair, *Arthroscopy* 7(1):115-117, 1991.
97. Sherman OH et al: Arthroscopy—no problem surgery, *J Bone Joint Surg* 68A:256-265, 1986.
98. Shuman WP et al: Double-constrast computered tomography of the glenoid labrum, *Am J Radiology* 141:581-584, 1983.
99. Simon WH: Soft tissue disorders of the shoulder, *Orthop Clin North Am* (2):521-539, 1975.
100. Simonet WT, Cofield RH: Prognosis in anterior shoulder dislocation, *Am J Sports Med* 12:19, 1984.
101. Sisk TD, Boyd HB: Management of recurrent anterior dislocation of the shoulder: DuToit-type or staple capsulorrhaphy, *Clin Orthop* 103:150, 1974.

102. Skyhar MJ, Altcheck DW, Warren RF: Tips of the trade: shoulder arthroscopy in the seated position, *Orthop Rev* 17(10):1003-1004, 1988.
103. Skyhar MJ et al: Shoulder arthroscopy with the patient in the beach-chair position, *Arthroscopy* 4(4):256-259, 1988.
104. Small NC: Complications in arthroscopic surgery performed by experienced arthroscopists, *J Arthroscopy Relat Surg* 4(3):215-221, 1988.
105. Small NC: Complications in arthroscopy: the knee and other joints, *Arthroscopy* 2:253-258, 1986.
106. Snyder SJ: Personal communication, 1991.
107. Snyder SJ et al: SLAP lesions of the shoulder, *Arthroscopy* 6(4):274-279, 1990.
108. Snyder SJ et al: Partial thickness rotator cuff tears: results of arthroscopic treatment, *Arthroscopy* 7(1):1-7, 1991.
109. Snyder SJ, Rames RD, Morgan CD: Anatomical variations of the glenohumeral ligaments, *Arthroscopy* 7(3):328, 1991.
110. Stein I: Managing frozen shoulder syndrome, *Orthop Rev* 5:92, 1976.
111. Tibone J, Ting A: Capsulorrhaphy with a staple for recurrent posterior subluxation of the shoulder, *J Bone Joint Surg* 72A:999-1002, 1990.
112. Tibone JE, Prietto C, Jobe FW: Staple capsulorrhaphy for recurrent posterior dislocation, *Am J Sports Med* 9:135-139, 1981.
113. Turek SL: The frozen shoulder, *J Int Coll Surg* 22:6-95, 1954.
114. Turkel SJ et al: Stabilizing mechanisms preventing anterior dislocation of the glenohumeral joint, *J Bone Joint Surg* 63A:1208-1217, 1981.
115. Uhthoff HK, Sarkar K: An algorithm for shoulder pain caused by soft tissue disorders, *Clin Orthop* 254(5):121-127, 1990.
116. Ward WG, Bassett FH III, Garrett WE Jr: Anterior staple capsulorrhaphy for recurrent dislocation of the shoulder: a clincal and biomechanical study, *S Med J* 83(5):510-518, 1990.
116a. Warner JP et al: Arthroscopic Bankart repair utilizing an absorbable cannulated fixation device. Paper presentation (#233) at the 1991 AAOS Annual Meeting, Anaheim, California.
117. Weber BG, Simpson LA, Hardegger F: Rotational humeral osteotomy for recurrent anterior dislocation of the shoulder associated with a large Hill-Sachs lesion, *J Bone Joint Surg* 66A:1443, 1984.
118. Weber SC, Caspari RB: A biomechanical evaluation of the restraints to posterior shoulder dislocation, *Arthroscopy* 5(2):115-121, 1989.
119. Wheeler JH, Ryan JB, Arciero RA, Molianan RN: Arthroscopic versus nonoperative treatment of acute shoulder dislocation in young athletes, *Arthroscopy* 5(3):213-217, 1989.
120. Wiley AM: Arthroscopic appearance of the frozen shoulder, *Arthroscopy* 7(2):138-143, 1991.
121. Wiley AM: Arthroscopy for shoulder instability and a technique for arthroscopic repair, *Arthroscopy* 4(10):25-30, 1988.
122. Wolf EM: Arthroscopic anterior shoulder capsulorrhaphy, *Techniques Orthop* 3(1):67-73, 1988.
123. Wolf EM: Arthroscopic anterior staple capsulorrhaphy, *Arthroscopy* 4(2):142, 1988.
124. Yoneda M et al: Arthroscopic stapling for detached superior glenoid labrum, *J Bone Joint Surg* 73B(5):746-750, 1991.
125. Zuckerman JD, Matsen FA: Complications about the glenohumeral joint related to the use of screws and staples, *J Bone Joint Surg* 66A:175, 1984.

CHAPTER

9 The Subacromial Space and Rotator Cuff Lesions

Arthroscopy provides a perspective heretofore not possible of the subacromial space and rotator cuff lesions, (Fig. 9-1, *A* and *B;* see also Fig. 9-5).[35] Arthroscopic surgery plays a major role in the management of impingement syndrome and rotator cuff tears. The benefits of the enhanced imaging of diagnostic arthroscopy and the microsurgical techniques of operative arthroscopy can be used to treat these types of shoulder problems.

CLINICAL ASSESSMENT

Refer to previous chapters in this text for the clinical assessment of the shoulder joint, including the subacromial space and rotator cuff. Consult other resources concerning the etiology, pathology, clinical diagnosis, physical examination, imaging tests, clinical evaluation, patient selection, conservative treatment, and open surgical management of impingement syndrome and rotator cuff tear.* Both the acromion and the coracoid process have been implicated in impingement.† This chapter will focus on the specific uses of arthroscopy in diagnosing and treating lesions in the subacromial space and rotator cuff.

The imaging tests of x-ray, CAT scan, magnetic resonance, and ultrasound provide only circumstantial evidence concerning shoulder problems.‡ Plain film x-rays may show os acrominale.[7,47,48] These tests are nevertheless important in the clinical investigation, especially in determining extraarticular disease and locating various shoulder lesions.[37,67,69] These imaging tests direct the surgeon's attention toward conditions to be inspected by arthroscopy. They also help the preoperative planning and direct the surgeon in choosing the method of surgical treatment.

*8, 27-29, 48, 50-56, 63, 65, 69, 70, 76
†6, 7, 25, 47, 48, 59, 64
‡4, 9, 12, 14-17, 31, 41, 44, 61, 74

Ultrasonography

When comparing sonography with arthroscopic findings, Pattee and Snyder[61] found sonography to be sensitive in 77% and specific in 65% of cases, with an accuracy of 73%. The predictive value of a positive sonogram was 82%. In another comparison of arthrography and ultrasonography in degenerative rotator cuff tears,[43] the diagnostic accuracy of arthrography was 87% and of sonography 37%. The diagnosis was confirmed at open surgery.

Sonography has the appeal of being noninvasive and relatively inexpensive, but interpretation requires regular practice and skill not generally available in most communities.[9,12,16,17]

Magnetic Resonance Imaging (MRI)

MRI has been demonstrated to have 83% sensitivity and 85% specificity in differentiating tendinitis from degeneration of the rotator cuff.[32] The method was 100% sensitive and 95% specific in the diagnosis of complete rotator cuff tears.[32] Magnetic resonance testing has been shown to be more accurate than computerized tomography (CT), arthrography, and ultrasonography in identifying partial rotator cuff lesions.[56]

In spite of the many good reports on the diagnostic accuracy of MRI, its major practical disadvantage is the high sensitivity and the "over reading" of tears in the official report (Fig. 9-2). Often, to the patient's consternation, small degenerative lesions are reported as tears. An extensive discussion is necessary to place the report and the actual size and site of the lesion in perspective concerning treatment.

Arthrogram

The arthrogram is most valuable when it shows a rotator cuff tear (Fig. 9-3), but false-negative arthrograms are common.[13,41,66] If the actual tear is small or filled with a

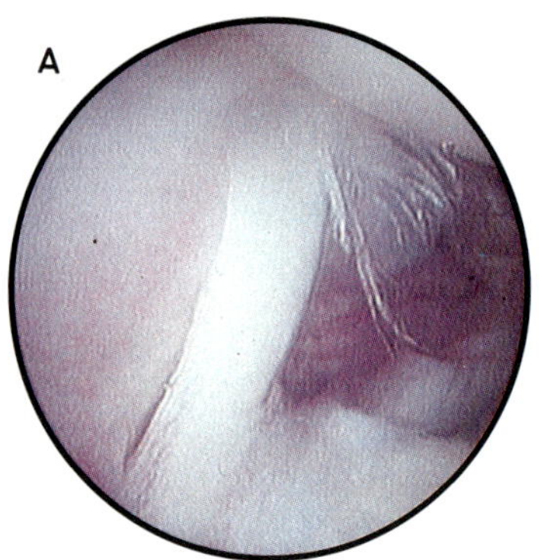

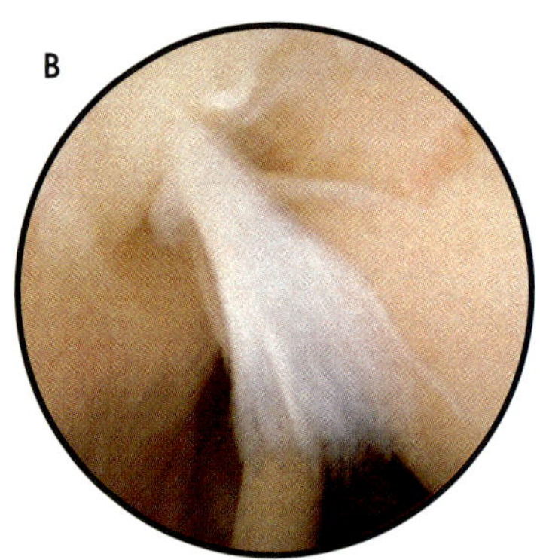

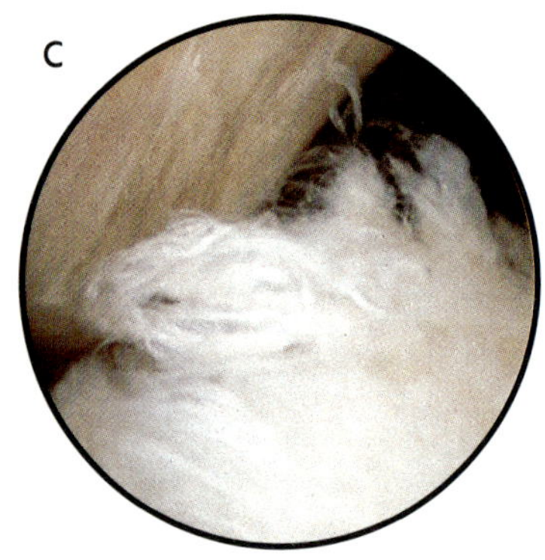

FIG. 9-1 Arthroscopic view demonstrates lesions not otherwise so easily demonstrated.

A Glenohumeral view: Arthroscopic view of biceps shows no separation from the rotator cuff indicating equalization of fluid pressure on each side of the cuff because of complete rotator cuff tear.

B Glenohumeral view: Small undersurface rotator cuff tear.

C Subacromial view: Superior surface rotator cuff tear with erosion under the acromion.

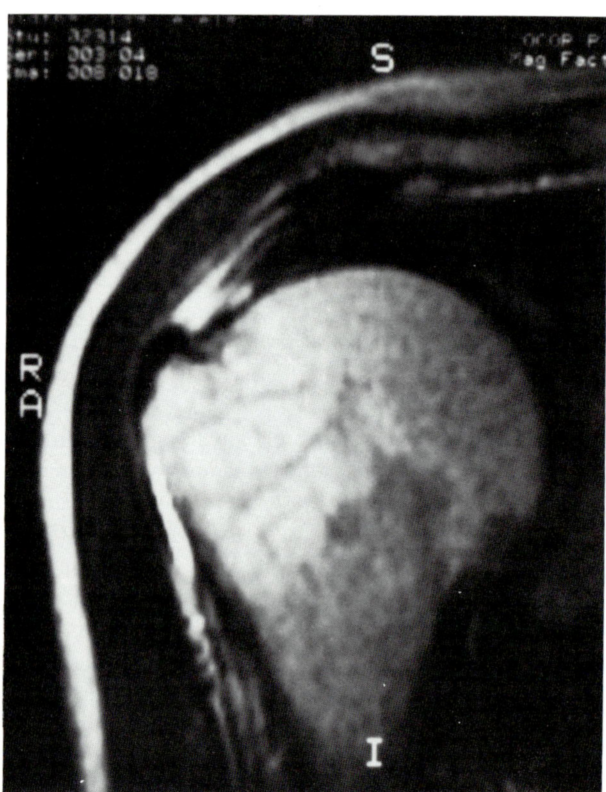

FIG. 9-2 Magnetic resonance imaging. MRI tends to over report rotator cuff tears because of its sensitivity.

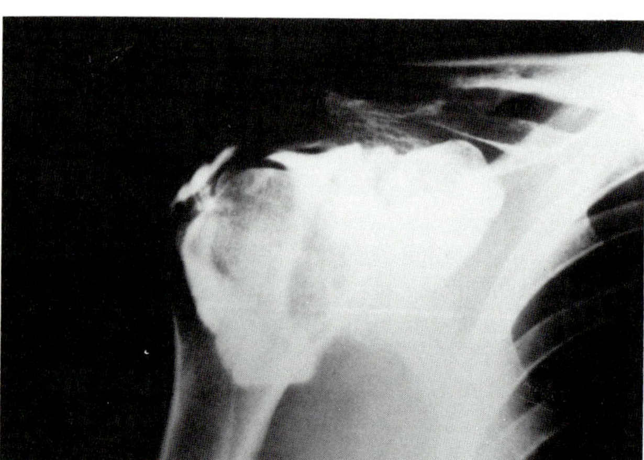

FIG. 9-3 This arthrogram shows extension of dye out of the glenohumeral joint into the layer between the capsular and tendinous portion of the rotator cuff.

clot, scar tissue, or a thin synovial covering, the flow of the dye is blocked. As in knee joint arthrography, the usefulness of shoulder arthrograms decreases as the clinician's arthroscopic skills improve.

Referred patients frequently have had arthrograms, but I rarely request the test when clinical signs indicate that an operative lesion is present.

Bone Scan

The bone scan is especially useful for patients who have had a failed treatment or medicolegal or workers compensation problems. These techniques have been widely used in orthopedics.[75] An excellent review of radionuclide techniques is in Chapter 14 of the Resnick and Niwayama textbook, *Diagnosis of Bone and Joint Disorders*.[67] Thomas et al have reported on the use of bone scan for preoperative screening in orthopedic patients with osteoarthritis of the knee.[75]

I have used radionuclide techniques in patients with shoulder problems. If the bone scan of a patient with chronic problems is negative and the history, physical examination, and x-ray results are negative, it is highly unlikely that an intraarticular pathological problem would be identifiable, let alone treatable. The bone scan may show whether the shoulder joint, the cervical spine, or the acromioclavicular (AC) area is involved. This exact localization of joint involvement is helpful in determining the extent of resection in debridement procedures (Fig. 9-4). Another example involves the AC joint (see Chapter 10). If the AC joint has a normal bilateral bone scan, then decompression of the acromion is restricted to the local area and coracoacromial (CA) ligament. If the AC joint shows increased uptake, then resection extends from the underside of the acromion and into the AC joint. In difficult diagnostic problems or previously operated joints, the benefit of bone scan localization is important.

DIAGNOSTIC ARTHROSCOPY

Diagnostic arthroscopy should precede or accompany every surgical intervention on this region of the shoulder. The interior structures of the glenohumeral joint, subacromial space, and AC joint are visualized by arthroscopy, thereby providing direct evidence of their status. The information gained by direct viewing of these anatomical areas is not possible by any other means (Fig. 9-5). Arthroscopy provides a more comprehensive view of the interior of these joints than the widest open surgical exposure, short of disarticulation or complete acromionectomy. An added benefit of arthroscopy is the inspection of anatomical structures in situ that is uninterrupted by the surgical dissection. Functional relationships can be appreciated with viewing while taking the shoulder through a range of motion. Arthroscopic probing of the various anatomical structures is still possible, even though the joint has not

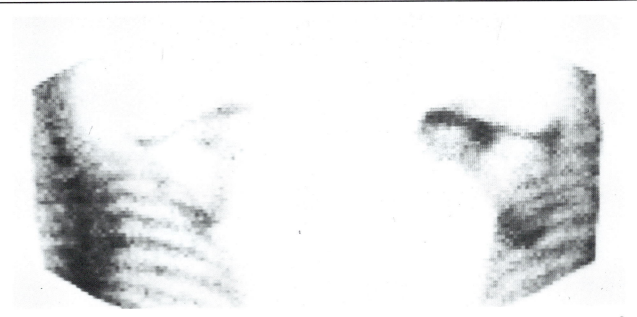

FIG. 9-4 Bone scan is helpful in localizing reactive area in shoulder region.

A Right shoulder has minimal reaction.

B Left shoulder shows increased uptake of radioisotope in coracoid process area and the acromion. No reaction is seen in the glenohumeral joint.

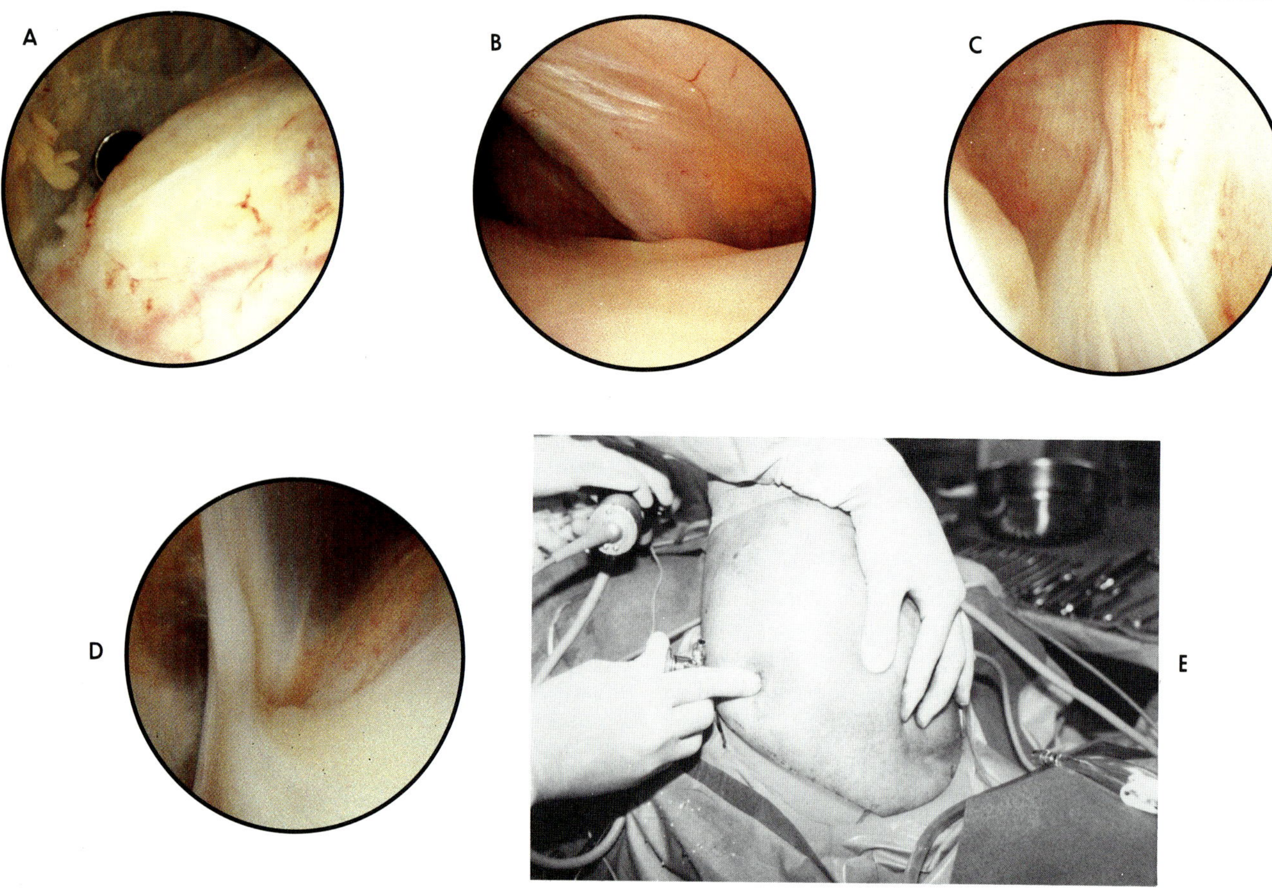

FIG. 9-5 Normal subacromial space.

A Vessels are seen on superior surface of the rotator cuff.

B The prominent normal CA ligament extends under the acromion.

C The free span of the CA ligament is covered with a thin normal fibrous band as it exits the space.

D Fibrous bands, very much like the plica in the knee, often span the space.

E Palpation of obturator under free span of normal CA ligament assists in finding normal bursa.

been opened (Fig. 9-6). Intraarticular documentation can be permanently recorded on videotape.

Diagnostic arthroscopy for impingement syndrome or rotator cuff disease must include inspection of both the glenohumeral joint and the subacromial space. This dual inspection rules out or confirms other intraarticular abnormalities. It also provides a means of visualizing both above and below the rotator cuff (see Fig. 9-1). The AC joint's juxtaposition to the subacromial space can be located with palpation or needle placement (see Fig. 9-27, *A*). Arthroscopic palpation is used to identify bony prominence of acromial spur and AC undersurface osteophytes.

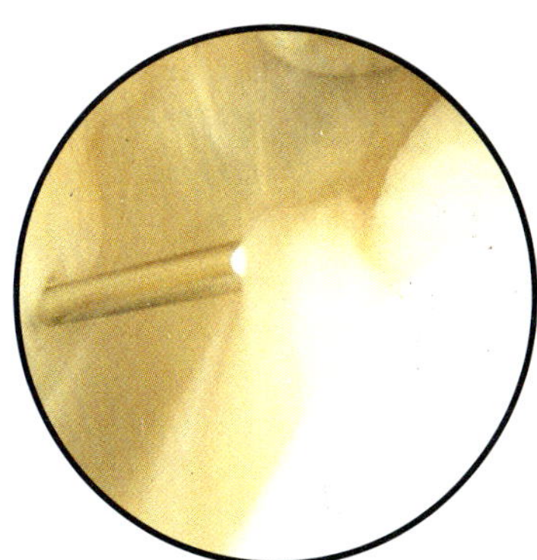

FIG. 9-6 Palpation. Palpation of the subacromial structures is possible with a needle (as shown here) or with a probe.

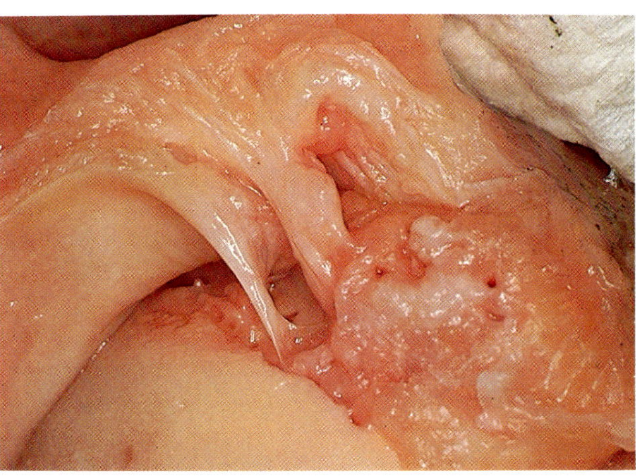

FIG. 9-7 Rotator cuff anatomy. This gross dissection shows the three layers: a synovial layer, capsule, and tendinous portion.

A

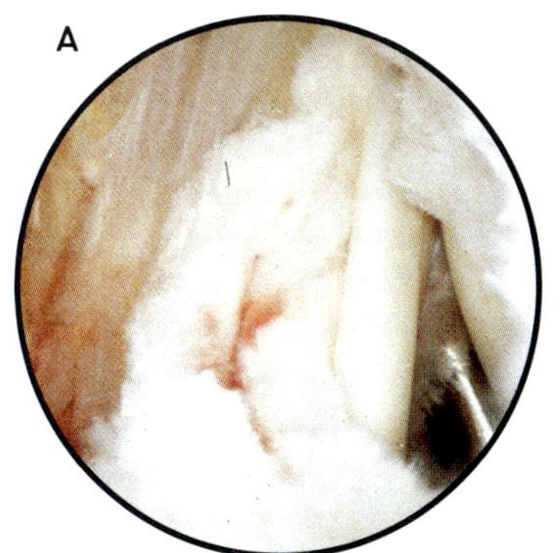

B

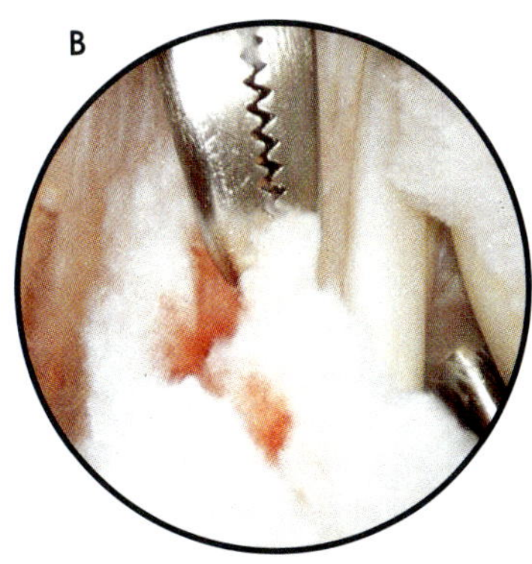

C

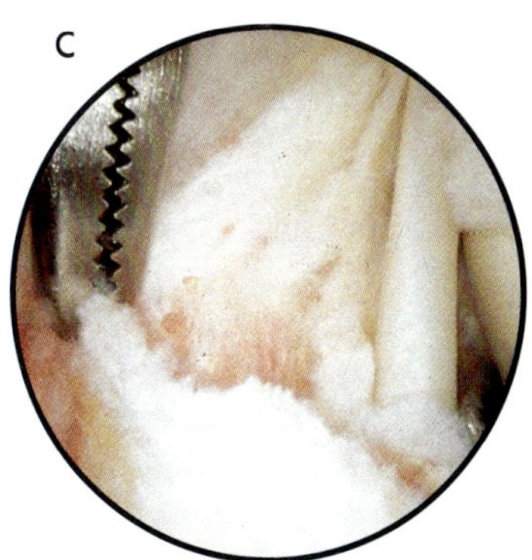

FIG. 9-8 Arthroscopic perspective of various layers of rotator cuff.

A Two portions of the rotator cuff with tendon to the left and capsule to the right. The biceps tendon is seen deep in the picture.

B Grasper pulling on the capsular portion.

C Grasper pulling on the tendinous portion.

Rotator Cuff Anatomy

An appreciation of normal arthroscopic anatomy is necessary to appreciate rotator cuff disease.[35] The rotator cuff is made up of three distinct layers that can be illustrated by anatomical dissection (Fig. 9-7). The synovial layer is to the joint side. A distinct capsular layer provides static stability. The tendon layer is superior. These layers are appreciated only if a rotator cuff tear is present (Fig. 9-8). A partial tear penetrates successively the synovial, capsular, and tendinous layers. The arthrogram may also demonstrate these layers when dye extravasates between the capsular and tendinous layers, but does not extend to the subacromial bursa (see Fig. 9-3).

To examine this area, the patient is positioned the same as for glenohumeral arthroscopy (see Chapter 8). A routine skin preparation and sterile drapes are applied to expose the surgical area. Television imaging and recording is routine.

A 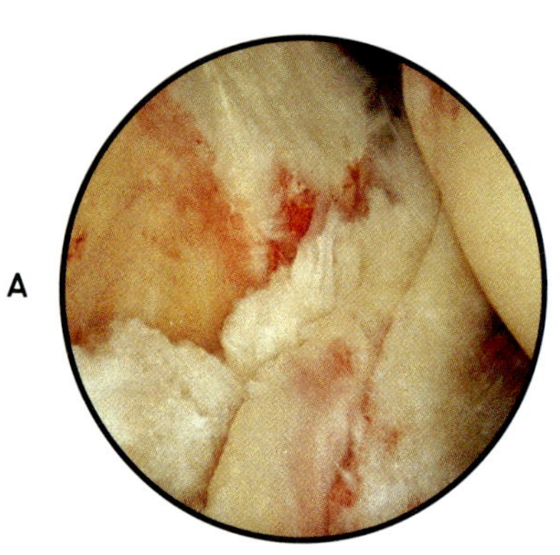

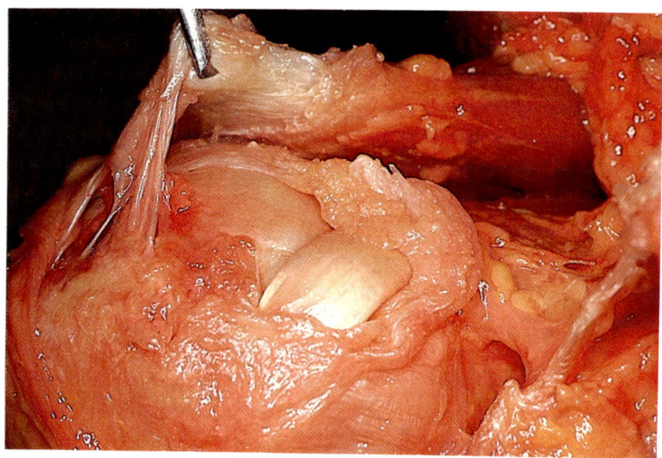 B

FIG. 9-9 Large rotator cuff tear.

A Arthroscopic view shows humerus to the right, biceps in center area, and large hole in cuff showing undersurface of the acromion.

B Gross dissection of cadaver specimen demonstrates exposed biceps tendon and the humeral head.

Glenohumeral Joint Inspection

Four glenohumeral joint observations are relevant to the rotator cuff. Inspection may show failure of the undersurface of the rotator cuff area to displace away from the biceps tendon, indicating a complete tear of the cuff (see Fig. 9-1, *A*). This occurs because of the equalization of fluid pressure on both sides of the cuff caused by the communication between the glenohumeral joint and the subacromial space.

Another glenohumeral joint finding is the partial-thickness undersurface rotator cuff tear (see Fig. 9-1, *B*). The small rotator cuff tear may be a complication of previous arthroscopy.[58]

A transverse thickening of the capsule under the rotator cuff tendon is a normal structure (see Fig. 6-19). The band is halfway from the glenoid to the tendinous attachment of the cuff to the humerus. It is a thickening in the capsular portion of the cuff and does not represent a rotator cuff tear. Anatomical dissection of the capsule shows the capsular thickenings.[12] The location of rotator cuff tears is lateral and distal to this structure.

A large rotator cuff tear is easy to identify by visualization (Fig. 9-9). In the large tear the arthroscope can enter the subacromial space from the glenohumeral joint.

The biceps tendon may be torn, fragmented, or ruptured (see Fig. 9-17).[53]

Subacromial Space Approach

The initial approach to the subacromial space uses the same skin puncture that was used for the glenohumeral arthroscopy (Fig. 9-10). The scope is removed from the glenohumeral joint. Preliminary distention of the bursae is not practical because its normal size is small and the synovial walls are not well-defined for palpation with a needle. One of the pathologic conditions found in the subacromial bursa is fibrous bands (see Fig. 9-14). In this case the space is not well visualized because of the many pathologic fibrous bands. In another pathologic condition, the bursa is large. In this case, entry is easy and attempting

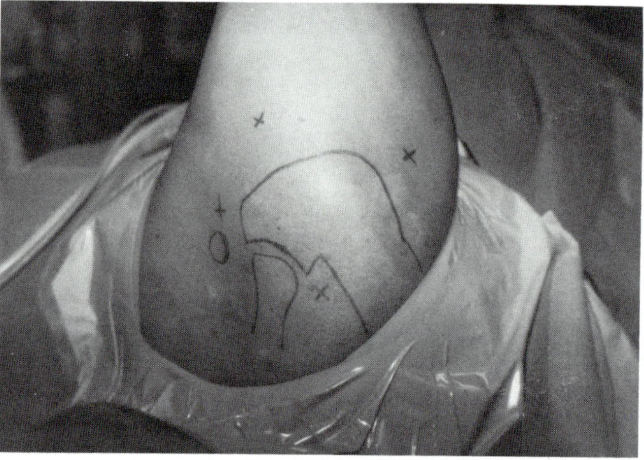

FIG. 9-10 Topographical location of bony structure and the anticipated portals. The outline on the skin shows the anticipated surgical portals marked with "X's" (right shoulder).

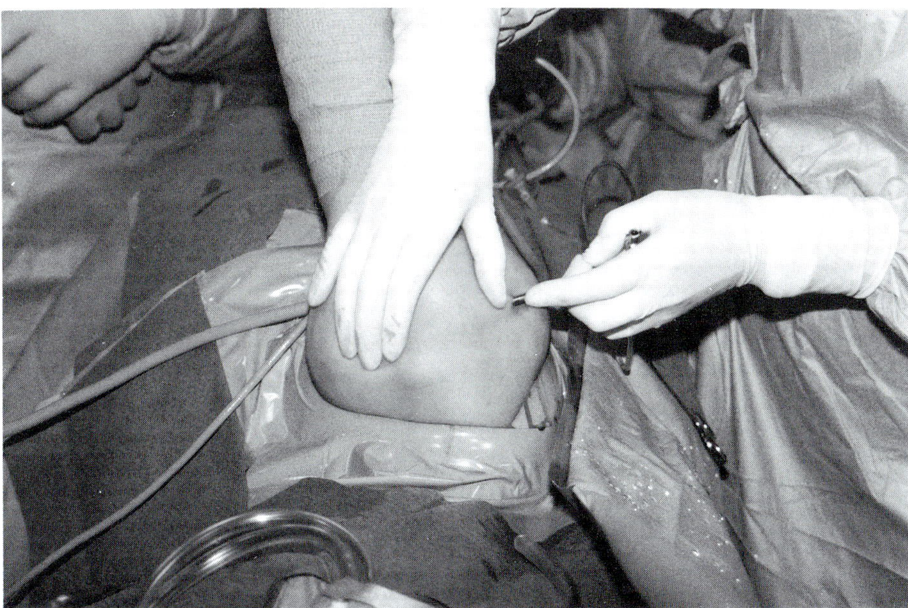

FIG. 9-11 Palpation. The surgeon places one hand on, in front, or on top of the acromion and the other on the cannula/obturator. The surgeon can palpate the underside of the acromion with the instrument or feel the tip of the obturator under the CA ligament on the right shoulder.

preliminary distention is unnecessary. In fact, in very large subacromial bursa, especially with a large rotator cuff tear, the bursa may be inadvertently entered during an attempt at glenohumeral penetration. This has happened to me in patients with rheumatoid arthritis with massive subacromial bursitis.

The entry cannula and obturator are redirected toward the underside of the acromion. The surgeon places one hand on in front or on top of the acromion and the other on the cannula/obturator. The surgeon can palpate the underside of the acromion with the instrument or feel the tip of the obturator under the CA ligament (Fig. 9-11).

Identification of the normal space is difficult because it is small. The normal subacromial bursal space is immediately under the free span of the CA ligament (see Fig. 9-5). For this reason the surgeon's free hand can palpate the obturator tip under the CA ligament as a topographical landmark (Fig. 9-5, *E*).

When entry into the subacromial bursa is difficult, three approaches are used to locate the bursa. The location under the CA ligament is first. Next is the approach under the acromion, with correlative palpation with the free hand. Finally, the arthroscope cannula and obturator aims toward the top of the rotator cuff on the humeral head. Humeral head palpation is assisted by rotation of the humerus and simultaneous palpation with the instrument.

Even with the surgeon's best effort, the normal bursa may not be entered. As a practical matter, I limit my entry tries to three times when clinical suspicion is low for subacromial bursal disease.

When suspicion of subacromial bursal disease is high, entry still may be difficult, especially for the inexperienced surgeon. The area under the acromion can be forcibly enlarged. I rarely resort to this measure because it results in false passage, distortion of normal anatomy, and extravasation of fluids and potentiates intraoperative complications. If you choose this method, entry may be facilitated by placing the cannula/obturator under the acromion by palpation and sweeping side to side, thereby developing a space. An arthroscopic debridement with motorized instrumentation may be required for adequate visualization in this "space." The iatrogenic disruption of tissues may lead to false-positive findings. Worse yet are intraoperative complications as a result of loss of position and "blind" surgical resection. I have consulted on a patient with nonunion created in mid-clavicule because of loss of orientation during arthroscopic acromioplasty (see Fig. 9-28).

Subacromial Space Anatomy

Normal. The normal subacromial bursa is small (see Fig. 9-5; see also Chapter 6).[42] It takes less than 10 ml of fluid. The synovial lining is flat and noninflamed. Folds may be evident across the bursa (Fig. 9-12, *A* and *B*). The folds are curved or circular and are not pathologic. The superior side of the rotator cuff (tendon covered with bursal synovium) may show blood vessels on the surface (see Fig. 9-5, *A*). The underside of the acromion is covered by an extension of the CA ligament (see Fig. 9-5, *B*). The ligament is white or yellow-white, and smooth. It is 1 cm wide, up to 4 cm long, and 0.5 cm in depth. The free span of the CA ligament is extra bursal (see Fig. 9-5, *C*). The normal AC joint is not seen or easily palpated from the subacromial bursa. Palpation of the structures in the subacromial space enhances the diagnostic evaluation. Identifying the underside of the AC joint may be assisted by placing a No. 18 spinal needle through the skin from superior into the joint and through into the subacromial bursa (Fig. 9-13).

Pathologic. The lining may be inflamed, with villus synovitis and prominent vascularity. The normal plica are often torn, appearing as fibrous bands (Fig. 9-14; see also Chapter 7).

Arthroscopic confirmation of impingement may be seen with erosion on the superior rotator cuff (tendon portion) or on the underside of the acromion with erosion or disruption of the CA ligament tissue (Fig. 9-15; see also Fig. 9-1, *C*). In more severe or larger rotator cuff tears, the CA ligament may be eroded, exposing the bone of the acromion (Fig. 9-16). I have not yet seen erosion or disruption of the free span of the CA ligament with impingement or in any other circumstance.[77]

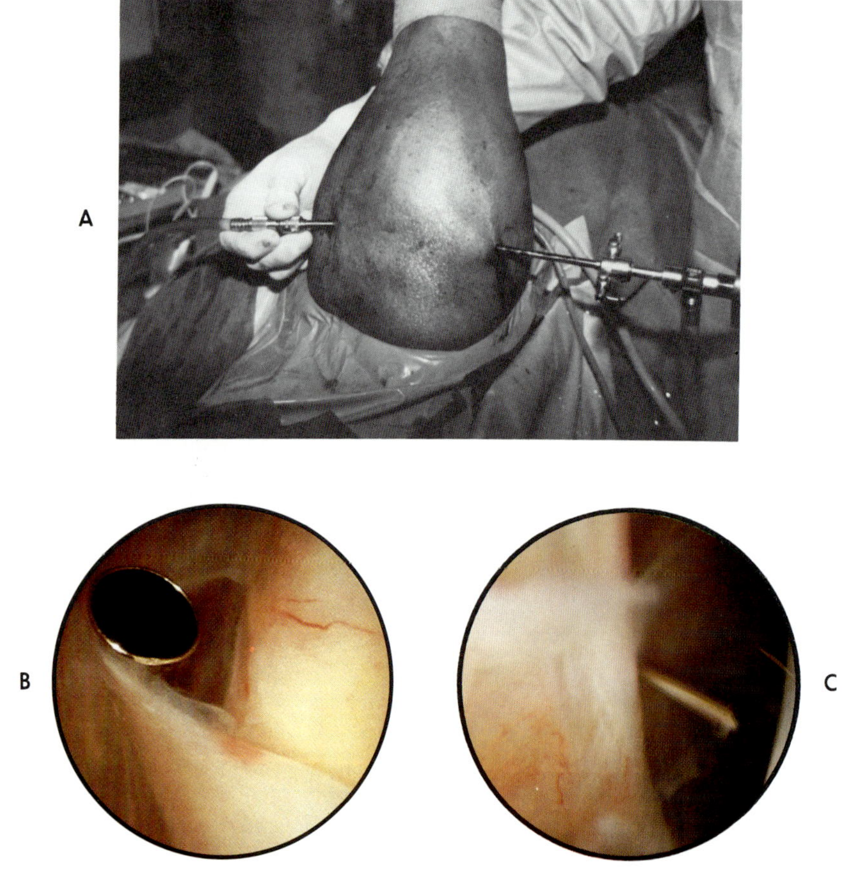

FIG. 9-12 Palpation in subacromial bursa.

A The scope is from posterior and the inflow cannula is to the left and anterior. Palpation is possible with the inflow cannula (right shoulder).

B Cannula under a normal fibrous band in the subacromial bursa.

C Needle in large bursa adjacent to CA ligament.

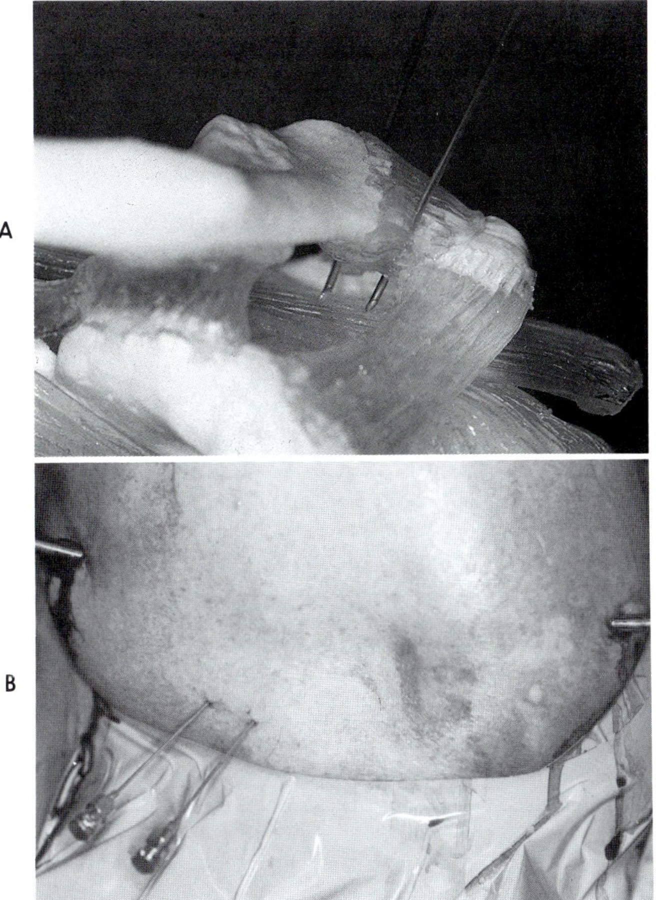

FIG. 9-13 Needle location of acromioclavicular joint.

A Needle placement shown on a plastic model.

B Outside view shows transcutaneous needle placement. The scope is to right, inflow to left (anterior) in right shoulder.

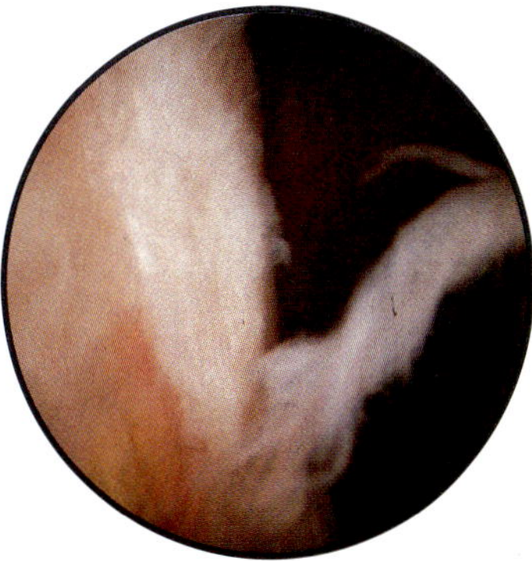

FIG. 9-14 Fragmentation and disruption of normal bursal fibrous bands occurs with impingement syndrome.

A 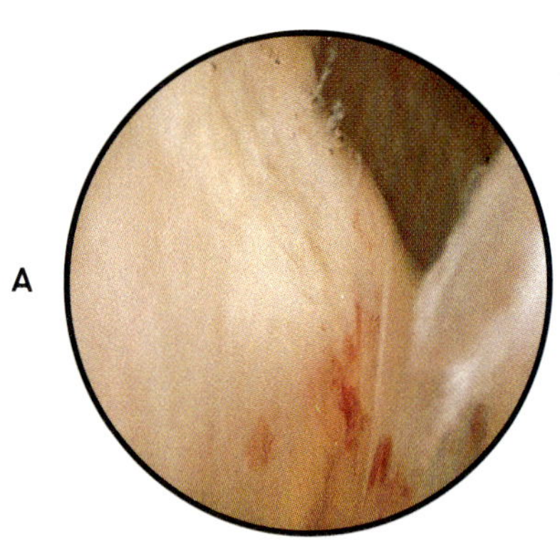

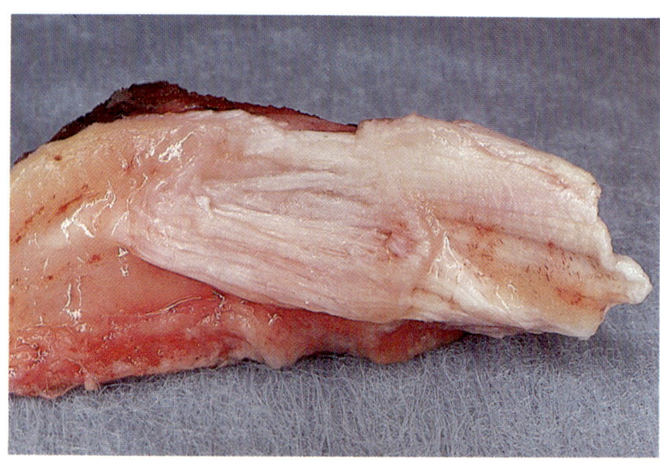 B

FIG. 9-15 Subacromial erosion of impingement.

A CA ligament eroded under the acromion. The red blood staining on the free span of the ligament was iatrogenic.

B Gross surgical specimen taken by open acromioplasty shows the junction of the uneroded free span of the ligament and the disrupted ligament in area of impingement.

A 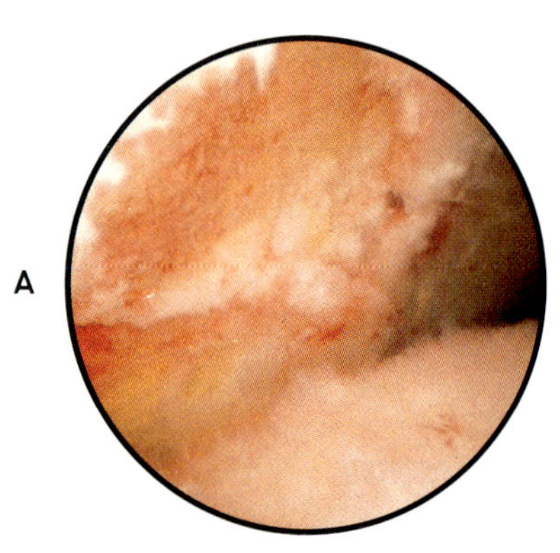

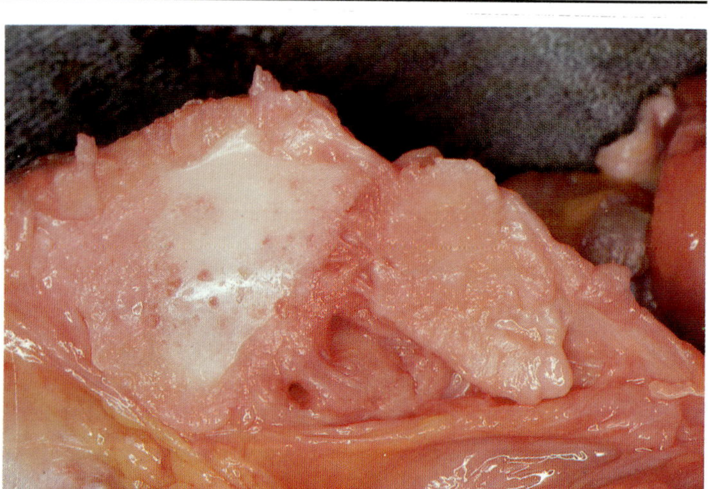 B

FIG. 9-16 Chronic impingement shows bone exposed on acromion.

A Erosion exposing bone under the acromion.

B Gross specimen of a similar condition shows exposed bone and extra osteophyte of the acromial spur to the right.

A large rotator cuff tear will expose the biceps tendon from above. The large opening will permit viewing down into the glenohumeral joint from above (Fig. 9-17, *A;* see also Fig. 9-8, *A*).

In severe long-standing rotator cuff disease, the humeral head and the underside of the acromion are in contact, resulting in bony erosion on both sides (see Fig. 9-16, *A*).

The biceps tendon may be exposed, permitting a grasping forceps to pull the tendon out of the groove and into the joint to evaluate the extent of tendon disruption.[53] The rotator cuff tendon and capsule may be separately identified (see Fig. 9-8, *A* and *B*). Grasping the layers of the cuff tear margins will demonstrate its mobility and evaluate the suitability for repair (see Fig. 9-8, *A* and *B*).

A rotator cuff tear may be partial or complete and small or large. The partial lesion may be only on the superior aspect (see Fig. 9-1, *B*). Probing will confirm the extent of most partial tears. Often debridement of the shaggy fragmentation adjacent to the tear is necessary to identify its size and extent (Fig. 9-18). In some cases the extent of the lesion can be determined only by injection of dilute methylene blue dye (Fig. 9-19).[26] The dye is injected into the glenohumeral joint while viewing from the superior side in the subacromial space. If communication exists, the dye injected under pressure will find its way to the subacromial space, thereby confirming the complete tear (Fig. 9-19, *B*).

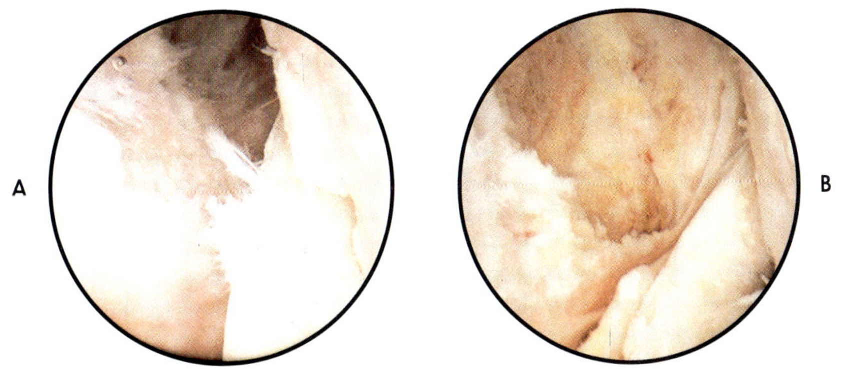

FIG. 9-17 Biceps exposed through large rotator cuff tear and seen from the bursal side.

A Kissing lesion of disrupted biceps tendon and the acromion.

B Post-acromioplasty status in same patient shows biceps cleaned of fragmentation and wider separation of acromion because of resection of bone.

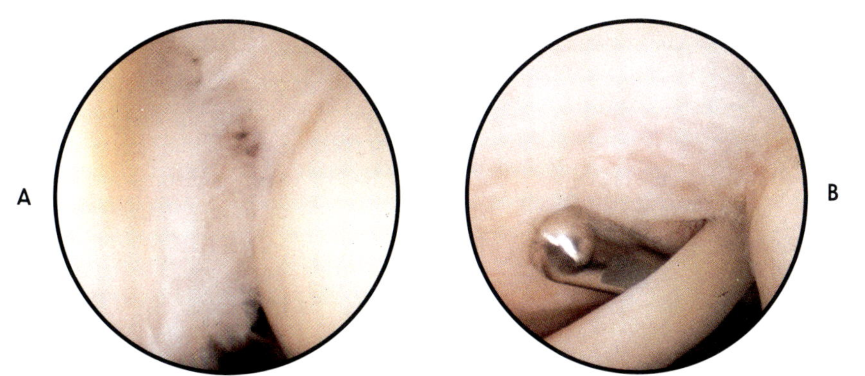

FIG. 9-18 Glenohumeral debridement.

A Arthroscopic view of shaggy undersurface tear of rotator cuff partial tear.

B Completion of debridement in same patient with use of motorized instrumentation.

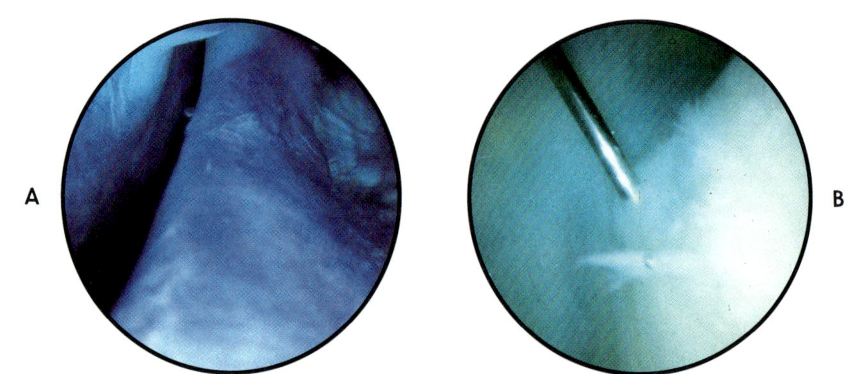

FIG. 9-19 Methylene blue dye injection exposes occult full thickness lesion.

A Arthroscopic view of glenohumeral joint shows biceps tendon.

B Simultaneous viewing within the subacromial bursa shows small leakage of dye near area of superior surface rotator cuff tear. Needle is palpating the superior cuff tear.

OPERATIVE ARTHROSCOPY

Arthroscopic operative procedures are adaptations of established open operations. The arthroscopic procedures are categorized as debridement, repair, acromioplasty, and reconstruction. The basic indications are the same as for the open procedures. The minimal morbidity of arthroscopy, coupled with the enhanced diagnostic sensitivity demonstrating smaller lesions, has resulted in earlier intervention and treatment of lesions of lesser magnitude.

Glenohumeral Joint Debridement Procedures Associated with Rotator Cuff or Subacromial Lesion

Glenohumeral debridement procedures are performed on small labrum tears, partial-thickness rotator cuff tears, partial-thickness biceps tendon tears, biceps tendon stumps, and coexistent synovial inflammation (see Fig. 9-18).[3] Loose bodies may be removed.

The glenohumeral techniques are more fully described in Chapter 8. The rotator cuff tear is debrided to determine the extent of the lesion or for therapeutic removal of the fragmentation. The partial-thickness undersurface rotator cuff defect should be debrided (see Fig. 9-18). In full-thickness lesions the margins are debrided before inspection from above. Other glenohumeral structures are also debrided (i.e., biceps tendon and labrum) (see Fig. 9-17).

Subacromial Bursa Debridement Procedures

Debridement procedures in the subacromial space include removing partial-thickness superior rotator cuff tears, resecting calcific tendonitis, clearing transbursal fibrosis, and bursectomy. Acromioplasty, AC joint resection, and clavicular bone removal are performed by arthroscopic debridement.

For all these procedures, the arthroscope is initially placed from posterior. If a communication exists between the glenohumeral joint and the subacromial space because of a complete rotator cuff tear, the anterior glenohumeral joint cannula is left in place for temporary inflow. This inflow will provide distention for subacromial bursal entry. If no communication exists between the joint and the bursa, then an anterior inflow will be established after arthroscope position is established.

After subacromial space entry is confirmed, an anterior portal is established lateral to the free span of the CA ligament by the Wissinger rod technique (see Fig. 9-12, *A*). A cannula is placed in this anterior portal for initial fluid inflow. The previously placed glenohumeral inflow cannula is not necessary and is removed.

The initial operative portal for the subacromial bursa is lateral (anterior). It is established with use of a No. 18 spinal needle (Fig. 9-20, *A*). A cannula for motorized instrumentation is placed along the same plane as the needle

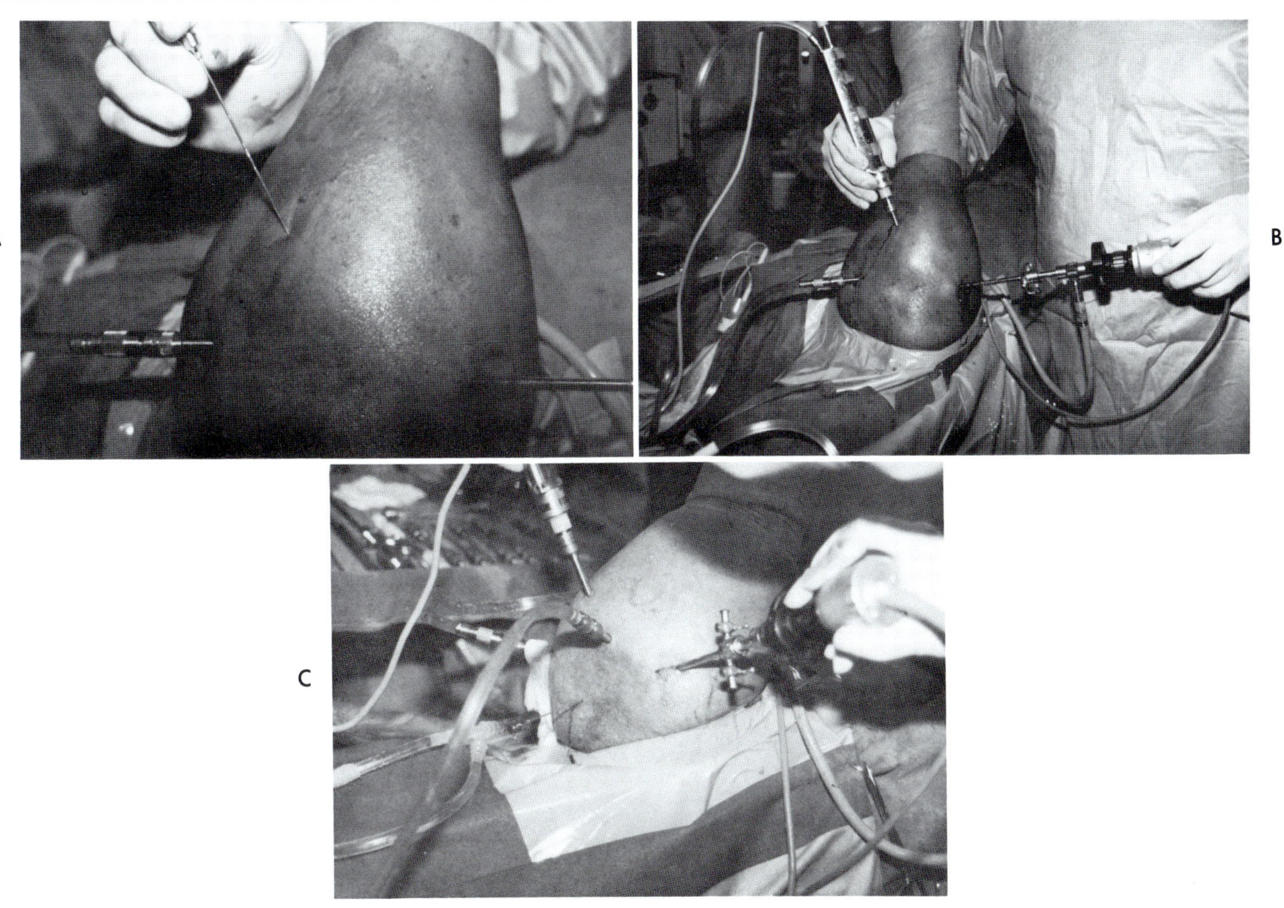

FIG. 9-20 Operative portal for arthroscopic acromioplasty.

A Location of needle placement during trial and error selection of topographical site for cannula placement (right shoulder).

B Arthroscope is placed posterior, the inflow is anterior, and the instrument portal is anterior and lateral (right shoulder).

C Alternate additional outflow is shown between arthroscope and motorized instrument portal. Needle locates AC joint. Inflow is from anterior (left shoulder).

(Fig. 9-20, *B*). Interchangability of these three portals is essential for both adequate arthroscopic visualization and surgery. The specifics will be discussed under each procedure.

Specific Procedures

Resection of Calcific Tendonitis. This is not a common surgical procedure. The condition is either self limiting or easily treated by an office procedure of transcutaneous needling and aspiration lavage. Either the calcium mass or the area of acute tenderness is easily palpable. Under sterile technique, the area is entered with a No. 18 needle and 20-ml syringe with 1% Lidocaine. When the area is entered, the calcium residue is washed out with intermittent ballotement with pushing on the syringe plunger (Fig. 9-21, *A*). This same method may be used under arthroscopic control to identify the lesion, before resection of a large calcific mass.

Surgical removal is indicated when a patient fails to resolve the painful symptoms of the calcium deposit with conservative treatment or when motion is restricted by a large mass.

If surgery is contemplated, then internal and external rotational plain film x-rays assist in locating the mass anteriorly in the supraspinatus tendon or posteriorly in the infraspinatus tendon (Fig. 9-21, *B* to *F*). The biceps tendon may be calcified in the bony bicipital groove. Calcium is sometimes seen in the subscapularis tendon. The latter two

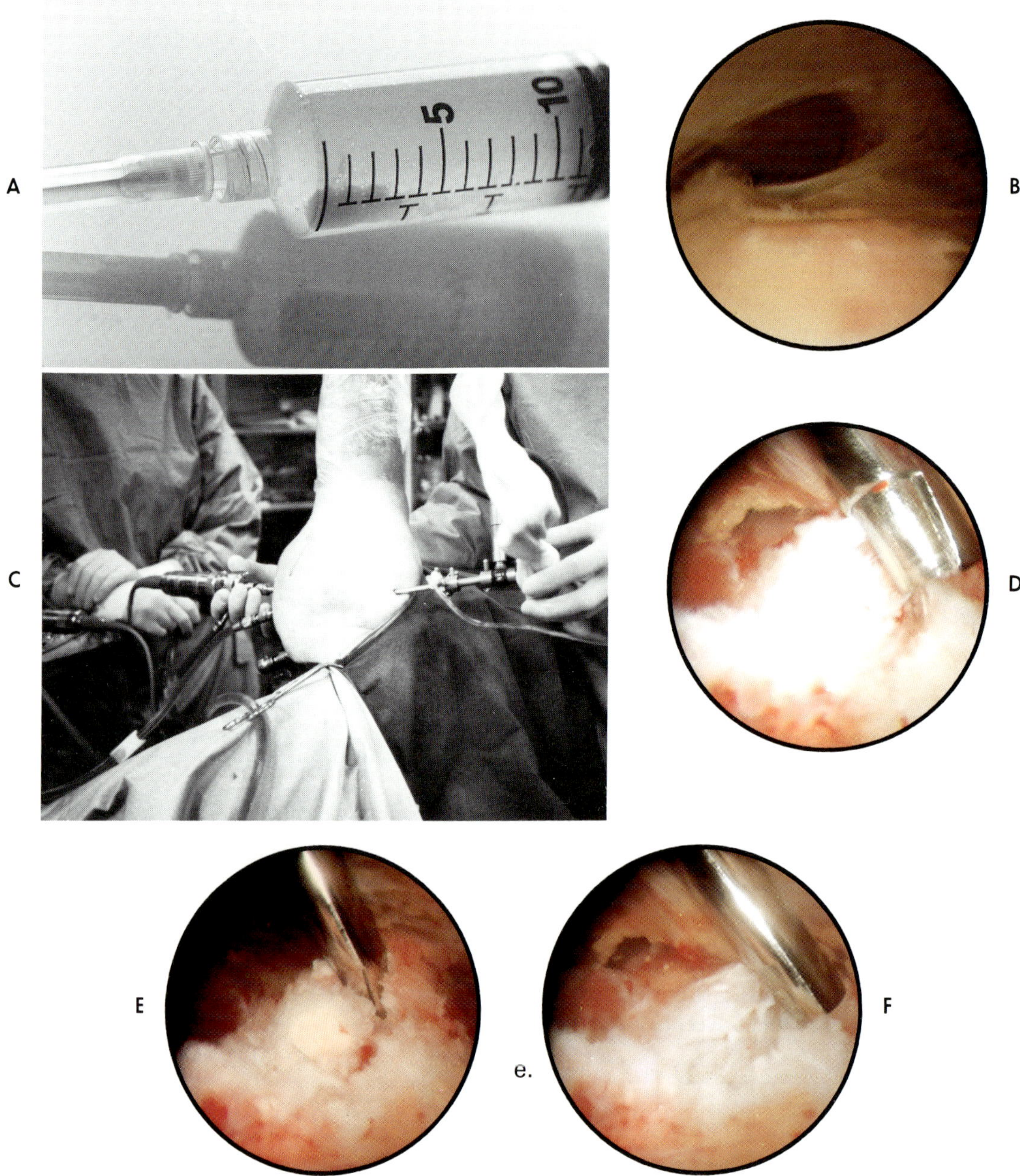

FIG. 9-21 Arthroscopic surgical treatment of calcific tendonitis.

A Calcium residue in syringe after wash out with ballotement irrigation technique as office procedure.

B Bursal space with calcific deposit seen in top of rotator cuff.

C Familiar arthroscopic environment with suspended upper extremity. Instruments are directed to subacromial bursae.

D Cutter in calcium deposit.

E Further resection of calcium mass.

F Small partial superior cuff defect after calcium removal.

locations may require open surgical exposure. The calcium mass in the infraspinatus or supraspinatus tendon is accessible to arthroscopic identification and debridement.

The standard arthroscopic approach to the subacromial space is used (Fig. 9-21, *C*). Entrance into the subacromial space does not expose the calcific deposit. Palpation of the cuff area may demonstrate a hard mass, but frankly, differentiating the humeral greater tuberosity and any calcium mass is difficult. For that reason, I prefer to use a No. 18 spinal needle for the probing, which permits penetrating the bursal lining and tendon. Entry into the calcium deposit is confirmed by a "crunchy" feel with the needle. Penetration may cause small calcium pieces to exit and float in the fluid medium in the subacromial space. On one occasion penetration of the mass resulted in extrusion of calcium in the form of paste. It looked similar to an extrusion of toothpaste. In a rare case, identification may require a superficial debridement of the bursal floor and the superior tendon. When I have had difficulty in locating the mass, it was more posterior than I expected. The surgical approach required the arthroscope to be moved to the anterior portal and the instrumentation to the posterior portal.

Once the area of the mass is confirmed, the mass is opened with a motorized instrument (Fig. 9-21, *D* to *F*). Weber[78] reported the use of intraoperative fluoroscopy to localize the calcium. This approach took an average of 2.2 minutes, which is faster than the hunt-and-peck, trial-and-error method.

The postoperative treatment is early mobilization. The results in my cases are good.

Snyder, Eppley, and Brewster[72] reported on 13 such shoulder surgeries in 12 patients (1 was bilateral). Immediate postoperative plain film x-rays showed complete removal of all calcium. They seldom performed a subacromial decompression. After 1- to 5-year follow-up, all patients had full range of motion. Three had no pain and 10 had slight pain with overhead strenuous activity. All patients had excellent to good results.

Weber[78] reported a series of 24 patients with calcium resection who had accompanying acromioplasty. The mean follow-up was 12.8 months. Using a UCLA scoring system, 20 patients had excellent results, 3 good, and 1 fair. No calcium was seen on subsequent x-ray films. No complications were reported.

Isolated Resection of Coracoacromial Ligament. Pujadas[64] presented a scientific exhibit at the American Academy of Orthopedic Surgeons in 1970 on the Coracoacromial Ligament Syndrome. He reported that the greater tuberosity does not impinge against the acromion, but rather against the free edge of the CA ligament. He recommended open resection of the ligament for chronic impingement syndrome.

The traditional clinical impression that the free span of this ligament is involved in impingement syndrome is not borne out by my arthroscopic observations.[34] The erosion is on the ligament as it extends under the acromion. I have yet to see the free span of the ligament have any sign of erosion or impingement. The misunderstanding of its involvement probably came from the clinical observation of pain production with palpation of the ligament. Simultaneous palpation of the ligament and arthroscopic viewing shows the impulse of the palpation to be transmitted through the free span of the ligament to the ligament attached to underside of the acromion. This transmission of impulse causes motion of the eroded CA ligament on the underside of the acromion and hence the production of pain. Resection of the free span of the ligament would not remedy the area of impingement under the acromion or of the prominant acromion. Thus it is not a surprise that resection of the CA ligament alone for impingement syndrome is no longer reported. In the past, I performed this procedure on a few occasions in the absence of impingement erosion on the acromion without subsequent patient benefit.

Additional evidence of the futility of isolated CA ligament resection is that in the few cases I have seen following this procedure, the ligament regrew with a fibrous band of tissue in the same area and the erosion was seen on the acromion. The isolated resection of the CA ligament is rarely indicated. The arthroscopic findings would support Neer's position of anterior acromial impingement (Fig. 9-22, *B*).

Arthroscopic Subacromial Bursectomy. The subacromial bursectomy is rarely performed as an isolated procedure. It is an essential part of any other surgery performed in this area. The debridement provides adequate visualization and removal of inflammed tissue.

For subacromial bursectomy, the surgical portals are positioned as illustrated in Fig. 9-20. It must be said that the initiation of debridement before identification of bursal entry is fraught with danger. After bursal entry, visualization may require debridement to clear the space of fibrous bands. Removal of the bursa enlarges the space for adequate viewing. An important area to be resected is posterior and adjacent to the arthroscope. The cleansed and enlarged bursa allows the arthroscope to be placed at a distance to gain an overview of this space.

Enlargement of space. In addition to improved viewing, the enlargement creates a larger space to hold fluid volume. The creation of a larger volume within the surgical site decreases the chance of decompression during suction with motorized instrumentation. Nevertheless, additional flow and volume are still needed and are supplied with the use of a Gravity Assist hand pump.

Avoidance of clogging of motorized instruments. Stephen Snyder has suggested an additional outflow and suction be used to remove fragments and reduce work stoppage (Fig. 9-20, *C*). The use of a separate cannula for discharge of acromial fragments has some advantages. It allows for continuous flow of fluids and fragmentation without concern over clogging of motorized instrumentation. This advantage is offset by several disadvantages.

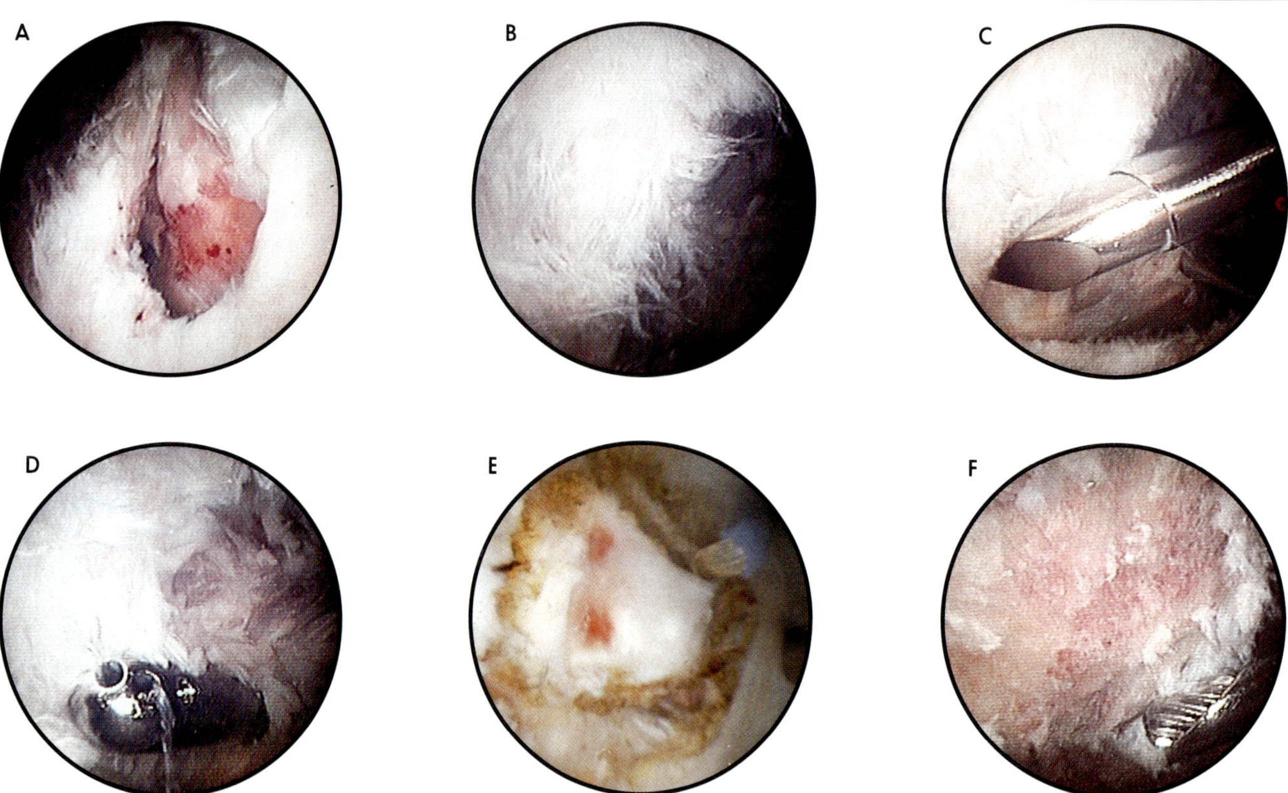

FIG. 9-22 Step-by-step approach to arthroscopic acromioplasty.

A Bursal view of 2 × 2 cm rotator cuff tear.

B Shaggy undersurface of the acromion demonstrates positive evidence of impingement.

C Arthroscopic cannula and trocar enters the joint from anterior and lateral portal in a plane that places it under acromion.

D Motorized instrumentation with whisker-cutting head cleans up shaggy synovium and minimizes bleeding.

E Electrocautery is used to outline the area of anticipated resection. This includes area of erosion.

F Acromionizer removing soft tissue and bone.

First and foremost is the disbursement of fragments throughout the subacromial space on their way to the outflow cannula. Many of the bone spicules will attach to the bursal lining, requiring subsequent debridement. In addition, special attention must be given to the motorized instrument end of this set-up. There must be double suction, one to instrument and one to outflow cannula. In this case the outflow lever on instrument must be shut off to avoid clogging. If one suction is used, it then must be switched from instrument to cannula and back. The outflow on the instrument must be closed. If acromionizer is switched to full radius resector, then suction must be reapplied to the motorized instrument. The multiple switching of outflow and suction is no faster in my hands than occasionally switching a clogged burr or acromionizer. I have two acromionizers in each set-up to facilitate this move.

The advantage of not having outflow cannula includes direct removal of debris from acromionizer that avoids disbursement of fragments. The second benefit is that the tissue is pulled up under tension for resection and removal, a basic principle of use of motorized instrumentation.

Hemostasis. Hemostasis in the subacromial space is

accomplished in several ways. Dilute adrenaline solution only during the diagnostic phase, intraoperative pressure of fluid distention, and electrocautery can be used. To protect against unmeasured infusion of adrenaline solution, I restrict its use to the diagnostic phase of the procedure. A mechanical means of increased flow and pressure to control bleeding increases the potential for extravasation of fluid, including massive swelling that will interfere with or conclude surgery. I use the manual Gravity Assist bulb to avoid unmonitored delivery of fluid. Electrocautery is provided by a standard Bovie system and an inexpensive coagulator (see Chapter 3). Electrocautery with this system requires a temporary change of fluid medium to sterile water to facilitate electroconductivity.

Electrocautery is the best method of hemostasis in this area. This technique accomplishes several tasks. First, it provides a landmark that would not otherwise be present once the acromioplasty is underway. The outlined landmark provides a guide to the amount of acromion to be resected (Fig. 9-22, *E*). The acromial attachment of the CA ligament is released with the electrocautery. This technique prophylactically stops bleeding in this area during subsequent resection.

Arthroscopic Acromioplasty. The pathologic evidence of erosion of the acromion should be present to confirm the diagnosis of impingement and to consider anterior-inferior acromioplasty. Acromioplasty is very amenable to arthroscopic methods. A radical acromioplasty is not indicated by either open or arthroscopic method.[55] A system of resection is important as orientation is difficult in the subacromial space. Once the resection of the acromion commences, visual orientation may become more difficult. The method of outlining the acromion with the electrocautery is important to maintaining future orientation (Fig. 9-22, *E*).

A systematic, step-by-step resection of bone is necessary (Fig. 9-22). The arthroscope is posterior, the inflow anterior, and the instrument portal lateral (see Fig. 9-20).

In step 1, the subacromial synovial bands are removed and the bursal space is carefully enlarged to enhance visualization (Fig. 9-22, *D*).

In step 2, electrocautery is used to outline the area of acromion to be resected (Fig. 9-22, *E*).

In step 3, soft tissue is cleaned off the acromion. Superficial material is removed with a whisker-cutting head to minimize debridement and bleeding (Fig. 9-22, *D*). The thicker soft tissue under the acromion in resected with a 5.5-mm cutter head. The instrumentation is changed to a full-thickness resector to clean off the underside of the bone. When the acromion is cleaned of soft tissue to the margins of the previously outlined area of anticipated resection, the cutting head is changed to the acromionizer (Fig. 9-22, *F*).

In step 4, the initial resection of acromion removes the bone anterior in line with the anterior clavicle. This step creates a vertical line from medial to lateral on the acromion, as set forth by Rockwood (Fig. 9-23, *A*).[69] Care must be taken not to resect beyond the bone and inadvertently release the deltoid fascia from the acromion in this anterior area. This bone/tendon junction is both visible and palpable during the resection of bone.

The acromial bone may extend into the AC ligament. If such a bone spur exists, resection should extend into the CA ligament. The junction of bone and ligament is differentially resected with a burr-type cutter on bone. The burr will not cut soft tissue. The soft tissue may be shredded; if so, it may be subsequently smoothed with a full-radius synovial resector.

In step 5, the anterior to posterior acromioplasty is performed (Fig. 9-23, *B*). The bony acromioplasty commences at the previous anterior margin of resection. The resection systematically extends from anterior to posterior. The anticipated plane of resection will be sloped from anterior to posterior, with the greatest depth anterior and the lesser depth posterior. The resection requires side-to-side motions of the motorized instrumentation (Fig. 9-24). The motion is a systematic "wiping." The bone should be removed "layer by layer," taking care not to create a concave surface during acromioplasty. Failure to attend to this detail may result in thinning of the bone in one area and a stress riser for a subsequent fracture (Fig. 9-23, *D*).

In step 6, inflow and instrumentation are interchanged. The first portal change I use is to interchange the inflow and the instrument portal. This maneuver places the cutting instrument anterior and in a plane that avoids creating a concavity of the acromion (Fig. 9-23, *D*). An additional benefit is that the anterior portal advantageously approaches the undersurface of the AC joint (Fig. 9-25). The undersurface of the acromion is leveled from the anterior portal, usually making optional step 7 unnecessary (see below). A final arthroscopic view from the lateral portal will show the smooth level undersurface of the acromion (see Fig. 9-23, *C*).

In step 7 (optional), the arthroscope is changed to the lateral portal and the instrumentation is moved to the posterior portal. Richard Caspari has advocated this positioning (Fig. 9-26). This is another step to avoid the potential acromial concavity that can occur when acromioplasty is performed from only the anterior-lateral portal (see Fig. 9-23, *C*). The posterior placement of the instrument places it parallel to the undersurface of the acromion. The lateral position of the arthroscope gives yet another perspective of the acromion.

A potential problem exists with the posterior instrument approach. It presumes the acromion is flat posterior; often it is arched and makes parallel placement impossible. If extravasation of fluids occurs, then the angle of approach from the original portal may not be parallel to the undersurface of the acromion.

In step 8 (surgical extension to AC joint), the resection continues to the AC joint. The isolated superior approach

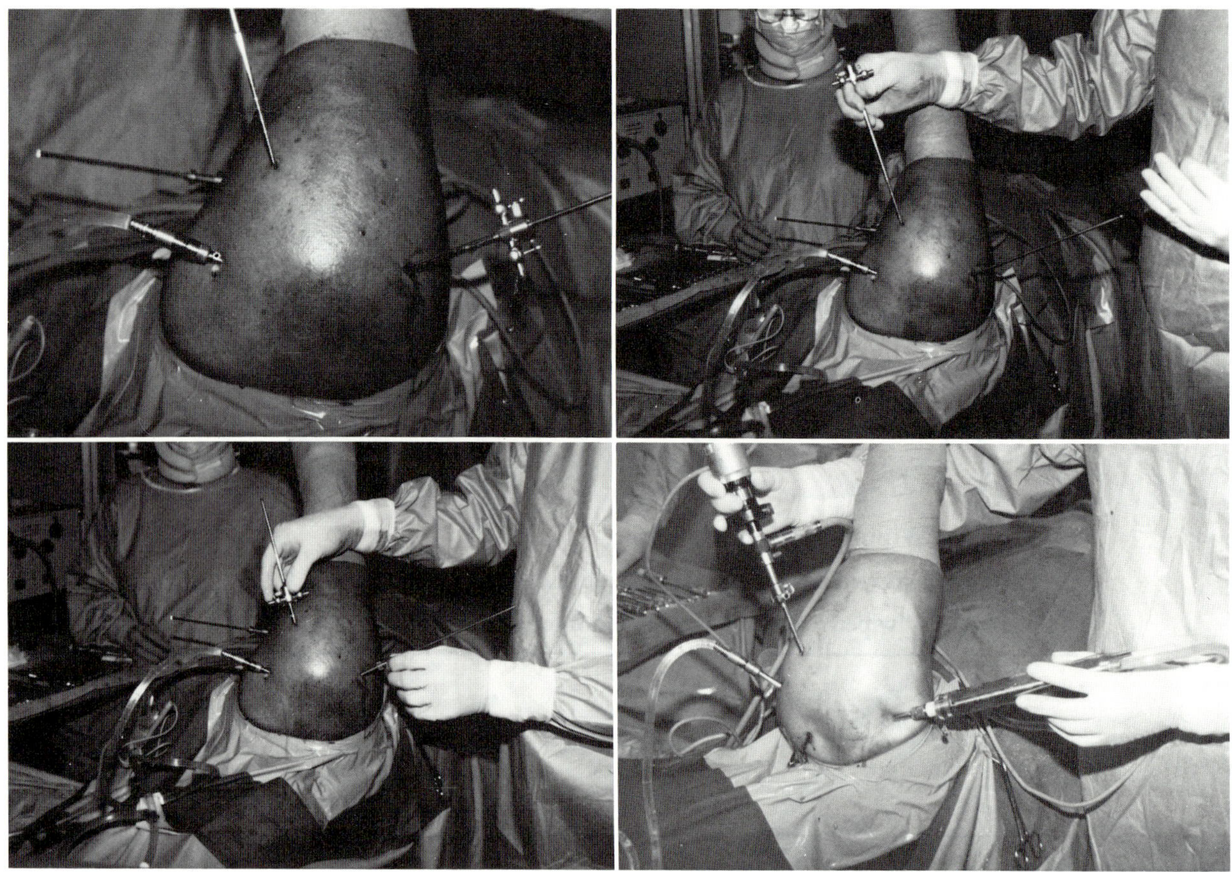

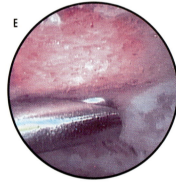

FIG. 9-26 Posterior surgical approach to acromioplasty (right shoulder).

A Outside view of inflow from anterior and switching sticks in place.

B Arthroscope is placed over lateral portal switching stick.

C Cannula is placed over the posterior portal switching stick.

D Arthroscope is placed anterior and lateral. The motorized instrumentation is placed posterior.

E Arthroscopic view shows the acromionizer approaching the acromion from left (posterior). A level undersurface contour is possible by this technique.

is unnecessary as it is combined with acromioplasty from beneath.[5] The indications for resection of this joint in combination with acromioplasty are a clinically painful AC joint, prominent underside osteophytes, and increased uptake by bone scan localized to the joint.

If resection of the AC joint is indicated, then the joint is best located with a No. 18 spinal needle from above (see Fig. 9-13). The resection instrumentation should be in the anterior portal for this step, because this position gives the best access to the AC joint. A change to the round-shaped burr, the abrader, is better suited for this maneuver. The needles outline the area of the joint (Fig. 9-27, *A*). After the acromioplasty has been performed, probing can help locate the undersurface of the AC joint (Fig. 9-27, *B*). The acromial bone

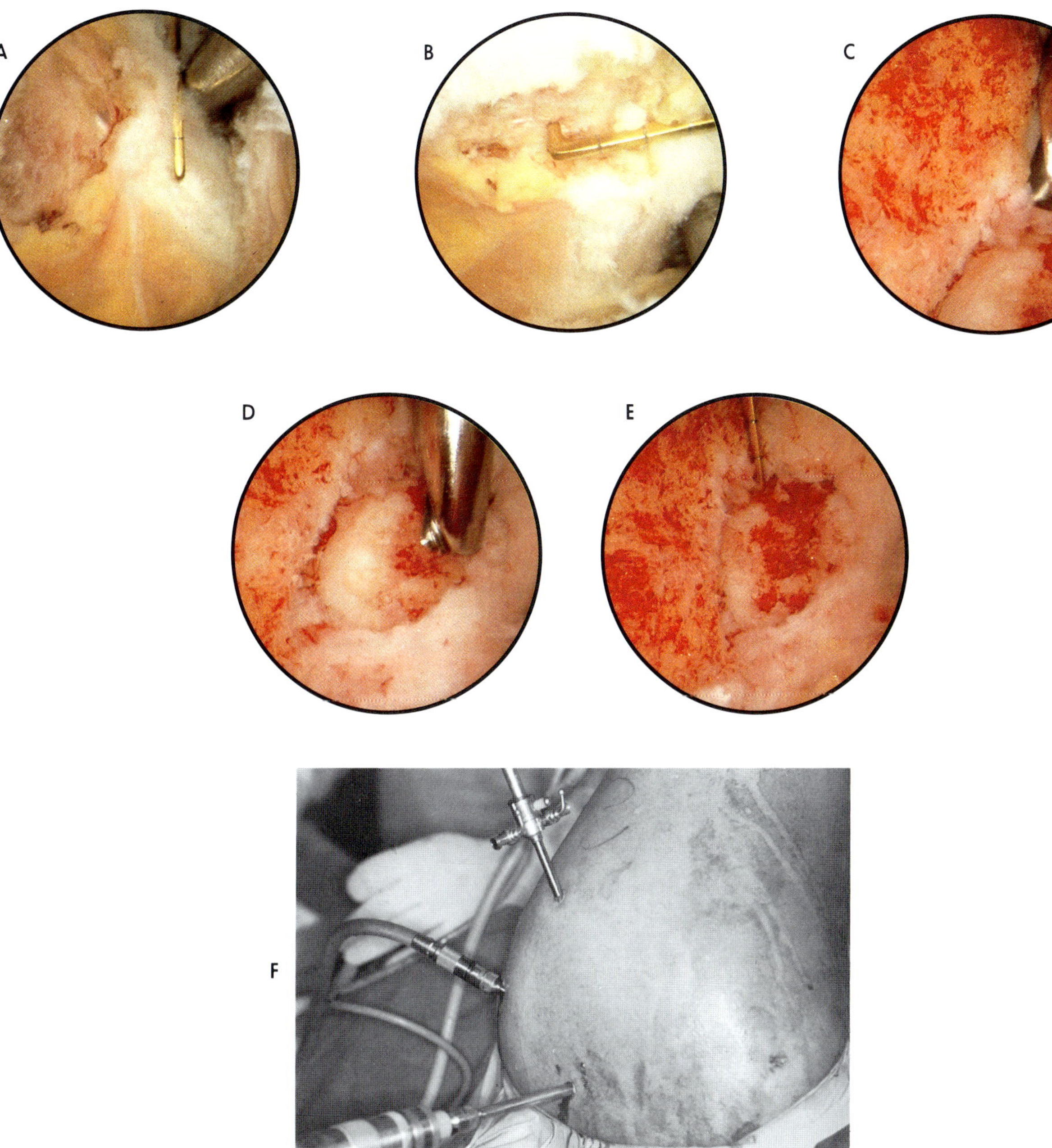

FIG. 9-27 **Needle location and probing identify the AC joint.**

A Bursal view shows acromioplasty complete and needle at end of resected CA ligament. Needle comes through the AC joint to enter the bursa.

B Probe is used to identify junction of acromion and the clavicle on the undersurface.

C Continuation of acromioplasty exposes AC joint.

D Motorized burr initiates resection of end of clavicle.

E AC joint is resected and the distal clavicle is excised in an oblique fashion in same plane as the acromioplasty.

F Superior approach to AC joint to complete resection. The scope is above in anterolateral portal. The inflow cannula is anterior to left. The motorized instrument comes from directly superior into the AC joint.

resection continues into this area. The lateral half of the joint (acromion) is resected, exposing the joint (Fig. 9-27, *C*). The meniscus is often disrupted or absent in chronic disease. If the meniscus is intact, a cartilaginous barrier exists to visualization of the outer end of the clavicle. Vascularity is abundant next to this joint and electrocautery is necessary to provide hemostasis.

After the soft tissue resection exposes the end of the clavicle, I perform a vertical resection of the articular surface (Fig. 9-27, *D*). At that point, I switch the cutting head to an acromionizer to create an oblique angle resection of the outer clavicle, leaving the superior AC ligaments intact to the acromion. Swelling may occur at this stage of the procedure, therefore reaching the AC joint from the original portal is not possible for two reasons: (1) the extravasation of fluid increases the distance, and (2) the swelling changes the angle of approach. If this occurs, I recommend creating a new approach to the AC joint from superior. A No. 18 spinal needle is placed through the skin to locate the proper portal position. This area of the shoulder is usually not swollen, and the AC joint has been partially resected and easily entered. This superior approach provides the opportunitiy for adequate resection on both sides of the joint (Fig. 9-27, *F*).

Probing is repeated at the conclusion of the resection to determine adequacy (Fig. 9-27, *E*). The question remains—what resection is adequate? Resection of the distal 1 centimeter of the clavicle is recommended from open surgery experience.[50] In practice I remove less than this amount. I remove the acromial side in the plane of the acromioplasty. The joint articular cartilage is resected. The undersurface of the clavicle is removed in an oblique manner in the plane of the acromioplasty. The instruments are positioned to remove bone at the superior aspect of the AC joint so that the entire articulation is resected. It may be shown that more bone resection is required, but to date this method has proven adequate for me.

Visualization and orientation are essential throughout the entire resection. Failure of basic arthroscopic principles may lead to erroneous bone resection during attempted acromioplasty or AC resection (Fig. 9-28).

Comparison of preoperative and postoperative arch view x-ray films demonstrate the adequacy of resection of the acromion (Fig. 9-29).

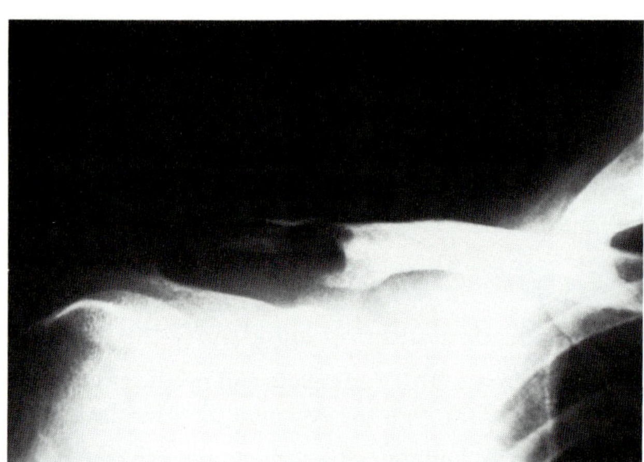

FIG. 9-28 Complication of acromioplasty. X-ray film shows nonunion of midclavicular area, probably caused by disorientation or loss of exposure.

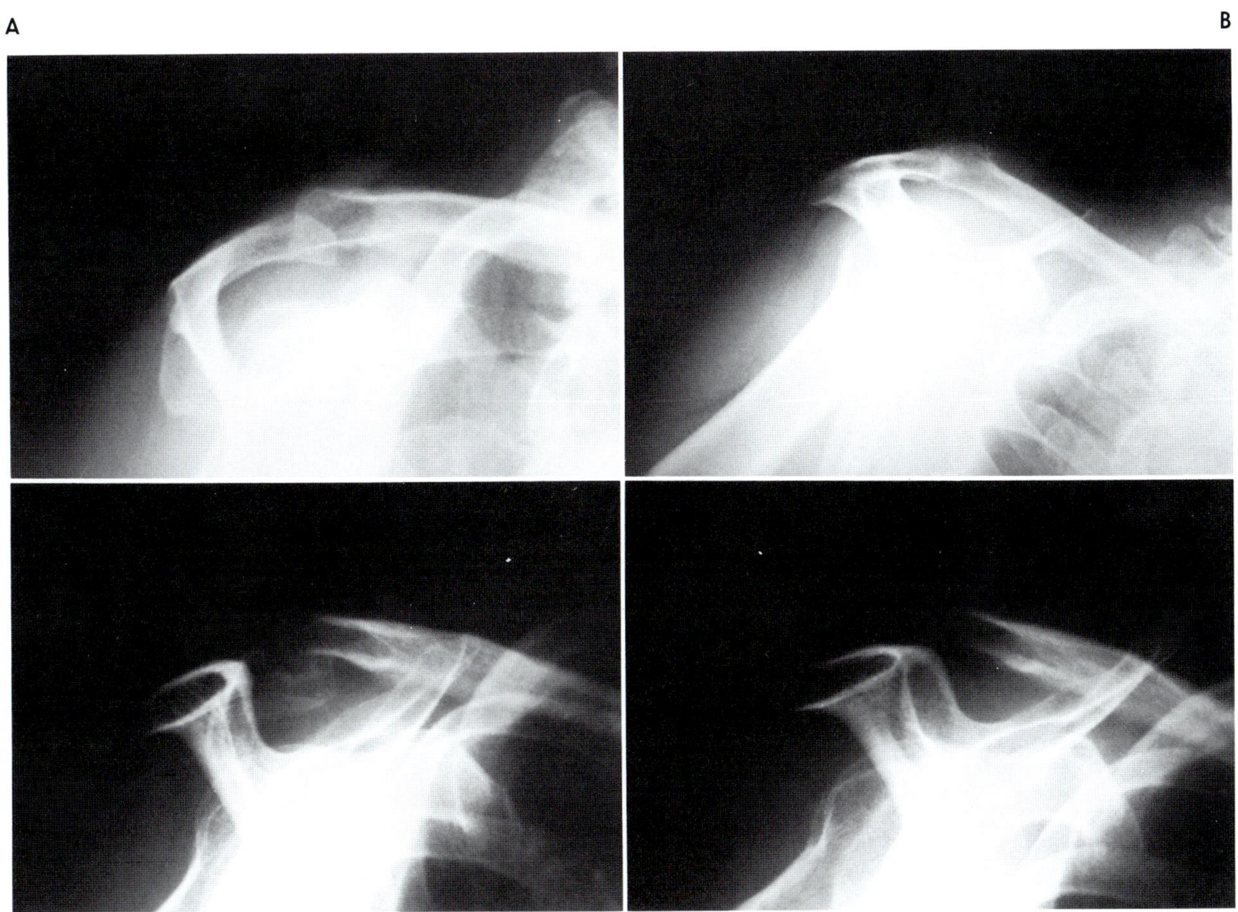

FIG. 9-29 Assessment of arthroscopic acromioplasty.

A Preoperative arch view in patient 1.

B Postoperative arch view in patient 1.

C Preoperative arch view in patient 2.

D Postoperative arch view in patient 2.

Continued.

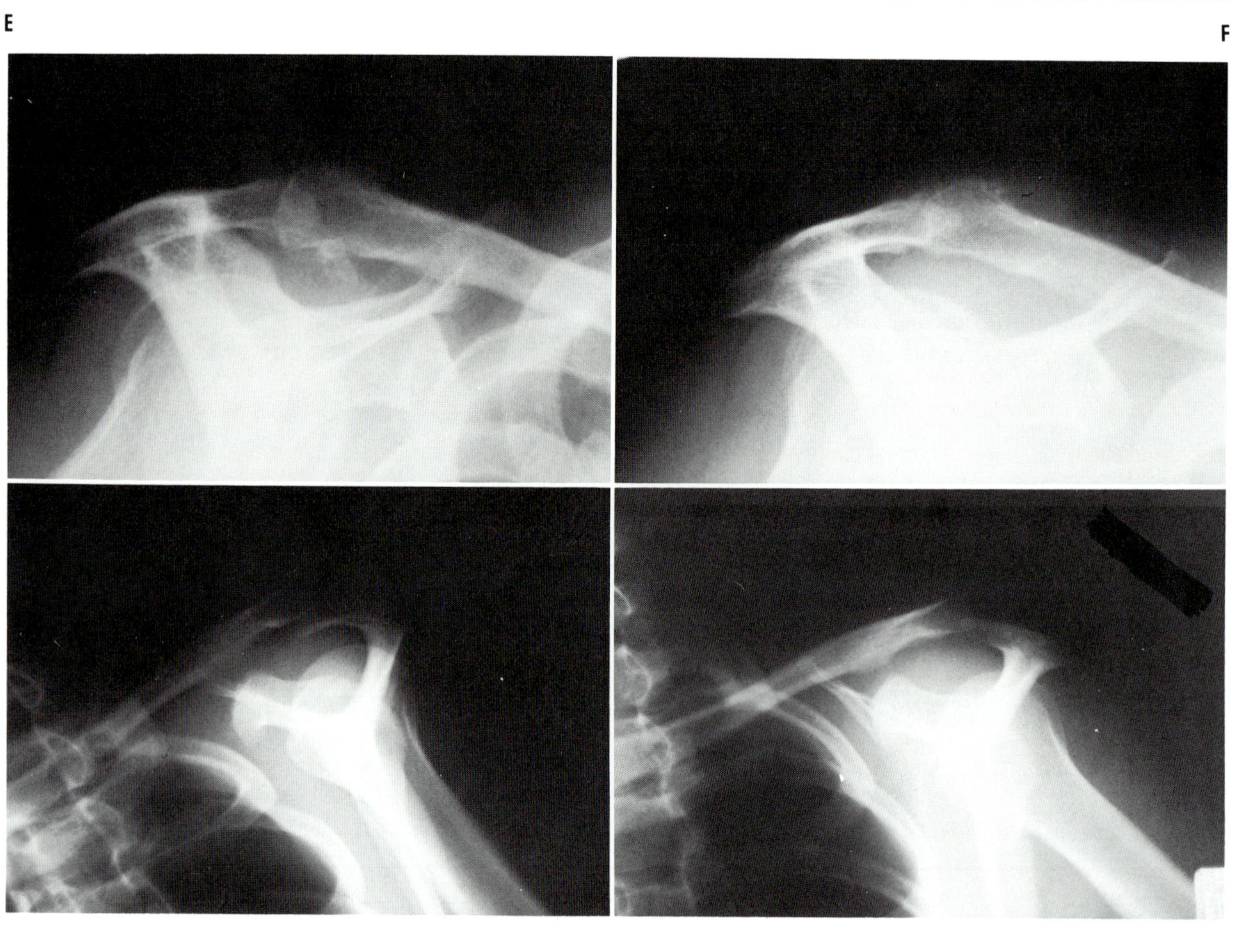

FIG. 9-29 *cont'd* **Assessment of arthroscopic acromioplasty.**

E Preoperative arch view in patient 3.

F Postoperative arch view in patient 3.

G Preoperative arch view in patient 4.

H Postoperative arch view in patient 4.

Mumford Procedure. Mumford described the resection of the outer end of the clavicle.[49] This procedure can be performed by arthroscopy. Patients with previous AC joint separations or degenerative arthritis with sufficient symptoms may be candidates for more extensive resection of the outer end of the clavicle. More extensive resection of the outer end of the clavicle may accompany the acromioplasty from the inferior approach just described or by superior approach. Chapter 10 describes isolated percutaneous AC joint resection from the superior approach.

Arthroscopic Acromioplasty Without Rotator Cuff Repair. Rockwood[68] has reported open acromioplasty without rotator cuff repair as a salvage procedure when the cuff tear was too large or contracted for reattachment (Fig. 9-30). His patients had a high percentage of reduction of preoperative pain and improved range of motion following this procedure. He emphasizes that the procedure should not be limited to the acromioplasty, but the debridement should include resection of the subacromial bursa and fragmented rotator cuff. He has not advocated ignoring the smaller, mobile reparable tears. The same procedure may be performed by arthroscopy.[39,73]

In my experience, arthroscopic subacromial bursal debridement with acromioplasty without cuff repair will decrease the patient's pain. As a result of pain reduction, the range of motion is improved. The patient still has weakness of external rotation and loss of over-the-head activity. Also, when my patients with small reparable lesions were compared those those who had lesions but did not have a repair, the repaired group has a greater sense of well being based on initial clinical subjective assessment. Those with the repair have same benefit of pain relief, but without increased strength and over-the-head activities. Therefore, I presently repair all reparable full-thickness rotator cuff tears.

Another approach to patient management could be to limit the surgery to arthroscopic acromioplasty for those patients who have acceptable motion and strength. This patient is often elderly or infirmed.

Arthroscopic acromioplasty without rotator cuff repair is best suited for the patient with a partial tear, usually on the undersurface of the cuff.[6] A small, partial-thickness superior surface tear may not require repair, but a large tear is tendinous in origin and should be approximated. An unrepaired large superior surface tear will result in postoperative symptoms of popping and pain (see Fig. 9-22, *A*).[71]

In my experience, if no evidence of acromial erosion is present, an acromioplasty for impingement syndrome yields poor results. The few worker's compensation patients in my practice have presented in this manner and experienced poor results following arthroscopic acromioplasty when no acromial erosion was identified.

Reports of others. Ellman was the first to report on arthroscopic subacromial decompression.[18-20] He reported on 50 cases, with a 1-year to 3-year follow-up.[19] He reported the procedure as technically demanding. He had two groups. Group 1 had stage II impingement without rotator cuff tear (40 patients), and Group 2 had a full-thickness rotator cuff tear (10 patients). Using the UCLA rating scale, he reported 88% of the cases satisfactory; 12% of the patients had fair or poor results. The results of Group 1 were not separated in this report. Those with full-thickness tears, 10 patients in Group 2 had 80% satisfactory results. There were patients in Group 2 in whom the tear was large and unreparable. He did not recommend arthroscopic acromioplasty alone for those patients with a reparable lesion.

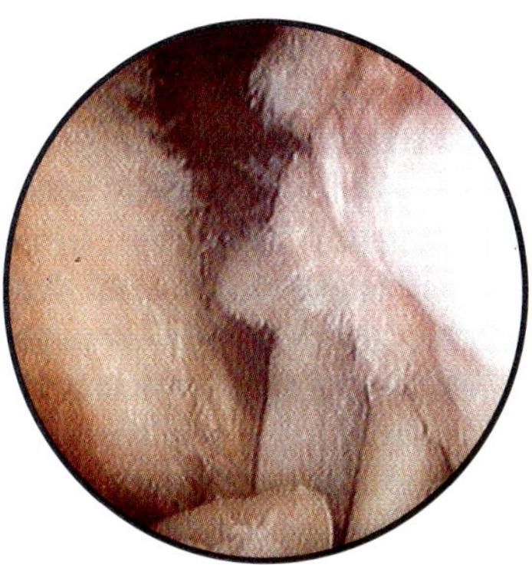

FIG. 9-30 Massive rotator cuff tear. Arthroscopic view of massive rotator cuff tear shows the humeral head to the right and the exposed acromion to the left. This is the only contracted cuff element inferior in the field.

Esch et al[21] evaluated results of arthroscopic acromioplasty according to the degree of rotator cuff tear in 71 patients available for follow-up at an average of 19 months following surgery. Eighty-two percent with stage II disease were satisfied; 82% were satisfied regardless of whether they had no rotator cuff tear (9 of 11) or had a partial tear (28 of 34) of the rotator cuff. Of those with stage II disease (complete cuff tears), 88% (23 of 26) were satisfied. An acceptable UCLA rating of 28 or above was seen in 82% of those without a tear, 76% with a partial tear, and 77% with a full-thickness tear. They concluded that the overall patient satisfaction rate of 85% and the objective success rate of 77% are within the range of that seen with open rotator cuff repair.

Gartsman[24] reported arthroscopic acromioplasty for lesions of the rotator cuff.[24] He operated on 165 patients. In Group 1, 100 patients were without a tear, but with stage II impingement syndrome. Seventy-eight patients were satisfied with the results; 73 patients had no pain; 81 patients had marked improvement in ratings of activities of daily living, work, and sports. Seven patients had subsequent open operation.

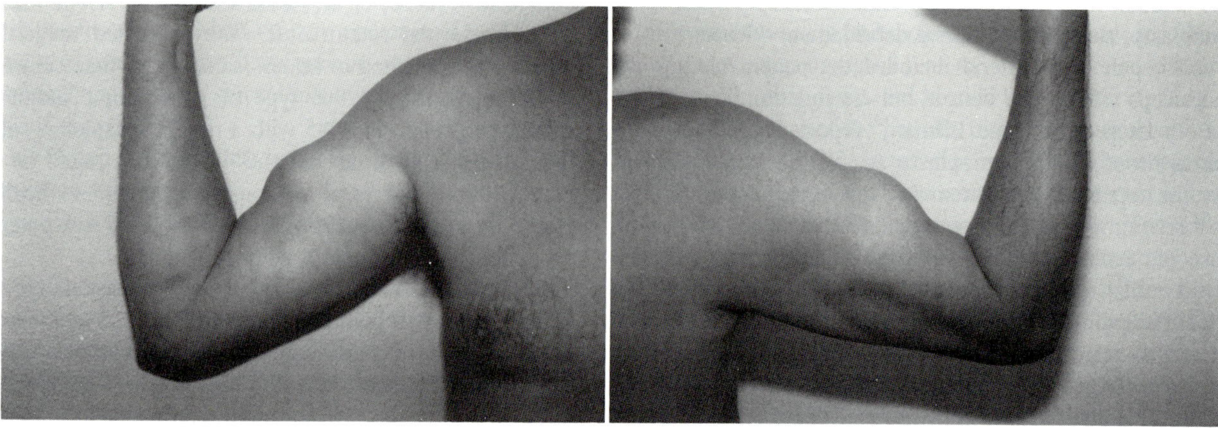

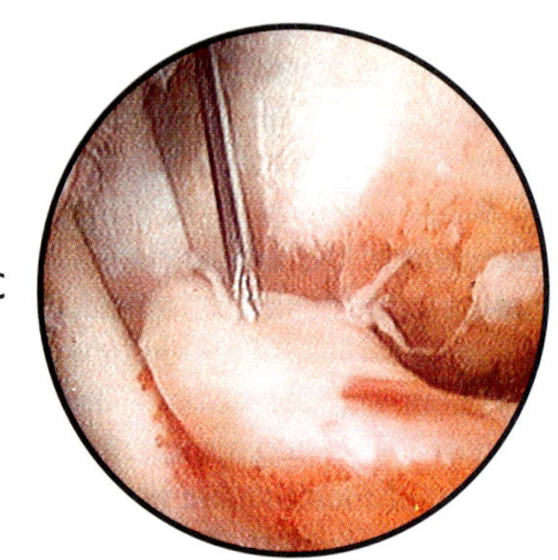

FIG. 9-32 Ruptured biceps tendon, long head.

A Photograph shows round, contracted long head of the biceps in the arm from anterior.

B Same patient with view from posterior.

C Arthroscopic view of stump of biceps tendon rounded off at superior glenoid. A needle points to the stump.

If the cuff is easily approximated, then only the superficial portion of the cortical bone of the greater tuberosity is removed. The area prepared is immediately distal to the articular cartilage margin (Fig. 9-33). The anterior portal provides the best approach for motorized instrumentation to accomplish this bone removal. Soft tissue is resected in this area with a full-radius resector. The superficial area of bone is removed with a burr. Care is taken not to remove the entire cortex because the underlying cancellous bone would not be adequate to hold the metallic staple.

The patient's arm remains in the suspended abducted position, but weights of countertraction are reduced to under 10 pounds to remove any distraction of the humerus.

The lateral portal is used to pass a meniscal (Schlesinger) forceps (Fig. 9-34, *A*). The rotator cuff is grasped. I prefer to pull on the capsular portion and allow the tendinous portion to trail along. If the tendon is pulled, then visualization of the underlying capsule is lost. Both portions should be advanced. The thickness of both tissues provides maximal tissue for staple insertion. Attention is given to where the cuff is grasped, either anterior or posterior. The best position by trial and error is chosen for an angle of pull to result in anatomical approximation.

Once the tendon is in place, the second assistant holds the grasper. (Fig. 9-34, *B*) The surgeon moves to the head of the table for staple insertion. A No. 18 spinal needle is used in a trial and error manner to determine the cutaneous portal that will give the best angle of approach for the staple (Fig. 9-34, *B*). There is no rule of thumb for an anterior or posterior approach; whichever superior portal works best is the route to use. Sometimes the acromion will

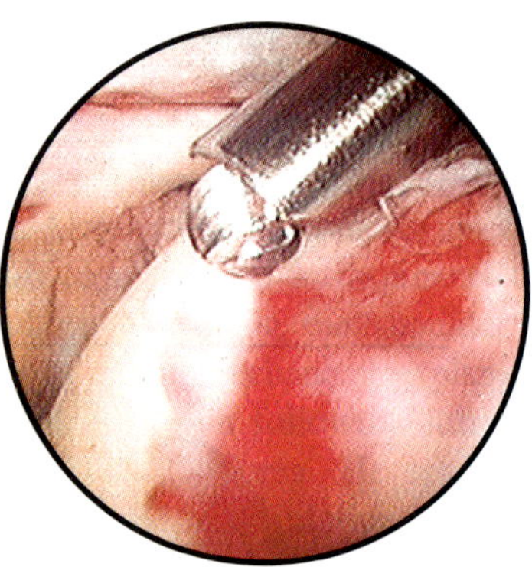

FIG. 9-33 Arthroscopic identification and preparation of the anticipated site of rotator cuff reattachment.

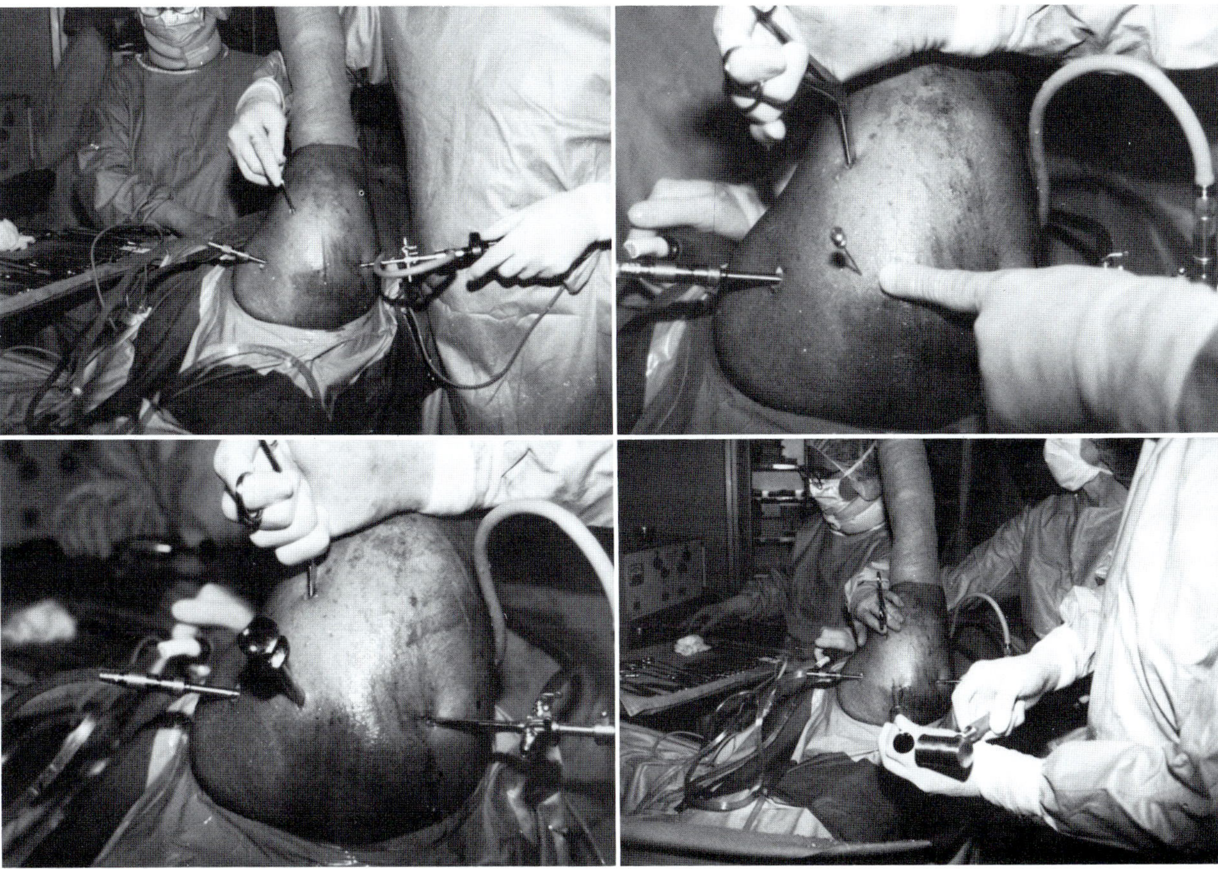

FIG. 9-34 Arthroscopic rotator cuff repair.

A Transcutaneous grasping of rotator cuff tear.

B Assistant holds tendon. Surgeon's finger points to the needle placement at site of anticipated staple delivery.

C LCR staple is in place and tendon is advanced with the grasper.

D Outside view of implantation of the metallic staple with driver and hammer.

block the angle of approach. On one occasion only, a supraspinatus superior portal would create the proper angle of approach. A trocar and cannula is placed along the previously decided angle of approach. This is changed with switching sticks to the larger LCR cannula (Fig. 9-34, *C*).

The rotator cuff repair is performed with a metallic staple(s) placed from superior device portal (Fig. 9-34, *D*). The large staple is used for maximal length to accommodate for thickness of the tendon and provide length for fixation to the humerus (Fig. 9-35).

The rotational position of the staple is important for protection of the tendon tissue (Fig. 9-35). The tines should be at right angles to the line of tension, which places the smooth and rounded edge of the tine towards the line of tension, resisting tearing. Positioning the tines along the line of tension results in cutting through the tendon, because each tine acts as a knife blade, which places the smooth and rounded edge of the tine toward the line of tension, resisting tearing.

A watertight seal is not necessary as proposed by the open surgical experience.[50,57] Postoperative inspections show that a biological, watertight seal occurs within 4 weeks (see Fig. 9-38).

A second staple may be necessary. If a third staple is

A
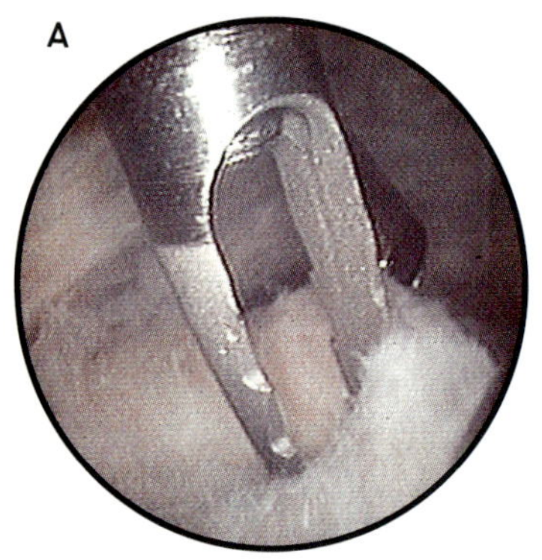
B
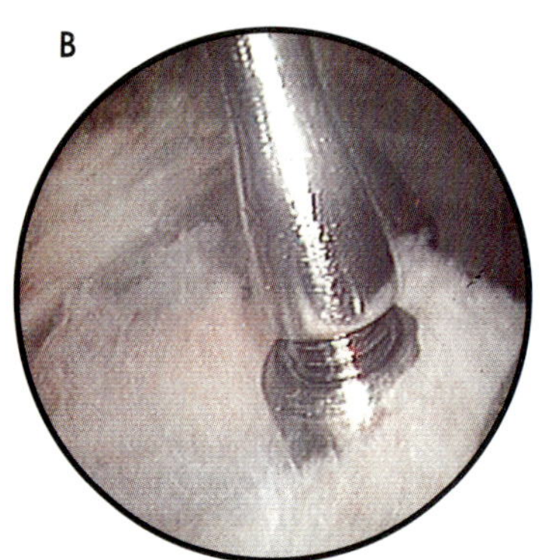
C
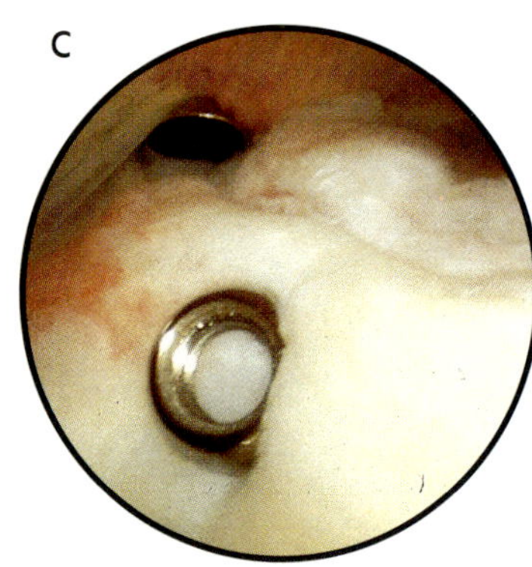

FIG. 9-35 Staple fixation.

A Staple is placed with wider portion of the tine accepting the tension of the advanced tendon.

B Staple is inserted with good cuff tissue captured in the crotch of the staple and tines long enough to secure tendon to bone.

C Immediate postoperative bursal view of rotator cuff repair.

needed, then an open repair should be considered; my only failure has been in the large tear requiring multiple staples. Using multiple small sutures attached to arthroscopically placed suture anchors may be better than using multiple large staples. The future will bring bioabsorbable devices for both staples and suture anchors for the arthroscopist (see Chapter 11).

Postoperative management. The surgery is performed on an outpatient basis. Those patients with significant medical conditions or severe pain are admitted to the hospital for 1 day following the operation.

The patient's upper extremity is placed in an abduction pillow for 6 weeks. He or she is encouraged to bend the elbow and use the hand to avoid swelling or atrophy (Fig. 9-36).

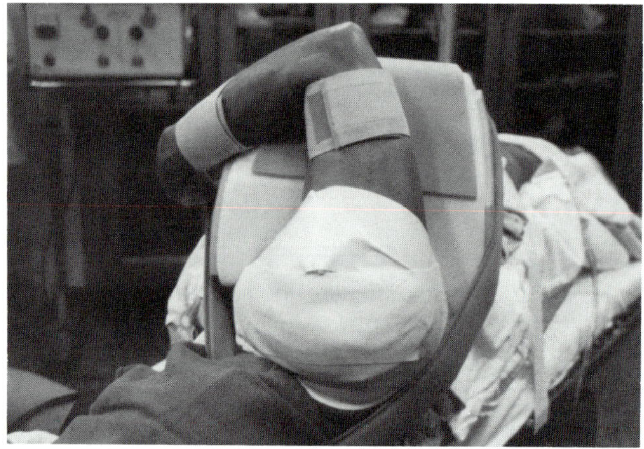

FIG. 9-36 Postoperative management includes use of abduction splint.

Routine postoperative plain film x-rays were taken to determine the position of the metallic staple (Fig. 9-37). The cloth abduction pillow is exchanged for a plastic pillow for showering. This can be accomplished by taking an empty bleach bottle and cutting a hole in the bottom to accommodate a rope that goes through the bottle and is tied around the neck. A plastic boat bumper would serve the same purpose.

Routine postoperative plain film x-rays are taken to determine the position of the metallic staple (Fig. 9-37).

Planned second procedure. A planned second surgery is necessary to remove the staple (Fig. 9-38, *A* and *B*). This is best performed with the patient under general anesthesia, because adhesiolysis may be necessary for exposure of the staple or staples. In one case using local anesthesia at the patient's request, I failed to identify or remove the staple. Although staples are intentionally left so the head is exposed, sometimes they are covered with fibrous tissue at the time of second look. In that case, palpation with a No. 18 spinal needle identifies the metal below the surface of the healed bursa.

The second procedure is a disadvantage but provides knowledge of healing time (4 to 6 weeks) and observation of the fate of a mechanically imperfect, watertight seal converting to biological seal by this time interval (Fig. 9-38).

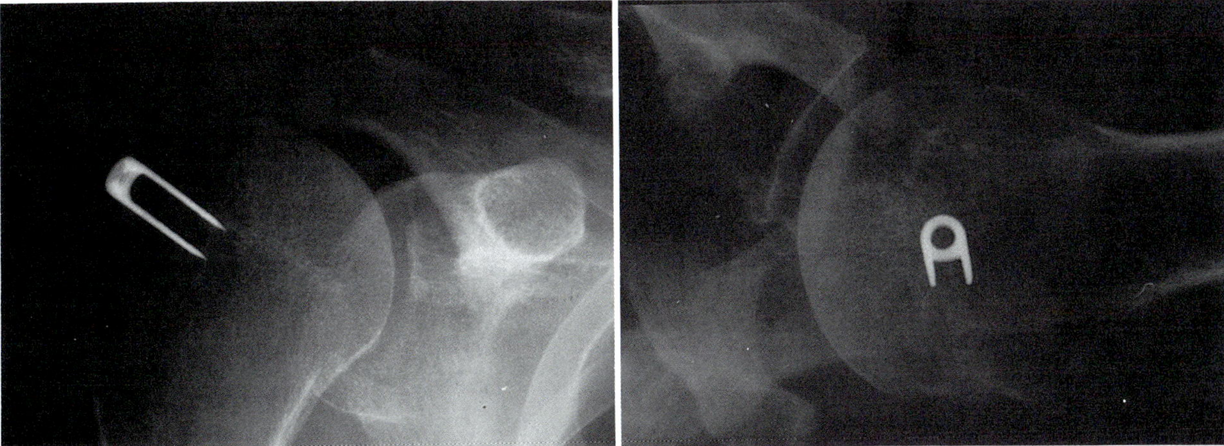

FIG. 9-37 **Postoperative X-ray film following arthroscopic rotator cuff repair.**

A Anterior-posterior plain film x-ray shows proper placement of staple in the greater tuberosity.

B Axillary view of same patient shows staple position.

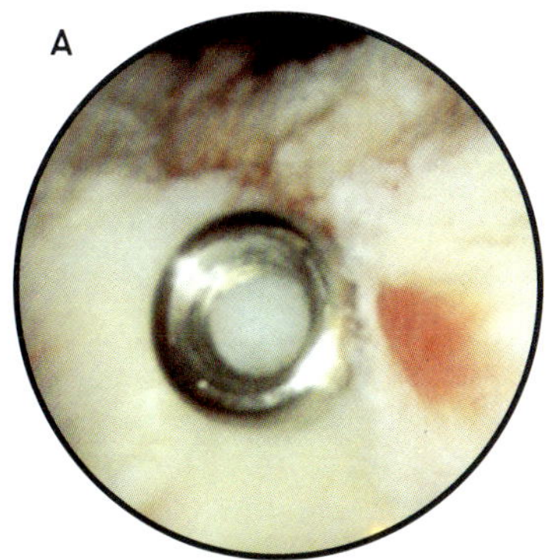

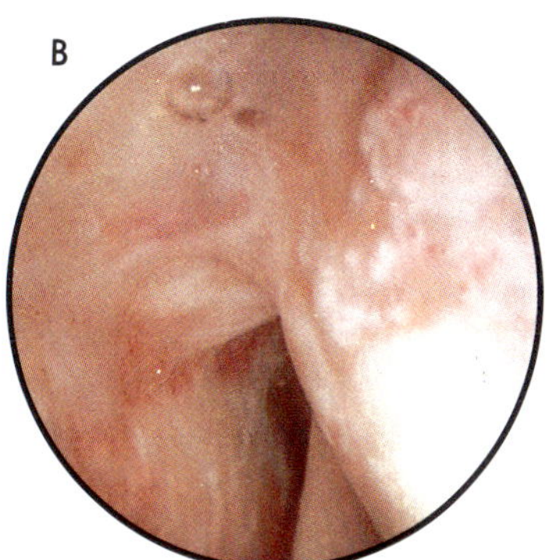

C

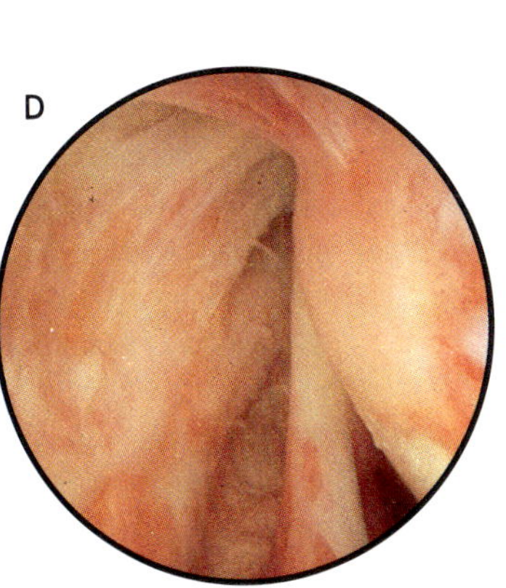

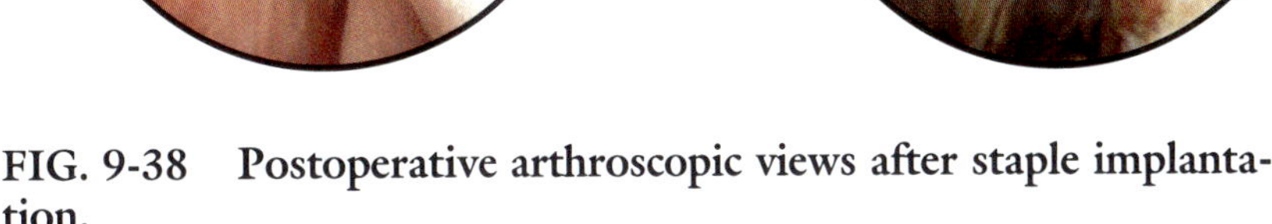
FIG. 9-38 **Postoperative arthroscopic views after staple implantation.**

A Arthroscopic bursal view eight weeks after implantation shows early healing.

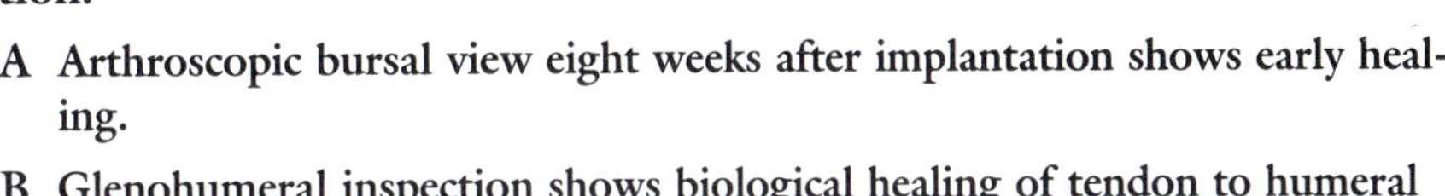
B Glenohumeral inspection shows biological healing of tendon to humeral head in same patient.

C Another case shows healing from bursal side. Notice the fibrous tissue ingrowth into the staple.

D Glenohumeral view in same patient as Fig. 9-37, *C,* shows biological seal to the humeral head.

Rehabilitation is initiated after staple removal. The patients start with pendulum exercises and advance slowly over 3 months to include strength exercises.

My metal staple series. Between May 5, 1985 and March 8, 1989, I performed 31 arthroscopic rotator cuff repairs on 25 men and 6 women. The average age was 57 years (range 36 to 76 years). The dominant arm was involved in 21 patients, and the nondominant arm was involved in ten. Preoperative plain film x-rays were taken on all patients. Thirteen patients had preoperative arthrogram. No patient had preoperative MRI.

A videotape was recorded and stored for every surgery. The medical record was computerized, storing essential data points for subsequent analysis.

All 31 patients were admitted as outpatients. If after surgery they needed medicinal control of pain from surgery or nausea and vomiting from anesthesia, they were admitted to the hospital. The average stay was less than 1 hospital day. The longest hospital stay was 1 day.

The follow-up included annual postcard questionnaires, a formal interval evaluation and examination at a minimum of 2 and 3 years after surgery.

Results. No intraoperative complications or aborted procedures resulted. One staple was used in most patients. Four was the most staples used, and those were used in one patient with the largest size tear in the group, 5 cm.

No postoperative complications of bleeding, infection, neurovascular injury, or thromboembolic phenomena occurred.

Twenty-nine of the 31 patients returned for a second look. The second look was recommended between 6 and 8 weeks, but for various reasons the patients returned between 1 and 60 months for this procedure. The mean was 4.7 months and the median was 2 months. Two patients declined the second look and staple removal.

In 3 of the 29 patients the cuff was healed but the staple was not identified at the initial second look and therefore not removed. A third attempt was made in one patient at a later date and the staple was removed.

Arthroscopic evidence of healing. The cuff healing was complete in 20 patients. When healing was complete the previous imperfect watertight seal became a watertight biological seal as early as 4 weeks.

The repair was incomplete in seven patients. In three patients the small defect (1 mm) was adjacent to the metal staple. This defect was presumed to be due to the stress riser effect of the metal staple. One patient (A.W.) returned at 4 months, having played golf in the interim. The staple was removed. He was improved at long-term follow-up. A second patient (M.G.) did not return for 60 months for staple removal; he returned at that time only to have the same surgery on the other shoulder. The previously operated shoulder was explored arthroscopically and a small defect was seen and the staple removed. He too is improved. The third patient in this group (D.L.) returned at 4 months for staple removal, and showed a small defect next to the staple. Only the staple was removed. The patient reports the same condition as preoperatively. All these patients had delayed metal staple removal.

Four patients showed a small unhealed area, but not next to the staple. In one patient the staples were loose. Two other patients were noncompliant with use of the abduction splint. No explanation for a small area of nonhealing was apparent in the fourth patient. Failure of fixation and/or noncompliance resulted in these small cuff separations, which were not closed. In long-term follow-up, one patient was improved, one the same, and two lost to follow-up.

Two patients had complete failure of cuff attachment at second look. One was seen at 2 months and the other at 3 months. The patient with an original 2 cm tear reported improvement at 4 years follow-up. The other patient had the largest tear in the series, 5 cm, and was not improved. A repeat open reconstructive surgery with shifting of the subscapularis and infraspinatus tendon failed to improve the patient's function.[10] Burkhart has given reasonable explanation for failure of this type of procedure. After this open reconstruction the patient had relief of pain, good deltoid muscle function, but lost mechanical advantage and useful independent arm elevation.

The reasons for failure were combinations of failure of compliance with either postoperative immobilization or optimal timing of staple removal.

Questionnaire follow-up. A questionnaire sent out early in the study, when patients were an average 2.9 years after surgery, showed high satisfaction with the method and outcome. The symptomatic outcome showed most patients satisfied with the treatment method at a minimum of 2 years (15 satisfactory, 2 unsatisfactory, 1 no answer). Most patients reported satisfaction with the treatment outcome at minimum 2 years (13 satisfactory, 3 unsatisfactory, 2 no answer).

This same questionnaire showed all patients had reduction in pain; 67% had no pain 3 years following surgery. Half of the patients experienced minimal loss of motion. Impairment occurred only at the extremes of motion (Figs. 9-39, 9-40, and 9-41). Strength was restored.

Long-term follow-up. At a mean of 4 years after surgery, another analysis was made of this series. The results were reviewed from the aspect of the subsequent healing of the tendon. One group (9 patients) showed complete healing at second look. Another group (3) had a small stress riser around the staple(s). The third group (4) had incomplete healing of the original tear. The fourth group (2) had no healing of the original tear.

The original repair was never mechanically watertight following staple repair. Nonetheless, nine patients available for follow-up had biological watertight seals (see Fig. 9-38).

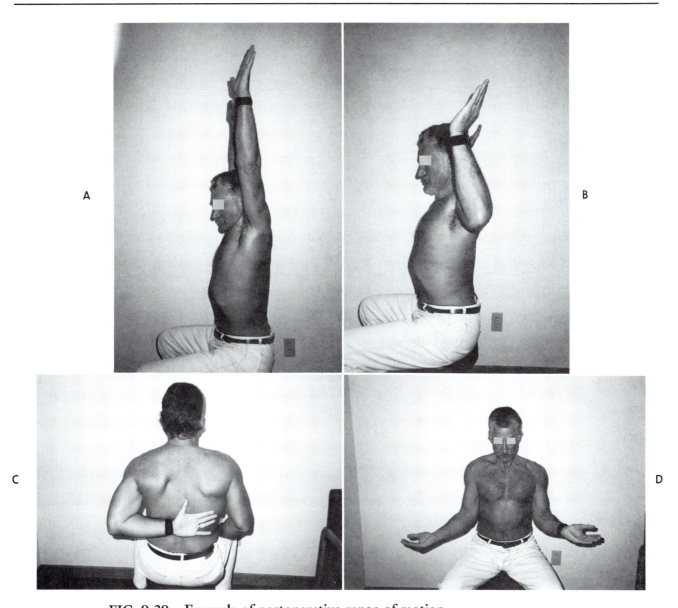

FIG. 9-39 Example of postoperative range of motion.

A. Elevation.

B Abduction and external rotation.

C Internal rotation.

D External rotation at the side.

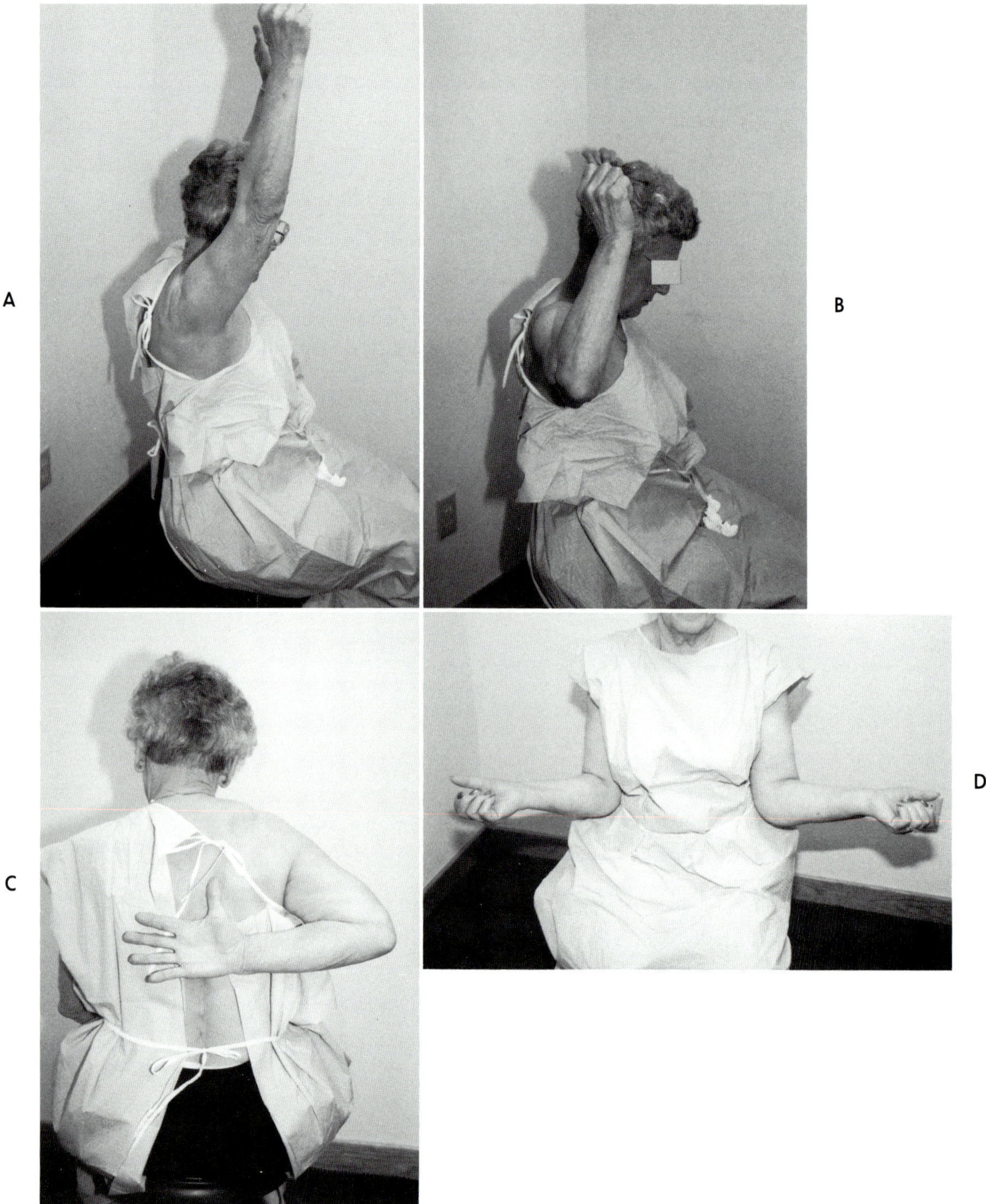

FIG. 9-40 Example of postoperative range of motion.

A Elevation.

B Abduction and external rotation.

C Internal rotation.

D External rotation.

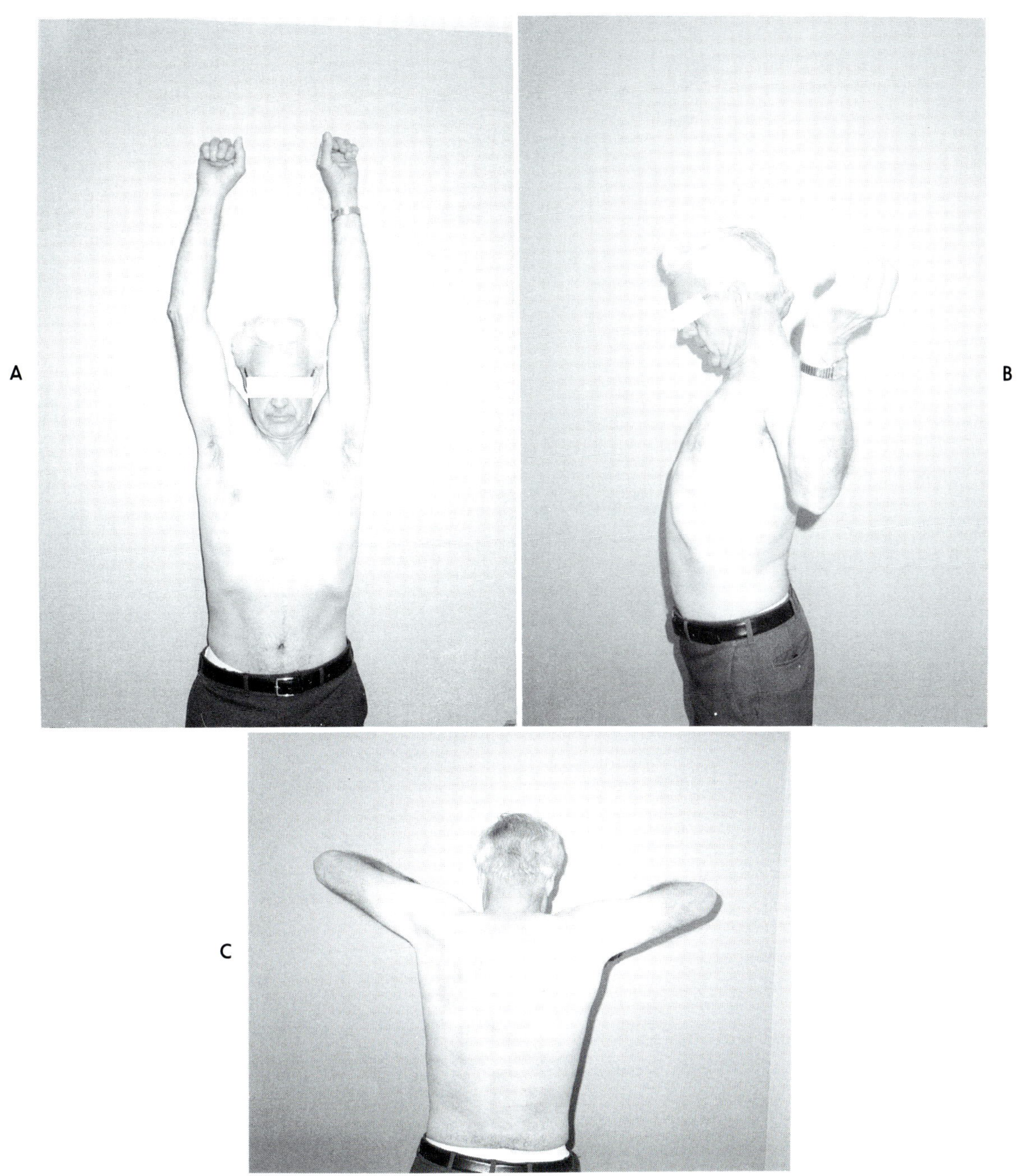

FIG. 9-41 Example of range of motion after long-term follow-up.

A Elevation.

B Abduction and external rotation.

C Abduction.

The three patients with incomplete healing caused by a stress riser around the staple returned at 4 months (2) and 60 months (1) for staple removal. All had been active with the shoulder. Two of these patients were improved and one reported no change.

Four patients had an incompletely healed tear. Two of these patients were noncompliant with the abduction pillow. One had partial backing out of two staples placed to hold the repair. One had no obvious explanation. These latter two were lost to follow-up. The two noncompliant patients said they were improved at 2 and 4 years of follow-up.

Two patients had no evidence of cuff repair at time of second look. One patient had a repair of a massive cuff tear with four staples under tension; this was the largest tear attempted in this series (4 cm). In this case the second look showed the tear was not only separated, but enlarged. This patient subsequently came to open rotator cuff repair, with rotation of the infraspinatus and subscapularis tendons to close the defect. Outcome for motion was poor. The other patient in this group had the staples removed and no subsequent repair. He reported improved status at 4 years following surgery.

Fifteen of these 18 patients returned for evaluation and physical examination at a minimum of 2 years after surgery. The shortest follow-up was 2 years, the longest was 5 years, and the mean was 3.8 years.

On physical examination the three groups were again divided for analysis. The nine patients with healed tendon had excellent range of motion and strength. The four patients with a small stress riser around the staple had good range of motion and strength. The two patients without repair showed that one with a large tear had ineffective motion or strength. The other, with a small tear, had good motion and good strength.

Present status. Although this series showed a potential for arthroscopic rotator cuff repair, it was just a precursor of a similar procedure using a biodegradable implant. Other methods of repair include arthroscopic suturing.

The arthroscopic repairs are limited to 1 to 2 cm defects that are easily mobilized and without tension when the arm is abducted.

It should be noted that little morbidity is associated with combining arthroscopic acromioplasty with a short longitudinal incision for the cuff repair.

An arthroscopic acromioplasty alone could be considered in patients with small rotator cuff tears based on results to date in the literature.[19, 21, 23]

The surgeon should use the method that is in the best interest of the patient. This includes the patient's request for cosmesis, which weighs the balance toward arthroscopy, or earlier mobilization, which is possible with an open repair and multiple suture method.

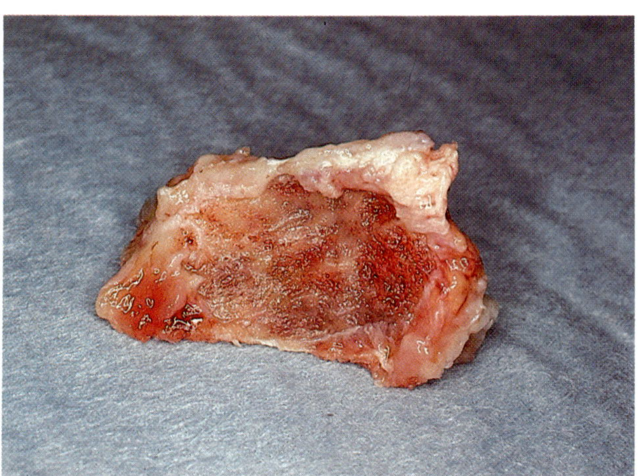

FIG. 9-42 Gross surgical specimen shows undersurface of the acromion was debrided over the same area as was resected by open surgery.

COMBINED ARTHROSCOPY AND OPEN PROCEDURES

Diagnostic arthroscopy should precede or accompany open surgery of the shoulder. On the other hand, arthroscopic surgery is not necessarily the best method of treatment in all shoulder problems.

Acromioplasty

If an acromioplasty is the only procedure indicated, then an arthroscopic method is preferred. Gartsman et al[24] has shown arthroscopic acromioplasty to be the technical equivalent of the open method. With improved surgical skills and perfected arthroscopic techniques, open acromioplasty will become less frequent. Early into my arthroscopic experience I would outline and debride the area under the acromion that would be excised if the procedure were performed by arthroscopy. I then would proceed with open acromioplasty and inspect the specimen (Fig. 9-42). The bone taken by open surgery showed the same resection margins as that of the arthroscopically marked undersurface.

Acromioplasty/Mini-Incision/Rotator Cuff Repair

The most common combined procedure is used when a full-thickness rotator cuff tear is identified. The glenohumeral joint is explored arthroscopically, followed by indicated debridement procedures. The arthroscope is redirected to the subacromial space. The bursectomy and acromioplasty is performed by arthroscopy. The AC joint may be included in the resection. The edges of the rotator cuff tear can be debrided by arthroscopy.

An important assessment is made of the potential for

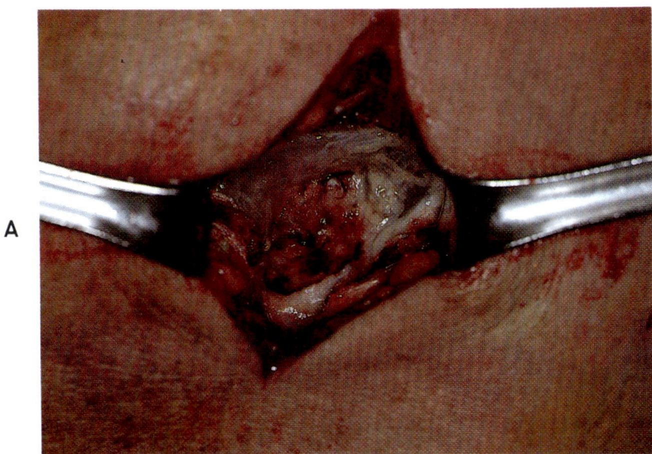

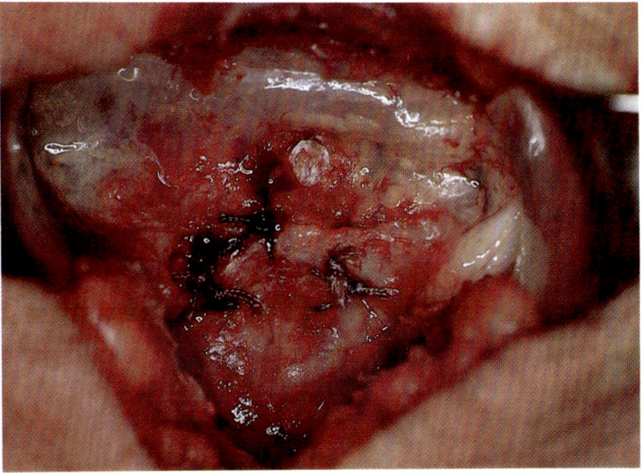

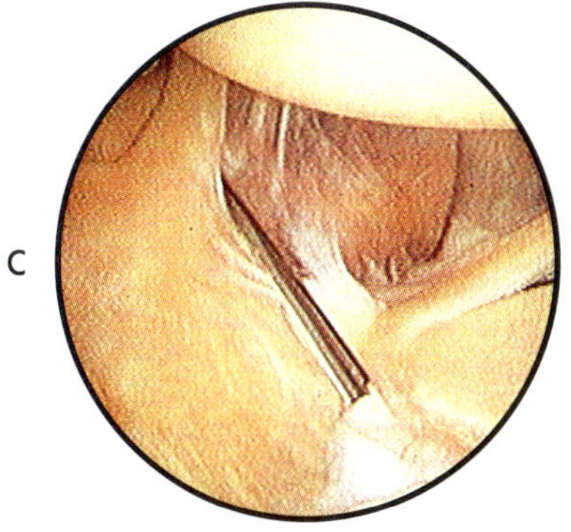

FIG. 9-43 Mini incision combined with arthroscopic acromioplasty.

A Short incision directly over the rotator cuff tear gives adequate exposure of the tear for repair.

B Close-up view shows completion of suture repair.

C Arthroscopic view of biceps tendon stump. The needle is on the biceps stump.

cuff advancement before committing to an open incision. The second benefit of the arthroscopic dimension is the ability to place a No. 18 spinal needle as a marker to choose the exact position of the subsequent skin incision.

Open exposure and repair of the rotator cuff tear is performed through a short (5 cm) longitudinal incision. (Fig. 9-43, *A*)[40] The incision is located anterior and lateral. The deltoid muscle fibers are split longitudinally. A minimal detachment of deltoid muscle from the acromial attachment may be required for adequate exposure. The undersurface of the acromion may be palpated to confirm adequacy of the arthroscopic acromioplasty.[30] The rotator cuff is repaired to bone with interrupted permanent sutures. The material should be at least No. 1 gauge or 1 mm cottony Dacron (Fig. 9-43, *B*). The cuff can be repaired to the decorticated greater tuberosity. The site could have been chosen and prepared during the arthroscopic portion of the procedure. If a trough is required in the greater tuberosity, it should be minimal in depth. The sutures are taken distal and lateral on the humerus for secure fixation over cortical bone.

Levy, Uribe, and Delaney[40] made a preliminary report of arthroscopic acromioplasty with open repair through a short incision. Of the 25 cases with minimum of 1-year follow-up, 80% of the patients had good to excellent results; 96% of patients were satisfied with the procedure. This is not much different than most arthroscopic reports on acromioplasty without repair of cuff tear.[21]

ARTHROSCOPIC TECHNIQUES THAT FACILITATE OPEN ROTATOR CUFF REPAIR

Arthroscopy affords several techniques to facilitate open rotator cuff repair.

Patient Positioning

The first benefit is that the lateral decubitus position with the arm in suspension is a perfect position for open rotator cuff surgery (Fig. 9-44). The arm is controlled by suspension, reducing the need for an assistance. The arm is abducted to remove tension on the anticipated repair. The arm is easily rotated for placing extreme anterior and posterior sutures without extending the incision.

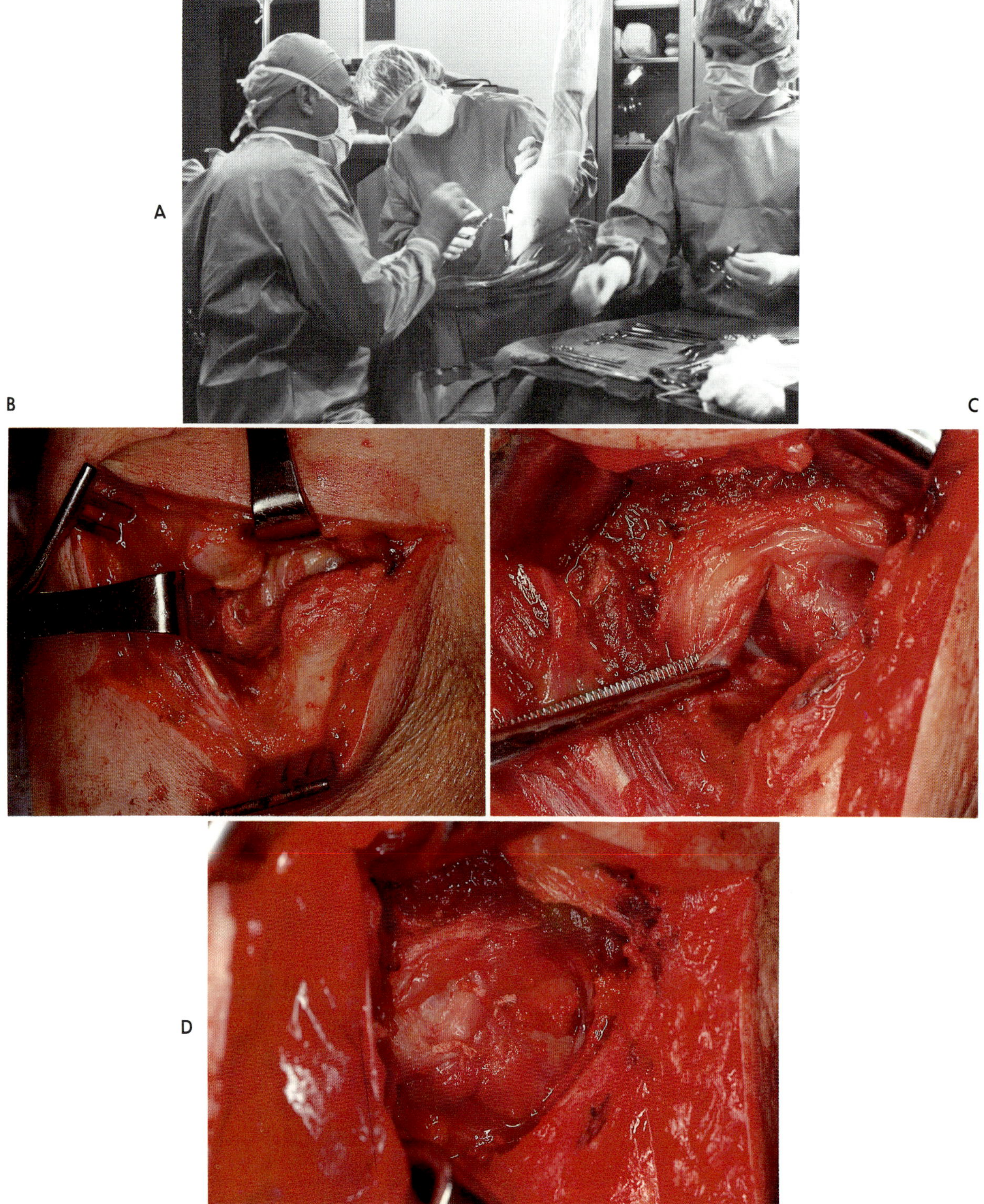

A B C D

FIG. 9-44 Combined procedure for open rotator cuff repair.

A The opposite lateral decubitus position for arthroscopy is unchanged and ideal for open surgical exposure.

B Surgical exposure shows retractors on deltoid muscle and the acute tear in the depth of the wound.

C The anterior acromioplasty is completed, yielding wider exposure of the tear. The clamp is on the anterior portion of the supraspinatus tear.

D Sutures are seen crossing the closure of the rotator cuff tear.

Arthroscopic Diagnosis and Debridement

Diagnostic arthroscopy includes the inspection of the glenohumeral joint and the underside of the rotator cuff. Lesions of the biceps tendon and subscapularis are identified. Labral and degenerative lesions are both identified and subject to arthroscopic debridement.

Arthroscopic trimming of tissues provides a clean operative field when the area is exposed by open incision.

Cuff Mobility

If after the diagnostic arthroscopy and debridement, open acromioplasty and rotator cuff is necessary, rotator cuff mobility can be assessed. A meniscus grasper is placed transcutaneously from the anterior-lateral portal (see Fig. 9-8, *B* and *C*, and Fig. 9-34). The humerus is in the 45-degree abducted position. The cuff tear is grasped and advanced to the greater tuberosity. This method of determining reparability before open incision avoids unnecessary, unfruitful open exploration in unreparable tears.

Cuff Mobilization

Another arthroscopic technique that facilitates open cuff repair is used in the patient in whom cuff mobility is compromised as determined by arthroscopy. In this case, the cuff is mobilized by arthroscopy. The synovial and capsular attachment to the superior glenoid may be released by electrocautery and blunt dissection. The mobility is reassessed. Freeing of superior adhesions by arthroscopic subacromial bursectomy may be helpful. Blunt dissection is performed on the superior surface of the cuff tendon and muscle. Mobility assessment is repeated. It has been my experience that results of the arthroscopic method of mobilization are equivalent to those possible by open surgery (except the extensive muscle sliding procedures).

Preliminary Coracoacromial Ligament Sectioning

Open surgical removal of the acromion is facilitated by preliminary arthroscopic resection or release of the CA ligament. When acromioplasty is performed without this preliminary release, the bone is cut, but difficult to mobilize because of the soft tissue attachments beneath the acromion. Open release of this attachment requires cutting deep in the wound, often without adequate visualization and with resultant bleeding. CA artery laceration may occur. These problems are avoided with a preliminary arthroscopic technique.

Preparation of Attachment Site

The area of anticipated attachment of the rotator cuff to the greater tuberosity can be selected and prepared by arthroscopic methods. The cuff is advanced according to the arthroscopic method described. The site is selected and can be prepared by arthroscopic debridement, including creating a bony groove for tendinous attachment by subsequent open surgery. This method decreases open surgical time and provides an accurate means of site selection and preparation.

Hemostasis

The hemostasis provided at arthroscopy is very effectively maintained during the open phase. This is especially true for acute tear repair (Fig. 9-44, *B* to *D*).

COMPLICATIONS

Fluid Extravasation

The most common intraoperative complication is the extravasation of fluid into the adjacent tissues.[38,60] The problem is not so much damage to muscle tissue as it is the increased mass to the shoulder area and depth of the tissue creating longer lever arms for the instrumentation. Extravasation is controlled by small, tight portals of entry around the cannulas, short operative time, and careful monitoring of fluid inflow pressures. The longer the procedure continues, the greater the chance of extravasation. In addition, I favor a gravity inflow system with intermittent increases in pressure and flow delivered by manual compression on a Gravity Assist bulb. The use of a mechanical pump creates a demand to ask for increased flow and pressure, as well as a loss of realizing that it has been turned up and is constantly pumping as time goes by. Morgan[46] believes that the mechanical pump is an expensive and complicated answer to a problem that does not exist. I agree.

Loss of Orientation

Care must be taken so as not to become disoriented or lose visualization. Disorientation has led to a complication of midclavicular resection and subsequent nonunion (see Fig. 9-28).

Local Anesthetic Injection

The postoperative injection of local anesthetic agents may cause cardiac problems. Kaeding et al[36] has shown that a 150 mg bolus infusion following knee arthroscopy is safe. The bolus remained in the joint for 32 minutes before saline infusion was initiated. Under these conditions the plasma levels peaked at 20 minutes. No toxic symptoms were seen, but levels of bupivacaine were higher in patients who had synovectomy. The postsurgical local circumstances are different following acromioplasty. Not only is soft tissue of the bursa exposed, but the exposed area of cancellous bone of the acromion and/or the clavicle have rich vascularity. The bone vascularity affords an immediate conduit to the vascular system. A recent report showed that 20 ml of 0.25% bupivacaine is safe.[33]

Two of my patients experienced immediate postbupivicaine hypotensive episodes following injection of this type dosage. I have since abandoned using local anesthetics after shoulder acromioplasty.

CHAPTER

10 The Acromioclavicular Joint

The acromioclavicular (AC) joint, although small, is amenable to arthroscopic inspection and surgery. This area of the shoulder region is affected by trauma and degenerative arthritis.

CLINICAL ASSESSMENT

This joint is most commonly injured by direct blows on the shoulder in a fall, resulting in either partial or complete separations. A prominence of the affected AC joint is common (Fig. 10-1). Most AC conditions are treated with conservative measures, including antiinflammatory medication and cortisone injection. Partial separations usually require no surgical intervention, but may result in degenerative changes and widening of the joint space (Figs. 10-2, *A* and 10-3, *A*). Persistent symptoms may be an indication for arthroscopic inspection, debridement, synovectomy, or resection of the distal end of the clavicle and acromion. Complete disruptions usually require open surgical restoration of the AC ligaments and/or resection of the outer end of the clavicle.[7,10,12]

Medical History

When this joint is affected, the most common complaint is pain. A bony prominence may also exist with an unreduced separation or degenerative arthritic spurring (Fig. 10-1). The patient may have limited shoulder elevation if the joint has developed ankylosis. A popping or catching sensation can occur when the small meniscal disc is torn.

Physical Examination

The superficial location of the joint provides access by physical examination (Fig. 10-4). Palpation of the affected joint will confirm the tenderness or mass. Motion restriction or popping sensation may be present. These abnormalities are discerned by inspection, palpation, manipulation, and auscultation (see Chapter 1).

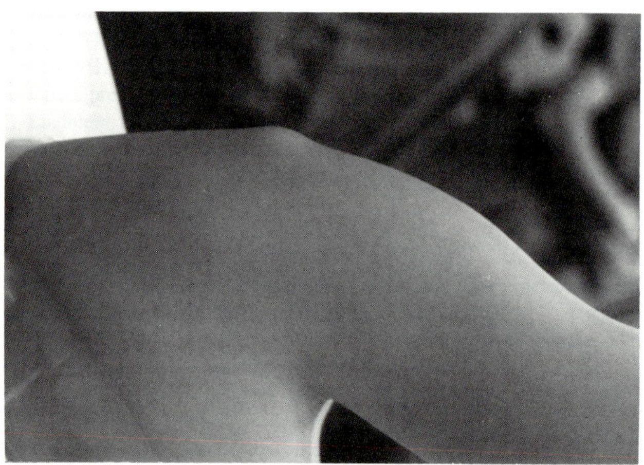

FIG. 10-1 Clinical presentation: Clinical photograph shows the typical prominence associated with AC disruption or degeneration. Note that some patients have normal prominences in which the bumps are bilateral.

Imaging

Plain film x-rays will demonstrate the various abnormalities. The degenerative joint shows both bone spurring and juxtaarticular cystic changes (Fig. 10-2, *A*). Osteolysis of this joint may follow trauma to the meniscus (Fig. 10-3), as often occurs in dedicated weight lifters.[2,8] The AC separation may be demonstrated by x-ray film, but disruption is more easily assessed by physical examination.

A bone scan is especially helpful in confirming the abnormality of this joint (Fig. 10-2, *B* and 10-3, *C*).[14] When this condition is associated with glenohumeral joint or impingement findings, determining exactly what area is producing the patient's symptoms may be difficult.[11] Another

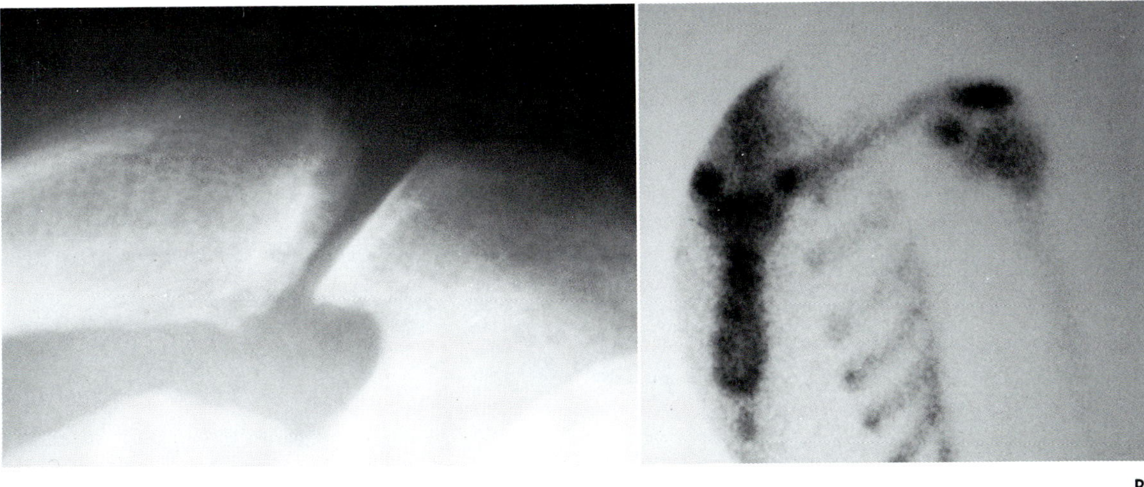

FIG. 10-2 Imaging of AC joint.

A Plain x-ray film shows degenerative arthritis with cystic changes.

B Bone scan shows increased uptake over the affected AC joint.

C Arthroscopy shows AC joint with degeneration and synovitis.

use of the bone scan is in surgical planning before acromioplasty. I use the preoperative bone scan in conjunction with the history and physical examination to determine the involvement of the AC joint. If this joint is clinically involved and demonstrates increased uptake of the radioisotope, then AC joint resection is included in the acromioplasty.

ACROMIOCLAVICULAR JOINT RESECTION

Diagnostic Arthroscopy

The diagnosis is usually established before arthroscopy. The joint is small, so there is no space to look around. The spectrum of diagnosis is narrow. Diagnostic arthroscopy confirms the meniscal or joint disruption. It may confirm the degenerative nature of the joint. The most important diagnostic observation would be the intraoperative recognition of juxtaarticular cysts and prominent osteophytes.

Indications

The clinical indications for exploration of this joint are few: torn meniscus, disruption of the joint, degenerative arthritis, and osteolysis (Fig. 10-2 and 10-3).[3,4,6,9,13] Rheumatoid arthritis may also be a rare indication.

Anatomy

Normal. The AC joint is immediately subcutaneous. It is surrounded with thick capsule and the end of each bone is covered with articular cartilage. The space is separated with fibrocartilaginous disc. The joint is immediately me-

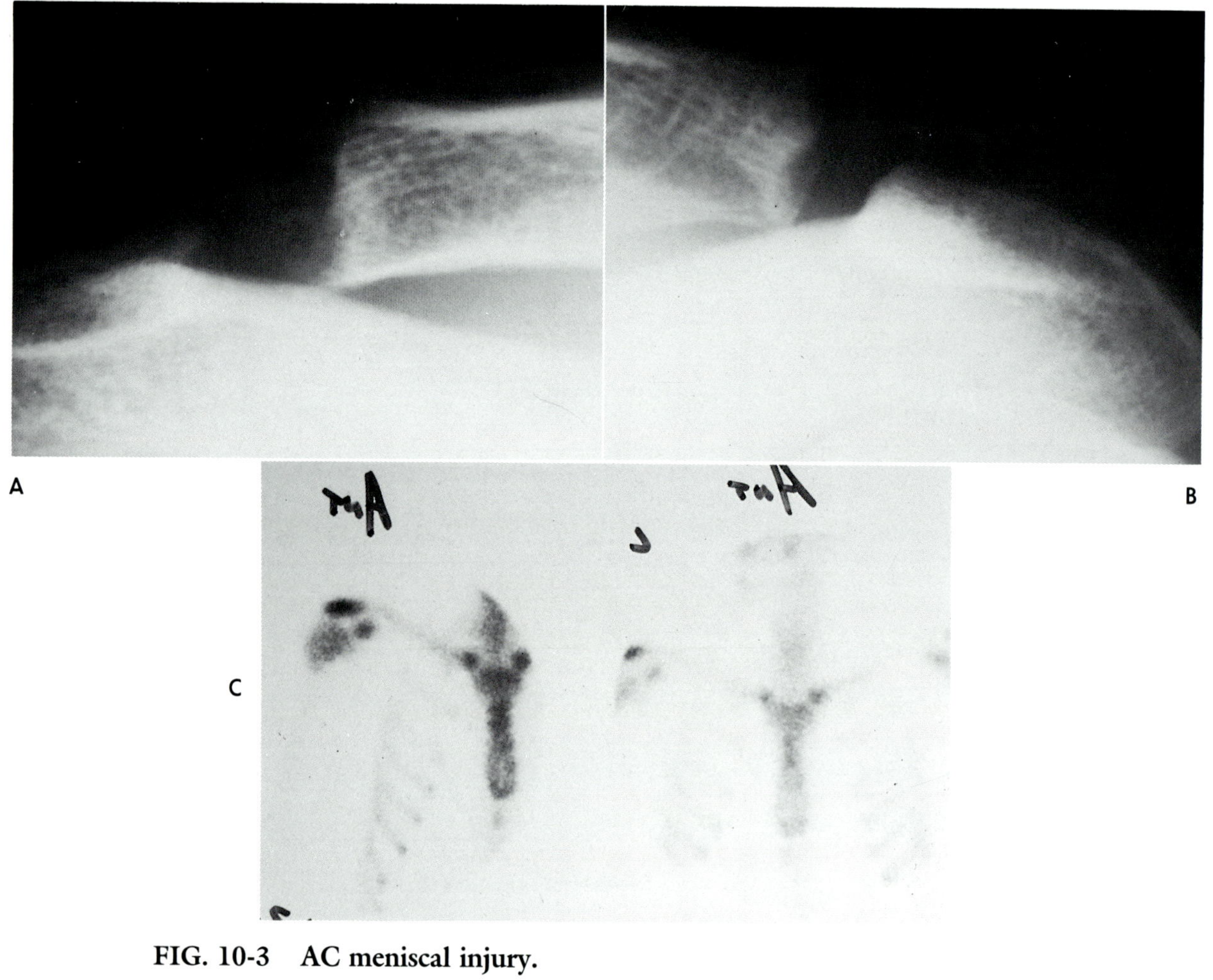

FIG. 10-3 AC meniscal injury.
A X-ray films show widened AC joint.
B View of normal opposite AC joint for comparison.
C Bone scan shows increased uptake in AC joint.

dial and superior to the subacromial bursa. The location makes this joint assessable from either the superior or the inferior approach (see also Chapters 6 and 9).

Pathologic. The normal joint space is so small that making an arthroscopic entry without injury to the joint would be difficult. Fortunately an indication for arthroscopy of the normal joint is rare. I have not seen the normal space arthroscopically, only by anatomical dissection (see also Chapter 7).

Osteolysis results in a wider joint space (Fig. 10-3).[2,8] Surgical access is possible even with a 4.0-mm diameter arthroscope and conventional instrumentation.

The other end of the pathological spectrum produces a narrow AC joint, even with osteophytes (see Fig. 10-2). Because this joint is already destroyed, arthroscopic penetration will not further injure the joint. Both a small diameter arthroscope and instrumentation may be required, especially at the beginning of the procedure.

In the diseased AC joint, the meniscus may be found intact, torn, or absent (see Fig. 10-2, *C*).

Surgical Techniques

This joint is approachable from superior or inferior. In some cases both approaches are necessary to accomplish

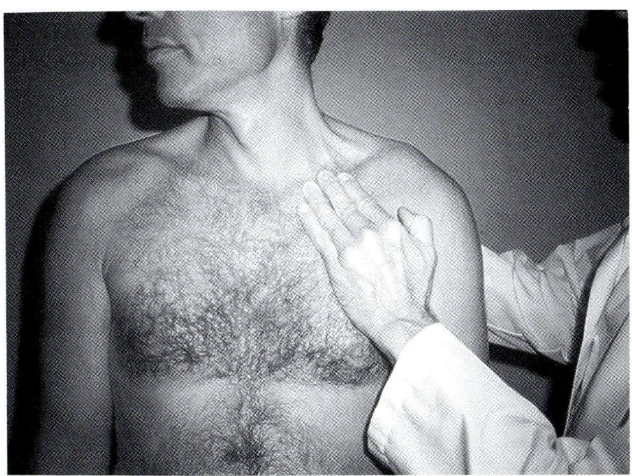

FIG. 10-4 Palpation of both the clavicle and the AC joint will assist in determining the location of the patient's complaint.

the intended resection (see Fig. 9-27, *F*).

The arthroscopic approach is technically difficult and requires a high level of arthroscopic skills. Neither the patient nor the surgeon should insist on this method when an open resection is technically easier and surer. If an arthroscopic approach is attempted but is intraoperatively unsuccessful, the procedure should be aborted and the joint opened.

The arthroscopic procedure includes resection of the joint debris; the synovium, meniscus, articular cartilage, and both ends of the acromial and clavicular bone.[5]

By either approach, preliminary needle identification is important to instrument placement (Fig. 10-5, *A*).

Subacromial Approach. This approach is technically easier than the superior approach. It is the more common approach because it is an extension of the acromioplasty. This approach could be used without acromioplasty if the subacromial bursal space were arthroscopically identifiable.

Surgical technique. This technique is discussed in Chapter 9.

Transcutaneous Superior Approach. This approach is technically challenging. The surgical time will probably be longer than the time needed for the same procedure by an open method. It has the benefit of cosmesis. In my experience it decreases neither the morbidity nor the recovery time when compared to open resection. Flatow et al[3] reported decreased morbidity and recovery time as compared to his open surgery. Disadvantages include limiting the visualization in the small space and assessing the accuracy of the amount of clavicle resected when compared to open surgical exposure.

Surgical technique. The patient is positioned as for any arthroscopic procedure of the shoulder. The joint is palpated to determine its position (Fig. 10-5, *A*). The angle is determined by palpating the osteophytes. The slope of the joint is determined by needle penetration and palpation. The AC joint is not parallel to any known outside topographical location.

A small needle is placed into the joint from posterior (Fig. 10-5, *B*). The joint is distended with pressure from a 60-ml syringe via a K-52 catheter. The space is small, and gravity or mechanical pump pressure and flows will not be sufficient.

Another needle is placed anterior to confirm the entry of the first needle by outflow of fluid through the second (Fig. 10-5, *C*).

This needle becomes the inflow site for arthroscope placement. A second check is made on flow by switching the inflow to the anterior needle and proving the outflow through the posterior needle (Fig. 10-5, *C*). This maneuver confirms both position and flow.

If the joint space is small, a small diameter arthroscope should be used to start the procedure. The smaller arthroscope is placed from posterior. Distention is maintained with inflow from the anterior needle portal. A larger scope is placed when the joint space is enlarged due to the patient's condition or surgical intervention. The larger scope provides a greater conduit for fluid delivery.

Confirmation of entry may be difficult because of the joint debris (Fig. 10-5, *E*). After the arthroscope is placed posterior, fluid flow out of the arthroscope cannula confirms entry (Fig. 10-5, *D*). Visualization of the anterior needle confirms the entry (Fig. 10-5, *F*).

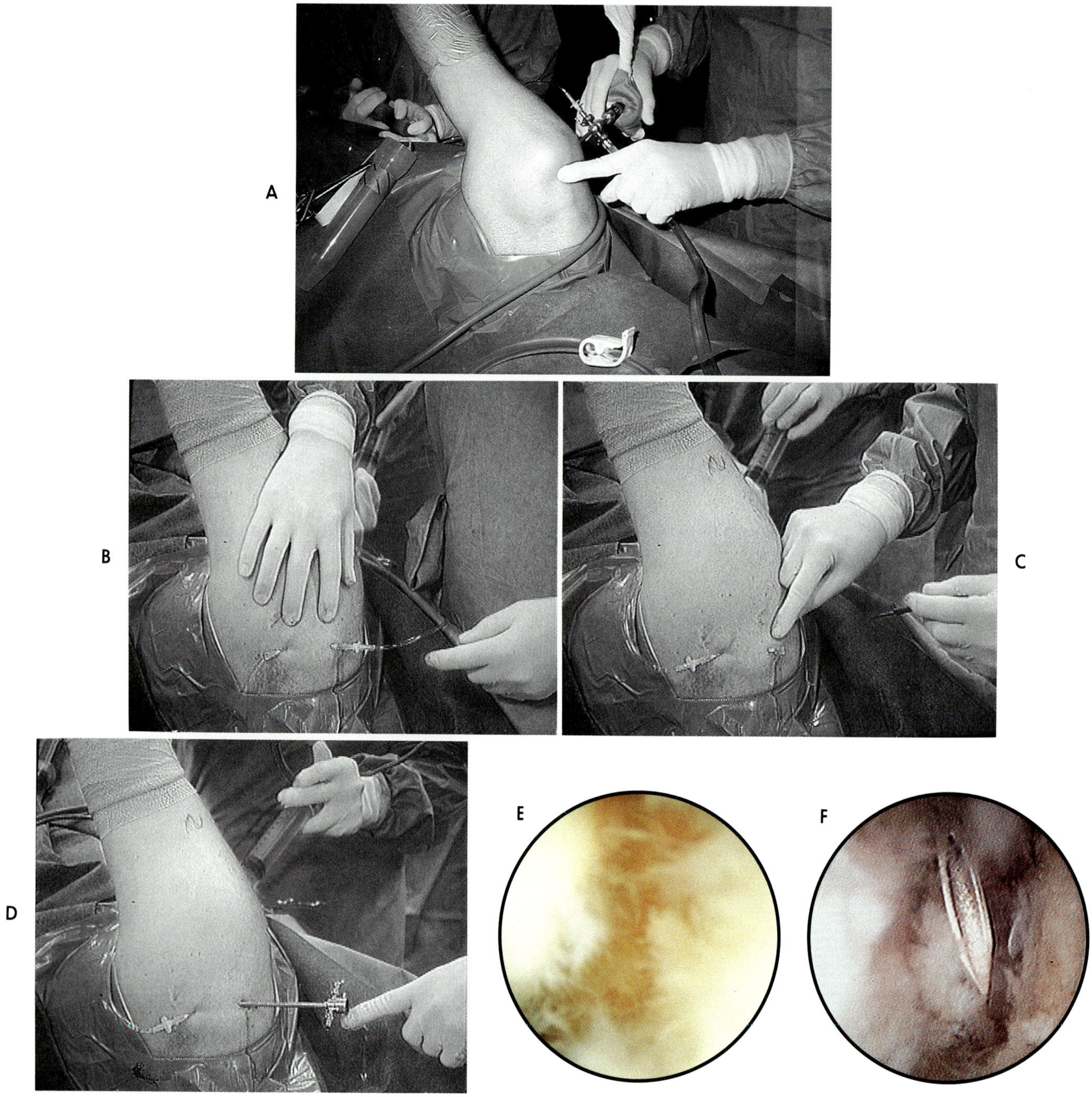

A

B

C

D

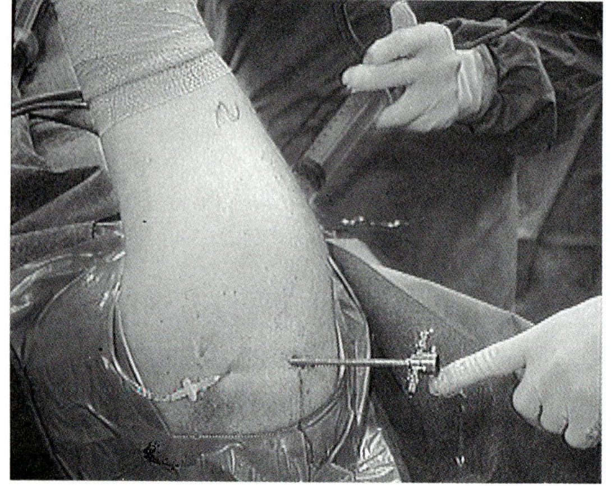

E

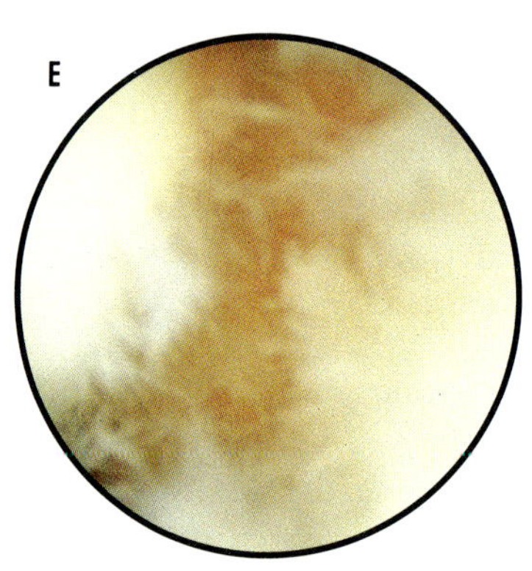

F

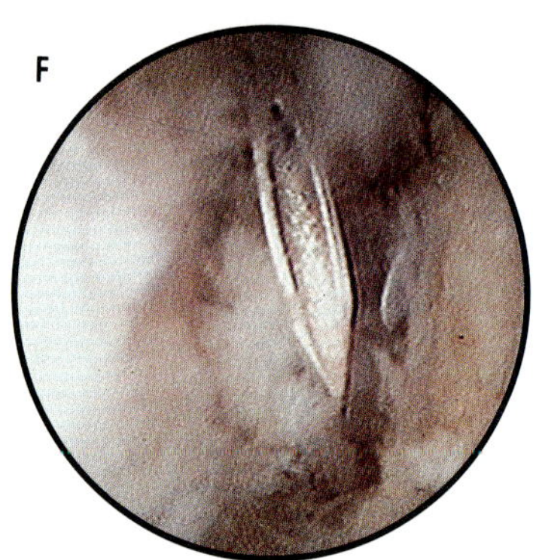

FIG. 10-5 Establishing AC joint entry and flow.

A Palpation of joint for location and angle.

B Needle placement for location and establishing flow. Flow comes out anterior.

C After interchange of inflow to anterior, needle flow comes out posterior needle.

D Arthroscope cannula is placed and flow comes out this cannula.

E Arthroscopic view confirmation may be difficult because of intraarticular debris.

F Location of the anterior inflow needle confirms the entry into the joint.

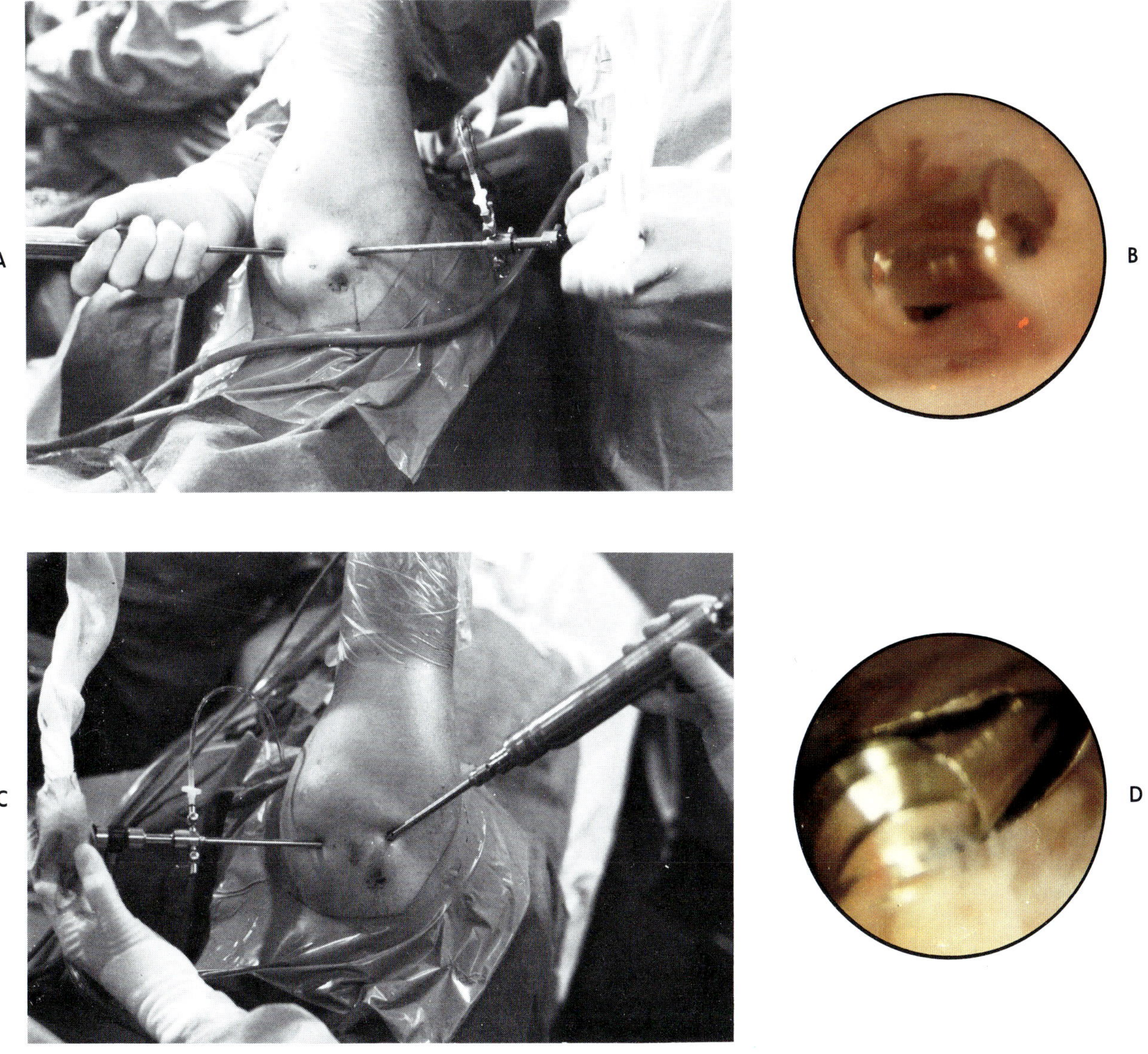

FIG. 10-6 Arthroscopic technique on AC joint.

A Arthroscope from posterior and instrument from anterior.

B Cutter head in AC joint.

C Instrumentation switched and arthroscope placed anteriorly.

D Arthroscope shows abrader entering from posterior AC joint.

Continued.

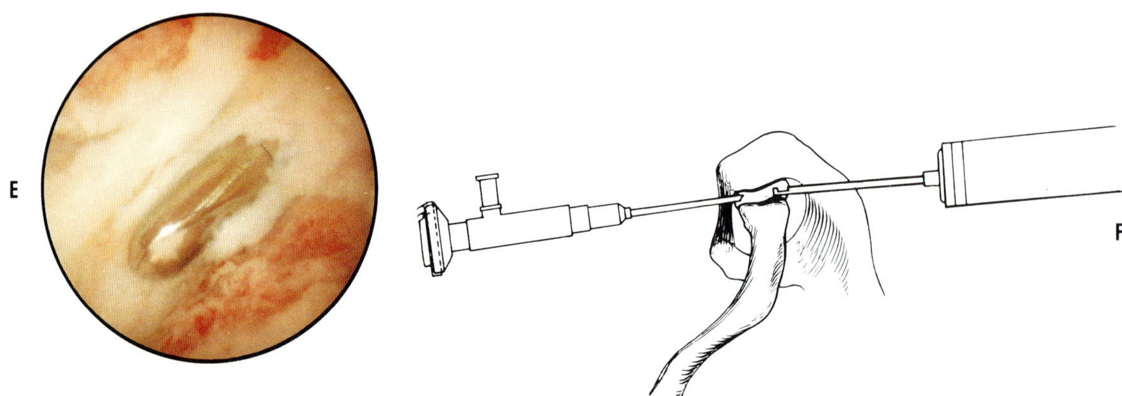

FIG. 10-6 *cont'd* **Arthroscopic technique on AC joint.**

E **Final arthroscopic view after meniscectomy and abrasion to exposed bone, both end of clavicle and acromion.**

F **Drawing of AC joint surgery.**

After entry is confirmed, the inflow system is transferred to the arthroscope spigot. Inflow is provided by intermittent boluses of saline via a 60-ml syringe and K-52 catheter. Surprisingly, the AC joint capsule provides an excellent seal, and no leakage occurs.

The anterior portal is established by the Wissinger rod method. The arthroscope is placed against the anterior joint wall. The scope is removed so a rod may be placed through the cannula and out the anterior joint. The skin is lacerated and an instrumentation cannula is retrograded over this rod. A cannula system is essential to maintaining access and for the interchangeability of portals.

AC joint debridement commences with soft tissue resection until the bone is exposed (Fig. 10-6, *A* and *B*). The meniscus tissue may be so large and tough that slicing with a small knife blade is necessary to reduce its size for resection by a motorized cutter. When the bone is exposed, switching sticks are used to interchange the cannula system with a large arthroplasty system cannula. A burr is used to resect the ends of the clavicle and acromion (Fig. 10-6, *D*). The final clean-up is performed with a small, full-radius resector (Fig. 10-6, *E*). An interchange of arthroscope and instrumentation is necessary to see the opposite side of this joint (Fig. 10-6, *A* and *C*).

When osteophytes exist, the burr is manipulated up and over the osteophyte. When cystic changes exist on x-ray film, their presence should be confirmed by arthroscopic exposure. Resection of the fibrocystic changes and adjacent bone removes this nidus of erosion (Fig. 10-7).

Results

Although I reported this method of AC arthroscopy in 1986, I have few case experiences.[6] In my experience, every patient has been an active sportsman who desires a vigorous life style. In fact, it was this life style that led to the AC joint condition. In spite of my cautioning them about the necessity of at least 3 months for fibrous tissue repair and reduction of symptoms, all patients have been unhappy with the slow recovery. Part of this is due to their expectations of less morbidity with the arthroscopic technique. Another problem is that the patient attempts vigorous over-the-head activities before the prescribed time for healing.

The initial pathological response to resection is blood clot formation. Eventually, this area fills in with fibrous tissue. The joint becomes stable and symptoms decrease.

Failure. Only one patient, an orthopedic surgeon, came to a second operation. The second procedure was performed for persistent pain and in his opinion inadequate excision of the clavicle. He reported the subsequent operating surgeon found an irregular regrowth of clavicle with fibrocartilage tissue. A pseudoarthrosis was present. The second procedure, an open resection, reduced his symptoms.

What is an adequate resection? This single experience has caused me to give more attention to the amount of clavicle to be resected. The standard amount resected by open surgery is 1 cm. The amount of space created between the two bones is one factor. The other factor is adequate removal of bone superior and inferior, especially the osteophytes. It would be possible to open a wide space between the bones and overlook the periphery of the joint that remains in contact. At present, it seems that at least 0.5 cm should be removed across the entire joint. Removal of greater than 1.0 cm is probably not necessary.

Flatow, Cordasco, and Bigliani[1,3] have reported their

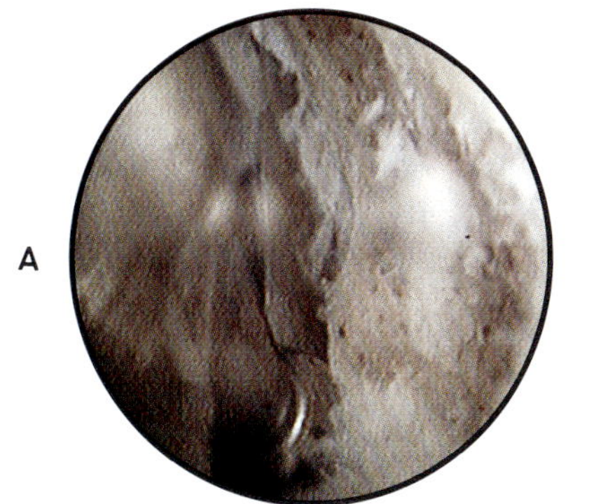

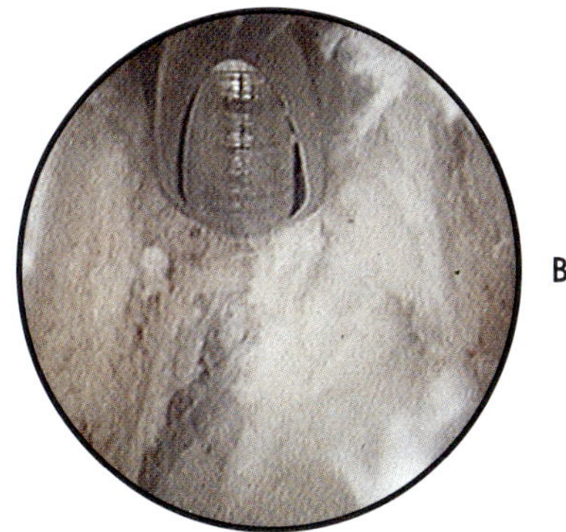

FIG. 10-7 Resection of osteophytes.

A Arthroscopic view of resection of osteophyte under capsular covering of the joint.

B Arthroscopic view of clean-up of site of previous osteophyte with full-radius resector.

experience with the superior approach for AC joint resection for osteolysis of the distal end of the clavicle. They reported the ability to remove 17 mm of the bone. This compared favorably with the 18 mm removed by open surgery. Pain relief was achieved 3.4 months earlier in the arthroscopic group. Hospital stay was shortened in the arthroscopic group as compared to the average 3 days for the open procedure patients.

MUMFORD TYPE PROCEDURE

Now that arthroscopic AC debridement is a reality, the potential for arthroscopic resection of the outer end of the clavicle exists. Patients with previous AC joint separations or AC degenerative arthritis and sufficient symptoms may undergo resection arthroplasty, including a small section of the outer end of the clavicle. The objective would be to produce an arthroscopic Mumford procedure.[7]

Caution should be taken with this approach because an important part of the open repair is the soft tissue closure and imbrication of the trapezius fascia. In addition, it may be recognized only at open surgery that the free end of resected clavicle is still floating and requires security by transferring the end of the CA ligament.

COMPLICATIONS

My patients have not experienced any complications. The main potential for complications unique to this procedure are technical: failure to enter the space or loss of orientation. These situations could result in injury to juxtaarticular neurovascular structures.

Either problem is a good reason to abort the procedure and proceed to open resection. The morbidity with open resection is only minimally greater, although cutaneous nerves are usually cut with the incision.

Care must be taken to avoid resection of clavicle beyond the stabilizing CA ligaments (see Fig. 9-28).

REFERENCES

1. Bigliani L et al: *The superior approach for arthroscopic resection of the distal clavicle.* Presented at American Academy of Orthopedic Surgeons Annual Meeting, March 1991.
2. Cahill BR: Osteolysis of the distal part of the clavicle in male athletes, *J Bone Joint Surg (Am)* 64:1053-1058, 1982.
3. Flatow EL et al: *Arthroscopic resection of the distal clavicle via a superior portal: a critical qualitative radiographic assessment of bone removal.* Presented at the American Orthopedic Association Residents Conference, Newport Beach, Calif, March 1990.
4. Fowler P: Swimmer problems, *Am J Sports Med* 7:141-142, 1979.
5. Gartsman GM et al: Arthroscopic AC joint resection: an anatomical study, *Am J Sports Med* 19:2-5, 1991.
6. Johnson LL: *Arthroscopic surgery: principles and practice,* St Louis, 1986, Mosby–Year Book.
7. Mumford EB: Acromioclavicular dislocation: a new operative treatment, *J Bone Joint Surg* 3:799-801, 1941.
8. Murphy OB et al: Post-traumatic osteolysis of the distal clavicle, *Clin Orthop* 109:108-114, 1975.
9. Myers JF: Arthroscopic debridement of the AC joint and distal clavicle resection. In McGinty JB et al, eds: *Operative arthroscopy,* New York, 1991, Raven.
10. Neer CS II: *Shoulder reconstruction,* Philadelphia, 1990, WB Saunders.
11. Resnick D: Shoulder arthrography, *Radiol Clin North Am* 19:243-252, 1981.
12. Rockwood CA Jr, Matsen FA III: *The Shoulder,* Philadelphia, 1990, WB Saunders.
13. Snyder SJ: Arthroscopic AC joint debridement and distal clavicle resection, *Techniques Orthop* 3:41-45, 1988.
14. Thomas RH et al: Compartmental evaluation of osteoarthritis of the knee: a comparative study of available diagnostic modalities, *Radiology* 116:585, 1975.

CHAPTER

11 The Future

Arthroscopy provided a technological advance in orthopedic surgery. It brought enhanced imaging, light source energy, television, miniature instrumentation, computer technology, changing surgical environment, and an entirely new way of thinking about orthopedic problems and their treatment. The future developments in orthopedic surgery will build on this foundation.

THE PRESENT

At present, the quality of the arthroscopic image is excellent. The arthroscopes are uniformly high quality. The television images are clear. Electronic documentation on tape, slides, and prints is good. The hand and motorized instrumentation is adequate for the procedures that are performed. Orthopedic surgeons are still developing their arthroscopic motor skills. The arthroscopic application has expanded beyond the glenohumeral joints to adjacent bursa. Debridement procedures (labrum resection, removal of loose body, and acromioplasty) are common place. Many procedures are performed in surgical centers under outpatient admission.

The future is nothing more than the fruition of the seed that we have already planted. The idea is conceived. The seed is often rejected because it does not resemble the fruit it is to bear. A dormant period is required for the seed. Soil preparation with plowing, fertilization, and weed control is necessary. Planting is finally performed. Watering and gardening are necessary. After some time and labor the seed becomes a fruit, the idea a reality. Everyone can recognize the value of the fruit.

The development of arthroscopy has followed this pattern. The idea (seed) was seen in the 1930s.[3] There was a long dormant period until the late 1960s.[5,7,11] The development required many surgeons' unappreciated efforts in the 1970s (see Chapter 1). Finally, the harvest was ready by the 1980s. The profession embraced arthroscopy as a standard method of treatment. In many ways this scenario reminds me of the nursery story of the Little Red Hen. The consumer's interest increases when the labor is over and the bread has just come out of the oven.

THE IMMEDIATE FUTURE

The future of shoulder arthroscopy in the 1990s will be a repeat of what was experienced in the knee joint in the 1980s. Most, but not all, shoulder surgery will be performed by arthroscopic methods. Not all surgeons have been in agreement with my perspective.[6]

On the other hand, open surgery of the shoulder will not pass away. As with knee surgery, some shoulder conditions can not be performed as well arthroscopically as by an open method. An extensive capsular shift for multidirectional instability is one present example.

The necessity remains, as in some knee surgery, to combine open procedures with arthroscopy, as in anterior cruciate ligament grafting. A similar situation exists in the shoulder. The subacromial space is debrided by arthroscopy including the acromioplasty, but is followed by mini-incision for rotator cuff repair.

Some knee surgery has not been performed by arthroscopy, but has been attempted. Caspari[4] has designed instruments for and performed a hemi-prosthetic replacement of one compartment in clinical trials. This procedure required laborious hours of surgery. The total shoulder remains an open procedure for the foreseeable future.

The immediate future will see the continued application of arthroscopic skills to shoulder problems. As orthopedic surgeons develop arthroscopic surgical skills, a diagnostic arthroscopy will precede or accompany most open shoulder surgeries for rotator cuff lesions. Variations of existing methods of surgical repair will be attempted for shoulder instability, labrum tears, and rotator cuff tears (see Chapters 8 and 9).[16]

Endoscopic Bone Surgery

The application of the endoscope to joints resulted in the term *arthroscopy*. The term *arthroscope* became clumsy when it was used to explore spaces other than joint (i.e., subacromial space). Such a procedure is called *bursoscopy*. Should the instrument be a bursoscope? What name should be applied to the arthroscope used for carpal tunnel release? Watanabe[15] suggests these procedures be called tunneling.

Eventually, we will see a change back to more generic naming, *endoscopy*. This is more than a nomenclature change; it is a conceptual change. The enhanced imaging of endoscopy has a potential application in all surgery, especially everything we do in orthopedics. It started with inspection of joints, hence arthroscopy. The widest application in orthopedics will be bone surgery. Andrews, Tedder, and Godbout recently reported on a distal tibial bone cyst debridement approached by ankle arthroscopy. The application of the endoscope to shoulder surgery has potential for treatment of nonunion of fractures and aseptic necrosis of the humeral head. I have personally also performed these bone techniques in the area of the knee and hip.

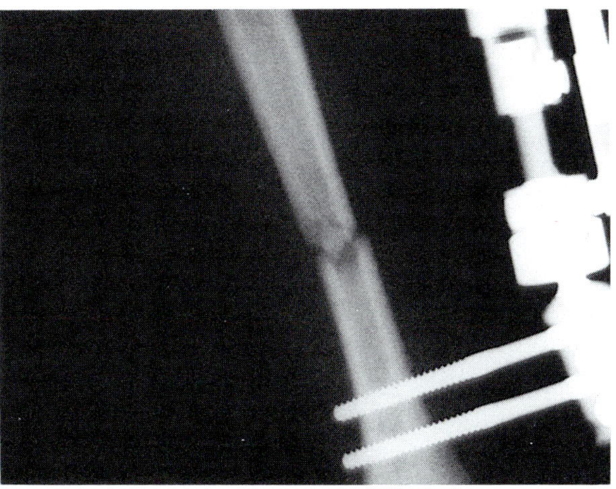

FIG. 11-1 Case 1. X-ray film of humerus at 5 months after injury. There is no evidence of healing. The external fixation is secure.

Transcutaneous Endoscopic Bone Grafting

Kenneth Morrison, one of my associates, and I have performed transcutaneous endoscopic bone grafting of delayed union of the humerus (Fig. 11-1).

Case 1. A 37-year-old white woman sustained an open fracture of her left humerus in an auto accident. There was bone loss and a radial nerve injury. The wound was debrided. The fracture was reduced. An external fixator device maintained the reduction.

After 3 months, the fracture site showed no signs of bony union (Fig. 11-1, *A*). A transcutaneous endoscopic bone grafting procedure was performed on the humerus.

The nonunion site was approached transcutaneously. The periosteum was stripped off the nonunion site. This area was distended with sterile, normal saline as in arthroscopy. The fracture site was easily visualized. An endoscopic debridement was performed with motorized instrumentation. Most of the fibrous nonunion was resected. A minimal debridement was performed on the bone.

The bone graft was harvested through a small incision from the iliac crest and delivered to the nonunion site with bone grafter (see Fig. 11-7).

The patient stayed in the hospital a total of 22 hours. The fracture united in 6 weeks (Fig. 11-2, *A*). The external fixation device was removed. By 6 months the patient had restoration of full elbow motion and upper extremity function (Fig. 11-2, *B*). The operative wounds were much smaller than the wound of the injury. The nonunion site continued to remodel (Fig. 11-3).

Case 2. A 24-year-old, white male sustained an open fracture of the left humerus among multiple other injuries. An open reduction, internal fixation was performed at another institution with plate, screws, and rod. After 7 months a nonunion of the proximal humerus was well established. A transcutaneous bone harvesting and grafting procedure was performed under endoscopic control. (Fig. 11-4, *A, B, C,* and *D*) The morbidity was minimal (Fig. 11-4, *E*). Postoperative x-ray films show an abundance of bone graft at the surgical site. (Fig. 11-5).

As a result of this humeral case and other experiences with transcutaneous endoscopic bone grafting procedures in other regions, we have developed the following protocol for grafting of nonunion of long bones.

INDICATIONS:

1. Established, delayed or nonunion of bone.
2. Compromised skin in area of fracture (previous skin or pedicle grafts).
3. Outrigger in place.

CONTRAINDICATIONS:

1. Active infection.
2. Lack of endoscopic experience.

BENEFITS:

1. Minimal trauma.
2. Short hospitalization (outpatient).
3. Fills defects with bone.
4. Provides marrow cells for osteogenesis potential.

Surgical Technique

Prophylactic antibiotics. Prophylactic intravenous antibiotics may be used at the discretion of the surgeon.

Patient position. The patient is positioned to expose the lateral iliac crest and approach to the long bone.

Tourniquet. Tourniquet control is recommended, if possible, because of the hyperemia in the area.

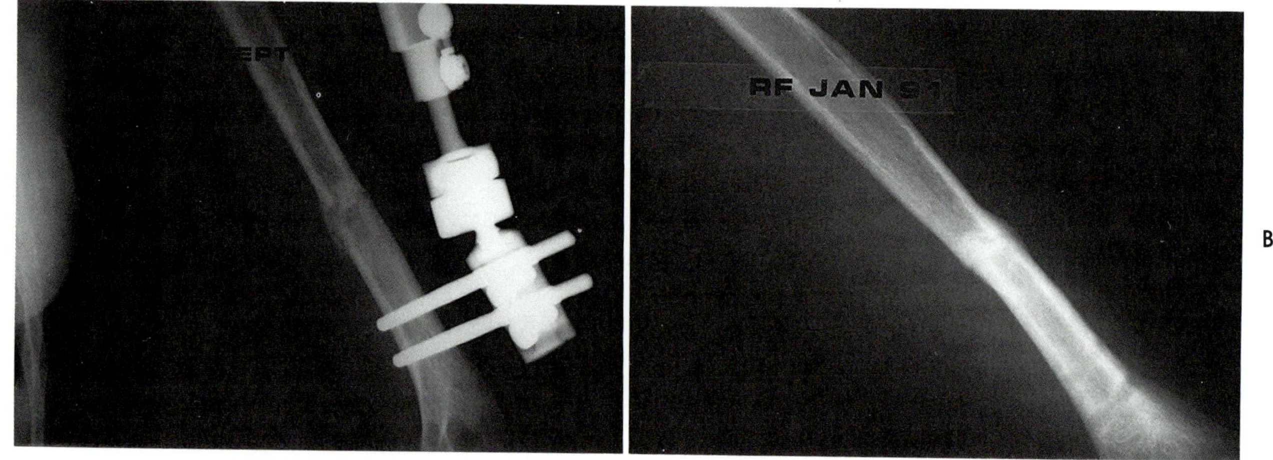

FIG. 11-2 Case 1.

A Postoperative bone graft x-ray film at 3 months shows union of humerus. External fixation device was removed.

B X-ray film at 1 year shows further remodeling of healed nonunion site.

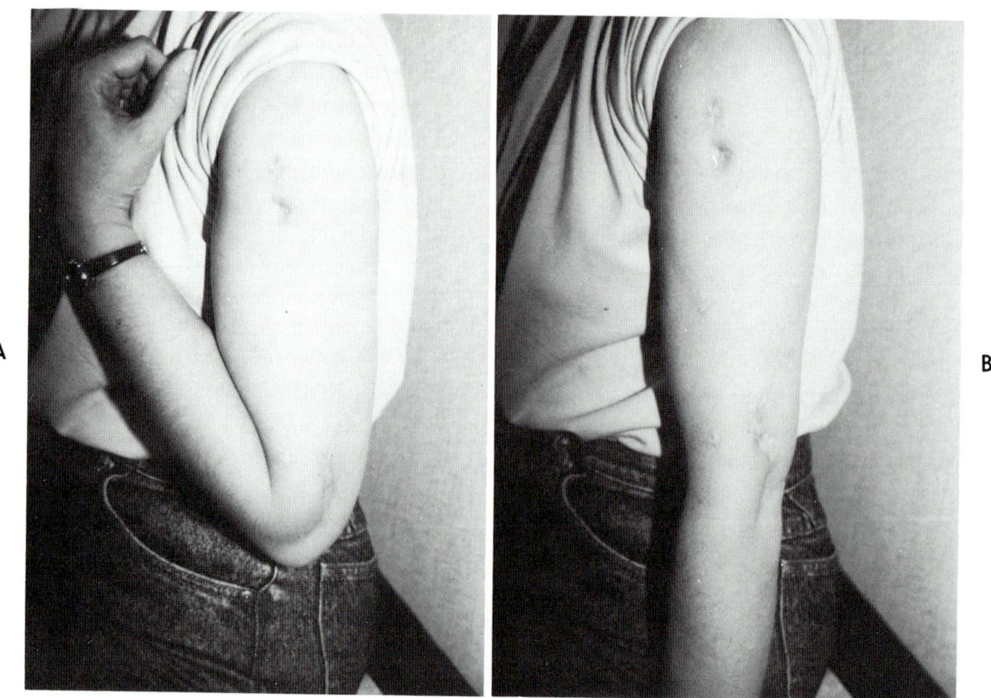

FIG. 11-3 Case 1. Clinical result: The incisions from the surgery are smaller than those of the injury on the posterior distal humerus and those of the external fixation device proximal and lateral. The patient has normal return of elbow range of motion.

A Elbow flexion is normal.

B Elbow extension is normal.

A

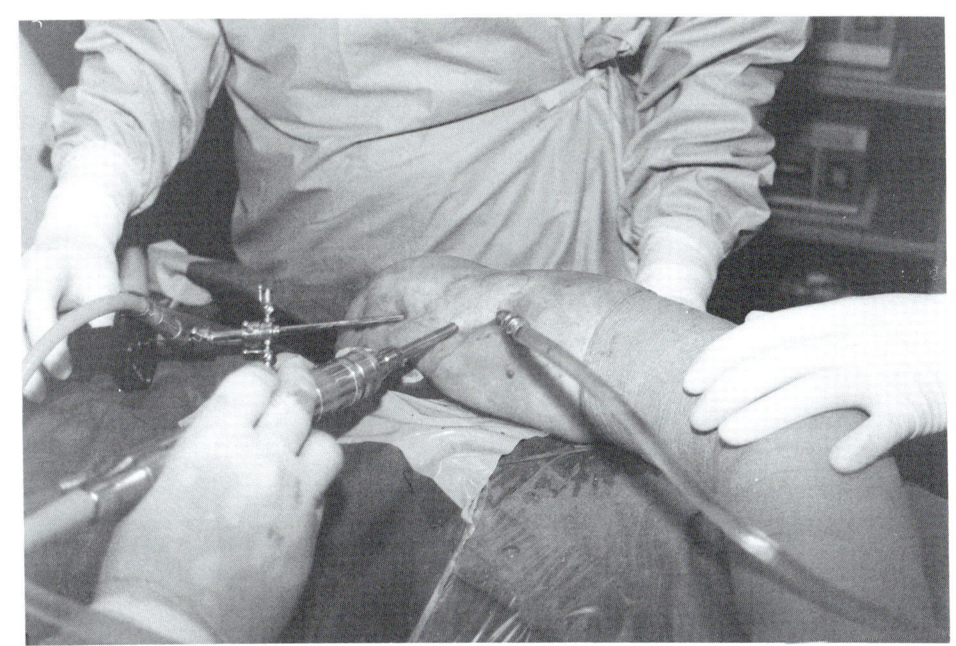

B

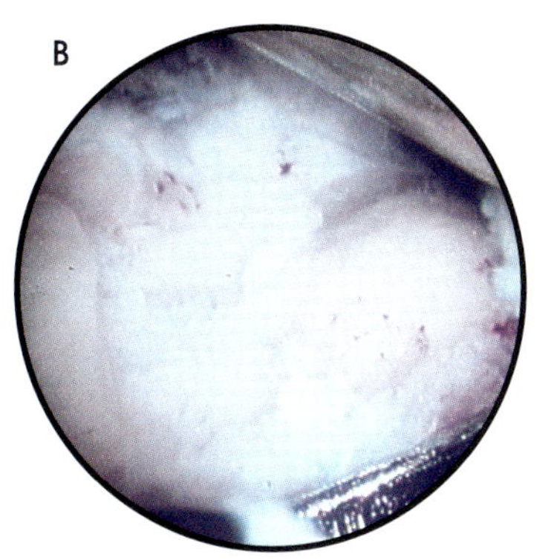

C

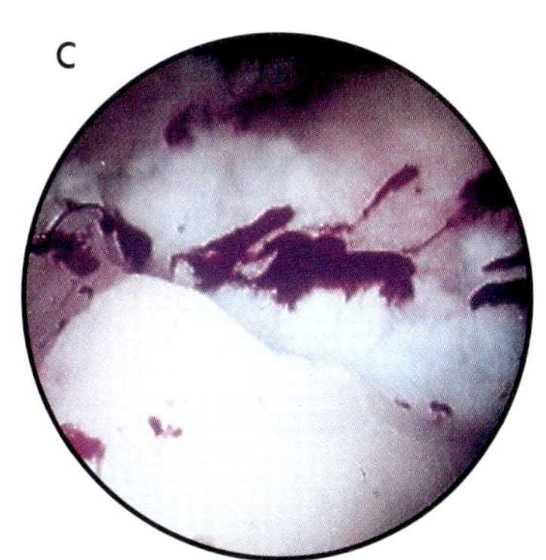

D

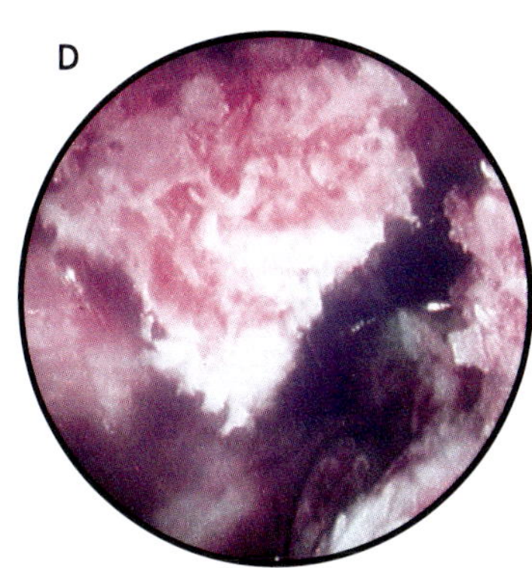

E

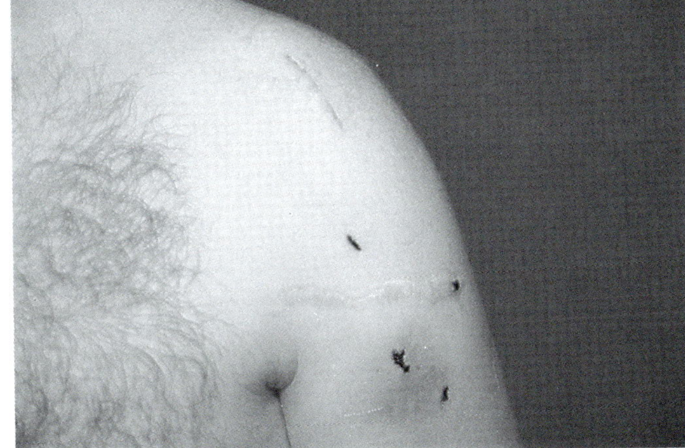

FIG. 11-4 Surgical exposure (Case 2).

A Transcutaneous exposure of fracture is with arthroscope to the left, inflow cannula to the right, and the motorized instrumentation placed over the nonunion site.

B Endoscopic view of the nonunion site. Note fibrous tissue between the two bone ends.

C Endoscopic view of nonunion site when space is decompressed. Note abundant vascularity.

D Endoscopic view of bone graft in place.

E Multiple small puncture wounds are healing at 1 week after surgery.

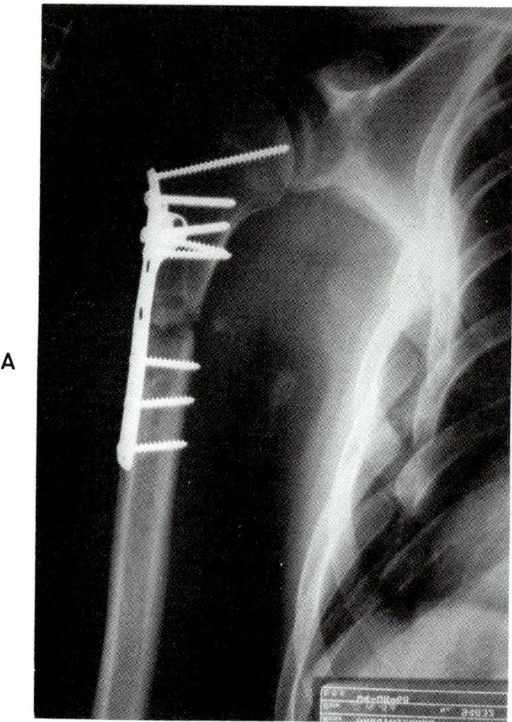

A

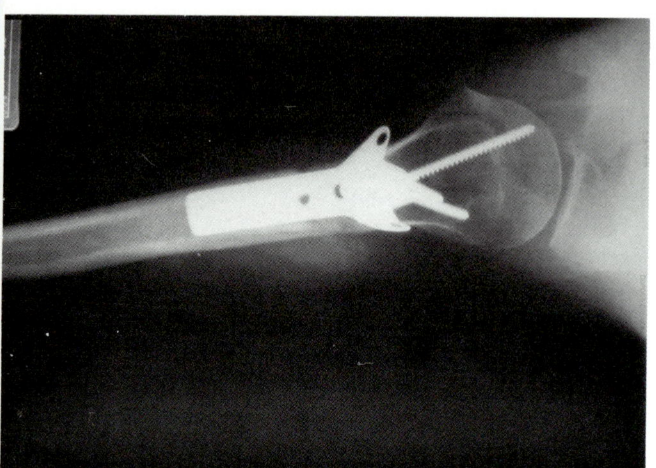

B

FIG. 11-5 Case 2. Post operative X-ray films.
A Anterior-posterior film: Note the bone graft in the resected non-union site.
B Lateral projection: Note the abundant graft along the humerus.

Fluid irrigation system. This is afforded by a large reservoir of fluid: 2 6-liter bags suspended at least 1 m above the patient.

An inflow cannula is recommended over inflow on the arthroscope. This system delivers more fluid and less motion in the tissues in front of the arthroscope.

A gravity assist hand pump is recommended. This pump allows both fluid and air to be delivered to the surgical area. This method of enhanced flow maintains surgical team consciousness of fluid delivery as compared to a continuous mechanical pump. Thus excessive amounts of fluid extravasation are avoided.

Control of fluid. The soft tissue envelope of the periosteal envelope is similar to a synovial joint. Excess fluid will leak from the wounds. Therefore, measures should be taken before surgery to control this problem. The draping should be placed to direct excess fluid leakage away from the surgical field and into a container (bucket) on the floor.

Sterile draping. The sterile draping should include covering the extremity with stockenette. An opening is made in the stockenette to expose the surgical area. Coban (3M) is used to wrap around the outrigger. Sterile plastic adhesive drape is used to cover the surgical area.

Surgical exposure (portals). The fixation on the x-ray film serves as landmark for the fracture site location and the subsequent incision sites.

The *first incision* should be proximal or distal to the long bone and parallel to the side of the bone to be exposed. This portal is used to strip the periosteum proximal and distal to the fracture site with a small bone elevator. This portal becomes the site of inflow cannula placement.

Subsequent portals. The subsequent portals accommodate interchangeability of the scope and the instrumentation (Fig. 11-4, *A*).

The *first interchangeable portal* should approach the fracture site at an angle that provides arthroscopic viewing. The *other interchangeable portal* should be in the same plane as the fracture so that the cutting instrument will pass easily into the fracture site for debridement.

Step By Step

Nonunion surgical exposure

1. Locate the fracture site in relation to the outrigger or other landmark with use of the x-ray film.
2. Use a pen to draw the fracture site from the perspective of anticipated surgical approach.
3. Use a pen to mark anticipated portal sites. These

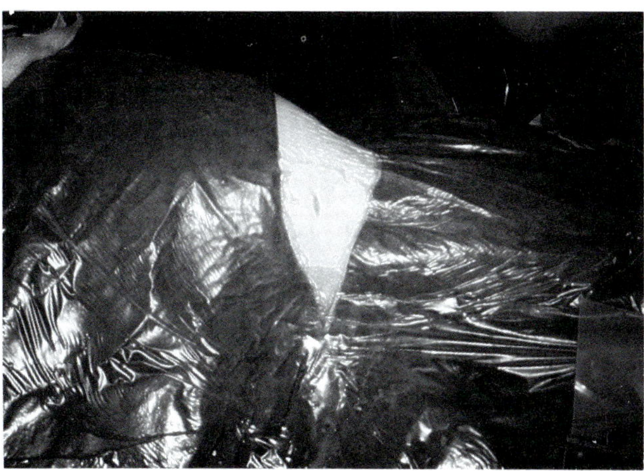

FIG. 11-6 Small incision over iliac crest provided access to bone graft donor site.

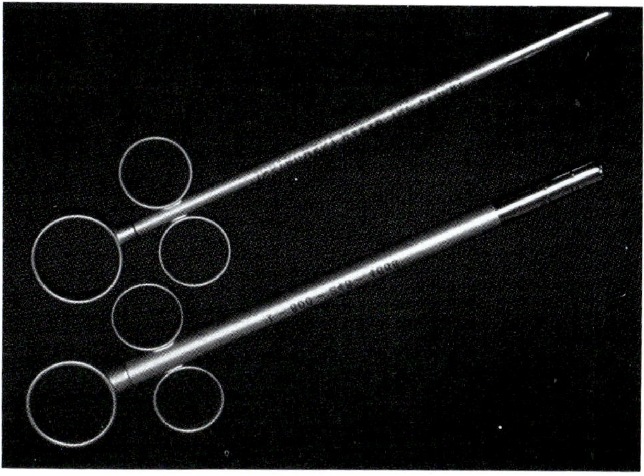

FIG. 11-7 Bone grafter instruments.

sites are described above. The skin portal should be removed from the fracture site so that sufficient soft tissue intervenes to prevent fluid leakage.

4. Establish the first portal (see above). A percutaneous subperiosteal stripping is accomplished.
   a. Place the inflow cannula.
   b. Establish the inflow.
5. Establish the second portal for the endoscope. Aim at the inflow cannula. Palpation of the bone and inflow cannula helps locate the envelope around the periosteum.
6. Establish the third portal. If the second portal is not ideal for the arthroscope, then attempt to make the third portal for the arthroscope and the second for the instruments. These portals will be interchangeable (Fig. 11-4, *A*).
7. The loose tissue in the envelope is removed with motorized instrumentation, such as a synovial resector.
8. The fracture site is identified.
   a. The nonunion tissue is white and firm (Fig. 11-4, *B*).
   b. The live bone is yellow-white and has small red vessels that are easily visualized.
9. The soft tissue is removed from the bone with motorized instrumentation (abrader tip).
10. A superficial debridement is performed on the ends of the bone. Care is taken to make this debridement superficial. The end point is the exposure of small red vessels in the bone. Blood supply to this area is good (Fig. 11-4, *C*).
11. The major portion of the soft tissue of the nonunion is removed. Some is maintained to control alignment of the bones.
12. The soft tissue is cleaned off each bone for at least 1 inch.

Harvesting the bone graft

1. Palpate the iliac crest for the area of greatest width.
2. Select the site of greatest width. This is usually 3 inches posterior from the anterior iliac spine. An alternate or additional site can be the anterior or posterior ilium.
3. Make a 1/2 inch incision over the crest (Fig. 11-6).
   a. Expose the crest.
   b. Excision of soft tissue may be necessary to palpate the bone.
   c. Create a divot on crest with rongeur into cancellous bone.
   d. Locate the space between the lamina with Kirschner wire. The is done by hand in order to not violate the inner or outer table.
   e. Over drill the K-wire with 1 cm cannulated drill.
4. Take the graft.
   a. Use the bone grafters to harvest by both 4-mm and 8-mm grafts (Fig. 11-7).
   b. The direction of harvest is both anterior and posterior.
   c. The instrument is used like a shovel against the inner wall of the ilium to scoop up cancellous bone. The free hand is placed on the ilium as directional guide.
   d. Start with 4-mm diameter bone grafter. As hole is enlarged change to 8-mm diameter.
   e. To take the graft, remove plunger from tube.
   f. To save time, one surgeon can use two instruments, taking the graft with one, while placing the graft with the other.
   g. Replace the plunger after graft is harvested.

Placing the bone graft

1. Place the grafts via the instrument site.
2. The bone grafter is placed through the skin with pressure and a stirring motion.
3. Watch the graft extrusion with endoscope.
4. Grafts can be manipulated into position with bone grafter or probe (Fig. 11-4, *D*).
5. Pack the nonunion site and areas of bone deficiency.
6. Lay graft proximal and distal to fracture site for 1 inch.
7. Take care not to wash bone grafts of marrow substance with irrigation flow.

Intraoperative complications. Intraoperative complications all have causes. The solution is either prevention or correction. Some of the complications are listed with cause, prevention, and correction measures.

1. *Extravasation of fluid*
   Cause: Ragged stripping of periosteum.
   Prevention: Single smooth periosteal stripping.
   Cause: Result of cannula out of view and in soft tissues.
   Correction: Find cannula and bring into pocket next to bone.
   Cause: Overdistention of pocket.
   Prevention: Do not pump against resistance.
2. *Bleeding*
   Cause: Hyperemic area.
   Prevention: Use fluid pressure to overcome.
   Correction: Use air to dry. Use electrocautery.
3. *Wrong surgical approach*
   Cause: Failure to properly triangulate.
   Correction: Change portals.
4. *Compartment syndrome*
   Cause: Extravasation of fluids.
   Prevention: Control of fluid inflow.
   Correction: Fasciotomy.

Postoperative management

1. A less than 1-day stay is customary. The morbidity is minimal and outpatient surgery is possible as experience is gained.
2. Postoperative pain is minimal. Surprisingly, the graft donor site is less painful than the surgical site. This is just the opposite of open surgical methods.
3. Postoperative x-ray films are taken at a minimum of two important intervals.
   a. Immediately after surgery (Fig. 11-5).
   b. 6 weeks postoperative.
4. Union is determined.
   a. Clinical absence of signs of inflammation.
   b. Mechanically solid to stress.
   c. X-ray evidence (Fig. 11-2).
   d. Return to function (Fig. 11-3).

Bone Grafting of Articular Defects. I have 6 years of experience with transcutaneous arthroscopic bone grafting of large articular defects of the knee femoral condyle because of osteochondritis dissecans and osteonecrosis. This procedure was based on observations I made during abrasion arthroplasty, bone grafting osteochondritis dissecans, and with postarthroscopic blood clot formation.[9,8] The similar defects of the humeral head or glenoid would be amenable to the same procedure. Traumatic defects would be another indication, especially on the glenoid surface following bursting fracture.

The transportation of this technology to the shoulder requires a skilled arthroscopist, simple instrumentation, and understanding of the healing process. The defect is debrided with motorized instrumentation. The edges are undercut similar to dentistry to hold the amalgam of the bone graft. The graft is harvested transcutaneously from the iliac crest through a small puncture wound (see above description). The graft is placed transcutaneously into the defect and is packed into place. Cancellous bone is like Velcro; its spicules are self-adhering to each other and to the acceptor site. A blood clot forms 5 to 7 minutes after surgery, resulting in fibrin deposition and further means of fixation.[9] I have not seen any of these types of grafts fall out in the knee. Second look into the knee cases with biopsy shows the formation and proliferation of fibrocartilage as early as 8 weeks and mature fibrocartilage by 10 months. The clinical outcomes have been good for reduction of pain and maintenance of joint space over several years.

I have not as yet performed such a procedure in the shoulder.

Bone Grafting of Osteonecrosis. Experience with the knee and the hip have shown it is possible to see and differentiate a live and dead bone by transcutaneous/intraosseous endoscopic methods. This same technology can be transported to the shoulder.

In the past, I have resected areas of osteonecrosis of the humeral head without grafting. In the future, small lesions will also be grafted endoscopically.

Tunneling Endoscopy

The concept of tunneling endoscopy was first written by Watanabe. The bone grafting procedure outlined above is one example of this concept. I also have used the transcutaneous method of endoscopy for resection of lipomas around the shoulder. My first experience was in 1985 in conjunction with an arthroscopic acromioplasty. The patient had a cosmetic, unacceptable subcutaneous lipoma on the same shoulder. This was approached with the arthroscope after the acromioplasty was completed. The area adjacent to the lipoma was approached with the arthroscope. The fluid distention separated the lipoma from the normal adjacent subcutaneous fat (Fig 11-8). The deltoid muscle was visualized deep in the operative field. Exposure was supplied by fluid distention. The tissue planes were easily defined. Resection was performed with motorized instru-

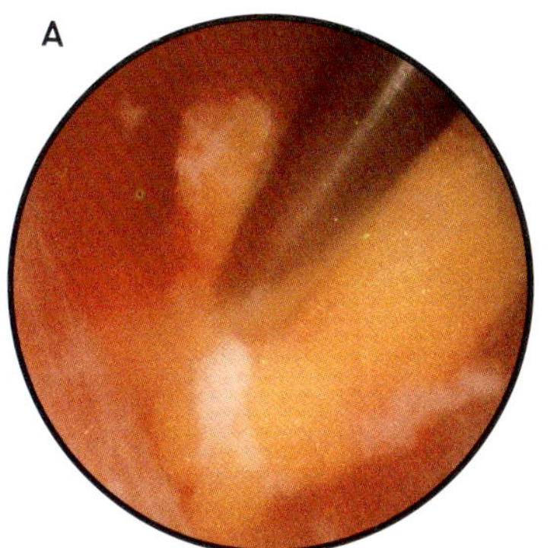

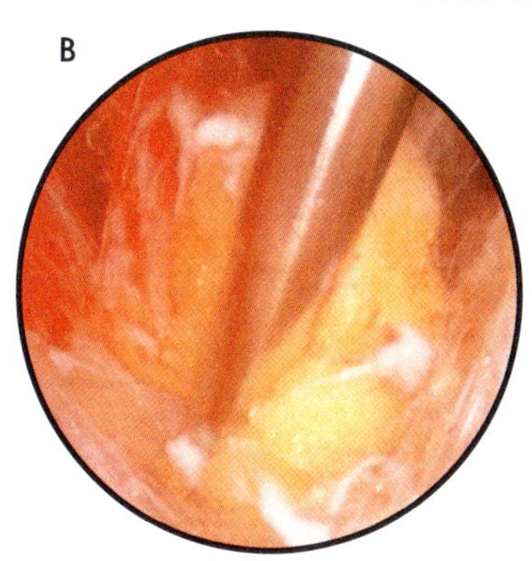

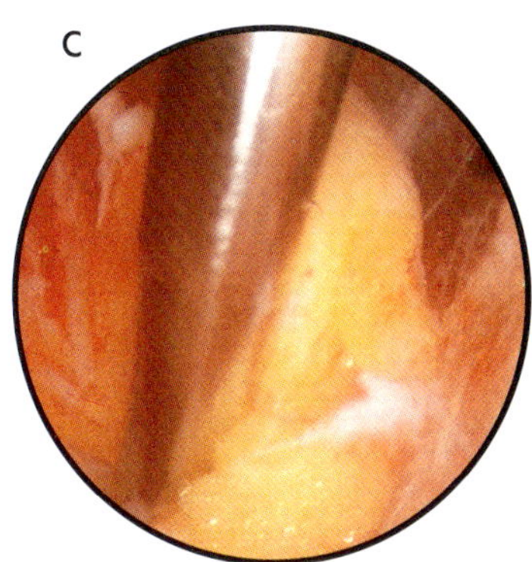

FIG. 11-8 Tunneling endoscopy.

A Endoscopic view of initial exposure to lipoma and motorized intruments in place. Yellow tissue is lipoma.

B Close-up view of lipoma and full radius resector.

C Endoscopic view near completion of resection. Notice the yellow lipoma, the red deltoid muscle in depth of wound, and the whiter subcutaneous fat to the right.

mentation. The removed tissue was collected in a separate cotton bag for pathological inspection.

Subsequently, I have performed the same procedure for lipoma over the shoulder area under local anesthesia. The injection of local anesthetic agent also served as initial fluid distention and disecting medium. Subsequent fluid distention in the operative site also provided subsequent adequate anesthesia.

This procedure is more refined than liposuction techniques of plastic surgery, in that the lesion is visualized and carefully dissected and resected.

Bioabsorbable Products

One of the next major technologic advancements in orthopedic surgery will be in the area of bioabsorbable products.[2] Arthroscopy will be the method of delivery.

Fixation Devices. The advent of biodegradable, implantable devices for holding tendons and ligaments about synovial joints will overcome the objections of metal implants next to joints. Russell Warren has reported 2-year follow-up with arthroscopic application of polyglycolide tack device for variety of shoulder instability cases.[13] This device is cylindrical, has transverse fins, a head, and is cannulated for transcutaneous control. This specific material is rapidly absorbed in a fluid environment. He subsequently changed to a polylactide material to overcome this disadvantage. Stephen Snyder heads an investigation team using polylactide device for arthroscopic shoulder repairs of a similar design as Warren.[12]

The polylactide devices have several disadvantages. They are glasslike and vulnerable to fracture. Their long degradation time when coupled with fragmentation results in joint irritation from effect of the loose body. This requires a second procedure for removal. Both Warren and Snyder have reported and abandoned polylactide. An ideal material is a combination of glycolic and lactic acid. The glycolic physical properties provide for resistance to breakage from impaction. The lactic acid properties provide slower absorption time. This is the chemical composition of the staple developed for the knee (Fig. 11-9).

At the time of this writing this staple has Food and Drug Administration (FDA) label approval for marketing in the knee and is commercially available. Application is under way for label approval in the shoulder. It may be important to point out that under United States law, the FDA does not "approve" anything other than how a company labels a product for use. This approval is based on demonstration of proofs that the product is safe and effective for this intended use. The FDA communications that grant this approval also state that this does not imply "FDA APPROVAL" beyond this legal confine. The FDA does not have jurisdiction over the practice of medicine. The state license to practice medicine gives the doctor the legal right to utilize various devices and methods at his own discretion in patient care.

The fixation devices will be produced in various shapes and sizes for use on biceps tendon tears, labrum tears, capsular injury, and rotator cuff repairs. The potential for use in labral tear repairs has been established by reports with use of metal staples.[16] My experience with the metal staple

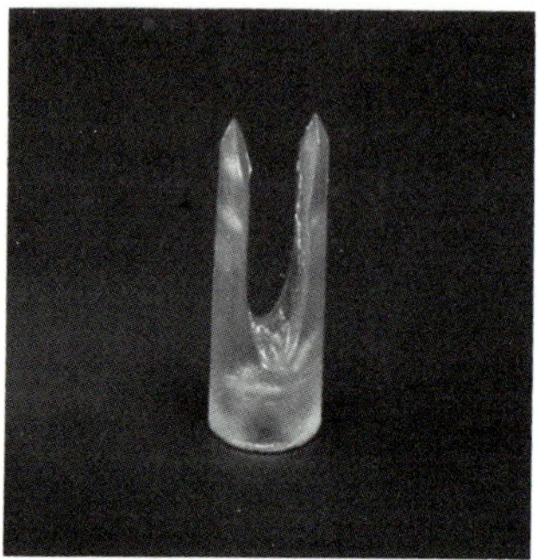

FIG. 11-9 Biodegradable staple for knee.

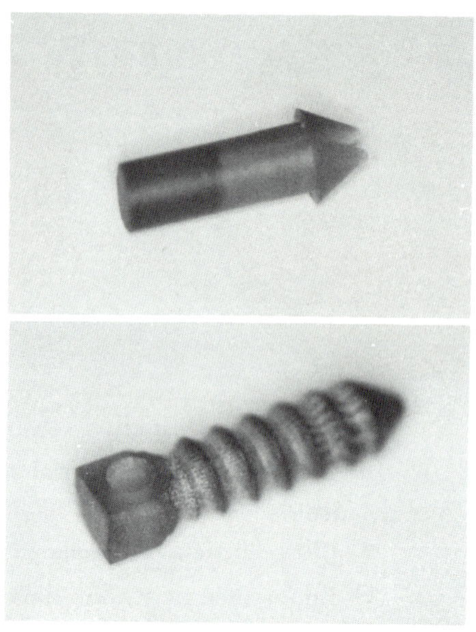

FIG. 11-10 Biodegradable suture anchor.
A Suture anchor staple.
B Screw-type anchor.

in the rotator cuff tears demonstrates great potential for bioabsorbable device use in this condition (see Chapter 9).

Suture Anchor Devices. Suture anchor devices, made of metal, were developed for the knee. They have been widely used in the shoulder for rotator cuff and anterior capsular repairs. They also have been used by arthroscopy for implantation for transcutaneous suturing methods (see Chapter 8). The device design does not always provide secure fixation, especially in osteoporotic cancellous bone. The metal is an objection, especially if subsequent surgery is required.

Bioabsorbable devices of this type are under development. One such device is the miniature staple (Fig. 11-10). This device is small and can be placed arthroscopically by cannula. The suture is held in the crotch of the staple. The hole is not drilled in the conventional way. It is created with a compaction drilling method that builds a thick wall to the sides of the hole without removal of bone. This is contrasted with conventional bone extraction drilling. Specialized instruments are necessary. The staple is placed in the hole. The external tines resist pullout. The head is flush with the surface of the bone. The suture selection type and size is at the discretion of the surgeon. It can be used for anchoring suture to both cancellous and cortical bone.

Bioabsorbable Vehicles. Bioabsorbable material has a wide spectrum of physical properties. It can be as hard and brittle as glass. It may be produced as a paste or putty consistency. In these various consistencies it can be used to transport material to stimulate cartilage or bone formation. The harder material could be used to fill a bone defect with MBF-2. The softer material can be mixed with the patient's own ground-up hyaline cartilage and delivered by arthroscopy to the articular defect. A combination of the two may be used to fill osteocartilaginous defects. An extension of this could be a future method of total joint resurfacing, as in the glenoid side of total joint.[14]

Suture Material. The first bioabsorbable suture material was 100% glycolic acid (Dexon). The second was 90% glycolic acid and 10% lactic acid (Vicryl). Both of these materials are rapidly absorbed. Biochemical variations result in stronger, longer-lasting threads that can be weaved, used for ligament and tendon substitution. This may revive the concept of filling large rotator tendon defects with absorbable mesh.

Screws and Rods. The use of biodegradable rods for fracture treatment is a reality.[2] Limitations do exist, however. The present material is rapidly absorbed. The techniques require additional external fixation.

Screws and various size rods of greater strength and slower absorption are now under clinical investigation (Fig. 11-11).

The very near future will see these devices used in fracture fixation in the shoulder.

THE FUTURE

The following discussion consists of patient management methods or technology I have seen in developmental stages.

Patient Management

The future holds a greater challenge for balance of high tech and high touch in patient care. The doctor-patient relationship will continue to erode. This has already occurred with designation of physician/surgeon as one of many "health care providers." Patients will not have direct access to a doctor of their choice.

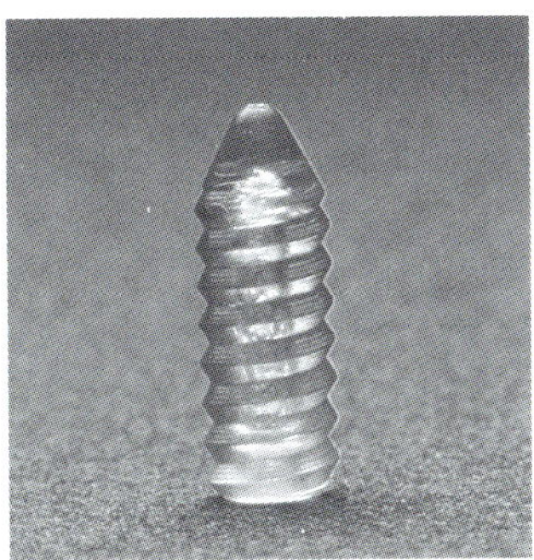

FIG. 11-11 Biodegradable screw (interference type).

Cost of Health Care

The cost of health care will continue to grow. The increases will be driven by demand and development of technology. The present method of cost shifting will fail when those few individuals paying their own way while subsidizing others will rebel. Those delivering health care will decrease their costs with employees replaced by automation. Health care costs will be eventually controlled by rationing.

Managed Health Care

Patient management will follow the golden rule of business: "He who has the gold makes the rules." The company or government agency that is paying the bills will determine patient referrals and ration the care they are to receive. This exists to some extent today.

The process of patient management may well follow this scenario. The patient will contact his or her insurance company–owned customer service center by telephone or their computer modem. The patient will register the shoulder complaint by computer-generated questionnaire to establish the anatomical region of complaint and severity. The computer data base will respond with a variety of patient options concerning time and place for their evaluation. The common referral choice will be to a diagnostic center for further evaluation of the shoulder problem.

Diagnostic Center

The present-day doctor's office will become a diagnostic center. These centers will use interactive video for collecting patient information and forming initial clinical impression. These centers will offer out patient diagnostic arthroscopy. Low radiation fluoroscopy will be available for shoulder motion evaluations.*

*Fluoroscan
HealthMate, Inc.
650 B Anthony Trail
Northbrook, IL 60062

The Initial Patient Encounter

The initial patient encounter will be with a television screen. They will not walk up to a desk and meet a live receptionist. As they pass into the room, a television will automatically come on. A friendly face on the television screen will welcome the patient and give directions to the next video station.

At the next station the patient will sit before an interactive video screen. The person on the computer screen will give instructions about documenting and recording the medical history. I envision interactive video as employee and doctor substitutes for collecting and documenting medical information. Interactive video also has the potential for performing the physical examination.

The doctor patient encounter will include a review of the medical history and confirm the physical findings. This data will be entered into the patient's computerized medical record. The indicated imaging and laboratory tests will be requested.

Computerized Medical Record

Computerization of the medical record will develop beyond what we know as artificial intelligence. The collected data base of medical history, physical examination, imaging, and laboratory tests results will be compared to a master data base. The clinical impression will be formulated with statistical probabilities.

The physician will review the computer-produced clinical impression to finalize the diagnosis. The doctor will review this information with the patient.

Patient Instructional Materials

Today, patient information is presented with combination of the printed page and television tapes. The future will expand on this concept.

The patient will be presented with a printout of clinical impressions, their probabilities, and treatment options from the computerized medical record and physician's opinion. Video instruction will provide the patient with illustrations and representative photographs of their suspected condition. If the patient desires more information on their condition, the video instruction would show graphics and/or videotape of arthroscopic view of exact diagnosis, a short version of the surgery, the postoperative management, and a "look" at the future condition of their body part for the specific surgery they choose. The probable outcomes will be presented for the specific surgeon and/or institution under consideration.

The patient would receive a printout and electronic-imprinted plastic card with their medical history, physical examination results, x-ray pictures, and reasons for the diagnosis, plus recommendations for treatment.

Patients will have the option to obtain a second opinion from the computer data base, without preceding with consultation or treatment.

Diagnostic Arthroscopy

The initial office evaluation will include diagnostic arthroscopy. The arthroscopic inspection of the subacromial bursa will be added to the present-day subacromial local anesthetic injection to determine status of the rotator cuff. The properly organized, office operating room environment will make this efficient for the surgeon and at a cost similar to the present-day arthrocentesis. Diagnostic arthroscopy will accompany or precede most shoulder surgery.

Operative Arthroscopy

The surgical techniques will expand in the numbers of surgeons performing and the spectrum of procedures possible. The further development of technology will have a positive impact on reducing medical costs. Outpatient surgery will expand for shoulder procedures. Anesthetic agents will be designed for this environment. Eventually, most debridement procedures and most repair procedures will be performed by arthroscopy. The fixation of soft tissue and bone with bioabsorbable devices will be routine by time of publication of this text (see above).

The Arthroscope

The single arthroscope may give way to multiple scopes in the shoulder. It would be possible for two small-diameter endoscopes placed into the same area coordinated electronically to produce a three-dimensional image on video screen. The three-dimensional image may be created by double barrel arthroscope similar to human eye placement.

Surgical Instrumentation

In the area of instrumentation, laser technology has always sparked the imagination. The miniaturization of the instrument has great appeal. When laser becomes cost effective it will be the cutting tool of choice. The ablation method of resection will enhance its usefulness. If and when the benefits of laser on articular cartilage healing occurs, its use and value will be established.[10] Operative procedures will include laser photochemical ablation.

Arthroscopically Delivered Biologic Treatments

Arthritis. Chemical synovectomy will be standard even for major joints like shoulder, but also every involved joint of the entire limb of a patient with rheumatoid arthritis. Joint lavage followed with hyaline cartilage healing medications will be used. The transcutaneous needle injection of bioabsorbable vehicles will generate articular fibrocartilage, perhaps even hyaline cartilage.[14]

Glenohumeral Instability. The treatment of subluxation and multidirectional instability will be accomplished under arthroscopic control with sclerosing agents injected into the capsular tissue for contracture. In cases of deficient capsular ligaments, the augmentation will be with a collagen-producing injectable to enhance the strength of the existing decompensated tissue.

Rotator Cuff Disease. Rotator cuff disease will be treated at the degenerative stage with laser ablation and collagen-promoting injectables.

Endoscopic Bone Surgery. Endoscopic bone surgery will be performed routinely for acute fracture treatment. The experience gained in anatomical replacement and internal fixation of avulsion fractures of humeral tuberosities will transfer to more complicated types of fractures. Transcutaneous bone grafting will be performed earlier in delayed union cases because of minimal morbidity of the procedure. Bone tumors will be treated with chemical or isotopic cellular labeling for identification, followed by endoscopic visualization and laser ablation.

Total Shoulder Replacement. The bionic total joint replacement we have known with implantable metal and plastics will give way to arthroscopically performed, biologic joint replacement. The procedure will consist of arthroscopic reshaping of the joint surface with biologically stimulating and replacement materials.

Sports Medicine. Complete diagnostic and operative facilities will be in major stadiums. The technology will provide for immediate exact diagnosis and minor surgical treatment for partial labrum, rotator cuff tears, and acromioclavicular meniscal tears.

I hope both the reader and I participate in development of this future.

REFERENCES

1. Andrews JR, Tedder JL, Godbout BP: Simple bone cyst of the distal tibia: a case for ankle arthroscopy, *Arthroscopy* 7(4):381-384, 1991.
2. Bostman OM: Absorbable implants for fixation of fractures, *J Bone Joint Surg* 73A(1):148-153, 1991.
3. Burman MS: Arthroscopy or the direct visualization of joints: an experimental cadaver study, *J Bone Joint Surg* 8:669-695, 1931.
4. Caspari RA: Personal communication, 1989.
5. Cassells SW: Arthroscopy of the knee joint: a review of 150 cases, *J Bone Joint Surg* 53A:287, 1971.
6. Cofield RH: The future of shoulder surgery, *Orthopedics* 11(1):179-181, 1988.
7. Jackson RW, Dandy DJ: *Arthroscopy of the knee,* New York, 1980, Grune and Stratton.
8. Johnson LL: Characteristics of the immediate post arthroscopic blood clot formation in the knee joint, *Arthroscopy* 7(1):14-23, 1991.
9. Johnson LL et al: Osteochondritis dissecans of the knee: arthroscopic compression screw fixation, *Arthroscopy* 6(3):179-189, 1990.
10. Miller DV et al: The use of the contact Nd:YAG laser in arthroscopic surgery: effects on articular cartilage and meniscal tissue, *Arthroscopy* 5(4):245-253, 1989.
11. O'Connor RL: *Arthroscopy,* Philadelphia, 1977, JB Lippincott.
12. Steve Snyder: Personal communication, 1991.
13. Warner JJP et al: Arthroscopic bankart repair utilizing an absorbable cannulated fixation device. Scientific paper presentation #233 at the annual meeting of AAOS, Anaheim, Calif, 1991.
14. Vacanti CA et al: Synthetic polymers seeded with chondrocytes provide a template for new cartilage formation, *Plastic Reconstructive Surgery* Nov:753-759, 1991.
15. Watanabe M: *Arthroscopy of small joints,* Tokyo/New York, 1985, Igakuu-Shoin.
16. Yoneda M et al: *Arthroscopic stapling for detached superior glenoid labrum, J Bone Joint Surg* 73B(5):746-750, 1991.

APPENDIX

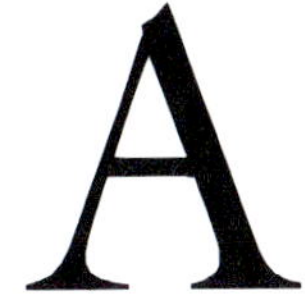

A Computerized Medical Record Forms

PATIENT INFORMATION QUESTIONNAIRE

Orthopedics

Maximum patient input contributes to the completeness of medical records and the quality of medical care.

Copies of this and other medical records produced from the information you provide are available for your personal files.

YOU NEED TO RETURN TO THE RECEPTIONIST IF:

√ More than one problem or condition exists (i.e. both knees or knee and shoulder). Tell the receptionist. She will give you the appropriate SUPPLEMENTAL FORMS.

INSTRUCTIONS

√ Fill out this form as accurately and completely as possible.

√ Answer each question as it applies to you TODAY. Include all conditions or body parts unaffected and unrelated to your present problem.

√ Attach copies of doctor's, hospital's, x-ray or surgical reports if available, but **not** as an alternative to completing this form.

If you need assistance of any type (including reading, writing, or explaining questions), the nurse or receptionist will be glad to help you. Feel free to call our office with any questions if you are completing this form at home.

Please return these forms to the receptionist. **If the forms are incomplete we will give them back to you for completion.**

Thank you for your cooperation.

PATIENT IDENTIFICATION:

Last name: Sample
First name: Martin
Middle name: ______
Title: Dr./Mr./Mrs./Ms. other: ______

FOR OFFICE USE: (we will fill in)

Patient number: ______

Universal Face Sheet

Patient's Form 100 (4.3)

2. **HAVE YOU EVER BEEN SEEN IN THIS OFFICE BEFORE?** NO/YES

3. **GENERAL INFORMATION:**
   1. Sex: (Male)/Female
   2. Date of birth: 10-26-47
   3. Marital status: single/married/divorced/separated/widowed

4. **SOCIAL SECURITY NUMBER:** 379-78-9468

5. **DRIVER'S LICENSE:** state: MI number: S 460 097 496 111

6. **HOME ADDRESS:**
   1. street address: 1240 Hill Street
   2. city: East Lansing 3. state: MI 4. zip code: 48823
   5. country (if not USA): ________

7. **TELEPHONE:**
   1. home: 517-339-8609
   2. daytime: ________

8. **PATIENT'S EMPLOYER:**
   1. name: Parts Manufacturing
   2. address: 5842 N. Clemens, Haslett, MI
   3. telephone: 517-347-1212

9. **WORK STATUS:**
   1. presently off work since: 12-20-87
   2. was off work from: __-__-____
   3. to: __-__-____
   4. off work due to a present orthopedic problem: Shoulder injury
   5. off work due to other problem: ________

10. **CURRENT TYPE OF JOB:**
    1. student
    2. homemaker
    3. sedentary (sit down)
    4. (physical (heavy labor,) lifting, walking, climbing)
    5. job name: tool room transport
    6. describe work activity: carrying and lifting heavy boxes
    7. retired from: ________

11. **REFERRING PHYSICIAN OR HEALTH CARE PROVIDER:**
    1. NONE
    2. name: Dr. Frank Williams
    3. address: 1278 Mt. Hope Road
    4. address: ________
    5. city-state: Lansing, MI 48970

Medical History: General Orthopedics

Patient's Form 300 (4.3)

FOR OFFICE USE: (we will fill in)	
Patient number:	1200
Problem number:	1
Date:	12-22-87

NAME: Martin Sample

DOCTOR'S NOTES

1. **AGE:** 40

2. **RACE OR GENETIC HERITAGE:** Caucasian

3. **HEIGHT:** 72 inches

4. **WEIGHT:** 220 pounds

5. **I AM:** (right handed)/left handed/truly ambidextrous

6. **MY DESIRED ACTIVITY LEVEL IS:**
   1. sedentary
   2. moderate
   3. (vigorous)

7. **PROBLEM AREAS FOR THIS EVALUATION:**

neck			back		
(shoulder)	(right)	left	pelvis		
arm	right	left	hip	right	left
elbow	right	left	thigh	right	left
forearm	right	left	knee	right	left
wrist	right	left	leg	right	left
hand	right	left	ankle	right	left
fingers			foot	right	left
other ________			toes		

8. **HAVE YOU HAD OTHER ORTHOPEDIC PROBLEMS?** (circle and/or add brief statement)

1. NO

1. rheumatism ________
2. arthritis ________
3. gout ________
4. joint swelling ________
5. loose body in joint ________
6. torn cartilage ________
7. torn ligaments ________
8. severe sprains ________
9. bone or joint infection ________
10. ________

1. neck ________
2. chest deformity ________
3. mid back problem ________
4. scoliosis ________
5. (low back problem) one episode, better with rest
6. sciatica ________
7. pelvis problem ________

2 - Medical History: General Orthopedics
Patient's Form 300

9. HAVE YOU HAD ANY OF THESE ORTHOPEDIC PROBLEMS?
1. soft bones ______
2. bone cyst ______
3. bone tumor or cyst ______
4. benign
5. malignant
6. osteoporosis ______
7. bursitis ______
8. tendonitis ______
9. torn tendon ______
(10. torn muscle) in low back
11. phlebitis ______
12. inherited bone joint disorder ______
13. injured or pinched nerve ______

10. HAVE YOU EVER FRACTURED ANY BONES? (1. NO) 2. yes
>M 1. bone: ______
2. treatment: ______
3. results: ______
4. date: ___-___-______

1. bone: ______
2. treatment: ______
3. results: ______
4. date: ___-___-______

1. bone: ______
2. treatment: ______
3. results: ______
4. date: ___-___-______

11. HAVE YOU EVER DISLOCATED ANY JOINTS? (1. NO) 2. yes
>M 1. joint: ______
2. treatment: ______
3. results: ______
4. date: ___-___-______

1. joint: ______
2. treatment: ______
3. results: ______
4. date: ___-___-______

Medical History: General Orthopedics - 3
Patient's Form 300

12. HAVE YOU HAD ARTHROSCOPIC SURGERY NOT RELATED TO PRESENT CONDITION?
>M (1. NO) 2. yes

1. joint: ______
2. diagnosis (problem): ______
3. type of surgery: ______
4. doctor: ______
5. hospital/city: ______
6. results: ______
7. date: __-__-____

1. joint: ______
2. diagnosis (problem): ______
3. type of surgery: ______
4. doctor: ______
5. hospital/city: ______
6. results: ______
7. date: __-__-____

13. HAVE YOU HAD OPEN ORTHOPEDIC SURGERY NOT RELATED TO PRESENT CONDITION?
>M (1. NO) 2. yes

1. body part: ______
2. diagnosis (problem): ______
3. type of surgery: ______
4. doctor: ______
5. hospital/city: ______
6. results: ______
7. date: __-__-____

1. body part: ______
2. diagnosis (problem): ______
3. type of surgery: ______
4. doctor: ______
5. hospital/city: ______
6. results: ______
7. date: __-__-____

14. HAVE YOU VISITED ANY DOCTOR IN THE PAST TWO YEARS? 1. NO (2. yes)
>M 1. diagnosis (problem): low back pain
2. doctor: William Nester, M.D.
3. hospital/city: Lansing, MI

1. diagnosis (problem): ______
2. doctor: ______
3. hospital/city: ______

15. WHEN WAS YOUR LAST COMPLETE PHYSICAL EXAM?
1. diagnosis (problem): ______
2. doctor: ______
3. hospital/city: ______
4. results: ______
5. date: __-__-____

4 - Medical History: General Orthopedics
Patient's Form 300

16. HAVE YOU HAD ANY OF THE FOLLOWING TESTS IN THE PAST 6 MONTHS?

Test name	Date	Results
1. CBC (blood count)	2. ___-___-______	3. ______________________
1. Urinalysis	2. ___-___-______	3. ______________________
1. Blood tests	2. ___-___-______	3. ______________________
1. Joint fluid analysis	2. ___-___-______	3. ______________________
1. Chest X-Ray	2. ___-___-______	3. ______________________
1. Electrocardiogram	2. ___-___-______	3. ______________________
1. Thyroid tests	2. ___-___-______	3. ______________________
1. (other) ____________	2. ___-___-______	3. ______________________
1. (other) ____________	2. ___-___-______	3. ______________________

17. HAVE YOU TAKEN ANY OF THE FOLLOWING MEDICATIONS IN THE PAST 6 MONTHS?

1. cortisone pills or shots
2. high blood pressure pills
3. water pills
4. heart medicine
5. insulin
6. tetanus immunization

Last two tetanus shot dates: ___-___-______ ___-___-______

18. PLEASE LIST THE MEDICATIONS YOU ARE CURRENTLY TAKING:

>M **Medication**	**Dosage** (tablets/capsules)	**Times/Day**
1. NONE		
1. ______________________	2. ______________	3. ________
1. ______________________	2. ______________	3. ________
1. ______________________	2. ______________	3. ________
1. ______________________	2. ______________	3. ________

19. ANY HOSPITALIZATIONS, OTHER THAN FOR SURGERY? (1. NO) 2. yes

>M 1. diagnosis (problem): ______________________
2. treatment: ______________________
3. doctor: ______________________
4. hospital/city: ______________________
5. results: ______________________
6. date: ___-___-______

1. diagnosis (problem): ______________________
2. treatment: ______________________
3. doctor: ______________________
4. hospital/city: ______________________
5. results: ______________________
6. date: ___-___-______

20. HAVE YOU HAD ANY NON-ORTHOPEDIC SURGERY? 1. NO 2. yes

>M 1. body part: ____________________
2. diagnosis (problem): ____________________
3. type of surgery: ____________________
4. doctor: ____________________
5. hospital/city: ____________________
6. results: ____________________
7. date: ___-___-______

1. body part: ____________________
2. diagnosis (problem): ____________________
3. type of surgery: ____________________
4. doctor: ____________________
5. hospital/city: ____________________
6. results: ____________________
7. date: ___-___-______

21. HAVE YOU RECEIVED OR BEEN GIVEN ANY BLOOD TRANSFUSIONS? 1. NO 2. YES

1. Date: ___-___-______
2. Date: ___-___-______

22. HEAD PROBLEMS: 1. NO 2. YES

1. unexplained hair loss
2. increased head size
3. headaches
4. migraines
5. (other) ____________________

23. NECK PROBLEMS: 1. NO 2. YES

1. stiff
2. thyroid trouble
3. pain
4. (other) ____________________

24. SKIN PROBLEMS: 1. NO 2. YES

1. infections
2. pimples
3. psoriasis
4. warts
5. skin lesions
6. skin cancers
7. dermatitis
8. (other) ____________________

25. EYE PROBLEMS: 1. NO 2. YES

1. loss or change in vision
2. pain
3. inflammation
4. excessive watering
5. double vision
6. glasses
7. contacts
8. cataracts
9. glaucoma
10. (other) ____________________

26. EARS-HEARING PROBLEMS: 1. NO 2. YES

1. loss of hearing
2. hearing aid
3. ringing or buzzing
4. infection
5. tubes
6. (other) ____________________

27. NOSE-THROAT PROBLEMS: 1. NO 2. YES

1. hoarseness
2. change in voice
3. nose bleeds
4. post nasal drip
5. blocked nasal passages
6. trouble swallowing
7. chronic infections/sore throat
8. (other) ____________________

6 - Medical History: General Orthopedics
Patient's Form 300

28. RESPIRATORY PROBLEMS: 1. NO 2. YES

1. asthma
2. wheezing
3. shortness of breath
4. pain with breathing
5. much sputum
6. bloody sputum
7. emphysema
8. bronchitis
9. (other) ____________________

29. CARDIOVASCULAR PROBLEMS: 1. NO 2. YES

1. chest pain
2. irregular or fast heartbeat
3. low blood pressure
4. high blood pressure
5. heart disease
6. leg cramps at night
7. leg cramps while walking
8. cold fingers or toes
9. sweating fingers or toes
10. leg or ankle swelling
11. (other) ____________________

30. GASTROINTESTINAL PROBLEMS: 1. NO 2. YES

1. stomach ulcer
2. nausea-vomiting
3. lack of appetite
4. stomach pain
5. stomach swelling
6. change in bowel habits
7. constipation
8. diarrhea
9. hemorrhoids
10. gall bladder trouble
11. pancreatitis
12. colitis
13. hepatitis
14. bloody stool
15. (other) ____________________

31. GENITAL URINARY PROBLEMS: 1. NO 2. YES

1. leakage
2. bloody urine
3. strong urine
4. frequent urination
5. night time urination
6. trouble starting/stopping/both
7. pain with urination
8. back pain
9. sores on genitalia
10. infections
11. discharge
12. herpes
13. AIDS
14. AIDS related complex
15. (other) ____________________

32. NEUROLOGIC PROBLEMS: 1. NO 2. YES

1. headaches
2. fainting
3. seizures-Epilepsy
4. stroke
5. paralysis of limbs
6. numbness/tingling
7. blackouts
8. severe head injury
9. (other) ____________________

33. EMOTIONAL PROBLEMS: 1. NO 2. YES

1. nervous breakdown
2. feel blue
3. frequent crying
4. anxious
5. tension
6. stress prone
7. cannot sleep
8. exhausted
9. drug abuse
10. alcohol abuse
11. (other) ____________________

34. BLEEDING DISORDER PROBLEMS: 1. NO 2. YES

1. anemia
2. bleeding problem
3. (other) ____________________

Medical History: General Orthopedics - 7
Patient's Form 300

35. METABOLIC PROBLEMS: (1. NO) 2. YES
1. diabetes
2. hypoglycemia
3. (other) ____________

36. GENETIC/INHERITED DISORDERS: (1. NO) 2. YES
1. ____________

37. FEMALE MEDICAL HISTORY:

Pregnant Now 1. yes/no/maybe 2. due date ___-___-______
Term Pregnancies 1. most recent ___-___-______ 2. total number _____
Miscarriages 1. most recent ___-___-______ 2. total number _____
Pregnancy Terminations 1. most recent ___-___-______ 2. total number _____
Endometriosis Problem 1. most recent ___-___-______ 2. total number _____
Birth Control Pills
1. YES/NO 2. type ____________ 3. presently 4. stopped ___-___-______
Last Menstrual Period 1. date ___-___-______ 2. nature ____________
Menopause 1. date ___-___-______ 2. nature ____________
IUD 1. name ____________ 2. reason ____________
Drugs during pregnancies: (DES, Thalidomide, etc.)
1. name ____________ 2. reason ____________
3. name ____________ 4. reason ____________
Complications of any above
1. ____________

38. FAMILY HISTORY:

>M	First name	Living/Deceased	Age	Medical condition or cause of death
Father:				
	1. *Charles*	2. (L)/D	3. *72*	4. *poor heart condition*
Mother:				
	1. *Shirley*	2. (L)/D	3. *70*	4.
Brothers:				
	1. *Byron*	2. (L)/D	3. *43*	4.
	1.	2. L/D	3.	4.
	1.	2. L/D	3.	4.
Sisters:				
	1. *Sandy*	2. (L)/D	3. *41*	4.
	1.	2. L/D	3.	4.
	1.	2. L/D	3.	4.
Children:				
	1. *Jenny*	2. (L)/D	3. *15*	4.
	1. *Judy*	2. (L)/D	3. *12*	4.
	1. *Dean*	2. (L)/D	3. *10*	4.
	1.	2. L/D	3.	4.

8 - Medical History: General Orthopedics
Patient's Form 300

39. FAMILY HISTORY (medical problems, please give details):

1. serious allergy: Y/N
2. describe: ____________

1. adverse reaction to anesthesia or surgery: Y/N
2. describe: ____________

1. high body temperature during surgery: Y/N
2. describe: ____________

40. LIFE STYLE:

	NOW amount	NOW how long	PAST amount	PAST how long
Coffee - Tea - Caffeine drinks	4	per day	yes - 8	per day
Alcoholic Beverages	one beer	per day	four beers	per day
Tobacco Products (circle all that apply)				
(cigarettes)	one pack	per day	one pack	per day
cigars				
snuff				
chewing				
Other Substances ____________				

Comments: ____________

41. PLEASE RATE YOUR OVERALL LEVEL OF PHYSICAL HEALTH:
(compare to others in your age group)

1. excellent
2. very good
3. (good)
4. fair
5. poor

42. DOCTOR'S NOTATIONS:
>M ____________

43. CERTIFICATION OF AUTHENTICITY:
I hereby certify that the above information is true and correct within the best of my ability.

Signed: Martin Sample **Date:** 12-22-87

Thank You

Please return this form to the receptionist

Version 4.3 May, 1990

Information Health Network
P.O. Box 23056
Lansing, Michigan 48909-3056
(800)443-0613 (517)351-1588

History Supplement: Shoulder

Patient's Form 501 (4.3)

NAME: *Martin Sample*

FOR OFFICE USE: (we will fill in)	
Patient number:	*1200*
Problem number:	*1*
Date:	*12-22-87*

1. THIS FORM APPLIES TO WHICH SHOULDER?
1. RIGHT (circled)
2. LEFT

2. MAJOR COMPLAINT: (the main reason you came to the doctor)
1. deformity
2. pain (circled)
3. aching - sore
4. numbness
5. stiffness
6. loss of motion (circled)
7. weakness
8. loss of strength (circled)
9. swelling
10. going out
11. locking
12. grinding
13. popping
14. makes noise
15. loss of work (circled)
16. loss of activities (circled)
17. (other) ______________________

3. NATURE OF MAJOR PROBLEM:
1. injury (circled)
2. fracture
3. dislocation
4. arthritis
5. infection
6. growth
7. developmental
8. congenital
9. tumor
10. (other) ______________________
11. do not know

4. ORIGINAL ONSET OF THE MAJOR PROBLEM (not just this episode):
1. Date of Onset: *12-20-87*

Nature of Problem:
1. gradual
2. sudden
3. injury while *lifting case of parts* (circled)
4. injury at work
5. injury in vehicle accident
6. reinjury of previous problem
7. (other) ______________________
8. do not know
9. without explanation

5. RECENT EPISODE OF THE MAJOR PROBLEM (if different from original onset):
1. Date of Onset: ___-___-______

Nature of Problem:
1. gradual
2. sudden
3. injury while ______________
4. injury at work
5. injury in vehicle accident
6. reinjury of previous problem
7. (other) ______________________
8. do not know
9. without explanation

6. (QUESTION 6 IS FOR DOCTOR'S NOTATIONS)

2 - History Supplement: Shoulder
Patient's Form 501

7. HAVE YOU EVER HAD THIS SHOULDER TREATED OR EXAMINED BEFORE?
1. NO - skip to question 17

2. YES - continue with next question

8. WERE THERE ANY INJURIES OR CONDITIONS OF THIS BODY PART THAT EXISTED BEFORE THIS PRESENT PROBLEM OCCURRED? 1. NO 2. yes (if yes, circle and/or add brief statement)
1. cut (laceration) ________
2. crush ________
3. ligament injury ________
4. fracture ________
5. dislocation ________
6. growth (tumor) ________
7. deformity ________
8. other ________

9. WERE YOU TREATED NON-SURGICALLY AT AN EMERGENCY ROOM FOR THIS PROBLEM?
>M 1. NO 2. yes

1. diagnosis (problem): ________
2. treatment: ________
3. doctor: ________
4. hospital/city: ________
5. results: ________
6. date: ___-___-______

1. diagnosis (problem): ________
2. treatment: ________
3. doctor: ________
4. hospital/city: ________
5. results: ________
6. date: ___-___-______

10. WERE YOU TREATED NON-SURGICALLY BY A REGULAR PHYSICIAN FOR THIS PROBLEM?
>M 1. NO 2. yes

1. diagnosis (problem): ________
2. treatment: ________
3. doctor: ________
4. hospital/city: ________
5. results: ________
6. date: ___-___-______ to ___-___-______

1. diagnosis (problem): ________
2. treatment: ________
3. doctor: ________
4. hospital/city: ________
5. results: ________
6. date: ___-___-______ to ___-___-______

History Supplement: Shoulder - 5
Patient's Form 501

16. WERE YOU EVER HOSPITALIZED FOR THIS PROBLEM (OTHER THAN SURGERY)?
>M 1. NO 2. yes

1. diagnosis (problem): ______
2. treatment: ______
3. doctor: ______
4. hospital/city: ______
5. results: ______
6. date: __-__-____ to __-__-____

1. diagnosis (problem): ______
2. treatment: ______
3. doctor: ______
4. hospital/city: ______
5. results: ______
6. date: __-__-____ to __-__-____

17. DID YOU HAVE REGULAR X-RAYS TAKEN FOR THIS PROBLEM? 1. NO 2. yes
>M 1. where: ______
2. body part: ______
3. results: ______
4. date: __-__-____

1. where: ______
2. body part: ______
3. results: ______
4. date: __-__-____

18. DID YOU HAVE SPECIAL X-RAYS OR TESTS FOR THIS PROBLEM? 1. NO 2. yes

>M	**Date**	**Body Part**	**Where**
1. Arthrogram	2. __-__-____	3. ______	4. ______
1. Tomogram	2. __-__-____	3. ______	4. ______
1. Bone Scan	2. __-__-____	3. ______	4. ______
1. CAT Scan	2. __-__-____	3. ______	4. ______
1. Magnetic Resonance	2. __-__-____	3. ______	4. ______
1. Ultrasound	2. __-__-____	3. ______	4. ______
1. Fluoroscopy	2. __-__-____	3. ______	4. ______
1. Stress X-Rays	2. __-__-____	3. ______	4. ______
1. ______	2. __-__-____	3. ______	4. ______

19. DO YOU HAVE SHOULDER PAIN?
1. NO - skip to question 26
2. YES - continue with next question

20. PLEASE RATE THE MAGNITUDE OF YOUR PAIN:
1. complete disability
2. marked
3. moderate
4. after unusual activity
5. slight
6. ______

6 - History Supplement: Shoulder
Patient's Form 501

21. LOCATION OF SHOULDER PAIN:

1. I cannot locate exact spot

I can locate exact spot at

2. front
3. back
4. arm pit
5. top side
6. deep inside
7. entire arm to hand
8. chest
9. neck
10. ________________________

22. FREQUENCY OF SHOULDER PAIN:

1. initially, but not now
2. occasionally
3. constantly
4. only recently
5. with activity
6. even when resting
7. ________________________

23. TIME OF DAY WHEN SHOULDER PAIN OCCURS:

1. morning
2. all day
3. end of the day
4. interrupts my sleep
5. ________________________

24. PAIN MADE WORSE WHEN:

1. resting
2. any shoulder motion
3. lifting only my arm
4. lifting any weight with arm
5. grasping with hand
6. throwing
7. physical therapy
8. doing my regular work as ____
9. ________________________

25. PAIN RELIEVED BY:

1. nothing
2. rest
3. activity
4. medicine--if so, what kind? ____
5. physical therapy
6. repositioning the shoulder
7. ________________________

26. SHOULDER APPEARANCE:
1. normal
2. swollen
3. shrunken
4. has lump I can feel
5. ______________________

27. SWELLING OF THE AFFECTED AREA:
1. none ever
2. originally, but not since
3. does not go away--swelling is constant
4. frequently
5. after going out
6. only after exercise or use of the shoulder
7. ______________________

28. SHOULDER JOINT MOBILITY:
1. same as ever
2. unable to elevate
3. unable to put hand behind back
4. unable to rotate
5. unable to lift objects
6. unable to throw
7. ______________________

29. HOW HIGH CAN YOU LIFT YOUR HAND ON AFFECTED SIDE?
1. not at all
2. to waist
3. to same shoulder
4. to opposite shoulder
5. to neck
6. top of head
7. above head
8. all the way up
9. ______________________

30. FUNCTION/ACTIVITIES:
(4 = normal, 3 = mild compromise, 2 = difficulty, 1 = with aid, 0 = unable, x = not available)

RT	LF		RT	LF	
0		use back pocket	2		dress
2		rectal hygiene	0		sleep on shoulder
2		wash opposite underarm	0		pulling
2		eat with utensil	0		use hand overhead
1		comb hair	0		throwing
0		use hand, arm at shoulder level	0		lifting
0		carry 10-15 lbs., arm at side	0		do usual work
		reach between shoulder blades (bra)	0		do usual sport

8 - History Supplement: Shoulder
Patient's Form 501

31. ACTIVITIES LIMITATIONS: 1. NONE

Inability to:
1. eat/feed myself
2. dress myself
3. comb hair
4. work at my job as tool transporter
5. housework
6. yard work
7. shop
8. sleep
9. sit
10. bend over
11. run
12. recreational activities
13. competitive sports
14. lift weights
15. musical instruments ________
16. hobbies ________
17. ________

Restricted ability to:
1. eat/feed myself
2. dress myself
3. comb hair
4. work at my job as ________
5. housework
6. yard work
7. shop
8. sleep
9. sit
10. bend over
11. run
12. recreational activities
13. competitive sports
14. lift weights
15. musical instruments ________
16. hobbies ________
17. ________

32. SPORTS ACTIVITIES:
1. equal performance at same sports as before
2. same sports, lower performance
3. active, but with different sports
4. significantly limited
5. no sports possible now
6. ________

33. SPECIFICALLY WHAT SPORTS ACTIVITY IS AFFECTED?

>M 1. recreational
2. competitive

1. walking
2. speed walking
3. jogging
4. running
5. aerobics
6. swimming
7. baseball
8. basketball
9. football
10. lacrosse
11. soccer
12. tennis
13. ________
14. ________

34. WHAT SPECIFIC POSITION OR ACTION IS LIMITED IN EACH ACTIVITY MENTIONED ABOVE?

>M 1. ________
2. ________
3. ________

35. OCCURRENCE OF JOINT STIFFNESS:
1. none
2. always
3. after activity
4. in the morning
5. end of the day
6. ______________________

36. GRATING, GRINDING, OR POPPING NOISES OR SENSATIONS IN THE JOINT:
1. none
2. feel with my hand
3. any motion
4. lifting
5. throwing
6. only when pushing or pulling
7. ______________________

37. LOCKING (GETTING STUCK) OF THE JOINT:
1. never
2. at first, but not now
3. just started
4. occasionally
5. frequently
6. constantly
7. ______________________

38. HAS SHOULDER GONE OUT OF JOINT (DISLOCATED)?
1. NO - skip to question 43
2. yes - continue with next question

39. TOTAL NUMBER OF TIMES (ESTIMATE): __________

40. WHERE SHOULDER GOES OUT:
1. front
2. back
3. arm pit
4. don't know
5. ______________________

41. SHOULDER WENT OUT OF JOINT (DISLOCATED):
1. first time on ___-___-______
2. how/doing what? ______________________
3. treatment ______________________

1. last time on ___-___-______
2. how/doing what? ______________________
3. treatment ______________________

42. HOW DOES SHOULDER GO OUT:
1. with major injury or stress
2. with simple movements of daily living
3. unexpectedly
4. I can do it myself at will
5. ______________________

10 - History Supplement: Shoulder
Patient's Form 501

43. NUMBNESS:

1. never
2. at first, not now
(3.) all the time
4. ______________________

Location:
1. shoulder
2. arm
3. hand
4. ______________________

44. SLEEPING POSITION:

(1.) on back
(2.) on stomach
3. on side of unaffected shoulder
4. on side of affected shoulder
5. affected arm up, shoulder between head and mattress
6. affected arm at side
7. ______________________

45. DOCTOR'S NOTATIONS: (validity of previous history, review of previous medical record, other...)
>M ______________________

46. CERTIFICATION OF AUTHENTICITY:
I hereby certify that the above information is true and correct within the best of my ability.

Signed: Martin Sample **Date:** 12-22-87

Thank You

Please return this form to the receptionist

Version 4.3 May, 1990

Information Health Network
P.O. Box 23056
Lansing, Michigan 48909-3056
(800)443-0613 (517)351-1588

PATIENT INFORMATION

Patient: 1200
Mr. Martin Sample
1240 Hill Street
East Lansing MI 48823
Home telephone: 517-339-8609

Patient's employer
Parts Manufacturing Co.
5842 N. Clemens
Work telephone: 517-347-1212

Sex: Male
Date of Birth: October 26, 1947
Social Security Number: 379-78-9468

Insurance Name: Employee Benefits Concepts
Group Number: 40902
Service Code: 4432-4AH3-77GH

This is a Worker's Compensation case.

This is not a legal or third person liability case.

This is not a no-fault insurance claim.

The responsible party for paying the bill and/or the insurance subscriber is:
Name: Parts Manufacturing Co.
Address: 5842 N. Clemens
City-State: Haslett, Mi

The bill should be sent to the patient's employer and the patient's insurance company.

The patient is presently working as a Laborer.
The patient is presently off work since December 20, 1987.
The patient is currently not working due to an orthopedic problem: shoulder injury.
The patient's job as tool room transport is of a physical nature.
The patient's typical work activity is carrying and lifting heavy boxes.

Referring physician or health care provider:
Name: Frank Williams M.D.
Address: 1278 Mt Hope Rd.
City-State: Lansing, Mi 48910

The patient has no allergies or adverse reactions to medication and/or anesthesia.

The date of the patient's first visit or treatment was 12-22-1987.

Re: Martin Sample / 1200
1240 Hill Street
East Lansing, Mi 48823
Worker's Compensation: Yes
Liability case: No

This 40-year-old Caucasian male was evaluated on December 23, 1987, having been referred by Frank Williams M.D.

The patient is 72 inches tall, weighs 220 pounds, and is right handed.

The patient's job as tool room transport is of a physical nature. The patient's typical work activity is carrying and lifting heavy boxes.

The patient is presently working as a Laborer.
The patient is presently off work since December 20, 1987.
The patient is currently not working due to an orthopedic problem: shoulder injury.

He desires a vigorous activity level.

The patient currently has problems with his right shoulder.

CHIEF COMPLAINT—RIGHT SHOULDER
The patient's major complaints are pain, loss of motion, loss of strength, loss of work, and loss of activities.

PRESENT HISTORY—RIGHT SHOULDER
His current orthopedic problem involves an injury to his right shoulder. The problem started after an injury while lifting a case of parts on December 20, 1987. The problem has resulted in the loss of work, restricted recreational sports, and an inability to sleep or dress himself.

He complained of pain and located the exact spot on the top of and deep inside of the shoulder and in the entire arm to the hand. The patient rated the magnitude of his pain as marked and causing complete disability. This pain occurs constantly and even when resting; typically occurring all day long and while sleeping. The pain is made worse when he uses any shoulder motion, lifts only his arm, grasps with his hand, and does his regular work as parts transporter. Nothing relieves the pain.

The shoulder appears normal and is never swollen.

The patient is unable to elevate, rotate, lift objects with, or throw with the affected shoulder or to put his hand behind his back. He is able to lift his hand to his waist.

With his right arm the patient had difficulty with rectal hygiene, washing his opposite underarm, eating with a utensil, and dressing. With his right arm the patient required aid to comb his hair. With his right arm the patient was unable to use his back pocket, use his hand with his arm at shoulder level, carry 10-15 lbs. with his arm at his side, sleep on his shoulder, pull, use his hand overhead, throw, lift, do his usual work, and play his usual sport.

The patient is unable to comb his hair, work at his job as tool transporter, do housework, do yard work, shop, participate in enjoyable recreational activities, or do weight lifting. The patient also is not able to participate in sports activities now.

Joint stiffness is experienced at all times and in the morning. Grating, grinding, or popping noises or sensations are felt with the patient's hand.

The patient's shoulder never goes out.

The patient experiences numbness all the time. The patient sleeps on his back and on his stomach.

The patient has not had this joint treated before.

PAST HISTORY
Within the past two years, the patient has visited William Nester M.D., in City General/Lansing, for low back pain.

ORTHOPEDIC HISTORY
In addition to the problem mentioned above, the patient has experienced the following orthopedic problems:
low back problem—one episode, better with rest
torn muscle—in low back

ALLERGY
The patient has no allergies or adverse reactions to medication and/or anesthesia.

MEDICATION
NO RESPONSES

HOSPITALIZATION FOR MEDICAL TREATMENT
None

SURGERY
The patient has not had previous arthroscopic surgery which was not related to his present problem. He has not had open orthopedic surgery which was not related to his present problem. The patient has not undergone any non-orthopedic surgery.

TRAUMA
He has never fractured any bones or dislocated any joints.

REVIEW OF SYSTEMS
The patient is experiencing the following problems:
NECK:
Stiff
EYES:
Glasses
NOSE-THROAT:
Post nasal drip
GASTROINTESTINAL:
Constipation
Hemorrhoids
NEUROLOGIC:
Headaches

FAMILY HISTORY

Father:				
	Charles	living	72	heart condition
Mother:				
	Shirley	living	70	
Brother:				
	Byron	living	43	
Sister:				
	Sandy	living	41	
Children:				
	Jenny	living	15	
	Judy	living	12	
	Dean	living	10	

HABITS
The patient consumes the following products regularly:

Coffee—Tea—Caffeine drinks at a rate of 4 per day now and 8 per day in the past.
Alcoholic Beverages at a rate of 1 beer per day now and 4 beers per day in the past.
Tobacco Products at a rate of 1 pack per day now and 1 pack per day in the past.

The patient rated his overall level of physical health as good.

He certified that the above information is true and correct to the best of his ability on this date December 22, 1987.

Edward M. Lowe, M.D.

Physical Examination: Shoulder - 3
Doctor's Form 502

18. PALPATION TENDERNESS-MUSCLE: 1. right/left

>M 1. anterior
2. posterior
3. superior
4. inferior
5. medial
6. lateral
7. axillary
8. ________

1. SCM
2. Trapezius
3. Levator scapulae
4. Rhomboids
5. Serratus anterior
6. Supraspinatus
7. Infraspinatus
8. Teres minor
9. Subscapularis
10. Pectoralis major
11. Pectoralis minor
12. Latissimus dorsi
13. Teres major
14. Deltoid
15. Biceps
16. long head
17. short head
18. Triceps
19. long head
20. lateral head
21. medial head
22. ________

Tenderness Located:
1. ________
2. ________
3. ________
4. ________
5. ________

19. MASS LOCATION: (1. NONE IDENTIFIED) 2. (right)/left

>M 1. subcutaneous tissue ________
BONE:
2. vertebra ________
3. ribs ________
4. scapula ________
5. clavicle ________
6. humerus ________
7. JOINT: ________
8. MUSCLE: ________
9. TENDON: ________
10. (other) ________

20. MASS SIZE: 1. right/left

>M ____ cm x ____ cm x ____ cm

21. MASS CHARACTERISTICS: 1. right/left

>M 1. non-tender
2. tender
3. ________

1. hard
2. firm
3. soft
4. ballottable
5. ________

1. fixed
2. moveable
3. ________

1. solid
2. translucent
3. ________

22. CIRCUMFERENTIAL MEASUREMENT: 1. N/T

RIGHT			LEFT		
1. arm	40	cm	1. arm	40	cm
2. elbow	28	cm	2. elbow	28	cm
3. forearm	____	cm	3. forearm	____	cm
4. wrist	____	cm	4. wrist	____	cm
5. hand	____	cm	5. hand	____	cm

4 - Physical Examination: Shoulder
Doctor's Form 502

23. DYNAMOMETER GRIP TEST: 1. N/T

	Right:	Left:
>M 1. Jamar/Preston	1. ______	1. ______
2. serial number ______	2. ______	2. ______
3. kg/lbs	3. ______	3. ______
4. 1 / 2 / 3 / 4 / 5	4. ______	4. ______
5. sequential (1-5)	5. ______	5. ______

24. RANGE OF MOTION: 1. NORMAL 2. Abnormal 3. N/T

>M **Body Position:**	**Reference Point:**	**Arm(s) Involved:**	**Measurements:**
1. sitting (circled)	1. spine	1. one	1. estimated
2. standing	2. coronal plane	2. both (circled)	2. measured (circled)
3. supine	3. sagittal plane	3. simultaneous (circled)	
4. prone	4. plumb line		

25. RANGE OF MOTION: 1. SITTING/STANDING

>M **Arm Starting Position:**	**(plus)**	**Motion Measured:**	ACTIVE RT	ACTIVE LF (circled)	PASSIVE RT	PASSIVE LF (circled)	LOCAL ANS RT	LOCAL ANS LF (circled)
side		elevation	45	170				
side		forward flexion	45	170				
side		abduction	30	90				
side		external rotation	0	30				
side		internal rotation						
90 abd	(0° external)	external rotation	45	+15				
90 abd	(______)	internal rotation						
90 abd	(______)	adduction						
90 abd	(______)	extension						
side		backward extension	30	45				

26. RANGE OF MOTION (SUPINE):

Arm Starting Position:	**(plus)**	**Motion Measured:**	ACTIVE RT	ACTIVE LF	PASSIVE RT	PASSIVE LF	LOCAL ANS RT	LOCAL ANS LF
side		elevation						
side		forward flexion						
side		abduction						
side		external rotation						
side		internal rotation						
90 abd	(______)	external rotation						
90 abd	(______)	internal rotation						
90 abd	(______)	adduction						
90 abd	(______)	extension						
side		backward extension						

27. RANGE OF MOTION (PRONE):

Arm Starting Position:	**(plus)**	**Motion Measured:**	ACTIVE RT	ACTIVE LF	PASSIVE RT	PASSIVE LF	LOCAL ANS RT	LOCAL ANS LF
90 abd	(______)	extension						
side		backward extension						

28. INTERNAL ROTATION:

Patient could reach to:	ACTIVE (circled) RT	ACTIVE LF	PASSIVE RT	PASSIVE LF	LOCAL ANS RT	LOCAL ANS LF
less than trochanter	O	O	O	O	O	O
trochanter (circled)	✗	O	O	O	O	O
gluteal	O	O	O	O	O	O
sacrum	O	O	O	O	O	O
vertebral level:		D5				

Physical Examination: Shoulder - 5
Doctor's Form 502

29. QUALITY OF MOTION: 1. NORMAL 2. N/T 3. (right)/left

>M	**NORMAL**	**slow**	**painful**	**painless**	**comment**
total elevation	O	X	X	O	
forward flexion	O	O	O	O	
abduction	O	O	O	O	
external rotation at side	O	O	X	O	
internal rotation at side	O	X	O	O	
90 deg abduct-ext rotation	O	O	O	O	
90 deg abduct-int rotation	O	O	O	O	
90 deg abduction-adduction	O	O	O	O	
90 deg abduction-extension	O	O	O	O	
backward extension	O	O	O	O	
hand behind back	O	O	O	O	
adduction	O	O	O	O	
waving	O	O	O	O	
circumduction	O	O	O	O	
pendulum exercise	O	O	O	O	

30. SHOULDER MOTION STRENGTH TESTS: 1. NORMAL 2. Abnormal 3. N/T
(Absent = 0, Trace = 1, Poor = 2, Fair = 3, Good = 4, Normal = 5)

	RIGHT	LEFT	COMMENTS
abduction-thumb down	4	5	
abduction-thumb up	4	5	
external rotation	3	5	painful
internal rotation	5	5	

31. MUSCULATURE TESTS: 1. NORMAL 2. Abnormal 3. N/T
(Absent = 0, Trace = 1, Poor = 2, Fair = 3, Good = 4, Normal = 5)

	RIGHT	LEFT	COMMENTS
sternocleidomastoid (C-2-3)			
trapezius (C-3-4)			
levator scapulae (C-3-4-5)			
rhomboids (C-5)			
serratus anterior (C-5-6-7)			
supraspinatus (C-5-6)			
infraspinatus (C-5-6)			
teres minor (C-5-6)			
subscapularis (C-5-6)			
pectoralis (C-5-T-1)			
other ______			

32. MUSCULATURE TESTS: (Absent = 0, Trace = 1, Poor = 2, Fair = 3, Good = 4, Normal = 5)

	RIGHT	LEFT	COMMENTS
latissimus dorsi (C-6-7-8)			
teres major (C-5-6)			
deltoid (C-5-6)			
anterior			
middle			
posterior			
biceps (C-5-6)	5	5	
triceps (C-7-8)			
brachioradialis (C-5-6)			
supinator (C-6)			
other ______			

6 - Physical Examination: Shoulder

Doctor's Form 502

33. AUSCULTATION: 1. SILENT 2. N/T 3. right/left

>M 1. crepitus — 1. with *internal rotation abduction* motion

2. popping — 2. suggesting *rotation cuff tear/impingement*

3. other ____________________

34. IMPINGEMENT TESTS: 1. NORMAL 2. Abnormal 3. N/T 4. right/left

>M

	N/T	neg.	pos.	painful	neg. with local anes.	produced crepitus	produced popping	not valid due to limited motion	comment
forward flexion:	O	O	●	●	●	O	O	O	______
resisted supination (Yergason's):	O	O	O	O	O	O	O	O	______
abduction/external rotation:	O	O	●	●	●	O	O	O	______
abduction/internal rotation:	O	O	●	●	●	●	O	O	______
adduction/external rotation:	O	●	O	O	O	O	O	O	______
adduction/internal rotation:	O	O	O	O	O	O	O	O	______
palm up:	O	O	O	O	O	O	O	O	______
palm down:	O	O	O	O	O	O	O	O	______

35. MANIPULATION: 1. NORMAL 2. N/T 3. right/left

>M

	STABLE	**SUBLUX**	**DISLOC**	**APPREHN**	**PAIN**
abd, ext rotation	1. Y/N	2. Y/N	3. Y/N	4. Y/N	5. Y/N
abd, downward force	1. Y/N	2. Y/N	3. Y/N	4. Y/N	5. Y/N
add flexion	1. Y/N	2. Y/N	3. Y/N	4. Y/N	5. Y/N
add flexion, post force	1. Y/N	2. Y/N	3. Y/N	4. Y/N	5. Y/N
fixed scapula, ant force	1. Y/N	2. Y/N	3. Y/N	4. Y/N	5. Y/N
fixed scapula, post force	1. Y/N	2. Y/N	3. Y/N	4. Y/N	5. Y/N

1. abd, ext rotation ____________________
2. abd, downward force ____________________
3. add flexion ____________________
4. add flexion, post force ____________________
5. fixed scapula, ant force ____________________
6. fixed scapula, post force ____________________

36. STABILITY WITH ARM AT SIDE: 1. NORMAL 2. N/T 3. right/left

>M **MANIPULATION DOWNWARD TRACTION**		**VOLUNTARY DOWNWARD FORCE**	
1. stable	______	1. stable	______
2. subluxation	______	2. subluxation	______
3. dislocation	______	3. dislocation	______
4. apprehension	______	4. apprehension	______

Physical Examination: Shoulder - 7
Doctor's Form 502

37. VOLUNTARY-ACTIVE INSTABILITY: 1. NORMAL 2. N/T 3. right/left

>M **ABDUCTION, EXTERNAL ROTATION**
1. stable ______
2. subluxation ______
3. dislocation ______
4. apprehension ______

ABDUCTION, DOWNWARD FORCE
1. stable ______
2. subluxation ______
3. dislocation ______
4. apprehension ______

ADDUCTION FLEXION
1. stable ______
2. subluxation ______
3. dislocation ______
4. apprehension ______

ADDUCTION FLEXION, POSTERIOR FORCE
1. stable ______
2. subluxation ______
3. dislocation ______
4. apprehension ______

FIXED SCAPULA, ANTERIOR FORCE
1. stable ______
2. subluxation ______
3. dislocation ______
4. apprehension ______

FIXED SCAPULA, POSTERIOR FORCE
1. stable ______
2. subluxation ______
3. dislocation ______
4. apprehension ______

38. STABILITY SUMMARY: 1.right/left

>M				
fixed dislocation	1. anterior	2. posterior	3. inferior	4.superior
fixed subluxation	1. anterior	2. posterior	3. inferior	4.superior
recurrent dislocation	1. anterior	2. posterior	3. inferior	4.superior
recurrent subluxation	1. anterior	2. posterior	3. inferior	4.superior
rare subluxation	1. anterior	2. posterior	3. inferior	4.superior
apprehension	1. anterior	2. posterior	3. inferior	4.superior
normal	1. anterior	2. posterior	3. inferior	4.superior

39. CIRCULATION: 1. NORMAL 2. N/T 3. right/left

>M **CAROTID**
1. present
2. diminished
3. absent
4. bruit

SUBCLAVIAN
1. present
2. diminished
3. absent
4. bruit

AXILLARY BRACHIAL
1. present
2. diminished
3. absent
4. bruit

ANTECUBITAL BRACHIAL
1. present
2. diminished
3. absent
4. bruit

RADIAL
1. present
2. diminished
3. absent
4. bruit
5. diminished with arm elevation

ULNAR
1. present
2. diminished
3. absent
4. bruit

RAYNAUD'S
1. present

RSD
1. present

SUDECK'S
1. present

EDEMA
1. present

1. Comments: ______

8 - Physical Examination: Shoulder
Doctor's Form 502

40. THORACIC OUTLET: 1. right/left

>M **WRIGHT'S HYPERABDUCTION MANEUVER**
1. normal pulse
2. diminished
3. absent
4. at _____ degrees elevation
5. other ________________________________

COSTOCLAVICULAR MANEUVER
1. normal pulse
2. diminished
3. absent
4. at _____ degrees elevation
5. other ________________________________

ADSON'S MANEUVER
1. normal pulse
2. diminished
3. absent
4. at _____ degrees elevation
5. other ________________________________

41. NEUROLOGIC: 1. right/left

>M **Sensation:** 1. NORMAL 2. Abnormal 3.N/T
1. ______________________ 1. dermatome
2. ______________________ 2. sensory nerve distribution

1. Comments: ________________________________

Proprioception: 1. NORMAL 2. Abnormal 3. N/T

Hoffmann test: 1. NEGATIVE 2. Positive 3. N/T

Babinski test: 1. NEGATIVE 2. Positive 3. N/T

1. Comments: ________________________________

DTR's: 1. EQUAL AND ACTIVE 2. Abnormal 3. N/T

1. diminished	1. biceps
2. absent	2. triceps
3. increased	3. wrist
	4. ______________________

1. Comments: ________________________________

42. STATUS OF ELBOW: 1. N/T 2. right/left

>M 1. asymptomatic 1. normal exam
2. symptomatic 2. abnormal exam

1. Comments: ________________________________

1. Diagnosis: ________________________________

Range of Motion: 1. FULL 2. Limited 3. N/T

43. ELBOW RANGE OF MOTION:

RIGHT		LEFT	
1. Flexion	______ deg	1. Flexion	______ deg
2. Extension	______ deg	2. Extension	______ deg
3. Pronation	______ deg	3. Pronation	______ deg
4. Supination	______ deg	4. Supination	______ deg

Physical Examination: Shoulder - 9
Doctor's Form 502

44. STATUS OF SPINE: 1. cervical/thoracic 2. N/T
>M 1. asymptomatic 1. normal exam
2. symptomatic 2. abnormal exam

1. Comments: ____________________

1. Diagnosis: ____________________

Range of Motion: 1. FULL 2. Limited 3. N/T

Flexion		1. Normal	2. Abnormal	3. ________
Extension		1. Normal	2. Abnormal	3. ________
Lateral rotation	1. R/L	2. Normal	3. Abnormal	4. ________
Lateral bending	1. R/L	2. Normal	3. Abnormal	4. ________

45. AMPUTATION LEVEL: 1. NONE 2. right/left
>M 1. forequarter
2. shoulder
3. arm
4. elbow
5. forearm
6. wrist
7. finger-thumb ____________________

Level:
1. above elbow
2. at elbow
3. below elbow
4. wrist
5. midcarpal

46. PATIENT COOPERATION:
1. GOOD
2. failed to relax
3. failed to cooperate
4. exam was not performed because ____________________
5. exam of ____________ considered unreliable because ____________

47. DOCTOR'S NOTATIONS: (Each observation will be printed as a paragraph)
>M ____________________

48. CLINICAL IMPRESSION OF PROBLEMATIC SHOULDER: 1. right/left
>M 1. rotator cuff tear
impingement syndrome
2. ____________________
3. ____________________

49. OPPOSITE SHOULDER CONDITION:
1. asymptomatic 1. normal exam
2. symptomatic 2. abnormal exam

1. Comments: ____________________

1. Diagnosis: ____________________

10 - Physical Examination: Shoulder
Doctor's Form 502

50. **ADDITIONAL COMMENTS:** (i.e. plan, tests, therapy, surgery)
>M (Each observation will be printed as a paragraph)

Doctor's Signature: Edward Lowe **Date:** 12-22-87

Patient name: Martin Sample
Patient number: 1200

Physician name: Edward Lowe, M.D.

Date of examination: December 22, 1987

PHYSICAL EXAMINATION

A physical examination was performed on December 22, 1987. The right shoulder was problematic.

The patient's right shoulder posture was normal. The patient avoided moving, lifting, reaching, pushing, and pulling with the right shoulder.

Right shoulder joint inspection revealed that the sternoclavicular, acromioclavicular, and glenohumeral joints were normal. Right shoulder inspection revealed that the clavicle, scapula, and humerus were normal.

The appearance, color, temperature, and texture of the skin of the patient's right shoulder appeared to be normal.

The right shoulder showed no skin scars.

The patient had the following circumferential measurements taken:

	RIGHT	LEFT
at deltoid insertion:	40 cm	40 cm
elbow:	28 cm	28 cm

The patient showed tenderness during palpation of the right anterior coracoacromial ligament. No masses were identified on the right side.

There was popping during internal rotation abduction motion which suggested rotation cuff tear/impingement.
The following impingement tests were negative:
- adduction/external rotation

The following impingement tests were positive:
- forward flexion
- abduction/external rotation
- abduction/internal rotation

The following impingement tests were painful:
- forward flexion
- abduction/external rotation
- abduction/internal rotation

The following impingement tests were negative with local anesthetic:
- forward flexion
- abduction/external rotation
- abduction/internal rotation

The following impingement tests produced crepitus:
- abduction/internal rotation

Manipulation, active voluntary movement, and stability with the patient's arm at his side were normal.

During range of motion testing, the body was in a sitting position. Bilateral and simultaneous arm measurements were taken with a goniometer.

RANGE OF MOTION:

ARM POSITION	MOTION MEASURED	ACTIVE RT	ACTIVE LF
side	elevation	45	170
side	forward flexion	45	170
side	abduction	30	90
side	external rotation	0	30
90 abd and 0 degrees	external rotation	45	+15
side	backward extension	30	45

INTERNAL ROTATION:

Patient could reach to:	ACTIVE RT	ACTIVE LF
trochanter	X	
a vertebral level of		D5

During range of motion testing on the right side, the effort in total elevation was slow and painful; external rotation at side was painful; and internal rotation at side was slow.

Shoulder motion strength tests have indicated the following musculature strength levels on a scale of 0 to 5 (0 = absent 1 = trace 2 = poor 3 = fair 4 = good 5 = normal strength):

	RIGHT	LEFT	COMMENT
abduction-thumb down	4	5	
abduction-thumb up	4	5	
external rotation	3	5	painful
internal rotation	5	5	

Musculature tests have indicated the following musculature strength levels on a scale of 0 to 5 (0 = absent 1 = trace 2 = poor 3 = fair 4 = good 5 = normal strength):

	RIGHT	LEFT
biceps	5	5

CIRCULATION:
Circulation appeared to be normal. The radial pulse circulation was present.

NEUROLOGICAL:
Sensation in the shoulder was normal.

The patient's cervical spine was asymptomatic and normal on examination.

The patient cooperated well.

CLINICAL IMPRESSION:
Right Shoulder
Rotator cuff tear.
Impingement syndrome.

The patient's opposite shoulder was asymptomatic and normal on examination.

Edward Lowe, MD

X-Ray Evaluation: Shoulder

Doctor's Form 503 (4.3)

Patient Name: Martin Sample
Patient Number: 1200
Problem Number: ___
Date: 12-22-87

1. NAME OF EVALUATING PHYSICIAN: Edward Lowe, M.D.

2. PHYSICIAN NUMBER: ___

3. PROBLEMATIC SHOULDER:
1. RIGHT (circled)
2. LEFT

4. PLAIN FILM PROJECTIONS:

>M	DATE		ELSEWHERE
1. AP Neutral (circled)	2. 12-23-87	3. here (circled)	4.
	__-__-	here	
1. AP Int Rotation (circled)	2. 12-23-87	3. here (circled)	4.
	__-__-	here	
1. AP Ext Rotation (circled)	2. 12-23-87	3. here (circled)	4.
	__-__-	here	
1. Axillary-rest- (circled)	2. 12-23-87	3. here (circled)	4.
	__-__-	here	
1. Active stress	2. __-__-	3. here	4.
	__-__-	here	
1. Passive stress	2. __-__-	3. here	4.
	__-__-	here	
1. Arch view (circled)	2. 12-23-87	3. here	4.
	__-__-	here	
1. Abduction	2. __-__-	3. here	4.
	__-__-	here	
1. Weighted	2. __-__-	3. here	4.
	__-__-	here	
1. Lateral: X-chest	2. __-__-	3. here	4.
	__-__-	here	
1. West Point view	2. __-__-	3. here	4.
	__-__-	here	
1. Stryker view	2. __-__-	3. here	4.
	__-__-	here	
1. ______	2. __-__-	3. here	4.
	__-__-	here	

SUMMARY

5. X-RAY INTERPRETATION:

>M 1. A-C joint degeneration
normal glenohumeral joint
beaked acromion

2 - X-Ray Evaluation: Shoulder

Doctor's Form 503

6. X-RAY DESCRIPTION:
>M 1. degenerative changes
2. osteophytes
3. joint space narrowing
4. loose bodies
5. calcification
6. demineralization
7. erosion
8. osteolytic lesion
9. osteoblastic lesion
10. osteonecrosis
11. osteochondritis
12. subluxation
13. dislocation
14. cuff tear arthropathy
15. Hill-Sach lesion

1. NO ABNORMALITIES
1. anterior
2. posterior
3. superior
4. inferior
5. medial
6. lateral
7. proximal
8. distal

1. clavicle
2. scapula
3. body
4. spine
5. acromion
6. coracoid
7. glenoid
8. humeral
9. head
10. neck
11. greater tuberosity
12. lesser tuberosity
13. shaft

1. sternoclavicular
2. acromioclavicular
3. glenohumeral

1. bursae
2. subacromial
3. subscapularis
4. tendon
5. rotator cuff
6. biceps

7. SC JOINT:
1. arthritis
2. separation
3. intra-articular fracture

8. AC JOINT:
1. arthritis
2. separation
3. grade I
4. grade II
5. grade III
6. grade IV
7. grade V

9. GH JOINT:
1. arthritis
2. glenohumeral dislocation
3. glenohumeral subluxation
4. inferior subluxation with ____ weight
6. Hill-Sach lesion

7. Glenoid rim:
8. fracture
9. bone reaction
10. Glenoid wear:
11. anterior
12. posterior
13. loose body(ies)
14. number ______
15. anterior
16. posterior
17. superior
18. inferior

10. IMPINGEMENT X-RAY FINDINGS:
1. anterior acromial spur
2. anterior acromial sclerosis
3. bone reaction greater tuberosity
4. inferior AC joint spurs
5. superior displacement humeral head

humeral head/acromion interval: ______ mm
unfused acromial epiphysis: pre _____ meso ____ meta ____ basi _____

Acromial morphology:
1. Type I (flat)
2. Type II (curved)
3. Type III (hooked)

11. CERVICAL SPINE X-RAY:

1. ______________________________

____

12. FOREIGN BODY OR IMPLANT: 1. NONE

>M 1. sternum
2. clavicle
3. scapula
4. humerus

Joint:
1. SC
2. AC
3. GH

Device:
1. prosthesis
2. screw
3. staple
4. nail
5. wire
6. total shoulder: ______________________________
7. (other) ______________________________

Position:
1. secure
2. loose
3. migrated
4. (other) ______________________________

13. DISLOCATION:

>M 1. NONE
2. recent
3. old

1. reduced
2. unreduced

Sternoclavicular:
1. anterior
2. posterior
3. superior
4. inferior

Acromioclavicular:
1. anterior
2. posterior
3. superior
4. inferior

Glenohumeral:
1. anterior
2. posterior
3. superior
4. inferior

14. FRACTURE:

>M 1. NONE
2. recent
3. old

1. open
2. closed

1. transverse
2. oblique
3. spiral
4. butterfly

1. sternum
2. clavicle
3. scapula
4. glenoid neck
5. glenoid rim
6. spine
7. body

1. humerus
2. greater tuberosity
3. lesser tuberosity
4. neck
5. shaft

1. undisplaced
2. displaced

1. angulated
2. rotated

1. simple
2. comminuted
3. avulsion

1. united
2. delayed union
3. malunion
4. pseudoarthrosis
5. post-reduction

4 - X-Ray Evaluation: Shoulder
Doctor's Form 503

15. FRACTURE POSITION:
1. acceptable
2. displaced
3. angulated
4. articular offset
5. ______________________________

16. SPECIAL TESTS:

Arthrogram 1. date ___-___-______ 2. where: ____________________
3. NORMAL Y/N 4. by report 5. by review
6. how: ____________________

Tomogram 1. date ___-___-______ 2. where: ____________________
3. NORMAL Y/N 4. by report 5. by review
6. how: ____________________

Bone Scan 1. date ___-___-______ 2. where: ____________________
3. NORMAL Y/N 4. by report 5. by review
6. how: ____________________

CAT Scan 1. date ___-___-______ 2. where: ____________________
3. NORMAL Y/N 4. by report 5. by review
6. how: ____________________

17. SPECIAL TESTS (continued):

Magnetic Resonance 1. date ___-___-______ 2. where: ____________________
3. NORMAL Y/N 4. by report 5. by review
6. how: ____________________

Ultrasound 1. date ___-___-______ 2. where: ____________________
3. NORMAL Y/N 4. by report 5. by review
6. how: ____________________

Fluoroscopy 1. date ___-___-______ 2. where: ____________________
3. NORMAL Y/N 4. by report 5. by review
6. how: ____________________

Stress X-Rays 1. date ___-___-______ 2. where: ____________________
3. NORMAL Y/N 4. by report 5. by review
6. how: ____________________

Doctor's Signature: Edward Lowe, M.D. **Date:** 12-23-87

Version 4.3 May, 1990

Information Health Network
P.O. Box 23056
Lansing, Michigan 48909-3056
(800)443-0613 (517)351-1588

Patient name: Martin Sample

Patient number: 1200

Physician name: Edward Lowe, M.D.

X-RAY EVALUATION

The right shoulder was problematic.

Plain film X-Rays were taken and/or reviewed in the following projections:

PROJECTION	DATE	PLACE
AP NEUTRAL	12-23-1987	here
AP INTERNAL ROTATION	12-23-1987	here
AP EXTERNAL ROTATION	12-23-1987	here
AXILLARY: RESTING	12-23-1987	here
ARCH VIEW	12-23-1987	here

X-RAY IMPRESSION:
The X-Ray impression was: A-C joint degeneration, Normal Glenohumeral joint, Beak acromion.

There were degenerative changes in the acromioclavicular joint.

The acromioclavicular joint showed signs of arthritis. Impingement X-rays showed an anterior acromial spur and anterior acromial sclerosis.

Edward M. Lowe, M.D.

Surgery Form: Shoulder

Doctor's Form 504 (4.3)

Note to Surgeons: The Surgery Form and Report do not handle cases aborted prior to any surgical intervention. If surgery is aborted before any surgical intervention actually takes place, you should dictate the surgery report instead of completing this Surgery Form.

Patient Name: Martin Sample

Patient Number: 1200
Problem Number: ___
Date: 1-10-88

1. **HOSPITAL NUMBER:** ________

2. **SHOULDER OPERATED ON:**
   1. RIGHT (circled)
   2. LEFT

3. **PATIENT STATUS:**
   1. outpatient/outpatient observation
   2. admitted before/after surgery (after surgery circled)
   3. on 1-10-88
   4. reason: pain control

4. **NAME OF SURGEON:** Edward Lowe, M.D.

5. **SURGEON NUMBER:** ________

6. **1ST ASSISTANT:** Ruth Jones, R.N.

7. **2ND ASSISTANT:** ________

8. **PHYSICIAN'S ASSISTANT:** ________

9. **ANESTHESIOLOGIST:** Eugene High, M.D.

10. **TYPE OF ANESTHETIC:**
    1. general (circled)
    2. endotracheal (circled)
    3. local ________
    4. block ________
    5. aborted - reason ________

11. **PATIENT POSITION:**
    1. supine
    2. prone
    3. right lateral decubitus
    4. left lateral decubitus (circled)
    5. other ________

    Secured by:
    1. Olympic Vac Pac (circled)
    2. mechanical means

12. **TYPE OF TABLE:**
    1. regular (circled)
    2. fracture

2 - Surgery Form: Shoulder

Doctor's Form 504

13. PAST SURGICAL HISTORY--OPEN:

>M **How many:**	**Procedure:**	
1. _____	arthrotomy	_____
1. _____	repair (dislocation)	_____
1. _____	repair (subluxation)	_____
1. _____	synovectomy	_____
1. _____	acromioplasty	_____
1. _____	CA ligament resection	_____
1. _____	rotator cuff repair	_____
1. _____	resection-repair AC joint	_____
1. _____	other _____	

Type of instability:
1. anterior
2. posterior
3. multidirectional

14. PAST SURGICAL HISTORY-DIAGNOSTIC ARTHROSCOPY:
1. how many: _______
2. last diagnosis: _______

15. PAST SURGICAL HISTORY-ARTHROSCOPIC SURGERY:

>M **How many:**	**Procedure:**	
1. _____	loose body	_____
1. _____	labrum resection	_____
1. _____	repair (dislocation)	_____
1. _____	repair (subluxation)	_____
1. _____	chondroplasty	_____
1. _____	rotator cuff debridement	_____
1. _____	synovectomy	_____
1. _____	bursectomy	_____
1. _____	acromioplasty	_____
1. _____	CA ligament resection	_____
1. _____	rotator cuff repair	_____
1. _____	AC resection	_____
1. _____	other _____	

Type of instability:
1. anterior
2. posterior
3. multidirectional

EXAM UNDER ANESTHESIA

16. RANGE OF MOTION (IN DEGREES): 1. N/T
1. NORMAL and equal to opposite, unaffected side

Arm Starting Position:	**(plus)**	**Motion Measured:**	**PASSIVE RIGHT**	**PASSIVE LEFT**
side		elevation	1. 170	2. 170
side		external rotation	1. 0	2. 50
side		abduction	1. _____	2. _____
side		internal rotation	1. _____	2. _____
90 abd	(_____)	external rotation	2. _____	3. _____
90 abd	(_____)	internal rotation	2. _____	3. _____
90 abd	(_____)	extension	2. _____	3. _____
side		forward flexion	1. _____	2. _____
side		backward extension	1. _____	2. _____

Surgery Form: Shoulder - 3
Doctor's Form 504

17. MANIPULATION: 1. N/T

>M **INVOLVED SHOULDER:**

1. STABLE	1. abduction	1. traction (axial)
2. subluxated	2. flexion (90 deg)	2. external rotation
3. dislocated	3. fixed scapula	3. internal rotation
4. popping		4. anterior force
5. catching	1. with arm free	5. posterior force
	2. in suspension	6. inferior force

OPPOSITE SHOULDER: 1. N/T

1. STABLE	1. abduction	1. traction (axial)
2. subluxated	2. flexion (90 deg)	2. external rotation
3. dislocated	3. fixed scapula	3. internal rotation
4. popping		4. anterior force
5. catching	1. with arm free	5. posterior force
	2. in suspension	6. inferior force

18. ARM POSITION: 1. free/secured

			# Pulleys:		
1. mechanical	1. suspended	1. apparatus	1. 1 / 2 / 3	1. 60	abduction
2. manual	2. traction	2. splint		2. 0	flexion
		3. sponge tape		3. ___	extension
		4. ace wrap			
		5. velcro straps			
		6. plastic foam gauntlet			

1. utilized 1. 16 lbs. for balanced suspension
2. was tied 2. ______

Second Suspension Device:

1. arm	1. anterior	1. suspension
2. forearm	2. posterior	2. traction
	3. superior	
	4. lateral	

19. PRE-OP DIAGNOSIS: — **DIAGNOSTIC ICD-9-CM CODE**

>M rotator cuff tear ______
impingement syndrome ______
______

20. POST-OP DIAGNOSIS: — **DIAGNOSTIC ICD-9-CM CODE**

>M 1. same
2. none made
3. additional labrum tear ______
5. different ______

DIAGNOSTIC ARTHROSCOPY

21. DIAGNOSTIC ARTHROSCOPY PERFORMED?
1. yes
2. no

22. SKIN PREPARATION:

1. Betadine	1. scrub
2. pHisoHex	2. paint
3. (other) ______	3. minutes ______

23. DRAPING:
1. J & J shoulder drape
2. (other) ______

24. PRE-INSERTION DISTENTION:

1. #18 spinal needle	1. anterior	1. ___ cc
2. cannula	2. posterior	2. ______ fluid
	3. superior	

4 - Surgery Form: Shoulder

Doctor's Form 504

25. JOINT FLUID:

	1. NORMAL	2. Abnormal	**Specimen:**	**Cleansed:**
1. minimal	1. yellow	1. mucinous	1. culture	1. serial washings
2. moderate	2. serosanguineous	2. purulent	2. cell count	2. continuous flow
3. massive	3. bloody	3. snowy (loose bodies)	3. cell block (path)	
		4. clear	4. laboratory analysis	

26. DISTENTION MEDIUM:

>M 1. initial	1. saline adrenaline	1. visualization
2. subsequent	2. saline	2. irrigation - lavage
3. continuous	3. Ringer's lactate	3. motorized instrumentation
4. intermittent	4. water	4. hemostasis
	5. air (room)	
	6. CO_2	
	7. adrenaline (1 mg/1000) cc solution	
	8. (other)____________________	

27. PRESSURE ON INFLOW:

>M 1. gravity	1. intermittent	1. pressure: _______ mm Hg
2. manual	2. variable	2. flow: _______ ml/min.
3. mechanical		
4. pump ____________________		

28. ARTHROSCOPE PORTAL:

>M 1. initially	1. anterior	1. routine	1. obesity
2. subsequently	2. posterior	2. difficult	2. scar
3. interchangeably	3. superior	3. following multiple attempts	3. previous surgery
		4. following _____ attempts	4. fluid extravasation
			5. technical problems

29. INFLOW:

>M 1. arthroscope	1. superior supraspinatus
2. separate needle	2. anterior
3. cannula system	3. lateral
	4. interchangeable locations

30. ARTHROSCOPY PERFORMED BY:

		Documentation:
1. direct vision	1. with	1. video monitor
2. television	2. without	2. video recording
		3. slide photography
		4. movie film
		5. Polaroid slides
		6. Polaroid prints

FINDINGS

GLENOHUMERAL JOINT

31. LOOSE BODIES: 1. NONE 2. Abnormal 3. N/V 4. present (number ________________)

>M 1. small	1. dispersed	1. anterior
2. medium	2. in joint	2. posterior
3. large	3. extrasynovial	3. superior
4. combination	4. synovial attached	4. inferior
		5. medial
		6. lateral

1. subscapularis bursae	1. cartilage
2. subacromial bursae	2. labral
3. recess	3. bony
4. humerus	4. synovial
5. glenoid	5. ligament
6. synovial lining	6. foreign body ____________________
7. rotator cuff ligament	7. surgical implant ____________________
8. glenohumeral ligaments	8. origin undetermined

Surgery Form: Shoulder - 5
Doctor's Form 504

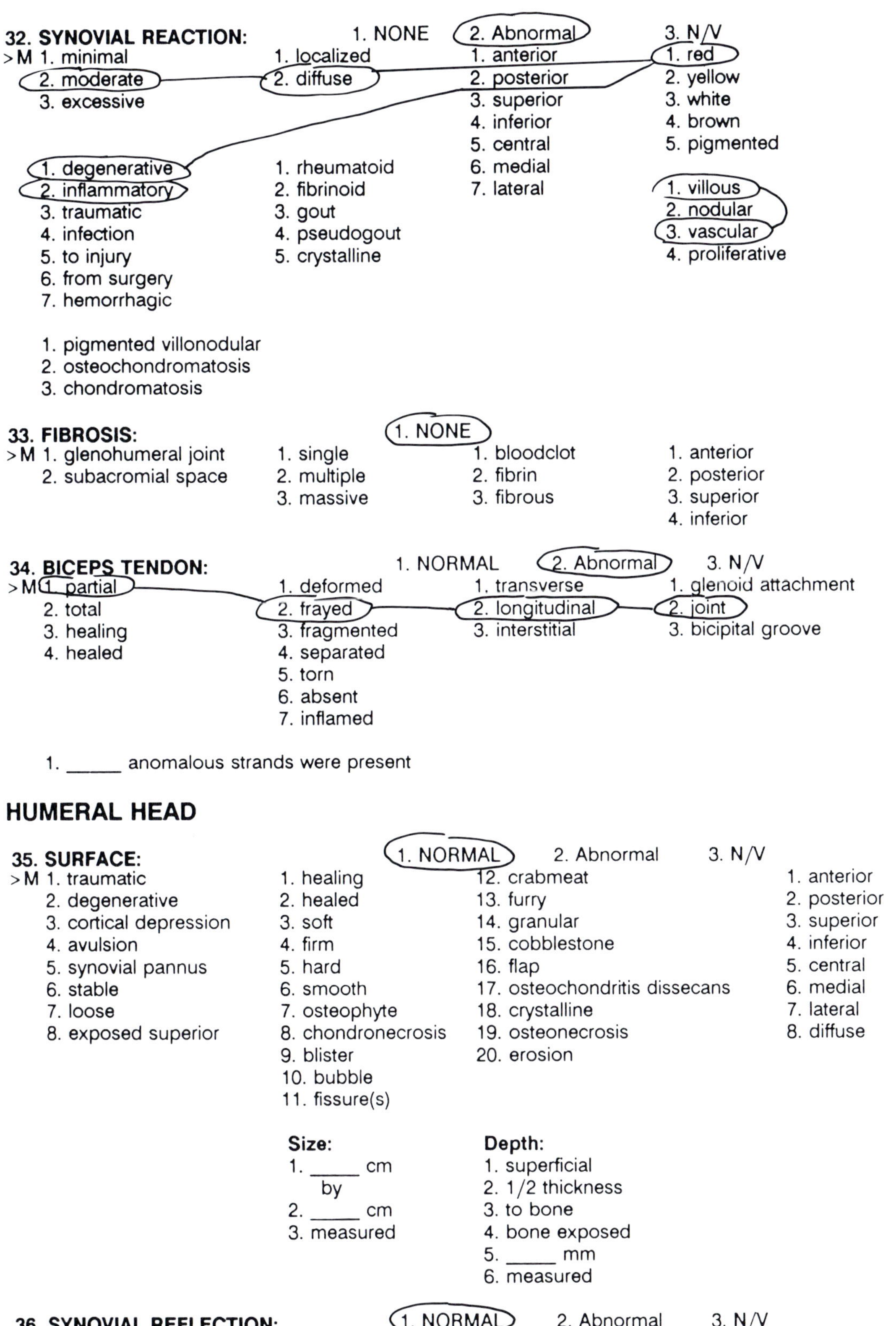

32. SYNOVIAL REACTION: 1. NONE 2. Abnormal 3. N/V

>M 1. minimal
2. moderate
3. excessive

1. localized
2. diffuse

1. anterior
2. posterior
3. superior
4. inferior
5. central
6. medial
7. lateral

1. red
2. yellow
3. white
4. brown
5. pigmented

1. degenerative
2. inflammatory
3. traumatic
4. infection
5. to injury
6. from surgery
7. hemorrhagic

1. rheumatoid
2. fibrinoid
3. gout
4. pseudogout
5. crystalline

1. villous
2. nodular
3. vascular
4. proliferative

1. pigmented villonodular
2. osteochondromatosis
3. chondromatosis

33. FIBROSIS: 1. NONE

>M 1. glenohumeral joint
2. subacromial space

1. single
2. multiple
3. massive

1. bloodclot
2. fibrin
3. fibrous

1. anterior
2. posterior
3. superior
4. inferior

34. BICEPS TENDON: 1. NORMAL 2. Abnormal 3. N/V

>M 1. partial
2. total
3. healing
4. healed

1. deformed
2. frayed
3. fragmented
4. separated
5. torn
6. absent
7. inflamed

1. transverse
2. longitudinal
3. interstitial

1. glenoid attachment
2. joint
3. bicipital groove

1. _____ anomalous strands were present

HUMERAL HEAD

35. SURFACE: 1. NORMAL 2. Abnormal 3. N/V

>M 1. traumatic
2. degenerative
3. cortical depression
4. avulsion
5. synovial pannus
6. stable
7. loose
8. exposed superior

1. healing
2. healed
3. soft
4. firm
5. hard
6. smooth
7. osteophyte
8. chondronecrosis
9. blister
10. bubble
11. fissure(s)

12. crabmeat
13. furry
14. granular
15. cobblestone
16. flap
17. osteochondritis dissecans
18. crystalline
19. osteonecrosis
20. erosion

1. anterior
2. posterior
3. superior
4. inferior
5. central
6. medial
7. lateral
8. diffuse

Size:
1. _____ cm
by
2. _____ cm
3. measured

Depth:
1. superficial
2. 1/2 thickness
3. to bone
4. bone exposed
5. _____ mm
6. measured

36. SYNOVIAL REFLECTION: 1. NORMAL 2. Abnormal 3. N/V

>M 1. smooth
2. pitted
3. pannus
4. erosion
5. hemorrhage

6 - Surgery Form: Shoulder

Doctor's Form 504

37. POSITION: 1. NORMAL 2. Abnormal 3. N/V

>M
1. reduced
2. subluxated
3. dislocated
4. reducible
5. displacable
6. stable

1. anterior
2. posterior
3. superior
4. inferior
5. medial
6. lateral

38. HILL-SACH LESION (ARTICULAR DEFECT): 1. NONE 2. N/V

>M
1. recent
2. old

Shape:
1. irregular
2. osteophyte
3. deformed
4. flattened
5. fragmented
6. loose body
7. depression
8. round
9. oval

1. anterior
2. posterior
3. superior
4. inferior
5. central
6. medial

Size:
1. _____ cm
by
2. _____ cm
3. measured

Depth:
1. superficial
2. 1/2 thickness
3. to bone
4. bone exposed
5. _____ mm
6. measured

GLENOID

39. GLENOID ARTICULAR SURFACE: 1. NORMAL 2. Abnormal 3. N/V

>M
1. traumatic
2. degenerative
3. cortical depression
4. avulsion
5. synovial pannus
6. stable
7. loose
8. exposed superior
9. central cartilage thin

1. healing
2. healed
3. soft
4. firm
5. hard
6. smooth
7. osteophyte
8. chondronecrosis
9. blister
10. bubble
11. fissure(s)

12. crabmeat
13. furry
14. granular
15. cobblestone
16. flap
17. osteochondritis dissecans
18. crystalline
19. osteonecrosis
20. erosion
21. disruption

1. anterior
2. posterior
3. superior
4. inferior
5. central
6. medial
7. lateral
8. diffuse

Size:
1. _____ cm
by
2. _____ cm
3. measured

Depth:
1. superficial
2. 1/2 thickness
3. to bone
4. bone exposed
5. _____ mm
6. measured

40. BONY GLENOID MARGINS: 1. NORMAL 2. Abnormal 3. N/V

1. fracture
2. osteophytes
3. degenerative changes
4. traumatic

1. anterior
2. posterior
3. superior
4. inferior

41. GLENOID ANTERIOR CENTRAL SULCUS: 1. NORMAL 2. Abnormal 3. N/V

1. prominent
2. traumatic
3. blood stained
4. fragmented
5. soft tissue flap

Surgery Form: Shoulder - 7
Doctor's Form 504

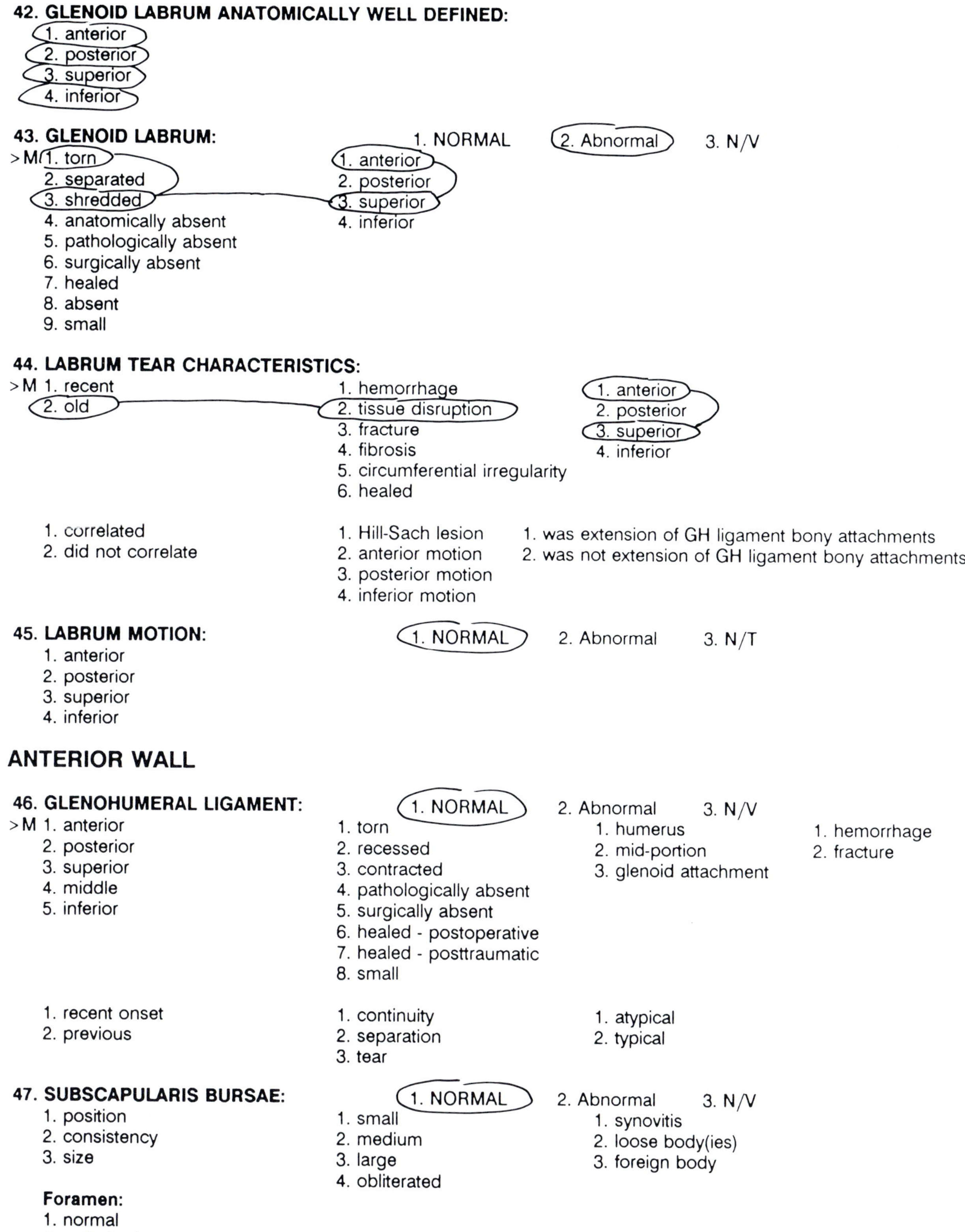

LABRUM

42. GLENOID LABRUM ANATOMICALLY WELL DEFINED:
1. anterior
2. posterior
3. superior
4. inferior

43. GLENOID LABRUM: 1. NORMAL 2. Abnormal 3. N/V

>M 1. torn
2. separated
3. shredded
4. anatomically absent
5. pathologically absent
6. surgically absent
7. healed
8. absent
9. small

1. anterior
2. posterior
3. superior
4. inferior

44. LABRUM TEAR CHARACTERISTICS:

>M 1. recent
2. old

1. hemorrhage
2. tissue disruption
3. fracture
4. fibrosis
5. circumferential irregularity
6. healed

1. anterior
2. posterior
3. superior
4. inferior

1. correlated
2. did not correlate

1. Hill-Sach lesion
2. anterior motion
3. posterior motion
4. inferior motion

1. was extension of GH ligament bony attachments
2. was not extension of GH ligament bony attachments

45. LABRUM MOTION: 1. NORMAL 2. Abnormal 3. N/T

1. anterior
2. posterior
3. superior
4. inferior

ANTERIOR WALL

46. GLENOHUMERAL LIGAMENT: 1. NORMAL 2. Abnormal 3. N/V

>M 1. anterior
2. posterior
3. superior
4. middle
5. inferior

1. torn
2. recessed
3. contracted
4. pathologically absent
5. surgically absent
6. healed - postoperative
7. healed - posttraumatic
8. small

1. humerus
2. mid-portion
3. glenoid attachment

1. hemorrhage
2. fracture

1. recent onset
2. previous

1. continuity
2. separation
3. tear

1. atypical
2. typical

47. SUBSCAPULARIS BURSAE: 1. NORMAL 2. Abnormal 3. N/V

1. position
2. consistency
3. size

1. small
2. medium
3. large
4. obliterated

1. synovitis
2. loose body(ies)
3. foreign body

Foramen:
1. normal
2. pathologic

8 - Surgery Form: Shoulder

Doctor's Form 504

48. SUBSCAPULARIS TENDON: 1. NORMAL 2. Abnormal 3. N/V

1. frayed
2. torn
3. not identified
4. absent
5. scarred over
6. completely exposed
7. healed - postoperative

1. congenital
2. traumatic
3. postoperative
4. pathologic
5. degenerative

49. INFERIOR SPACE: 1. NORMAL 2. Abnormal 3. N/V

1. labrum tear
2. arcuate portion inferior glenohumeral ligament
3. loose body(ies)
4. synovitis
5. fibrosis

50. POSTERIOR SPACE: 1. NORMAL 2. Abnormal 3. N/V

1. labrum tear
2. loose body(ies)
3. capsule disruption
4. synovitis
5. fibrosis

SUPERIOR SPACE

51. UNDERSIDE ROTATOR CUFF: 1. NORMAL 2. Abnormal 3. N/V

>M 1. synovitis
2. thickening
3. encroachment on joint
4. adhesion to biceps
5. healed

Tear
1. partial
2. complete

1. transverse
2. longitudinal
3. horizontal
4. oval

1. anterior
2. posterior
3. proximal
4. distal

1. recent origin
2. previously existed

1. red
2. yellow
3. white

1. flap
2. frayed
3. rounded

1. humerus
2. tendon substance
3. capsule
4. synovial lining

1. ______ cm by ______ cm
1. ______ cm by ______ cm

52. CHARACTER CUFF DEFECT:

>M **Communication to Subacromial Space:**

1. visualization
2. flow

1. possible
2. not possible

1. movable
2. fixed

Approximation Defect:
1. does not
2. does

53. GLENOHUMERAL INSTABILITY COMPOSITE FINDINGS:

>M 1. subluxation
2. dislocation

1. anterior
2. posterior
3. superior
4. inferior
5. multidirectional

Identified by:
1. history
2. physical exam
3. X-Ray
4. exam under anesthesia
5. during arthroscopy
6. traction-external rotation
7. Bankart lesion
8. Hill-Sach lesion
9. sulcus sign

Surgery Form: Shoulder - 9
Doctor's Form 504

SUBACROMIAL SPACE

54. SUBACROMIAL SPACE: 1. NORMAL 2. Abnormal 3. N/V 4. not attempted

>M 1. via rotator cuff tear
2. via redirection of scope
3. not entered although attempted
4. normal small space without inflammation

1. well developed	1. synovitis	1. superior surface tear
2. pathologic	2. fibrous bands	2. biceps tendon
3. not pathologic	3. loose body(ies)	3. acromium
4. ________	4. erosion	4. coracoacromial ligament
	5. tear	
	6. inflammation	
	7. calcification	
	8. ________	

ACROMIOCLAVICULAR JOINT

55. ACROMIOCLAVICULAR JOINT: 1. NORMAL 2. Abnormal 3. N/V 4. not attempted

>M 1. palpation	1. transcutaneous	1. osteophytes	1. anterior	1. palpation
2. needle location	2. subacromial space	2. synovitis	2. posterior	2. inspection
3. arthroscope entry		3. meniscal disruption	3. superior	
4. surgical exposure		4. cystic changes	4. inferior	

OPERATIVE ARTHROSCOPY

56. SURGERY PERFORMED:
1. YES
2. NO

>M 1. anterior	1. glenohumeral
2. posterior	2. subacromial space
3. superior	3. AC joint
4. lateral	
5. multiple	
6. interchangeable	

GLENOHUMERAL JOINT

58. SYNOVECTOMY:

1. limited synovectomy	1. anterior	1. rotator cuff
2. major synovectomy	2. posterior	2. biceps tendon
3. limited debridement	3. superior	3. biceps groove
4. major debridement	4. middle	4. labrum
	5. inferior	5. sulcus
		6. subscapularis tendon
		7. bone
		8. glenohumeral ligament

59. LOOSE BODY REMOVAL:
>M **Number:**

1. ______	1. attached	1. cartilage	1. anterior	1. lavage
	2. loose	2. labrum	2. posterior	2. suction
	3. unremoved	3. bony	3. superior	3. forceps
		4. synovial	4. inferior	4. motorized instruments
		5. foreign body ________		5. ________
		6. surgical implant of ________		

10 - Surgery Form: Shoulder

Doctor's Form 504

60. CHONDROPLASTY:

>M 1. limited
2. partial
3. full thickness abrasion

1. anterior
2. posterior
3. superior
4. inferior
5. central

1. glenoid
2. humerus

Size:
1. _____ cm 2. by ______ cm
1. _____ cm 2. by ______ cm

61. LABRUM RESECTION:

>M 1. small
2. moderate
3. large
4. _____ cm

1. anterior
2. posterior
3. superior
4. inferior

1. full
2. partial

1. preserving
2. sacrificing
3. dissecting

1. anterior
2. posterior

1. glenoid
2. superior GH
3. middle GH
4. inferior GH
5. subscapularis tendon
6. biceps tendon
7. posterior inferior (ligament)

62. ROTATOR CUFF DEBRIDEMENT (undersurface):

>M 1. anterior
2. posterior
3. proximal
4. distal
5. under surface
6. edge

Extent:
1. limited
2. superficial
3. expanded lesion
4. extension

Exposing:
1. vascularity
2. healthy tendon
3. subacromial space
4. acromion

63. GLENOHUMERAL JOINT RECONSTRUCTION: NARRATIVE 1. Inserted 2. Attached

>M **Site prep included:**
1. anterior synovectomy
2. labrum resection partial
3. labrum resection total
4. labrum dissection
5. bony glenoid decortication

Number/Type:
1. staple ________________
2. suture ________________
3. graft ________________
4. implant ________________

Portal:
1. established
2. new

Repair included:
1. anterior GH ligaments
2. posterior GH ligaments
3. superior GH ligaments
4. middle GH ligaments
5. inferior GH ligaments
6. labrum
7. subscapularis superior tendon slip

Advanced:
1. to glenoid
2. superiorly
3. medially
4. to reestablished labrum

Placement confirmed by:
1. direct visualization
2. scapular motion
3. palpation

SUBACROMIAL SPACE SURGERY

64. SURGICAL EXPOSURE:

>M **Exposed via:**
1. initial portal
2. redirection
3. replacement

1. anterior
2. posterior
3. superior
4. lateral
5. multiple approaches

Inflow via:
1. initial portal
2. anterior
3. posterior
4. superior
5. lateral
6. various portals

65. DEBRIDEMENT PROCEDURES:

1. bursectomy
2. coracoacromial ligament
3. superior rotator cuff
4. acromioplasty
5. acromioclavicular joint
6. AC joint osteophytes
7. resection calcific deposit

Surgery Form: Shoulder - 11
Doctor's Form 504

66. CA LIGAMENT:

1. resection
2. release
3. sectioned

1. acromion
2. middle
3. coracoid

67. ROTATOR CUFF DEBRIDEMENT (superior surface):

>M 1. anterior
2. posterior
3. proximal
4. distal
5. under surface
6. edge
7. superior space

Extent:
1. limited
2. superficial
3. expanded lesion
4. extension

Exposing:
1. vascularity
2. healthy tendon
3. humeral head
4. acromion
5. calcific deposits
6. ______________________________

68. ACROMIOPLASTY:

>M 1. partial
2. full

1. anterior
2. lateral
3. medial

1. ligament
2. bone
3. osteophytes

1. oblique
2. transverse

1. Adequate space was developed between acromion and rotator cuff

69. AC JOINT:

1. osteophyte removal
2. meniscectomy
3. resection clavicular end
4. resection acromial side

1. anterior
2. posterior
3. superior
4. inferior

70. HUMERAL HEAD:

1. synovectomy of pannus
2. osteophyte resection
3. smoothed surface

71. BICEPS TENDON:

1. synovectomy
2. resection

1. debridement
2. stabilization

1. K-wires
2. staple

72. ROTATOR CUFF RECONSTRUCTION:

NARRATIVE: 1. Inserted 2. Attached

Suitability:
1. mobility
2. tissue integrity
3. tissue viability
4. tendon length

Site Preparation:
1. bony
2. soft tissue

1. intracortical
2. cancellous

FIXATION DEVICE
Number/Type
1. staple ______________________________
2. screw ______________________________
3. suture ______________________________

Via:
1. insertion device
2. drill hole
3. screw driver

73. BIOPSY:

>M 1. intra articular
2. extra articular

1. anterior
2. posterior
3. superior
4. inferior
5. medial
6. lateral

1. biceps
2. subscapularis
3. rotator cuff

1. synovial
2. labral
3. cartilage
4. ligament
5. tendon

1. humerus
2. glenoid
3. acromion
4. clavicle

14 - Surgery Form: Shoulder

Doctor's Form 504

89. TELEVISION RECORDING DONE:

>M	1. inside	1. teaching value
	2. outside	2. research value
	1. continuous	1. 1/2 inch Beta
	2. edited	2. 3/4 inch cassette
		3. VHS
		4. disc

90. SLIDE PHOTOGRAPHY DONE:

>M	1. inside	1. regular	1. teaching value
	2. outside	2. Polaroid	2. research value
			3. for text book

1. lesion ______________________________

91. MOVIE RECORDING DONE:

>M	1. inside	1. teaching value
	2. outside	2. research value
	1. 16 mm	1. lesion ______________________________
	2. 35 mm	

92. PHOTOGRAPHIC PRINTS DONE:

>M	1. inside	1. teaching value
	2. outside	2. research value
	1. black & white	1. lesion ______________________________
	2. color	
	3. Polaroid	

PATHOLOGY

93. GROSS SPECIMEN PHOTO TAKEN:

>M	1. slide	1. lesion ______________________________
	2. video	
	3. movie	

94. MICROSCOPIC SECTION REQUESTED:

>M	1. H & E	1. teaching value
	2. special stain	2. research value
	3. electron microscopy	3. textbook

1. lesion ______________________________
2. pathology number ______________

POSTOPERATIVE MANAGEMENT

95. GENERAL STATEMENTS:

1. ALL of the following
2. sterile dressing applied
3. suspension released
4. circulation returned immediately
5. tolerated procedure well
6. delivered to recovery room in good condition
7. ______________________________

96. PATIENT INSTRUCTION SHEET PROVIDED:

1. YES
2. no

Surgery Form: Shoulder - 15
Doctor's Form 504

97. MEDICATION PRESCRIPTION PROVIDED:
1. NO
2. Tylenol # 3 (circled)
3. Percodan
4. (other) ______

98. POST OP MANAGEMENT:
>M 1. sling
2. immobilizer
3. brace
4. abduction splint (circled)
5. casted

For:
1. ______ days
2. 3 weeks
3. ______ months

Exercises:
1. none (circled)
2. pendulum
3. below waist
4. over head

1. ______ times per day

1. at home
2. at physical therapy
3. until office visit (circled)

99. FOLLOW-UP RECOMMENDATIONS:
>M Call for return appointment:
1. our office (circled)
2. referring Dr. office

In:
1. ______ days
2. / weeks
3. ______ months

Off work:
1. ______ days
2. ______ weeks
3. 3 months
4. N/A

100. COMMENTS/ELABORATION:
>M 1. ______

101. TECHNICAL PROBLEMS:
>M 1. ______

102. SPECIAL VIEWING OR SURGICAL APPROACHES:
>M 1. ______

103. MEDICAL RECOMMENDATIONS:
>M 1. ______

104. PROGNOSIS:
1. excellent
2. good (circled)
3. fair
4. poor
5. medical condition not stationary

Reason:
1. *good anatomical repair of cuff*

16 - Surgery Form: Shoulder
Doctor's Form 504

105. COPY OF REPORT TO:
>M Type of Report:
1. operative report
2. composite letter

1. coach
2. company physician
3. disability agency
4. employer (circled) — Parts Manufacturing
5. government agency
6. insurance company (circled) — Employee Benefit Concepts
7. lawyer
8. other physician
9. parent/guardian
10. patient (circled)
11. physical therapist
12. referring physician (circled) — Dr. Frank Williams
13. rehabilitation agency
14. trainer
15. other
16. all of these

106. DRAWING (below):
1. YES
2. no

Doctor's Signature: Edward Lowe, M.D. **Date:** 1-10-88

Version 4.3 May, 1990

Information Health Network
P.O. Box 23056
Lansing, Michigan 48909-3056
(800)443-0613 (517)351-1588

RE: Martin Sample

CHART: 1200

DIAGNOSTIC AND OPERATIVE ARTHROSCOPIC SURGERY REPORT

Date of Operation	January 10, 1988
Date of Documentation:	January 10, 1988
Joint operated on:	RIGHT shoulder
Patient status:	Admitted after surgery on January 10, 1988 Reason: pain control
Surgeon:	Edward Lowe, M.D.
First assistant:	Ruth Jones, R.N.
Anesthesiologist:	Eugene High, M.D.
Type of anesthesia:	general and endotracheal

PRE-OPERATIVE DIAGNOSIS: rotator cuff tear impingement syndrome

POST-OPERATIVE DIAGNOSIS: (in addition to the preoperative diagnosis) Labrum tear

RANGE OF MOTION
The patient showed the following ranges of motion (in degrees):

ARM POSITION	MOTION MEASURED	PASSIVE	
		Right	Left
	elevation	170	170
	external rotation	0	50

MANIPULATION:
The involved shoulder was stable. The opposite shoulder was stable.

ARM POSITION:
The arm was secured with an apparatus, a splint, sponge tape, ace wrap, and velcro straps and was suspended mechanically over 2 pulleys placing the upper extremity at 60 degrees abduction and 0 degrees flexion. The suspension apparatus utilized 16 lbs for balanced suspension.

OPERATIVE ARTHROSCOPIC procedure(s) performed:

GLENOHUMERAL JOINT DEBRIDEMENT limited	29822
ROTATOR CUFF DEBRIDEMENT	29823
BURSECTOMY (extensive debridement)	29823
CORACOACROMIAL LIGAMENT RESECTION	23415
SUPERIOR ROTATOR CUFF	29823
ACROMIOPLASTY	23130
ACROMIOCLAVICULAR JOINT	23106
osteophytes	23106
BICEPS TENDON	29823
ROTATOR CUFF RECONSTRUCTION	23420

OPEN SURGERY procedure(s) performed:

ROTATOR CUFF REPAIR	23420

DIAGNOSTIC ICD-9-CM CODES

JOINT FLUID	
yellow	719.0
SYNOVIAL REACTION	
degenerative	715.21
pigmented villonodular	719.2
BICEPS TENDON	
partial	727.62
GLENOID LABRUM	
torn	726.21
LABRUM TEAR CHARACTERISTICS	
old	726.21
ROTATOR CUFF APPEARANCE	
torn-complete	727.611
SUBACROMIAL SPACE	
synovitis	726.192
acromial erosion	726.191

PREPARATION
A satisfactory general and endotracheal anesthetic was administered, the patient was placed in the left lateral decubitus position on a regular table, and was secured by an Olympic Vac Pac. A Betadine skin preparation was performed by painting and a J & J shoulder drape was used to expose the shoulder.

Saline-adrenaline solution (1 mg/1000 cc) was used initially as a distension medium for visualization. Ringer's lactate was used subsequently and continuously as a distension medium for motorized instrumentation.

The joint fluid was abnormal in amount, color, and consistency. A minimal amount of yellow fluid was identified.

The inflow pressure was by gravity.

The arthroscope portal initially was posterior and entry was routine. Inflow was via a cannula system from the anterior portal. Diagnostic arthroscopy was performed by television and documented with a video monitor and video recording.

Arthroscopically, no loose bodies were found. The synovial reaction was abnormal. There were moderate; diffuse; red; and villous and vascular degenerative changes and inflammatory reaction in the synovium.

There was no fibrosis in the joint.

The biceps tendon was abnormal and partially frayed in the longitudinal plane in the area spanning the joint. The humeral head surface was normal.

The synovial reflection was normal. The position of the humeral head was abnormal and subluxated on the anterior and inferior sides.

The glenoid articular surface demonstrated a central cartilage thinning lesion.

The bony glenoid margins were normal.

The glenoid anterior central sulcus was normal. The anterior, posterior, superior, and inferior glenoid labrum was anatomically well defined. The glenoid labrum was abnormal. It was torn and shredded at the anterior and superior position. The labrum tear showed evidence of an old tissue disruption at the anterior and superior position. The labrum motion was normal to probing.

The glenohumeral ligaments were normal.

The subscapularis bursae were normal. The subscapularis tendon was normal.

The inferior glenohumeral space was normal. The posterior glenohumeral space was normal. The rotator cuff was abnormal and showed encroachment on the joint and/or a complete transverse tear in the distal portion. It was pre-existing and yellow and white in color with frayed edges in the tendon substance, in the capsule, and in the synovial lining.

Communication to the subacromial space was possible by visualization and flow from the glenohumeral joint. The character cuff defect was movable with probing or grasping and provided for approximation to the humerus. The subacromial space was abnormal. The subacromial space was entered via the rotator cuff tear and with redirection of the scope. The subacromial space was well developed and pathological. It showed synovitis and acromial erosion.

The acromioclavicular joint was abnormal. The acromioclavicular joint was identified by needle location and surgical exposure from the subacromial space. The pathological observations showed osteophytes and meniscal disruption.

OPERATIVE ARTHROSCOPY
Arthroscopic surgery was performed.

Surgical portals were established at anterior aspects of the glenohumeral joint and subacromial space. The portals established during the diagnostic phase were utilized, as well as the aforementioned ones. Arthroscopic surgical procedures were performed using television with a video monitor and video recording.

GLENOHUMERAL JOINT
A limited debridement was performed on the anterior and superior portions of the labrum of the glenohumeral joint.

The distal area and under surface of the rotator cuff were debrided with the extent of the resection being expansion of the lesion and exposing vascularity, healthy tendon, and subacromial space.

SUBACROMIAL SPACE
Exposure of the subacromial space was via redirection posteriorly. Inflow to the subacromial space was via the anterior portal. The debridement procedures performed included the subacromial bursa, the coracoacromial ligament, the superior rotator cuff, an acromioplasty, the acromioclavicular joint, and the acromioclavicular joint osteophytes.

The coracoacromial ligament was released at the acromion.

The superior portion of the rotator cuff was debrided distally with the extent of the resection being expansion of the lesion and exposing vascularity, healthy tendon, and the humeral head.

The acromioplasty consisted of a partial thickness resection of the anterolateral acromion including the ligament, bone, and osteophytes. The resection was performed in an oblique fashion.

ACROMIOCLAVICULAR JOINT
Acromioclavicular joint resection included inferior osteophyte removal, meniscectomy, resection on the clavicular end, and resection on the acromial side.

A resection and debridement were performed on the biceps tendon.

Rotator cuff reconstruction suitability was determined by mobility, tissue integrity, tissue viability, and tendon length. Site preparation was by bony and soft tissue removal which used intracortical bony exposure.

Motorized instrumentation was used for debridement of the labrum, degeneration, and tendons.

OPEN SURGERY
Open surgery was performed. The patient position was unchanged from the arthroscopic suspension.

Letter Input Form - 2
Doctor's Form 200

8. PHYSICAL EXAMINATION
1. Positive impingement signs. No strength loss after local anesthetic injection

9. LABORATORY TESTS
1. ______

10. X-RAYS
1. Acromialspur

11. LIGAMENT TESTS
1. ______

12. OPERATIVE REPORTS
1. ______

13. VIDEO TAPES
1. ______

14. OTHER:
1. ______

15. NO APPARENT EXPLANATION
1. for your ______ symptoms

16. TREATMENT RENDERED DURING OFFICE VISIT:
1. ______

17. INVESTIGATIONAL RECOMMENDATIONS:
1. Blood Test(s): ______
2. X-Ray: ______
3. Arthrogram: to rule out complete rotator cuff tear
4. Myelogram: ______
5. Tomogram: ______
6. Bone Scan: ______
7. CAT Scan: ______
8. Magnetic Resonance: ______
9. Ultrasound: ______
10. Neurological Tests: ______
11. Vascular Tests: ______
12. (other) ______

Letter Input Form - 3
Doctor's Form 200

18. REFERRAL/CONSULTATION APPOINTMENT: 1. referral 2. consultation

>M 1. diagnostic tests: ______________________________
2. definitive treatment: ______________________________
3. coordinated care: ______________________________
4. bracing: ______________________________
5. physical therapy: ______________________________

1. name: ______________________________
2. address: ______________________________
3. address: ______________________________
4. city-state: ______________________________
5. phone: ______________________________

1. on ___-___-______
2. at _____ o'clock
3. AM/PM
4. You should arrange for your own appointment
5. You should contact ______________________________
6. to arrange an appointment with ______________________________

REFERRAL/CONSULTATION APPOINTMENT: (continued) 1. referral 2. consultation

>M 1. diagnostic tests: ______________________________
2. definitive treatment: ______________________________
3. coordinated care: ______________________________
4. bracing: ______________________________
5. physical therapy: ______________________________

1. name: ______________________________
2. address: ______________________________
3. address: ______________________________
4. city-state: ______________________________
5. phone: ______________________________

1. on ___-___-______
2. at _____ o'clock
3. AM/PM
4. You should arrange for your own appointment
5. You should contact ______________________________
6. to arrange an appointment with ______________________________

19. RECOMMENDATION:

>M **1. Medication:** ______________________________

1. ________ days	1. after tests
2. ________ weeks	2. after surgery
3. ________ months	3. as necessary

Letter Input Form - 4
Doctor's Form 200

20. RECOMMENDATION:
>M **1. Bracing:** ____________________

1. ________ days	1. after tests
2. ________ weeks	2. after surgery
3. ________ months	3. as necessary

21. RECOMMENDATION:
>M **1. Physical therapy:** ____________________

1. ________ days	1. after tests
2. ________ weeks	2. after surgery
3. ________ months	3. as necessary

22. RECOMMENDATION:
1. Weight loss: ____________________
2. Stop smoking: ____________________
3. Caffeine restrictions: ____________________

23. RECOMMENDATION:
>M **1. Other:** ____________________

1. ________ days	1. after tests
2. ________ weeks	2. after surgery
3. ________ months	3. as necessary

24. ACTIVITY WITHIN LIMITATIONS OF:
1. pain
2. discomfort
3. motion
4. strength
5. balance
6. general health
7. (other) ____________________

25. MODIFICATION OF PHYSICAL ACTIVITY:

>M **Starting:**	**For:**
1. now	1. _______ days
2. on ___-___-______	2. _______ weeks
3. after surgery	3. _______ months
	4. until surgery
	5. ____________________

1. temporarily eliminating: ____________________
2. permanently eliminating: ____________________

26. REPEAT OFFICE EVALUATION:

>M 1. ____ days	1. after tests
2. ____ weeks	2. after surgery
3. ____ months	3. as necessary

4. ____________________

Letter Input Form - 5
Doctor's Form 200

27. SURGICAL INDICATIONS:
>M 1. include 2. are not present 3. could develop

1. presence/persistence of:

1. pain
2. swelling
3. locking
4. giving out
5. instability
6. stiffness
7. scar tissue
8. contracture
9. fracture
10. dislocation
11. malalignment
12. numbness
13. weakness
14. ____________________

1. deformity
2. tumor
3. infection
4. implant
5. loosening
6. migration
7. __________

Loss of:
1. motion
2. strength
3. sleep
4. daily activities
5. work
6. sports activities
7. ____________________

Lack of improvement after:
1. medication
2. conservative treatment
3. previous surgery
4. ____________________

28. SURGICAL INDICATIONS FROM:
1. Laboratory tests indicating ____________________
2. X-Rays showing acromial spur
3. Special test of ____________________
4. showing ____________________
5. (other) ____________________

29. SURGERY:
>M 1. was scheduled
2. will be scheduled
3. is medically indicated
4. is a future consideration
5. is not medically indicated
6. please call our office if you wish to schedule surgery

On your:
1. right
2. left

1. knee
2. shoulder
3. (other) _______
4. (other) _______

30. SURGERY SCHEDULED:

1. on ___-___-______

2. at _____ o'clock

3. AM/PM

1. Please see enclosed instructions
2. Call our office for confirmation
3. Follow instructions given by our office

Letter Input Form - 6
Doctor's Form 200

31. OPERATIVE TREATMENT TO INCLUDE: DIAGNOSTIC ARTHROSCOPY	**CPT CODE - MODIFIER**
>__________	#_____ ____
OPERATIVE ARTHROSCOPY	
>__________	#_____ ____
>__________	#_____ ____
> acromioplasty	#_____ ____
>__________	#_____ ____
>__________	#_____ ____
OPEN SURGERY (by second incision)	
>__________	#_____ ____
>__________	#_____ ____
>__________	#_____ ____
>__________	#_____ ____
>__________	#_____ ____

32. SURGICAL FEE:

1. I [am not/am] a participating Medicare physician
2. Estimation of surgical fee: $ 1500
3. Medicare will probably reimburse you: $________
4. We will accept insurance as payment [./in full/plus the deductible]
5. (circled) Fee may exceed the amount you are reimbursed
6. Fee probably not a benefit covered by your insurance company
7. (circled) Check with your insurance company
8. Check with your government agency
9. (circled) Fee includes 3 months of follow-up office visits
10. Other ____________________

33. UTILIZED:	1. now/following surgery		
>M 1. (simple dressing)	2. (for)/up to	3. 2	4. (days)/weeks/months
1. cast	2. for/up to	3. ___	4. days/weeks/months
1. brace	2. for/up to	3. ___	4. days/weeks/months
1. splint	2. for/up to	3. ___	4. days/weeks/months
1. crutches	2. for/up to	3. ___	4. days/weeks/months
1. walker	2. for/up to	3. ___	4. days/weeks/months
1. (sling)	2. (for)/up to	3. 1	4. days/(weeks)/months
1. immobilizer	2. for/up to	3. ___	4. days/weeks/months
1. physical therapy	2. for/up to	3. ___	4. days/weeks/months
1. medication	2. for/up to	3. ___	4. days/weeks/months
1. (other) ________	2. for/up to	3. ___	4. days/weeks/months

Letter Input Form - 7
Doctor's Form 200

34. ANTICIPATED HOSPITALIZATION STATUS:
1. outpatient 2. possibly will be inpatient 3. inpatient

1. Name of medical facility: Central Hospital

Starting:
1. the day before/after surgery

For:
1. ____ days
2. ____ weeks
3. ____ months

REASON:
1. Medical condition of ____
2. Magnitude of surgical procedure
3. Post surgical pain control
4. Intensive physical therapy
5. Continuous passive motion
6. IV antibiotics
7. Residence ____ miles away
8. (other) ____

35. PRE-OPERATIVE INFORMATION:
1. Cell saver use
2. Consider donating ________ units of your own blood
3. Additional instructions: ____

36. COMPLICATIONS:
1. **Those of anesthesia including potential:**
   2. stoppage of heart
   3. stoppage of breathing
   4. adverse drug reaction to anesthesia
   5. high temperature during or after anesthesia that could threaten life

37. COMPLICATIONS:
1. **Those related to surgery including potential:**
   2. injury to nerves
   3. disruption of a nerve repair
   4. injury to blood vessels
   5. disruption of a vessel repair
   6. bleeding
   7. blood clots in extremity
   8. blood clots in lung
   9. infection
   10. bone infection
   11. fat embolus
   12. swelling
   13. stiffness
   14. loss of motion
   15. fracture
   16. degenerative arthritis
   17. dislocation
   18. subluxation
   19. tourniquet injury
   20. numbness
   21. impaired muscle function

1. A blood transfusion is unlikely/possible/probable/certain

Letter Input Form - 8
Doctor's Form 200

38. COMPLICATIONS (surgical) CONT'D:

1. implant problems:
2. breakage
3. loosening
4. migration
5. deterioration
6. removal
7. malfunction
8. loosening of artificial joint
9. continued loosening of joint
10. instrument breakage
11. painful or unsightly scar
12. impaired function
13. cosmetic or functional deformity
14. growth deformity
15. reinjury to repaired tissue
16. failure of procedure
17. loss of a digit or limb
18. incomplete relief of pain
19. incomplete return of motion
20. incomplete return of strength
21. incomplete healing
22. additional surgery

39. OTHER COMPLICATIONS:

1. ____

____

____

40. TREATMENT DEFERRAL:

>M 1. possible/(probable)

1. gradual improvement in condition or symptom
2. continuance of same condition or symptoms
(3.) progression of condition or symptoms
4. future complications
5. more extensive surgery
6. (other possibilities/probabilities) ______________________

41. ANTICIPATED TIME NEEDED FOR CONVALESCENCE AND REHABILITATION:

1. ____ days
2. ____ weeks
3. _3_ months

Letter Input Form - 9
Doctor's Form 200

42. WORK RECOMMENDATIONS:
>M 1. off work
2. print separate "off work" sheet

Return to:
3. work
4. (regular duty)
5. light work
6. left-handed work
7. right-handed work
8. gym or physical education
9. with restrictions: ____________________
10. print separate "return to work" sheet

Starting:
1. now
2. on ___-___-______
(3.) day of surgery

For (estimated):
1. ____ days
2. _3_ weeks
3. ____ months

1. comments: ____________________

43. DISABILITY:
>M 1. (temporary)
2. permanent

1. partial
2. (total)

For:
1. sedentary work
2. (heavy labor)
3. (other) ____________________

1. comments: ____________________

44. PROJECTED TIME FOR RETURN TO:
>M 1. school
2. (recreation)
3. competitive sports
4. other ____________________

In:
1. ____ days
2. ____ weeks
3. _6_ months

45. PROGNOSIS:
>M 1. In general,
2. (without surgery)
3. after surgery
4. even with surgery
5. possible/probable permanent impairment of function or activities

1. excellent
2. good
3. (fair)
4. poor
5. medical condition not stationary

1. The reason for the above prognosis ____________________
____

Letter Input Form - 11
Doctor's Form 200

50. INSURANCE COMPANY:

(1.) requires a second opinion — (1.) make your own arrangements
2. call insurance company for a referral
3. call our office for a referral

51. APPROVAL OF ANTICIPATED SURGERY:

>M 1. telephone — 1. as outpatient
2. written — 2. with ______ days hospitalization

1. Spoke with: ____________________
2. Obtained by: ____________________

52. OFFICE INFORMATION:

1. Letter was signed in doctor's absence
2. Input by: ____________________

53. FORMS FOR PATIENT AUTHORIZATION (signature):

1. Informed consent
2. Sending all information to others
3. Direct payment from insurance company to doctor
4. Patient agreement to pay balance of bill
5. Retrieval of previous medical records to this office
6. Photographic consent-clinical records
7. Photographic consent-publication
8. All of the above

The 1. signed 2. dated release form(s) were received on ___-___-______

54. P.S. TO PATIENT:

1. ____________________
____
____

55. P.S. TO REFERRING DOCTOR:

1. ____________________
____
____

Doctor's Signature: ____________________ **Date:** ___-___-______

Information Health Network
P.O. Box 23056
Lansing, Michigan 48909-3056
(800)443-0613 (517)351-1588

January 10, 1988

Martin Sample
1234 Hideway St.
St. Clair, MI 44886

Dear Martin Sample:
Thank you for the opportunity to participate in your health care. This letter should serve to clarify my opinion and recommendations.

My clinical impression was:

	DIAGNOSTIC ICD-9-CM CODES
Impingement syndrome; rt. shoulder	726.2

This clinical impression was based upon information reviewed on January 10, 1988 and an examination on January 10, 1988. This impression was also based upon the following information:

Present medical history: Persistent pain worse at night and at extremes of motion. It is unrelieved by physical therapy and medicine.

Family history: non-contributory.

Review of systems: normal.

Allergies: none.

Bleeding tendencies: none.

Physical examination: There are positive impingement signs. There was no loss of strength after local anesthetic injection.

X-Rays: An acromial spur is present.

I suggest that the following tests be obtained:
Arthrogram: to rule out complete rotator cuff tear.

Surgery is medically indicated and is a future consideration for the right shoulder. Indications for surgery include the persistence of pain as well as the loss of motion, daily activities, and work. Surgery is indicated on the basis of X-rays showing acromial spur. You should call our office if you desire to have surgery scheduled.

The operative treatment is to include the following:
Operative arthroscopy:

	CPT CODE
acromioplasty	23130

You will be admitted as an outpatient at Central Hospital.

Typically, after this surgery, a simple dressing will be applied for 2 days and you will use a sling for one week. The amount of time needed for convalescence and rehabilitation is approximately 3 months. It is anticipated that you will return to regular work starting the day of surgery and continuing for approximately 3 weeks. You will need to take a temporary total disability leave from heavy labor. You may return to recreational activities in approximately 6 months.

The estimated surgical fee is $1500.00. The estimate is based on current fees for the anticipated procedure. The actual fee would change only if a significantly different procedure is required. This fee includes 3 months of follow-up office visits. This fee may exceed the amount you are reimbursed by your insurance company. You may wish to check the reimburse-

January 10, 1988

RE: Martin Sample
Patient number: 1200

Tom Jones, M.D.
4456 Mt. Hope
St. Clair, MI 44886

Dear Dr. Jones:

This report regarding your patient, Martin Sample, is for your information and may be used for your records.

My clinical impression was:

	DIAGNOSTIC ICD-9-CM CODES
Impingement syndrome; rt. shoulder	726.2

This clinical impression was based upon information reviewed on January 10, 1988 and an examination on January 10, 1988. This impression was also based upon the following information:

Present medical history: Persistant pain worse at night and at extremes of motion. It is unrelieved by physical therapy and medicine.

Family history: non-contributory

Review of systems: normal.

Allergies: none.

Bleeding tendencies: none.

Physical examination: There are positive impingement signs. There was no loss of strength after local anesthetic injection.

X-rays: An acromial spur is present.

I suggest that the following tests be obtained:
Arthrogram: to rule out complete rotator cuff tear.

Surgery is medically indicated and is a future consideration for the right shoulder. Indications for surgery include the persistence of pain as well as the loss of motion, daily activities, and work. Surgery is indicated on the basis of X-Rays showing acromial spur. You should call our office if you desire to have surgery scheduled.

The operative treatment is to include the following:
Operative arthroscopy:

	CPT CODE
acromioplasty	23130

He will be admitted as an outpatient at Central Hospital.

It is probable that a deferral in the recommended treatment will result in a progression of the patient's condition or symptoms.

The amount of time needed for convalescence and rehabilitation is approximately 3 months. The patient's prognosis without surgery should be fair.

I have requested that the following materials be sent for the patient's information:
Patient Medical Information Report
Physical Exam Report
X-Ray Report

Thank you for the opportunity to care for your patient.

Sincerely,

Lanny L. Johnson, MD

January 25, 1987

RE: Martin Sample
Patient number: 1200
Date of operation: 01-10-1987

Frank Williams M.D.
1278 Mt Hope Rd.
Lansing, Mi 48910

Dear Dr. Williams:

This report is for your information and may be used for your records.

CLINICAL EVALUATION:

Martin Sample was examined on December 23, 1987. The patient's major complaint is pain, loss of motion, loss of strength, loss of work, as well as loss of activities. His current orthopedic problem involves an injury to his right shoulder.

During range of motion testing the body was in a sitting position. Bilateral and simultaneous arm measurements were taken with a goniometer.

During active internal rotation the patient could reach to the trochanter.

The patient showed tenderness during palpation of the anterior coracoacromial ligament. No masses were identified.

There was popping during internal rotation abduction motion which suggested rotator cuff tear-impingement. The forward flexion impingement test was positive, painful, and relieved by local anesthetic. The abduction/internal rotation impingement test was positive, painful, relieved by local anesthetic, and crepitus producing. The abduction/external rotation impingement test was positive, painful, and relieved by local anesthetic. The adduction/external rotation impingement test was negative.

Manipulation, active voluntary movement, and stability with arm at side were normal.

Circulation on the affected side appeared to be normal. The radial circulation was present.

Neurological sensation in the affected shoulder was normal.

The status of the patient's neck was normal.

The patient cooperated well.

X-RAY

The X-ray impression was: A-C joint degeneration, Normal Glenohumeral joint, Beak acromion.

CLINICAL IMPRESSION:

The clinical impression was: Rotator cuff tear and Impingement syndrome.

SURGERY:

Arthroscopic surgery was performed on January 10, 1987 under a satisfactory general and endotracheal anesthetic administered by Eugene High, M.D..

PRE-OPERATIVE DIAGNOSIS: rotator cuff tear impingement syndrome

POST-OPERATIVE DIAGNOSIS: (in addition to the preoperative diagnosis) Labrum tear

A DIAGNOSTIC ARTHROSCOPIC procedure was performed.

OPERATIVE ARTHROSCOPY

The following procedures were performed in the glenohumeral joint:

glenohumeral joint limited debridement
rotator cuff debridement (undersurface)

The following procedures were performed in the subacromial space:

debridement
rotator cuff debridement (superior surface)
acromioplasty
CA ligament:
  release
biceps tendon:
  resection
rotator cuff reconstruction

AC joint resection included superior osteophyte removal, meniscectomy, resection on the clavicular end, and resection on the acromial side.

OPEN SURGERY

The following open reconstruction procedures were performed.

Rotator cuff repair

RECOMMENDATIONS:

The patient was placed in an abduction splint for 3 weeks and he is to perform no exercises until the next office visit.

It was recommended that the patient call our office for a return appointment in one week and remain off work for 3 months.

Prognosis: The prognosis is good. The reason for the prognosis is that there was good anatomical repair of cuff.

Thank you for the opportunity to care for your patient.

Sincerely,

Edward M. Lowe, M.D.

RE: Martin Sample
ID: A110121505

MEDICAL HISTORY (draft)

This 51-year-old caucasian male was evaluated on January 10, 1988.

He gave the following medical history.

The patient states that he is 71 inches tall, weighs 200 pounds, and is right handed.

The patient's job as welder is of a physical nature.

He desires a vigorous activity level.

The patient states that he currently has problems with his right shoulder.

PRESENT COMPLAINT

In response to specific questions regarding the patient's complaints and problems, the patient stated the following:

CHIEF COMPLAINT—RIGHT SHOULDER
The patient's major complaint is aching and soreness.

PRESENT HISTORY—RIGHT SHOULDER
The patient did not know the nature of the problem. The patient maintains that the problem originally started gradually in June 1987.

He complained of pain and located the exact spot in the front of and on the top of the shoulder. The patient rated the magnitude of his pain as causing complete disability (0). This pain occurs constantly; typically occurring all day long. The pain is made worse when he performs any shoulder motion. Nothing relieves the pain.

The patient stated that the shoulder appears swollen and is swollen constantly.

The patient states that he is unable to rotate the affected shoulder. He says that he is not able to lift his hand.

The patient rated his ability to perform specific functions referable to the shoulder as listed below (4 = normal 3 = mild compromise 2 = difficulty 1 = with aid 0 = unable x = information not available):

FUNCTION/ACTIVITY	RIGHT LEFT	FUNCTION/ACTIVITY	RIGHT LEFT
use back pocket	2	dress	2
rectal hygiene	2	sleep on shoulder	0
wash opposite underarm	2	pulling	2
eat with utensil	2	use hand overhead	0
comb hair	0	throwing	0
use hand, arm at shoulder level	2	lifting	1
		do usual work	2
carry 10-15 lbs. arm at side	2	do usual sport	0
reach between shoulder blades	2		

The patient maintains that he is unable to do weight lifting. He maintains that he is restricted in his ability to feed himself, dress himself, comb his hair, work at his job, do yard work, sleep, or participate in enjoyable recreational activities. The patient is not able to participate in sports activities now.

Joint stiffness is experienced at all times. The patient feels no grating, grinding, or popping noises or sensations in the joint. The joint never locks or gets stuck.

The patient's shoulder never goes out.

The patient experiences numbness sometimes in the arm. The patient sleeps on the side of his affected shoulder.

The patient has had this joint treated or examined before.

DOCTOR'S NOTATIONS:

The patient had no injuries or conditions of the right shoulder before the present problem.

He was treated non-surgically at an emergency room by Dr. Kohen in St. Joseph in July 1987. The problem was diagnosed as soreness and swelling, the treatment consisted of ultrasound and hotpacks, and the results were Unsatisfactory.

He was treated non-surgically by a general physician, Tom Jones, M.D., in St. Clair in August 1987. The treatment consisted of physical therapy and Tylenol and the results were unsatisfactory.

Previous regular X-rays were taken of the right shoulder at St. Joseph in July 1987 which showed neg.

He has not had any special X-rays or tests performed.

PAST HISTORY
His last complete physical exam was performed by Dr. Johnson, of St. Joseph, in May 1987 and had the following results: Satisfactory. He was diagnosed as Good health. The patient stated that he has not visited any doctor in the past two years.

In the past six months, the patient states that he has undergone the following tests:
CBC (blood count) in May 1987; results were neg.
Blood tests in May 1987; results were neg.
Chest X-ray in May 1987; results were neg.

ORTHOPEDIC HISTORY
In response to specific questions regarding the patient's complaints and problems, the patient stated the following:

In addition to the problem mentioned above, the patient has experienced the following orthopedic problems:
torn ligaments
severe sprains
low back problem
tendonitis
torn tendon

ALLERGY
The patient maintains that he has no allergies or adverse reactions to medication and/or anesthesia.

MEDICATION
The patient states that he is not currently on any medication nor has he had any in the past six months. The patient is currently taking the following medications:
Tylenol 3; 1 tablet 3 times per day

HOSPITALIZATION FOR MEDICAL TREATMENT
NONE

SURGERY
The patient has not had previous arthroscopic surgery unrelated to his present problem. He has not had open orthopedic surgery unrelated to his present problem. The patient has not undergone any non-orthopedic surgery. The patient has not undergone non-orthopedic surgery unrelated to his present problem.

TRAUMA
He has never fractured any bones or dislocated any joints.

The patient states that he has not received any blood transfusions.

REVIEW OF SYSTEMS

The patient stated that he had no problems with his head, neck, skin, eyes, ears or hearing, nose or throat, respiratory system, cardiovascular system, gastrointestinal system, urogenital system, or neurologic system and he has no emotional problems, bleeding disorders, metabolic problems, or genetic disorders.

FAMILY HISTORY

Father:			
Ted	deceased	83	Cancer
Mother:			
Margaret	deceased	74	heart attack
Child:			
Joseph	living	20	Good

FAMILY MEDICAL HISTORY
The patient states that his family has no history of serious allergies, adverse reaction to anesthesia or surgery, or hyperthermia during surgery.

LIFE STYLE
NO RESPONSES

The patient rated his overall level of physical health as very good compared to others in his age group.

DOCTOR'S NOTATIONS:

PATIENT'S CERTIFICATION OF AUTHENTICITY:
I hereby certify that the above information is true and correct within the best of my ability.

Signed: ______________________________ Date: __-__-______

East Lansing Orthopedic Association

SAMPLE POSTCARD: SHOULDER

Patient name ______________________ # __________ Year ________ Shoulder ________

TREATMENT METHOD ☐ SATISFACTORY ☐ UNSATISFACTORY

TREATMENT OUTCOME ☐ SATISFACTORY ☐ UNSATISFACTORY

PAIN? ☐ NO ☐ YES ☐ WITH ACTIVITY ☐ AT REST ☐ AT NIGHT

PAIN INTENSITY? ☐ SLIGHT ☐ MODERATE ☐ SEVERE

PAIN RELIEF? ☐ NONE ☐ LITTLE ☐ SOME ☐ A LOT ☐ COMPLETE

MEDICATION? ☐ NO ☐ YES TYPE? ______________________

LOSS OF MOTION? ☐ NO ☐ YES HOW? ______________________

UNDER DOCTOR'S CARE? ☐ NO ☐ YES WHO? ______________________

ARE YOU: ☐ RIGHT HANDED ☐ LEFT HANDED ☐ TRULY AMBIDEXTROUS

Has shoulder problem recurred? ☐ NO ☐ YES

WHEN WAS 1ST TIME? ______________________

WHAT CAUSED IT? ______________________

HOW MANY TIMES IN ALL? ______________________

Have you had any surgeries on this joint after the year listed above?

☐ ARTHROSCOPIC SURGERY? ☐ OPEN SURGERY?

HOW MANY? __________ HOW MANY? __________

YEAR(S) __________ YEAR(S) __________

WHERE? __________ WHERE? __________

Your Current Address

____
Street

____
City State

____
Zip

____
Phone

4.3
2/17/90

Research Follow-up History: Shoulder

Patient's Form 505

FOR OFFICE USE: (we will fill in)
Patient number: ____________
Problem number: ____
Date: ____-____-______

NAME: ____

DOCTOR'S NOTES

1. THIS FORM APPLIES TO WHICH SHOULDER?
1. right
2. left

FOLLOWING SHOULDER SURGERY:

2. HOW LONG WAS YOUR SHOULDER IMMOBILIZED? 1. NONE
1. in sling for ______ weeks 2. ____ days
1. in brace for ______ weeks 2. ____ days

3. HOW LONG BEFORE YOU:
1. returned to work ______ weeks
2. returned to sports ______ weeks
3. returned to unrestricted activities ______ weeks

4. DID YOU USE FORMAL POST-OPERATIVE PHYSICAL THERAPY?
1. YES
2. no

5. ANY COMPLICATIONS: (ask the office staff for any explanations)
1. NONE
2. yes (see below)

1. infection
2. thrombophlebitis
3. pulmonary embolism
4. hemorrhage-bleeding
5. bleeding in joint
6. effusion
7. fistula
8. atelectasis
9. pneumonia
10. urinary retention
11. ileus
12. extremity neurovascular problem
13. ligament injury
14. redislocation

6. PATIENT HAS PRESENT COMPLAINT: 1. YES 2. no

7. GENERAL DESCRIPTION OF SURGICAL RESULT:
1. improved 2. same 3. worse 4. N/A

IF YOU HAVE A PRESENT COMPLAINT, CONTINUE WITH QUESTION 8.
IF YOU HAVE NO PRESENT COMPLAINT, SKIP TO QUESTION 48.

Research Follow-up History: Shoulder - 2
Patient's Form 505

8. MAJOR POST-OPERATIVE COMPLAINT: (please circle just ONE)

1. deformity
2. pain
3. aching - sore
4. numbness
5. stiffness
6. loss of motion
7. weakness
8. loss of strength
9. swelling
10. going out
11. locking
12. grinding
13. popping
14. makes noise
15. loss of work
16. loss of activities
17. (other) ______________________________

9. NATURE OF PROBLEM:

1. injury
2. fracture
3. dislocation
4. arthritis
5. infection
6. growth
7. developmental
8. tumor
9. (other) ______________________________
10. do not know

10. ORIGINAL ONSET OF THE POST-OPERATIVE PROBLEM (not just this episode):

1. Date of Onset: ___-___-______

Nature of Problem:

1. gradual
2. sudden
3. injury while ______________
4. injury at work
5. injury in vehicle accident
6. reinjury of previous problem
7. (other) ______________________________
8. do not know

11. RECENT EPISODE OF THE POST- OPERATIVE PROBLEM (if different from the original onset):

1. Date of Onset: ___-___-______

Nature of Problem:

1. gradual
2. sudden
3. injury while ______________
4. injury at work
5. injury in vehicle accident
6. reinjury of previous problem
7. (other) ______________________________
8. do not know

12. HAVE YOU HAD THIS SHOULDER TREATED OR EXAMINED BEFORE?

1. NO - skip to question 22
2. YES- continue with next question

13. WERE THERE ANY INJURIES OR CONDITIONS OF THIS BODY PART THAT EXISTED BEFORE THIS PRESENT PROBLEM OCCURRED? 1. NO 2. yes (if yes, circle and/or add brief statement)

1. cut (laceration) ______________________________
2. crush ______________________________
3. ligament injury ______________________________
4. fracture ______________________________
5. dislocation ______________________________
6. growth (tumor) ______________________________
7. deformity ______________________________
8. other ______________________________

Research Follow-up History: Shoulder - 3
Patient's Form 505

14. WERE YOU TREATED NON-SURGICALLY AT AN EMERGENCY ROOM FOR THIS PROBLEM?
>M 1. NO 2. yes

1. diagnosis (problem): ____________
2. treatment: ____________
3. doctor: ____________
4. hospital/city: ____________
5. results: ____________
6. date: ___-___-______

1. diagnosis (problem): ____________
2. treatment: ____________
3. doctor: ____________
4. hospital/city: ____________
5. results: ____________
6. date: ___-___-______

15. WERE YOU TREATED NON-SURGICALLY BY A REGULAR PHYSICIAN FOR THIS PROBLEM?
>M 1. NO 2. yes

1. diagnosis (problem): ____________
2. treatment: ____________
3. doctor: ____________
4. hospital/city: ____________
5. results: ____________
6. date: ___-___-______ to ___-___-______

1. diagnosis (problem): ____________
2. treatment: ____________
3. doctor: ____________
4. hospital/city: ____________
5. results: ____________
6. date: ___-___-______ to ___-___-______

16. WERE YOU EVER TREATED WITHOUT SURGERY (CONSERVATIVELY) BY A SPECIALIST FOR THIS PROBLEM? 1. NO 2. yes

>M 1. diagnosis (problem): ____________
2. treatment: ____________
3. doctor: ____________
4. hospital/city: ____________
5. results: ____________
6. date: ___-___-______ to ___-___-______

1. diagnosis (problem): ____________
2. treatment: ____________
3. doctor: ____________
4. hospital/city: ____________
5. results: ____________
6. date: ___-___-______ to ___-___-______

Research Follow-up History: Shoulder - 4
Patient's Form 505

17. WERE YOU EVER TREATED BY A PHYSICAL THERAPIST FOR THIS PROBLEM? 1. NO 2. yes

>M 1. diagnosis (problem): ____________________
2. treatment: ____________________
3. physical therapist: ____________________
4. hospital/city: ____________________
5. results: ____________________
6. date: ___-___-______ to ___-___-______

1. diagnosis (problem): ____________________
2. treatment: ____________________
3. physical therapist: ____________________
4. hospital/city: ____________________
5. results: ____________________
6. date: ___-___-______ to ___-___-______

18. DID YOU HAVE ARTHROSCOPIC SURGERY PERFORMED FOR THIS PROBLEM? 1. NO 2. yes

>M 1. diagnosis (problem): ____________________
2. type of surgery: ____________________
3. doctor: ____________________
4. hospital/city: ____________________
5. results: ____________________
6. date: ___-___-______

1. diagnosis (problem): ____________________
2. type of surgery: ____________________
3. doctor: ____________________
4. hospital/city: ____________________
5. results: ____________________
6. date: ___-___-______

1. diagnosis (problem): ____________________
2. type of surgery: ____________________
3. doctor: ____________________
4. hospital/city: ____________________
5. results: ____________________
6. date: ___-___-______

Research Follow-up History: Shoulder - 5
Patient's Form 505

19. DID YOU HAVE OPEN ORTHOPEDIC SURGERY PERFORMED FOR THIS PROBLEM?
>M 1. NO 2. yes

1. diagnosis (problem): ______
2. type of surgery: ______
3. doctor: ______
4. hospital/city: ______
5. results: ______
6. date: ___-___-______

1. diagnosis (problem): ______
2. type of surgery: ______
3. doctor: ______
4. hospital/city: ______
5. results: ______
6. date: ___-___-______

1. diagnosis (problem): ______
2. type of surgery: ______
3. doctor: ______
4. hospital/city: ______
5. results: ______
6. date: ___-___-______

20. DID YOU HAVE OPEN SURGERY PERFORMED FOR THIS PROBLEM BY A SURGEON OTHER THAN AN ORTHOPEDIST (i.e. PLASTIC SURGEON, VASCULAR SURGEON, ETC...)?
>M 1. NO 2. yes

1. diagnosis (problem): ______
2. type of surgery: ______
3. doctor: ______
4. hospital/city: ______
5. results: ______
6. date: ___-___-______

1. diagnosis (problem): ______
2. type of surgery: ______
3. doctor: ______
4. hospital/city: ______
5. results: ______
6. date: ___-___-______

Research Follow-up History: Shoulder - 6
Patient's Form 505

21. WERE YOU EVER HOSPITALIZED FOR THIS PROBLEM (OTHER THAN SURGERY)?
>M 1. NO 2. yes

1. diagnosis (problem): ______________________
2. treatment: ______________________
3. doctor: ______________________
4. hospital/city: ______________________
5. results: ______________________
6. date: ___-___-______ to ___-___-______

1. diagnosis (problem): ______________________
2. treatment: ______________________
3. doctor: ______________________
4. hospital/city: ______________________
5. results: ______________________
6. date: ___-___-______ to ___-___-______

22. DID YOU HAVE REGULAR X-RAYS TAKEN FOR THIS PROBLEM? 1. NO 2. yes
>M 1. where: ______________________
2. body part: ______________________
3. results: ______________________
4. date: ___-___-______

1. where: ______________________
2. body part: ______________________
3. results: ______________________
4. date: ___-___-______

23. DID YOU HAVE SPECIAL X-RAYS OR TESTS FOR THIS PROBLEM? 1. NO 2. yes

>M	**Date**	**Body Part**	**Where**
1. Arthrogram	2. ___-___-______	3. __________	4. __________
1. Tomogram	2. ___-___-______	3. __________	4. __________
1. Bone Scan	2. ___-___-______	3. __________	4. __________
1. CAT Scan	2. ___-___-______	3. __________	4. __________
1. Magnetic Resonance	2. ___-___-______	3. __________	4. __________
1. Ultrasound	2. ___-___-______	3. __________	4. __________
1. Fluoroscopy	2. ___-___-______	3. __________	4. __________
1. Stress X-Rays	2. ___-___-______	3. __________	4. __________
1. __________	2. ___-___-______	3. __________	4. __________

24. PLEASE RATE THE MAGNITUDE OF YOUR PAIN:
1. complete disability
2. marked
3. moderate
4. after unusual activity
5. slight
6. ______________________

Research Follow-up History: Shoulder - 7
Patient's Form 505

25. LOCATION OF SHOULDER PAIN:
1. I cannot locate exact spot

I can locate exact spot at
2. front
3. back
4. arm pit
5. top side
6. deep inside
7. entire arm to hand
8. chest
9. neck
10. ______________________

26. FREQUENCY OF SHOULDER PAIN:
1. initially, but not now
2. occasionally
3. constantly
4. only recently
5. with activity
6. even when resting
7. ______________________

27. TIME OF DAY WHEN SHOULDER PAIN OCCURS:
1. morning
2. all day
3. end of the day
4. interrupts my sleep
5. ______________________

28. PAIN MADE WORSE WHEN:
1. resting
2. any shoulder motion
3. lifting only my arm
4. lifting any weight with arm
5. grasping with hand
6. throwing
7. physical therapy
8. doing my regular work as ____
9. ______________________

29. PAIN RELIEVED BY:
1. nothing
2. rest
3. activity
4. medicine--if so, what kind? ____
5. physical therapy
6. repositioning the shoulder
7. ______________________

Research Follow-up History: Shoulder - 10
Patient's Form 505

39. OCCURRENCE OF JOINT STIFFNESS:
1. none
2. always
3. after activity
4. in the morning
5. end of the day
6. ____________________

40. GRATING, GRINDING, OR POPPING NOISES OR SENSATIONS IN THE JOINT:
1. none
2. feel with my hand
3. any motion
4. lifting
5. throwing
6. only when pushing or pulling
7. ____________________

41. LOCKING (GETTING STUCK) OF THE JOINT:
1. never
2. at first, but not now
3. just started
4. occasionally
5. frequently
6. constantly
7. ____________________

42. HAS SHOULDER GONE OUT OF JOINT SINCE SURGERY?
1. NO - skip to question 47
2. yes - continue with next question

43. TOTAL NUMBER OF TIMES (ESTIMATE): _____

44. WHERE SHOULDER GOES OUT:
1. front
2. back
3. arm pit
4. don't know
5. ____________________

45. SHOULDER WENT OUT OF JOINT SINCE SURGERY:
1. first time on ___-___-_____
2. how ____________________
3. treatment ____________________

1. last time on ___-___-_____
2. how ____________________
3. treatment ____________________

46. HOW DOES SHOULDER GO OUT:
1. with major injury or stress
2. with simple movements of daily living
3. unexpectedly
4. I can do it myself at will
5. ____________________

47. NUMBNESS:

1. never
2. at first, not now
3. all the time
4. ____________________

Location:

1. shoulder
2. arm
3. hand
4. ____________________

48. SLEEPING POSITION:

1. on back
2. on stomach
3. on side of unaffected shoulder
4. on side of affected shoulder
5. affected arm up, shoulder between head and mattress
6. affected arm at side
7. ____________________

49. DOCTOR'S NOTATIONS: (validity of previous history, review of previous medical record, other...)
>M ____
____
____
____
____

Thank You

Please return this form to the receptionist

4.3
2/17/90

Research Follow-up Exam: Shoulder

Doctor's Form 506

Patient Name: ______________________ **Patient Number:** ________
Problem Number: ___
Date: ___-___-___

1. PHYSICIAN INFORMATION:
1. Name of evaluating physician ______________________
2. Physician number ______________________

2. # OF YEARS: _____

3. HEIGHT: 1. _______ cm/inches

4. WEIGHT: 1. _______ lbs./kgs.

5. BLOOD PRESSURE: 1. ____/_____

6. TEMPERATURE: 1. _______ degrees Fahrenheit/Celsius

7. PULSE: 1. _______ beats per minute

8. RESPIRATION: 1. _______ per minute

9. PROBLEMATIC SHOULDER:
1. RIGHT
2. LEFT
3. BOTH 1. R > L 2. R < L 3. R = L

10. POSTURE: 1. NORMAL 2. right/left
>M 1. winged scapula
2. protracted scapula
3. retracted scapula
4. hunched
5. droops
6. adducted
7. abducted
8. in sling
9. bandaged
10. held by other hand
11. other ______________________

11. USAGE: 1. NORMAL 2. right/left
>M 1. avoids 1. moving
2. difficulty 2. lifting
3. unable 3. reaching
4. unwilling 4. pushing
5. pulling
6. (other) ______________________

12. INSPECTION OF JOINTS: 1. right/left
>M SC Joint 1. NORMAL 2. prominent 3. ______________
AC Joint 1. NORMAL 2. prominent 3. ______________
Glenohumeral 1. NORMAL 2. prominent 3. ______________

Research Follow-up Exam: Shoulder - 2
Doctor's Form 506

13. INSPECTION OF BONES: 1. right/left

>M Clavicle	1. NORMAL	2. deformity	3. ______
Scapula	1. NORMAL	2. deformity	3. ______
Humerus	1. NORMAL	2. deformity	3. ______

14. SKIN: 1. right/left

>M Appearance:	1. NORMAL	2. Abnormal	how: ______
Color:	1. NORMAL	2. Abnormal	how: ______
Temperature:	1. NORMAL	2. Abnormal	how: ______
Texture:	1. NORMAL	2. Abnormal	how: ______
Atrophy:	1. ABSENT	2. Present	site: ______

15. SKIN SCARS: 1. NONE 2. right/left

>M 1. arthroscopic	1. single	1. healing	1. tender
2. open	2. multiple	2. healed	2. swollen
3. surgical		3. open	3. reddened
4. stretch marks		4. draining	4. widened
5. ______			

16. SITE OF INCISION/SCAR: 1. right/left

>M 1. anterior	1. vertical	1. length ______ cm
2. posterior	2. horizontal	2. width ______ cm
3. superior	3. transverse	
4. inferior	4. saber type	1. length ______ cm
5. medial	5. curvilinear	2. width ______ cm
6. lateral	6. oblique	
7. axillary	7. ______	

1. Comment: ______

17. PALPATION TENDERNESS: 1. NONE 2. right/left

>M **Position:**	**Bone:**
1. anterior	1. Sternum ______
2. posterior	2. Clavicle ______
3. superior	3. Humerus ______
4. inferior	4. greater tuberosity ______
5. medial	5. lesser tuberosity ______
6. lateral	6. Scapula ______
7. axillary	7. acromion ______
8. diffuse	8. coracoid process ______
9. proximal	9. spine of scapula ______
10. middle	10. Vertebra spine ______
11. distal	11. Rib # ______
12. ______	12. Paraspinal area ______
	13. ______

Bursa:	**Joint:**	**Ligament:**
1. subdeltoid ______	1. SC ______	1. CA ______
2. subacromial ______	2. AC ______	2. CC ______
3. scapulothoracic ______	3. GH ______	
4. subcoracoid ______	4. ______	
5. ______		

18. PALPATION TENDERNESS-MUSCLE: 1. right/left

>M 1. anterior
2. posterior
3. superior
4. inferior
5. medial
6. lateral
7. axillary
8. ______________

1. SCM
2. Trapezius
3. Levator scapulae
4. Rhomboids
5. Serratus anterior
6. Supraspinatus
7. Infraspinatus
8. Teres minor
9. Subscapularis
10. Pectoralis major
11. Pectoralis minor

12. Latissimus dorsi
13. Teres major
14. Deltoid
15. Biceps
16. long head
17. short head
18. Triceps
19. long head
20. lateral head
21. medial head
22. ______________

Tenderness Located:
1. ______________________
2. ______________________
3. ______________________
4. ______________________
5. ______________________

19. MASS LOCATION: 1. NONE IDENTIFIED 2. right/left

>M 1. subcutaneous tissue ______________________
BONE:
2. vertebra ______________________
3. ribs ______________________
4. scapula ______________________
5. clavicle ______________________
6. humerus ______________________
7. JOINT: ______________________
8. MUSCLE: ______________________
9. TENDON: ______________________
10. (other) ______________________

20. MASS SIZE: 1. right/left

>M _____ cm x _____ cm x _____ cm

21. MASS CHARACTERISTICS: 1. right/left

>M 1. non-tender
2. tender
3. ______________

1. hard
2. firm
3. soft
4. ballottable
5. ______________

1. fixed
2. moveable
3. __________

1. solid
2. translucent
3. __________

22. CIRCUMFERENTIAL MEASUREMENT: 1. N/T

RIGHT
1. arm ______ cm
2. elbow ______ cm
3. forearm ______ cm
4. wrist ______ cm
5. hand ______ cm

LEFT
1. arm ______ cm
2. elbow ______ cm
3. forearm ______ cm
4. wrist ______ cm
5. hand ______ cm

Research Follow-up Exam: Shoulder - 4
Doctor's Form 506

23. DYNAMOMETER GRIP TEST: 1. N/T

>M 1. Jamar/Preston
2. serial number ______________
3. kg/lbs
4. 1 / 2 / 3 / 4 / 5
5. sequential (1-5)

	Right:	Left:
1.	____________	____________
2.	____________	____________
3.	____________	____________
4.	____________	____________
5.	____________	____________

24. RANGE OF MOTION: 1. NORMAL 2. Abnormal 3. N/T

>M **Body Position:**	**Reference Point:**	**Arm(s) Involved:**	**Measurements:**
1. sitting	1. spine	1. one	1. estimated
2. standing	2. coronal plane	2. both	2. measured
3. supine	3. sagittal plane	3. simultaneous	
4. prone	4. plumb line		

25. RANGE OF MOTION: 1. SITTING/STANDING

>M **Arm Starting Position:**	**(plus)**	**Motion Measured:**	**ACTIVE RT**	**ACTIVE LF**	**PASSIVE RT**	**PASSIVE LF**	**LOCAL ANS RT**	**LOCAL ANS LF**
side		elevation	___	___	___	___	___	___
side		forward flexion	___	___	___	___	___	___
side		abduction	___	___	___	___	___	___
side		external rotation	___	___	___	___	___	___
side		internal rotation	___	___	___	___	___	___
90 abd	(____________)	external rotation	___	___	___	___	___	___
90 abd	(____________)	internal rotation	___	___	___	___	___	___
90 abd	(____________)	adduction	___	___	___	___	___	___
90 abd	(____________)	extension	___	___	___	___	___	___
side		backward extension	___	___	___	___	___	___

26. RANGE OF MOTION (SUPINE):

Arm Starting Position:	**(plus)**	**Motion Measured:**	**ACTIVE RT**	**ACTIVE LF**	**PASSIVE RT**	**PASSIVE LF**	**LOCAL ANS RT**	**LOCAL ANS LF**
side		elevation	___	___	___	___	___	___
side		forward flexion	___	___	___	___	___	___
side		abduction	___	___	___	___	___	___
side		external rotation	___	___	___	___	___	___
side		internal rotation	___	___	___	___	___	___
90 abd	(____________)	external rotation	___	___	___	___	___	___
90 abd	(____________)	internal rotation	___	___	___	___	___	___
90 abd	(____________)	adduction	___	___	___	___	___	___
90 abd	(____________)	extension	___	___	___	___	___	___
side		backward extension	___	___	___	___	___	___

27. RANGE OF MOTION (PRONE):

Arm Starting Position:	**(plus)**	**Motion Measured:**	**ACTIVE RT**	**ACTIVE LF**	**PASSIVE RT**	**PASSIVE LF**	**LOCAL ANS RT**	**LOCAL ANS LF**
90 abd	(____________)	extension	___	___	___	___	___	___
side		backward extension	___	___	___	___	___	___

28. INTERNAL ROTATION:

Patient could reach to:	**ACTIVE RT**	**ACTIVE LF**	**PASSIVE RT**	**PASSIVE LF**	**LOCAL ANS RT**	**LOCAL ANS LF**
less than trochanter	O	O	O	O	O	O
trochanter	O	O	O	O	O	O
gluteal	O	O	O	O	O	O
sacrum	O	O	O	O	O	O
vertebral level:	___	___	___	___	___	___

Research Follow-up Exam: Shoulder - 5
Doctor's Form 506

29. QUALITY OF MOTION: 1. NORMAL 2. N/T 3. right/left
>M

	NORMAL	**slow**	**painful**	**painless**	**comment**
total elevation	O	O	O	O	______
forward flexion	O	O	O	O	______
abduction	O	O	O	O	______
external rotation at side	O	O	O	O	______
internal rotation at side	O	O	O	O	______
90 deg abduct-ext rotation	O	O	O	O	______
90 deg abduct-int rotation	O	O	O	O	______
90 deg abduction-adduction	O	O	O	O	______
90 deg abduction-extension	O	O	O	O	______
backward extension	O	O	O	O	______
hand behind back	O	O	O	O	______
adduction	O	O	O	O	______
waving	O	O	O	O	______
circumduction	O	O	O	O	______
pendulum exercise	O	O	O	O	______

30. SHOULDER MOTION STRENGTH TESTS: 1. NORMAL 2. Abnormal 3. N/T
(Absent = 0, Trace = 1, Poor = 2, Fair = 3, Good = 4, Normal = 5)

	RIGHT	LEFT	COMMENTS
abduction-thumb down	____	____	______
abduction-thumb up	____	____	______
external rotation	____	____	______
internal rotation	____	____	______

31. MUSCULATURE TESTS: 1. NORMAL 2. Abnormal 3. N/T
(Absent = 0, Trace = 1, Poor = 2, Fair = 3, Good = 4, Normal = 5)

	RIGHT	LEFT	COMMENTS
sternocleidomastoid (C-2-3)	____	____	______
trapezius (C-3-4)	____	____	______
levator scapulae (C-3-4-5)	____	____	______
rhomboids (C-5)	____	____	______
serratus anterior (C-5-6-7)	____	____	______
supraspinatus (C-5-6)	____	____	______
infraspinatus (C-5-6)	____	____	______
teres minor (C-5-6)	____	____	______
subscapularis (C-5-6)	____	____	______
pectoralis (C-5-T-1)	____	____	______
other ________	____	____	______

32. MUSCULATURE TESTS: (Absent = 0, Trace = 1, Poor = 2, Fair = 3, Good = 4, Normal = 5)

	RIGHT	LEFT	COMMENTS
latissimus dorsi (C-6-7-8)	____	____	______
teres major (C-5-6)	____	____	______
deltoid (C-5-6)	____	____	______
anterior	____	____	______
middle	____	____	______
posterior	____	____	______
biceps (C-5-6)	____	____	______
triceps (C-7-8)	____	____	______
brachioradialis (C-5-6)	____	____	______
supinator (C-6)	____	____	______
other ________	____	____	______

Research Follow-up Exam: Shoulder - 6
Doctor's Form 506

33. AUSCULTATION: 1. SILENT 2. N/T 3. right/left
>M 1. crepitus 1. with ______________________ motion
2. popping 2. suggesting ______________________
3. other ______________

34. IMPINGEMENT TESTS: 1. NORMAL 2. Abnormal 3. N/T 4. right/left
>M

	N/T	neg.	pos.	painful	neg. with local anes.	produced crepitus	produced popping	not valid due to limited motion	comment
forward flexion:	O	O	O	O	O	O	O	O	________
resisted supination (Yergason's):	O	O	O	O	O	O	O	O	________
abduction/external rotation:	O	O	O	O	O	O	O	O	________
abduction/internal rotation:	O	O	O	O	O	O	O	O	________
adduction/external rotation:	O	O	O	O	O	O	O	O	________
adduction/internal rotation:	O	O	O	O	O	O	O	O	________
palm up:	O	O	O	O	O	O	O	O	________
palm down:	O	O	O	O	O	O	O	O	________

35. MANIPULATION: 1. NORMAL 2. N/T 3. right/left
>M

	STABLE	SUBLUX	DISLOC	APPREHN	PAIN
abd, ext rotation	1. Y/N	2. Y/N	3. Y/N	4. Y/N	5. Y/N
abd, downward force	1. Y/N	2. Y/N	3. Y/N	4. Y/N	5. Y/N
add flexion	1. Y/N	2. Y/N	3. Y/N	4. Y/N	5. Y/N
add flexion, post force	1. Y/N	2. Y/N	3. Y/N	4. Y/N	5. Y/N
fixed scapula, ant force	1. Y/N	2. Y/N	3. Y/N	4. Y/N	5. Y/N
fixed scapula, post force	1. Y/N	2. Y/N	3. Y/N	4. Y/N	5. Y/N

1. abd, ext rotation ______________________
2. abd, downward force ______________________
3. add flexion ______________________
4. add flexion, post force ______________________
5. fixed scapula, ant force ______________________
6. fixed scapula, post force ______________________

36. STABILITY WITH ARM AT SIDE: 1. NORMAL 2. N/T 3. right/left

>M **MANIPULATION DOWNWARD TRACTION**
1. stable ______________
2. subluxation ______________
3. dislocation ______________
4. apprehension ______________

VOLUNTARY DOWNWARD FORCE
1. stable ______________
2. subluxation ______________
3. dislocation ______________
4. apprehension ______________

Research Follow-up Exam: Shoulder - 7
Doctor's Form 506

37. VOLUNTARY-ACTIVE INSTABILITY: 1. NORMAL 2. N/T 3. right/left

>M **ABDUCTION, EXTERNAL ROTATION**
1. stable ________
2. subluxation ________
3. dislocation ________
4. apprehension ________

ABDUCTION, DOWNWARD FORCE
1. stable ________
2. subluxation ________
3. dislocation ________
4. apprehension ________

ADDUCTION FLEXION
1. stable ________
2. subluxation ________
3. dislocation ________
4. apprehension ________

ADDUCTION FLEXION, POSTERIOR FORCE
1. stable ________
2. subluxation ________
3. dislocation ________
4. apprehension ________

FIXED SCAPULA, ANTERIOR FORCE
1. stable ________
2. subluxation ________
3. dislocation ________
4. apprehension ________

FIXED SCAPULA, POSTERIOR FORCE
1. stable ________
2. subluxation ________
3. dislocation ________
4. apprehension ________

38. STABILITY SUMMARY: 1.right/left

>M fixed dislocation	1. anterior	2. posterior	3. inferior	4.superior
fixed subluxation	1. anterior	2. posterior	3. inferior	4.superior
recurrent dislocation	1. anterior	2. posterior	3. inferior	4.superior
recurrent subluxation	1. anterior	2. posterior	3. inferior	4.superior
rare subluxation	1. anterior	2. posterior	3. inferior	4.superior
apprehension	1. anterior	2. posterior	3. inferior	4.superior
normal	1. anterior	2. posterior	3. inferior	4.superior

39. CIRCULATION: 1. NORMAL 2. N/T 3. right/left

>M **CAROTID**
1. present
2. diminished
3. absent
4. bruit

SUBCLAVIAN
1. present
2. diminished
3. absent
4. bruit

AXILLARY BRACHIAL
1. present
2. diminished
3. absent
4. bruit

ANTECUBITAL BRACHIAL
1. present
2. diminished
3. absent
4. bruit

RADIAL
1. present
2. diminished
3. absent
4. bruit
5. diminished with arm elevation

ULNAR
1. present
2. diminished
3. absent
4. bruit

RAYNAUD'S
1. present

RSD
1. present

SUDECK'S
1. present

EDEMA
1. present

1. Comments: ________________________________

Research Follow-up Exam: Shoulder - 8
Doctor's Form 506

40. THORACIC OUTLET: 1. right/left

>M **WRIGHT'S HYPERABDUCTION MANEUVER**
1. normal pulse
2. diminished
3. absent
4. at _____ degrees elevation
5. other ______________________________

COSTOCLAVICULAR MANEUVER
1. normal pulse
2. diminished
3. absent
4. at _____ degrees elevation
5. other ______________________

ADSON'S MANEUVER
1. normal pulse
2. diminished
3. absent
4. at _____ degrees elevation
5. other ____

41. NEUROLOGIC: 1. right/left

>M **Sensation:** 1. NORMAL 2. Abnormal 3.N/T
1. ________________________ 1. dermatome
2. ________________________ 2. sensory nerve distribution

1. Comments: ____

Proprioception: 1. NORMAL 2. Abnormal 3. N/T

Hoffmann test: 1. NEGATIVE 2. Positive 3. N/T

Babinski test: 1. NEGATIVE 2. Positive 3. N/T

1. Comments: ____

DTR's: 1. EQUAL AND ACTIVE 2. Abnormal 3. N/T

1. diminished	1. biceps
2. absent	2. triceps
3. increased	3. wrist
	4. ____________________

1. Comments: ____

42. STATUS OF ELBOW: 1. N/T 2. right/left

>M 1. asymptomatic 1. normal exam
2. symptomatic 2. abnormal exam

1. Comments: ____

1. Diagnosis: ____

Range of Motion: 1. FULL 2. Limited 3. N/T

43. ELBOW RANGE OF MOTION:

RIGHT		LEFT	
1. Flexion	______ deg	1. Flexion	______ deg
2. Extension	______ deg	2. Extension	______ deg
3. Pronation	______ deg	3. Pronation	______ deg
4. Supination	______ deg	4. Supination	______ deg

44. STATUS OF SPINE: 1. cervical/thoracic 2. N/T
>M 1. asymptomatic 1. normal exam
2. symptomatic 2. abnormal exam

1. Comments: ______________________________

1. Diagnosis: ______________________________

Range of Motion:		1. FULL	2. Limited	3. N/T
Flexion		1. Normal	2. Abnormal	3. ______
Extension		1. Normal	2. Abnormal	3. ______
Lateral rotation	1. R/L	2. Normal	3. Abnormal	4. ______
Lateral bending	1. R/L	2. Normal	3. Abnormal	4. ______

45. AMPUTATION LEVEL: 1. NONE 2. right/left
>M 1. forequarter **Level:**
2. shoulder 1. above elbow
3. arm 2. at elbow
4. elbow 3. below elbow
5. forearm 4. wrist
6. wrist 5. midcarpal
7. finger-thumb ______________________________

46. PATIENT COOPERATION:
1. GOOD
2. failed to relax
3. failed to cooperate
4. exam was not performed because ______________________________
5. exam of ______________ considered unreliable because ______________

47. DOCTOR'S NOTATIONS: (Each observation will be printed as a paragraph)
>M ______________________________

48. CLINICAL IMPRESSION OF PROBLEMATIC SHOULDER: 1. right/left
>M 1. ______________________________
2. ______________________________
3. ______________________________

49. OPPOSITE SHOULDER CONDITION:
1. asymptomatic 1. normal exam
2. symptomatic 2. abnormal exam

1. Comments: ______________________________

1. Diagnosis: ______________________________

Research Follow-up Exam: Shoulder - 10
Doctor's Form 506

50. ADDITIONAL COMMENTS: (i.e. plan, tests, therapy, surgery)
>M (Each observation will be printed as a paragraph)

____
____
____
____
____
____

Doctor's Signature: ______________________ **Date:** ___-___-_____

4.3
2/17/90

Follow-up X-Ray Evaluation: Shoulder

Doctor's Form 508

Patient Name: ______________________________ **Patient Number:** __________
Problem Number: ___
Date: ___-___-___

1. NAME OF EVALUATING PHYSICIAN: ______________________________

2. PHYSICIAN NUMBER: __________

3. PROBLEMATIC SHOULDER:
1. RIGHT
2. LEFT

4. PLAIN FILM PROJECTIONS:

>M	**DATE**		**ELSEWHERE**
1. AP Neutral	2. ___-___-______ ___-___-______	3. here here	4. ______________ ______________
1. AP Int Rotation	2. ___-___-______ ___-___-______	3. here here	4. ______________ ______________
1. AP Ext Rotation	2. ___-___-______ ___-___-______	3. here here	4. ______________ ______________
1. Axillary-rest-	2. ___-___-______ ___-___-______	3. here here	4. ______________ ______________
1. Active stress	2. ___-___-______ ___-___-______	3. here here	4. ______________ ______________
1. Passive stress	2. ___-___-______ ___-___-______	3. here here	4. ______________ ______________
1. Arch view	2.___-___-______ ___-___-______	3. here here	4. ______________ ______________
1. Abduction	2. ___-___-______ ___-___-______	3. here here	4. ______________ ______________
1. Weighted	2. ___-___-______ ___-___-______	3. here here	4. ______________ ______________
1. Lateral: X-chest	2. ___-___-______ ___-___-______	3. here here	4. ______________ ______________
1. West Point view	2. ___-___-______ ___-___-______	3. here here	4. ______________ ______________
1. Stryker view	2. ___-___-______ ___-___-______	3. here here	4. ______________ ______________
1. __________	2. ___-___-______ ___-___-______	3. here here	4. ______________ ______________

SUMMARY

5. X-RAY INTERPRETATION:

>M 1. ____
____

Follow-up X-Ray Evaluation: Shoulder - 2
Doctor's Form 508

6. X-RAY DESCRIPTION:

>M 1. degenerative changes
2. osteophytes
3. joint space narrowing
4. loose bodies
5. calcification
6. demineralization
7. erosion
8. osteolytic lesion
9. osteoblastic lesion
10. osteonecrosis
11. osteochondritis
12. subluxation
13. dislocation
14. cuff tear arthropathy
15. Hill-Sach lesion

1. NO ABNORMALITIES
1. anterior
2. posterior
3. superior
4. inferior
5. medial
6. lateral
7. proximal
8. distal

1. clavicle
2. scapula
3. body
4. spine
5. acromion
6. coracoid
7. glenoid
8. humeral
9. head
10. neck
11. greater tuberosity
12. lesser tuberosity
13. shaft

1. sternoclavicular
2. acromioclavicular
3. glenohumeral

1. bursae
2. subacromial
3. subscapularis
4. tendon
5. rotator cuff
6. biceps

7. SC JOINT:
1. arthritis
2. separation
3. intra-articular fracture

8. AC JOINT:
1. arthritis
2. separation
3. grade I
4. grade II
5. grade III
6. grade IV
7. grade V

9. GH JOINT:
1. arthritis
2. glenohumeral dislocation
3. glenohumeral subluxation
4. inferior subluxation with ____ weight
6. Hill-Sach lesion

7. Glenoid rim:
8. fracture
9. bone reaction
10. Glenoid wear:
11. anterior
12. posterior
13. loose body(ies)
14. number ______
15. anterior
16. posterior
17. superior
18. inferior

10. IMPINGEMENT X-RAY FINDINGS:
1. anterior acromial spur
2. anterior acromial sclerosis
3. bone reaction greater tuberosity
4. inferior AC joint spurs
5. superior displacement humeral head

humeral head/acromion interval: ______ mm
unfused acromial epiphysis: pre _____ meso ____ meta ____ basi _____

Acromial morphology:
1. Type I (flat)
2. Type II (curved)
3. Type III (hooked)

Follow-up X-Ray Evaluation: Shoulder - 3
Doctor's Form 508

11. CERVICAL SPINE X-RAY:
1. ____________________

12. FOREIGN BODY OR IMPLANT: 1. NONE

>M	1. sternum 2. clavicle 3. scapula 4. humerus	**Joint:** 1. SC 2. AC 3. GH
	Device: 1. prosthesis 2. screw 3. staple 4. nail 5. wire	**Position:** 1. secure 2. loose 3. migrated 4. (other) ____________

6. total shoulder: ____________
7. (other) ____________

13. DISLOCATION:

>M	1. NONE 2. recent 3. old	1. reduced 2. unreduced	
	Sternoclavicular: 1. anterior 2. posterior 3. superior 4. inferior	**Acromioclavicular:** 1. anterior 2. posterior 3. superior 4. inferior	**Glenohumeral:** 1. anterior 2. posterior 3. superior 4. inferior

14. FRACTURE:

>M	1. NONE 2. recent 3. old	1. open 2. closed	1. transverse 2. oblique 3. spiral 4. butterfly
	1. sternum 2. clavicle 3. scapula 4. glenoid neck 5. glenoid rim 6. spine 7. body	1. humerus 2. greater tuberosity 3. lesser tuberosity 4. neck 5. shaft	1. undisplaced 2. displaced
	1. angulated 2. rotated	1. simple 2. comminuted 3. avulsion	1. united 2. delayed union 3. malunion 4. pseudoarthrosis 5. post-reduction

Follow-up X-Ray Evaluation: Shoulder - 4
Doctor's Form 508

15. FRACTURE POSITION:

1. acceptable
2. displaced
3. angulated
4. articular offset
5. ______________________________

16. SPECIAL TESTS:

Arthrogram 1. date ___-___-______ 2. where: ____________________
3. NORMAL Y/N 4. by report 5. by review
6. how: ______________________________

Tomogram 1. date ___-___-______ 2. where: ____________________
3. NORMAL Y/N 4. by report 5. by review
6. how: ______________________________

Bone Scan 1. date ___-___-______ 2. where: ____________________
3. NORMAL Y/N 4. by report 5. by review
6. how: ______________________________

CAT Scan 1. date ___-___-______ 2. where: ____________________
3. NORMAL Y/N 4. by report 5. by review
6. how: ______________________________

17. SPECIAL TESTS (continued):

Magnetic Resonance 1. date ___-___-______ 2. where: ____________________
3. NORMAL Y/N 4. by report 5. by review
6. how: ______________________________

Ultrasound 1. date ___-___-______ 2. where: ____________________
3. NORMAL Y/N 4. by report 5. by review
6. how: ______________________________

Fluoroscopy 1. date___-___-______ 2. where: ____________________
3. NORMAL Y/N 4. by report 5. by review
6. how: ______________________________

Stress X-Rays 1. date___-___-______ 2. where: ____________________
3. NORMAL Y/N 4. by report 5. by review
6. how: ______________________________

Doctor's Signature: ______________________________ **Date:** ___-___-______

4.3
4/15/91

Clinical Research: Primary Selection

PRIMARY SELECTION: This is the computer function of pulling selected charts and making initial inquiries from ONE (1) form.

NAME OF THE PRIMARY SELECTION:

1. **I CALL THIS STUDY:** ________________
   THE DESCRIPTION IS:

PULLING THE CHARTS:

2. **THE TIME PERIOD I DESIRE FOR THIS STUDY:**
   1. begins on ___-___-_____
   2. and ends on ___-___-_____

3. **I WANT TO LOOK AT FORM:** (enter the number) _________
   I understand I am limited to this form for the primary selection criteria to be listed in question #5.

4. **I WANT TO USE ONE OF THE FOLLOWING TO COMBINE THE CRITERIA IN QUESTION #5:**
   1. AND - requires that all criteria listed below must exist in the form
   2. OR - requires that at least one of the criteria listed below exists in the form

5. **MY PRIMARY SELECTION WILL CONSIST OF THE FOLLOWING CRITERIA:**

>M key (line 4 below) = (M)atching, (E)qual to, (L)ess than, (G)reater than

INCLUDING:

question #	group #	response #	key	fill in or optional text
1. ________	2. ________	3. ________	4. ___	5. ________________
1. ________	2. ________	3. ________	4. ___	5. ________________
1. ________	2. ________	3. ________	4. ___	5. ________________

EXCLUDING:

1. ________	2. ________	3. ________	4. ___	5. ________________
1. ________	2. ________	3. ________	4. ___	5. ________________
1. ________	2. ________	3. ________	4. ___	5. ________________

If you wish to extract additional information on these patients from the above form, continue with the next question. If you want the charts pulled now, continue with these steps:

STEPS TO PULL CHARTS: Press the ESC key. The next screen shows the Query Menu. Move to the "Fetch" option and press the ENTER key. This action will start the search of your entire data base for the charts you want pulled. After a period of time, the totals will appear on the screen with a prompt to press the ENTER key to see the results.

OPTIONAL INITIAL INQUIRY OF PRIMARY SELECTION CHARTS:

6. I WANT TO REVIEW THESE PATIENTS FROM THE FOLLOWING STANDPOINT:
>M I understand I cannot use this primary selection to make inquiries about different forms.

1. The form date. 2. The problem number.

question #	group #	response #
1. ______	2. ______	3. ______
1. ______	2. ______	3. ______
1. ______	2. ______	3. ______
1. ______	2. ______	3. ______
1. ______	2. ______	3. ______
1. ______	2. ______	3. ______

When completed with this question, take the steps to pull the charts as directed in question #5. The additional information you requested in this question will be produced for each chart pulled. The listing will indicate either negative (blank) or positive (an entry) responses.

Information Health Network
P.O. Box 23056
Lansing, Michigan 48909-3056
(800)443-0613 (517)351-1588

4.3
4/15/91

Clinical Research: Secondary Selection

SECONDARY SELECTION: This process is necessary to interrogate data from ONE (1) form. This selection process provides access to any previous primary or secondary case groups.

NAME OF THIS SECONDARY SELECTION:

1. **I CALL THIS STUDY:** ______________
   THE DESCRIPTION IS:

2. **THE NAME OF THE PREVIOUS SELECTION I WANT TO USE AS A BASE (FROM QUESTION #1 OF THE PREVIOUS PRIMARY OR SECONDARY SELECTION FORM) IS:** ____________

PULLING THE CHARTS:

3. **I WANT TO LOOK AT FORM:** (enter the number) _________
   I understand I am limited to this form for the secondary selection criteria to be listed in question #5.

4. **I WANT TO USE ONE OF THE FOLLOWING TO COMBINE THE CRITERIA IN QUESTION #5:**
   1. AND - requires that all criteria listed below must exist in the form
   2. OR - requires that at least one of the criteria listed below exists in the form

5. **THIS SECONDARY SELECTION WILL CONSIST OF THE FOLLOWING CRITERIA:**

>M key (line 4 below) = (M)atching, (E)qual to, (L)ess than, (G)reater than

INCLUDING:

question #	group #	response #	key	fill in or optional text
1. _________	2. _________	3. _________	4. ___	5. ____________________
1. _________	2. _________	3. _________	4. ___	5. ____________________
1. _________	2. _________	3. _________	4. ___	5. ____________________

EXCLUDING:

1. _________	2. _________	3. _________	4. ___	5. ____________________
1. _________	2. _________	3. _________	4. ___	5. ____________________
1. _________	2. _________	3. _________	4. ___	5. ____________________

If you wish to extract additional information on these patients from the above form, continue with the next question. If you want the charts pulled now, continue with these steps:

STEPS TO PULL CHARTS: Press the ESC key. The next screen shows the Query Menu. Move to the "Fetch" option and press the ENTER key. This action will start the search of the base you selected in question #2 for the charts you want pulled. After a period of time, the totals will appear on the screen with a prompt to press the ENTER key to see the results.

Clinical Research: Secondary Selection - 2

OPTIONAL INITIAL INQUIRY OF SECONDARY SELECTION CHARTS:

6. I WANT TO REVIEW THESE PATIENTS FROM THE FOLLOWING STANDPOINT:
>M I understand I cannot use this secondary selection to make inquiries about different forms.

1. The form date. 2. The problem number.

question #	group #	response #
1. __________	2. __________	3. __________
1. __________	2. __________	3. __________
1. __________	2. __________	3. __________
1. __________	2. __________	3. __________
1. __________	2. __________	3. __________
1. __________	2. __________	3. __________

When completed with this question, take the steps to pull the charts as directed in question #5. The additional information you requested in this question will be produced for each chart pulled. The listing will indicate either negative (blank) or positive (an entry) responses.

Information Health Network
P.O. Box 23056
Lansing, Michigan 48909-3056
(800)443-0613 (517)351-1588

4.3
4/15/91

Clinical Research: Study Profile

STUDY PROFILE: This option provides standard research data on specific prior case selections, either primary or secondary.

1. THE DESCRIPTION OF THIS PROFILE IS:

2. THE NAME OF THE PREVIOUS SELECTION I WANT A PROFILE OF (FROM QUESTION #1 OF THE PREVIOUS PRIMARY OR SECONDARY SELECTION FORM) IS: ______________

I WANT TO SEE THE FOLLOWING STANDARD DATA (check each one desired):
(question #16 provides options)

3. FROM THE UNIVERSAL FACE SHEET (100):

1. ID Number
2. First Name
3. Last Name
4. Title
5. Street Address
6. City
7. State
8. Zip Code
9. Country

1. Home Phone
2. Work Phone
3. Phone During the Day
4. Sex
5. Workers Compensation Case (yes or no)
6. Legal or Third Party Case (yes or no)
7. No-fault Insurance Case (yes or no)

4. FROM THE MEDICAL HISTORY FORM (300):

1. Age
2. Race or Genetic Heritage
3. Height
4. Weight
5. Dominant Hand
6. Problem Areas For Evaluation
7. Rating of Health

5. FROM THE KNEE HISTORY SUPPLEMENT FORM (401):

1. Date of Examination
2. Problematic Side
3. Date of Onset

6. FROM THE SHOULDER HISTORY SUPPLEMENT FORM (501):

1. Date of Examination
2. Problematic Side
3. Date of Onset

7. FROM THE GENERAL ORTHOPEDIC HISTORY SUPPLEMENT FORM (301):

1. Date of Examination
2. Main Problem Area For Evaluation
3. Date of Onset

8. **FROM THE ELBOW HISTORY SUPPLEMENT FORM (601):**
    1. Date of Examination
    2. Problematic Side
    3. Date of Onset

9. **FROM THE SPINE HISTORY SUPPLEMENT FORM (801):**
    1. Date of Examination
    2. Area of Spine (neck, thoracic, low back)
    3. Date of Onset

10. **FROM THE KNEE SURGERY FORM (404):**
    1. Date of Surgery
    2. Side Operated On
    3. Diagnostic Codes
    4. Procedures Performed

11. **FROM THE SHOULDER SURGERY FORM (504):**
    1. Date of Surgery
    2. Side Operated On
    3. Diagnostic Codes
    4. Procedures Performed

12. **FROM THE ELBOW SURGERY FORM (604):**
    1. Date of Surgery
    2. Side Operated On
    3. Diagnostic Codes
    4. Procedures Performed

13. **FROM THE ANKLE SURGERY FORM (1204):**
    1. Date of Surgery
    2. Side Operated On
    3. Diagnostic Codes
    4. Procedures Performed

14. **FROM THE MEDICOLEGAL FORM (1002):**
    1. Date of Examination
    2. Date of Most Recent Contact

15. **FROM THE PROGRESS NOTES FORM (901):**
    1. All Progress Notes

I WOULD ALSO LIKE TO SEE IN THIS PROFILE SOME ADDITIONAL SPECIFIC DATA.

16. THE SPECIFIC INQUIRIES TO ADD TO THIS STUDY PROFILE ARE:
>M (Multiple observations allow for more than one form number)

The Form I want to use is: (enter the number) __________

1. The form date and problem number.

question #	group #	response #
1. __________	2. __________	3. __________
1. __________	2. __________	3. __________
1. __________	2. __________	3. __________
1. __________	2. __________	3. __________
1. __________	2. __________	3. __________
1. __________	2. __________	3. __________
1. __________	2. __________	3. __________
1. __________	2. __________	3. __________
1. __________	2. __________	3. __________
1. __________	2. __________	3. __________

17. OUTPUT FORMAT: regular/WordPerfect

Information Health Network
P.O. Box 23056
Lansing, Michigan 48909-3056
(800)443-0613 (517)351-1588

APPENDIX

B American Shoulder and Elbow Surgeons Shoulder Assessment Form (Draft)

SHOULDER ASSESSMENT FORM (DRAFT) AMERICAN SHOULDER AND ELBOW SURGEONS				
Patient Name:			**Date:**	
PHYSICIAN ASSESSMENT				
RANGE OF MOTION	**RIGHT**		**LEFT**	
	Active	**Passive**	**Active**	**Passive**
Flexion (maximum forward elevation)				
Abduction				
External rotation (arm at side)				
External rotation (arm at 90°)				
Internal rotation (arm at side)				
Internal rotation (arm at 90°)				

STABILITY		
0 = none; 1 = mild; 2 = moderate; 3 = severe		
Direction	**Right**	**Left**
Anterior	0 1 2 3	0 1 2 3
Anterior apprehension	0 1 2 3	0 1 2 3
Posterior	0 1 2 3	0 1 2 3
Posterior apprehension	0 1 2 3	0 1 2 3
Inferior	0 1 2 3	0 1 2 3

OTHER SIGNS (record if present)		
SIGN	**Right**	**Left**
Impingement sign	0 1 2 3	0 1 2 3
Subacromial crepitus	0 1 2 3	0 1 2 3
Power (MRC) Grade)		
Flexion	1 2 3 4 5	1 2 3 4 5
External Rotation	1 2 3 4 5	1 2 3 4 5
Internal Rotation	1 2 3 4 5	1 2 3 4 5

PATIENT SELF-EVALUATION		
Do you have pain in your shoulder at night (circle response)?	Yes	No
Do you take pain medication?	Yes	No
Do you take narcotic pain medication (codeine or stronger)?	Yes	No
How many pills do you take each day (average)?	# pills	
How bad is your pain today (mark line)? [________________________________] No pain at all — Pain as bad as it can be		

Mark where your pain is on this diagram:

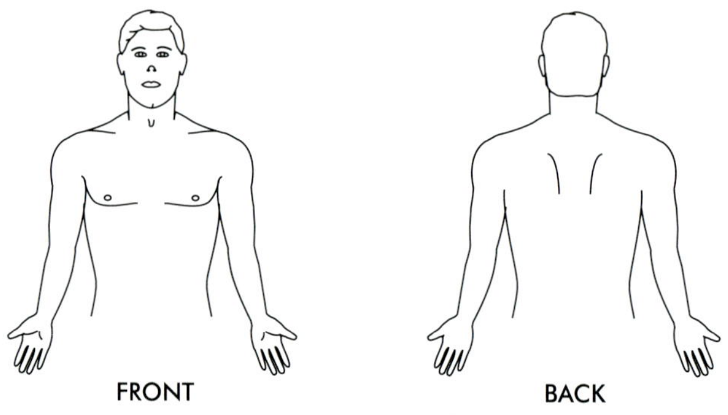

Circle the number in the box that indicates your ability to do the following activities: 0 = **Unable** to do; 1 = **Very** difficult; 2 = **Somewhat** difficult; 3 = **Not** difficult		
Activity	**Right Arm**	**Left Arm**
Lift heavy objects	0 1 2 3	0 1 2 3
Put on a coat	0 1 2 3	0 1 2 3
Manage toiletting	0 1 2 3	0 1 2 3
Sleep on your side	0 1 2 3	0 1 2 3
Wash back/do up bra	0 1 2 3	0 1 2 3
Comb hair	0 1 2 3	0 1 2 3
Reach a high shelf	0 1 2 3	0 1 2 3
Eat with utensil	0 1 2 3	0 1 2 3
Do usual work—List:	0 1 2 3	0 1 2 3
Do usual sport—List:	0 1 2 3	0 1 2 3

APPENDIX

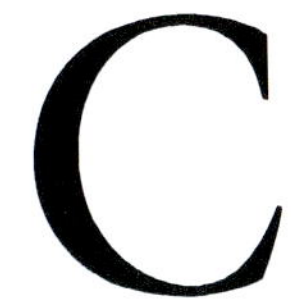

C Instruments for Shoulder Arthroscopy

Supplier Name	Instruments	Catalog No.
Abbott Laboratories P.O. Box 1140 North Chicago, IL 60064 Phone: 1-800-222-6883	Large-bore Y-Irrigation Set	6599-01
Baxter Hospital Supply 2320 McGaw Road Obetz, OH 43207 Phone: 1-800-456-0044	Gomoco rubber stopper #12 two hole Pharmaseal K-52 (sterile) Novex Three-way stopcock with 20 inch extension tube	65650-250 PK-52
Baxter Scientific Products 30500 Cypress Romulus, MI 48174 Phone: 1-800-876-3747	5-gallon glass jug	B7600-5
Bearse Manufacturing 3815 N. Courtland Chicago, IL 60647 Phone: 1-312-235-8710	4×6 Drawstring specimen bag	
Roudolph Beaver, Inc. 411 Waverly Oaks Rd. Waltham, MA 02154 Phone: 1-800-225-1482	Becton Dickinson Knife Handle	4320
Biomet Inc. State Rd. 15 South Box 587 Warsaw, IN 46581 Phone: 1-219-267-6639 1-800-348-9500	OEC shoulder foam abduction splint Small Medium Large	 667110 667115 667120
Blickman Health Industries P.O. Box 48820-21 201 Wagaraw Rd. Fair Lawn, NJ 07410 Phone: 1-800-247-5070	Four-Hook IV pole	7789-55-4

Supplier Name	Instruments	Catalog No.
Codman and Shrutleff Inc. Randolph, MA 02368 Phone: 1-800-255-0640	Cushing Dressing Forcceps (bayonet shape)	30-1155
	Crile Hemostatic Forceps (straight 6¼ inches)	34-4040
Davis & Geck American Cynamed Co. Cranbury, CT 06810 Phone: 1-800-225-5341	0 Tycron	3008-61
Deknatel 600 Airport Rd. Fall River, MA 02722-2980 Phone: 1-508-677-6600	Cottony-II Dacron 1 mm with HC5 taper needle	X 4323
Delacher Associates, Inc. 4054 Summit View N.E. Grand Rapids, MI 49505 Phone: 1-800-942-9852	Sling and Swath	
	Small	0205-03
	Medium	0205-04
	Large	0205-05
	X-Large	0205-06
DePuy P.O. Box 988 Warsaw, IN 46580 Phone: 1-219-267-8143	Ace Wrap 6 inches X 11 yards	3775-12
Instrument Makar 2950 East Mt. Hope P.O. Box 329 Okemos, MI 48864 Phone: 1-800-248-4668	Regular Blade Set	10001-S
	Retrograde Blade Set	10007
	3.2 Gold probe with 3 mm gradations	10014-G
	Heavy Duty Meniscal Grasper (4.2 mm)	10019
	Meniscal Grasper (3.2 mm)	10020
	IM Jaws	10027
	Bone Grafter	10080
	Golden Retriever	10100
	Switching Sticks	10150
	Wissinger Rod	10151
	Shoulder Suspension System	10209
	Cloud 9 Absorbant Mat	10227
	Gravity Assist	10235
	IM Disposable Face Shields	
	Full Face Shield	10500
	½ Face Shield	10505
	Disposable O.R. Boots	
	Small Size	10503-S
	Medium Size	10503-M
	Large Size	10503-L
	Complete LCR System	10750
	Original Staples	
	Small Staple	10751
	Medium Staple	10757
	Large Staple	10753
	Profile '90 Staples	

Supplier Name	Instrument	Catalog No.
Instrument Makar, *cont'd*	Medium Staple	10757-NP
	Large Staple	10753-NP
	Bio-Absorbable Staple™	12056
	Instrumentation set for Bio-Absorbable Staple™	12015
	IM Mini Cannulated Screw Set	60000
	Hand-Controlled Coagulators	
	90° Push/Pull Tip	10789
	90° Paddle Tip	10794
	Hook Tip	10798
	Foot Controlled Coagulators	
	90° Push/Pull tip	10788
	90° Paddle Tip	10791
	Hook Tip	10797
Olympic Medical Corp. 5900 1st. Ave. S. Seattle, WA 98108 Phone: 1-800-426-0353 1-206-624-0426	Surgical Positioning System Olympic Vac Pac	51630
PRN Services, Inc. 1551 E. Lincoln Ave. Madison Heights, MI 48701 Phone: 1-800-543-2776	Yamshidi Biopsy Needle 3½ inch 13-gauge	DJ3513
Smith & Nephew Dyonics, Inc. 1600 Dascomb Road Andover, MA 01810 Phone: 1-800-343-8386	Medi Mech Video Cart	3500
	13″ Sony Monitor (high resolution RGB monitor)	3594
	Auto Brite illuminator II	3180
	Metal Halide Arc Lamp	2974
	DyoCam 750 Camera Control Unit	4164
	DyoCam Video Camera System with dual C-mount camera head	3945
	PS 3500 Control Unit	3478
	PS 3500 foot switch	3498
	PS 3500 Motor Drive	3476
	Cannulas, trocar, obturator, inflow connector 4.5	3709
	Cannulas, trocar, obturator, inflow connector 5.5	3112
	Reusable Blades for PS 3500 Motor	
	3.5 Cutter	3457
	4.5 Cutter	3458
	5.5 Cutter	3459
	3.5 Full-Radius Synovial Resector	3461
	4.5 Full-Radius Synovial Resector	3462
	5.5 Full-Radius Synovial Resector	3463
	3.5 Full-Radius Whisker	3468
	5.5 Full-Radius Whisker	3469
	4.0 Abrader	3464
	5.5 Abrader	3465
	5.5 Gemini Universal Cable	2140
	Dyonics/Wolf Adapter	2147
	Storz/Olympus Adapter	2143
	Drilling System with Key 450 Drill with ¼-inch Chuck	2851

Supplier Name	Instrument	Catalog No.
Smith & Nephew Dyonics, Inc., *cont'd*	Drill Bit Set (1 each 9 sizes)	2873
	Sagittal Saw	2855
	Saw Blade	
	standard	3701
	short	3703
	800 Wire Driver	2856
	2 Pac II Power Packs	2863
	NPC IV Charger	3082
Jamner Surgical Instruments Inc. 9 Skyline Dr. Hawthorne, NY 10532 Phone: 1-914-592-9050	Richardson Retractors	
	Baby 3/4 inch	202-155
	Small 1 inch	202-156
	Medium 1½ inch	202-157
	Appendix Retractors	202-160
	Kelly 2 inch Retractors	202-166
Johnson & Johnson Medical Inc P.O. Box 130 Arlington, TX 76004 Phone: 1-800-433-5170	Barrier Shoulder Pack	1216
Medical Surgical Div. ℅ 3M St Paul, MN 55144 Customer Help Number 1-800-228-3957	Steri-Drape U-Shaped (120 × 130 cm)	1015
Smith & Nephew Richards 1450 Books Rd. Memphis, TN 38116 Phone: 1-800-238-7538	Houston Suture Retriever	111579
	Angular Rongeur	28-2582
	Stille-Ruskin Rongeur	28-2620
	Richards Bone Curettes	
	Size 1	11-1384
	Size 2	11-1385
	Size 3	11-1386
	Size 4	11-1387
	3-inch Spreader Block	16-0963
Sparta Surgical 26602 Corporate Ave. Hayward, CA 94545 Phone: 1-800-277-0674	Gezog Mallet	44-810

Supplier Name	Instrument	Catalog No.
Karl Stortz Endoscopy-America Inc. 1101 W. Jefferson Blvd. Culver City, CA 90232-3578 Phone: 1-800-252-2008 1-800-421-0837	30° Storz Scope 4mm × 17.5 cm 70° Storz Scope 90° Storz Scope Cannula, obturator, trocar (2-stopcock)	7200B 7200C 7200D 28124B
George Tiemann & Co. 84 Newtown Plaza Plainview, NY 11830 Phone: 1-516-694-6283	Fukuda Style Retractor Small Fukuda Style Retractor Large Taylor Spinal Retractor (sharp) 1¼ × 2⅜ inch 1¼ × 3 inch Weitlaner Self Retaining Retractor Sharp 5½ inch Gelpi Self Retaining Retractor 5½ inch	80-1869S 80-1869SL 80-1929S 80-1930S 80-1955S 80-1772
Zimmer Inc. P.O. Box 708 Warsaw, IN 46581-0708 Phone: 1-800-348-2759	2- Small Rake Retractor, Sharp 2-Volkman Rake Retractor Sharp 1-Langenbeck Periosteal Elevator (narrow) Kiene Bone Tamp 000-Brun Bone Currette (regular handle) 000-Brun Bone Currette (angled cup) Trinklc Bracc Brace Extension Screwdriver Handle with Snap Lock Chuck Lever-type Screwdriver Counter Sink Jacobs Chuck with Trinkle Shank Hollow Mill Screwdriver Woodruff Bit Screwdriver Single Slot Screwdriver (Phillips) Mayo-Collins (Army-Navy) Retractor Bent Mayo-Collins (Army-Navy) Retractor Flex Foam Traction Bandage 3 inches × 35 yards Key Periosteal Elevators ¼ inch blade width ½ inch blade width	2970-03 3011-04 3650 958 3675-00-01 3676-00-01 1085-01 1085-03 1085-02 1282-01 1085-09 1085-18 60002-14 85-1280-04 85-1280-13 sp. order. 3008 3008SP 3861-02 2910-02 2910-04

Index